Immunology: A Systems Biology Perspective

Immunology: A Systems Biology Perspective

Edited by Katie Murphy

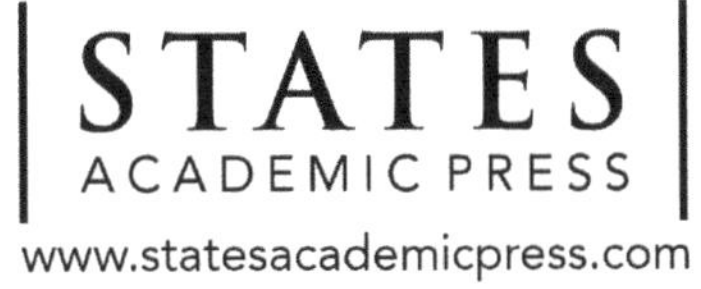

States Academic Press,
109 South 5th Street,
Brooklyn, NY 11249, USA

Visit us on the World Wide Web at:
www.statesacademicpress.com

ISBN: 978-1-63989-780-3

Cataloging-in-Publication Data

Immunology : a systems biology perspective / edited by Katie Murphy.
p. cm.
Includes bibliographical references and index.
ISBN 978-1-63989-780-3
1. Immune system. 2. Systems biology. 3. Immunology. 4. Immune response--Molecular aspects. I. Murphy, Katie.
QR181 .I46 2023
616.079--dc23

Table of Contents

Preface

Every book is initially just a concept; it takes months of research and hard work to give it the final shape in which the readers receive it. In its early stages, this book also went through rigorous reviewing. The notable contributions made by experts from across the globe were first molded into patterned chapters and then arranged in a sensibly sequential manner to bring out the best results.

The branch of biology and medicine that focuses on the study of immune systems in all organisms is termed as immunology. The basic purpose of studying the immune systems is to chart, measure and describing the functioning of the immune system in the state of health and disease. The study of immunology has a wide range of applications in different fields of medicine such as bacteriology, parasitology, psychiatry, oncology and organ transplantation. Immunological disorders can lead to immunodeficiency and autoimmune diseases. Immunodeficiency is a condition in which the organism's ability to fight infectious diseases and cancer is absent or is highly compromised. Autoimmune diseases are a result of abnormal immune response to a functioning part of the body. This book contains some path-breaking studies in the field of immunology. From theories to research to practical applications, case studies related to all contemporary topics of relevance to this field have been included herein. The book aims to serve as a resource guide for students and experts alike and contribute to the growth of the discipline.

It has been my immense pleasure to be a part of this project and to contribute my years of learning in such a meaningful form. I would like to take this opportunity to thank all the people who have been associated with the completion of this book at any step.

Editor

1

Quantitative Measurement of Naïve T Cell Association with Dendritic Cells, FRCs and Blood Vessels in Lymph Nodes

Humayra Tasnim[1†], G. Matthew Fricke[1,2†], Janie R. Byrum[3†], Justyna O. Sotiris[1], Judy L. Cannon[3,4,5] and Melanie E. Moses[1,6,7]*

[1] *Moses Biological Computation Laboratory, Department of Computer Science, The University of New Mexico, Albuquerque, NM, United States,* [2] *UNM Center for Advanced Research Computing (CARC), The University of New Mexico, Albuquerque, NM, United States,* [3] *The Cannon Laboratory, Molecular Genetics & Microbiology, The University of New Mexico, Albuquerque, NM, United States,* [4] *Department of Pathology, The University of New Mexico, Albuquerque, NM, United States,* [5] *Autophagy, Inflammation, and Metabolism Center of Biomedical Research Excellence, The University of New Mexico, Albuquerque, NM, United States,* [6] *Biology Department, The University of New Mexico, Albuquerque, NM, United States,* [7] *Santa Fe Institute, Santa Fe, NM, United States*

***Correspondence:**
Judy L. Cannon
jucannon@salud.unm.edu

[†] *These authors have contributed equally to this work.*

T cells play a vital role in eliminating pathogenic infections. To activate, naïve T cells search lymph nodes (LNs) for dendritic cells (DCs). Positioning and movement of T cells in LNs is influenced by chemokines including CCL21 as well as multiple cell types and structures in the LNs. Previous studies have suggested that T cell positioning facilitates DC colocalization leading to T:DC interaction. Despite the influence chemical signals, cells, and structures can have on naïve T cell positioning, relatively few studies have used quantitative measures to directly compare T cell interactions with key cell types. Here, we use Pearson correlation coefficient (PCC) and normalized mutual information (NMI) to quantify the extent to which naïve T cells spatially associate with DCs, fibroblastic reticular cells (FRCs), and blood vessels in LNs. We measure spatial associations in physiologically relevant regions. We find that T cells are more spatially associated with FRCs than with their ultimate targets, DCs. We also investigated the role of a key motility chemokine receptor, CCR7, on T cell colocalization with DCs. We find that CCR7 deficiency does not decrease naïve T cell association with DCs, in fact, CCR7$^{-/-}$ T cells show slightly higher DC association compared with wild type T cells. By revealing these associations, we gain insights into factors that drive T cell localization, potentially affecting the timing of productive T:DC interactions and T cell activation.

Keywords: mutual information, T cells, dendritic cells, FRCs, CCR7, lymph nodes

1. INTRODUCTION

The adaptive immune response depends on T cell interactions with dendritic cells (DCs) in the paracortex, or T cell zone, of lymph nodes (LNs). The rate at which naïve T cells sample DCs determines how fast the immune system can mount a response to infection (1). The development of imaging methods such as two-photon microscopy (2PM) and histocytometry have enabled direct observation of cell locations in tissues. Many studies showing the relative location of T cells and DCs suggest that they are both positioned in the LN to maximize the likelihood of T:DC interactions (2, 3). Despite advances in the ability to image and observe T cells in LNs, few studies make direct quantitative comparisons of how closely T cells associate with multiple other cells types in LNs.

T cells enter the paracortex of the LN from small post-capillary blood vessels termed high endothelial venules (HEVs). T cells, DCs, and fibroblastic reticular cells (FRCs) occupy this region along with blood vessels (BVs). T cells move among DCs, FRCs, and other T cells to interact with DCs presenting antigen. FRCs are stromal cells that encapsulate a collagen fiber conduit network which allows for transport of lymph fluid carrying soluble antigen and chemokines (4–7). FRCs produce the chemokine CCL21, which has an established role in naïve T cell homing into the paracortex from blood vessels (8, 9). FRCs also provide structural support required for efficient T cell activation (10). Bajenoff et al. showed the FRC network is closely associated with naïve T cells moving within the paracortex, suggesting that FRCs may provide a network on which T cells migrate (11).

There are several hypotheses regarding the role of individual cell types in mediating T:DC interactions. HEVs are the entry points for T cells entering the LN. Girard et al. suggests that DCs gather near HEVs to maximize their contact rate with incoming T cells (12). Others have suggested that DCs may congregate at the intersections of the FRC network, allowing T cells that travel along the edges of the network to encounter DCs at an increased rate (13–16). Spatial interactions between T cells and blood vessels, FRCs, and DCs are important if they change how T cells move through the paracortex and the timing of encounters with antigen-presenting DCs, the key step in T cell activation and the initiation of the adaptive immune response.

In addition to structural and cellular cues, chemical mediators, including chemokines, contribute to T cell motion and T:DC contacts in the LN. For example, the signaling molecule LPA produced by FRCs has been shown to mediate rapid T cell motion in LNs (17). In addition, C–C chemokine receptor type 7 (CCR7), the receptor recognizing CCL21, is important for high speed T cell motility in the LN (18, 19). While CCR7 increases T cell movement speed in LNs, whether CCR7 impacts T:DC contacts has not been investigated.

Understanding the contribution of cellular and structural LN components to T cell localization requires a quantitative metric that allows direct comparisons of spatial associations of multiple cell types. Several other groups have reported spatial relationships between cells and structures using methods such as visual inspection (12, 20) and comparison of turning angles of T cell movements with structures (11, 21). However, none of these directly compare associations between multiple cell types or structures with a consistent quantitative metric.

In this study, we use both the Pearson correlation coefficient [PCC (22, 23)] as well as Mutual Information [MI (24)] to compare the spatial association of multiple cell types and structures. PCC measures the covariance of homologous pixel intensities, and has been often used to determine colocalization, particularly of fluorescent proteins, in multiple biological systems including the study of T cells (25, 26). PCC and MI can be calculated without the need to identify individual cell boundaries which can be difficult for 2PM images.

MI is an application of Shannon entropy (which measures the amount of uncertainty about the value of a random variable in bits) originally defined to understand limitations on signal processing and communication (27). MI quantifies the reduction in uncertainty about one variable when one knows the value of another variable. In analyzing spatial associations, we measure the reduction in uncertainty about the location of one cell type given the location of another cell type. MI has been successfully used in other biomedical image processing applications, particularly in measuring image similarity in X-rays and MRIs for automated image registration (28–31). Furthermore, MI and other information theoretic measures are increasingly recognized as powerful tools for analysis of non-linear complex systems, including complex biological systems such as the immune system (32, 33). In this article, we use MI to quantify the spatial association of T cells with other cell types (e.g., DCs or FRCs). We use MI as a measure of spatial association that is independent of specific types of cells or structures. In addition, MI is theoretically insensitive to coarse graining (34). Thus, MI can measure the amount of spatial dependence of one fluorescent marker on another while minimizing observational bias. MI, unlike distance measures such as nearest-neighbor analysis, is parsimonious, since it does not require extensive image processing to remove photon noise and determine cell boundaries. Instead, MI can operate on the image directly without the introduction of thresholds. In preliminary work we used MI to quantify the association of T cells and DCs and found less correspondence between T cell and DCs than expected (35).

However, MI is not comparable across images with different sizes and amounts of fluorescence. In this study, we use NMI to normalize MI to be between 0 and 1 (36–39), which allows quantitative comparisons of spatial associations between cells fluorescing in one color channel and another cell type fluorescing in a different color channel across experiments. Since PCC and NMI are both pixel-based methods that do not correspond to cell sizes, we create regions within the images that match cellular scales and apply PCC and NMI. Analyzing regions as well as pixels allows these methods to capture associations at biologically relevant scales. Both regional PCC and NMI analyses show T cells associate much less with their ultimate targets, DCs, than with FRCs. Our results also show that CCR7 does not increase T cell association with DCs.

2. MATERIALS AND METHODS

2.1. Mice and Reagents

Experiments were performed with C57BL/6 mice (Jackson Laboratories), B6.Ubiquitin-GFP mice (Jackson Laboratories), B6.CCR7$^{-/-}$ mice (Jackson Laboratories) and B6.Cg-Tg(Itgax-Venus)1Mnz/J mice (Jackson Laboratories). Both female and male mice were used between 8 and 20 weeks of age. Breeding, maintenance, and use of animals used in this research conform to the principles outlined by the Institutional Animal Care and Use Committee (IACUC). The IACUC at the University of New Mexico approved the protocol for animal studies (protocol number 16-200497-HSC). Anesthesia via ketamine and xylazine was performed during mouse injections, and euthanasia was administered via isofluorane overdose followed by cervical dislocation. For blood vessel staining, DyLight 594 labeled *Lycopersicon esculentum* (tomato) lectin (Vector Laboratories) was used at a dose of 70 μg per mouse. To isolate naïve T cells, Pan T Cell Isolation Kit II (mouse, Miltenyi Biotec, 130-095-130) was used according to manufacturer's instructions. To fluorescently label naïve T cells, CellTracker™Orange (5-(and-6)-(((4-chloromethyl)benzoyl)amino) tetramethylrhodamine) (CMTMR) Dye (ThermoFisher Scientific, C2927) was incubated with naïve T cells at a final concentration of 5 μm at 37°C for 30 min before being washed. Labeled naïve T cells were then immediately adoptively transferred into recipient mice.

2.2. Mouse Procedures

For all images: 10^7 naive T cells were adoptively transferred into mice 14–16 h prior to LN harvest for imaging by 2PM. For T:DC images: T cells from naïve wild type (WT) mice were labeled with orange vital dye CMTMR and adoptively transferred into naïve CD11c-yellow fluorescent protein (YFP) mice in which all CD11c$^+$ DCs are YFP$^+$. For T:BV images: T cells from naïve Ubiquitin-green fluorescent protein (GFP) mice were adoptively transferred into naïve C57Bl/6 recipient mice. DyLight 594-labeled *L. esculentum* (tomato) lectin was injected intravenously into the recipient mice 5 min before harvesting the LNs for imaging. The fluorescent lectin binds to glycoproteins on blood vessel endothelial cells and emits red fluorescence. For T:FRC images: T cells from naïve WT mice were labeled with CMTMR and adoptively transferred into Ubiquitin-GFP recipient mice that were lethally irradiated (10 Gy). The mice were reconstituted with C57Bl/6 bone marrow 4 weeks prior to T cell adoptive transfer. In this chimeric mouse model, the stromal cell populations fluoresce GFP while the hematopoietic cell populations are non-fluorescent.

2.3. Two-Photon Microscopy Setup

Two-photon microscopy was performed using either a ZEISS LSM510 META/NLO microscope or Prairie Technologies UltimaMultiphoton microscope from Bruker.

Prairie Technologies UltimaMultiphoton microscope from Bruker: A Ti-Sapphire (Spectra Physics) laser was tuned to either 820 nm for excitation of CMTMR or 850 nm for simultaneous excitation of YFP and CMTMR, GFP and DyLight 594, or GFP and CMTMR excitation. The Prairie system was equipped with Galvo scanning mirrors and an 801 nm long pass dichroic to split excitatory and emitted fluorescence. Emitted fluorescence was separated with a 550 nm long-pass dichroic mirror. Fluorescence below 550 nm was split using a 495 nm dichroic and filtered with 460/60 and 525/50 nm filters before amplification by photomultiplier tubes. Fluorescence above 550 nm was split with a 640 nm long-pass dichroic mirror before passing through 590/50 and 670/50 nm filters before amplification by GaAsP photomultiplier tubes. AUMPlanFLN 20× water immersion objective (0.5 numerical aperture) was used. Prairie View 5.4 software (Prairie Technologies) was used to acquire time-lapse z-stacks.

ZEISS LSM510 META/NLO: Chameleon Ti:Sapphire laser tuned to 850 nm (Coherent) was used for excitation of either GFP and CMTMR, YFP and CMTMR, or Dylight 594 and GFP. A 560 nm dichroic mirror and 500–550 and 575–640 nm band pass filters were used for detection of fluorophores. Movies were captured with the ZEN user interface (Zeiss). In both imaging systems, z-stacks with step size of 4 μm were repeatedly imaged over time to obtain movies of 10–45 min in duration. All analyses were performed on 2D image z-stacks captured by 2PM.

2.4. Lymph Node Preparation for Live Imaging

After euthanasia, LNs from mice were surgically dissected and transferred to a Chamlide AC-B25 imaging chamber (Live Cell Instruments) with a customized coverslip platform to allow flow beneath the LN. The LN was stabilized with a tissue slice harp (Warner Instruments) and superfused with oxygenated Dulbecco's Modified Eagle's Medium (Gibco, 21063-045) and maintained at 37°C. For experiments in which blood vessels were imaged in conjunction with T cells or DCs, with 70 μg DyLight 594-labeled lectin (from *L. esculentum*, Vector Laboratories) was intravenously administered by tail vein injection 5 min before euthanasia.

2.5. Calculation of Mutual Information

MI measures how much the value of one variable tells us about the value of another variable. In this study, MI is used to quantify how much the locations and color intensities of DCs, FRCs and blood vessels reveal about the locations and color intensities of T cells. We calculate the MI of color intensities resulting from 2PM imaging of two cell types. Each image is composed of a sequence of 2-color 3D images. In these images one cell type is dyed red and another green. We calculate the MI of the red and green channels from every image to determine the association of the corresponding cell types for that image.

The 2PM images contain red, blue and green channels. For every time step, we extract the red and green channels into two separate 3D images r and g.

The MI calculation procedure can be summarized in the following 3 steps:

1. We calculate the entropy of color intensities in image r and image g: H(r) and H(g). This measures the uncertainty of the color intensity in each image.
2. We calculate the joint entropy H(r, g) which measures the uncertainty about the color intensities in corresponding positions in both images.
3. We calculate MI as the sum of the entropies of the individual images H(r) and H(g) minus the joint entropy of the two images H(r, g). This reveals how much uncertainty about the color intensity and location of one cell type (i.e., T cells) is reduced when we know the color intensity and locations of the other cell type.

2.5.1. Entropy

Entropy measures the amount of information in the probability distribution of a random variable (24). It indicates the uncertainty in the outcome of an event. Entropy can be understood by considering a coin toss. The probability of heads is $p(x)=\frac{1}{2}$ and the probability of tails is $p(y)=\frac{1}{2}$. The entropy H is $-\left(\frac{1}{2}\times\log_2\left(\frac{1}{2}\right)+\frac{1}{2}\times\log_2\left(\frac{1}{2}\right)\right)$. Since $\log_2\left(\frac{1}{2}\right)=-1$, H=1 bit.

The formula for calculating entropy is:

$$H(r)=-\sum_{r}p(r)\log_2 p(r), \tag{1}$$

where H(r) is the entropy of variable r and $p(r)$ is the probability of r occurring. Here, we use $\log_2$ so that entropy is measured in bits, the unit of information. The expression is negated because the $\log_2$ of probabilities (which are always less than or equal to 1) is always negative or 0.

Entropy is maximized for a random event in which the probabilities of all outcomes are equally likely (all N possible outcomes have a probability of occurrence of $1/N$) leading to an entropy of $\log_2(N)$ bits. Entropy is minimized for a completely predictable event in which one outcome has a probability of occurrence equal to 1, and all other outcomes have 0 probability of occurrence, leading to an entropy of 0.

We calculate the entropy of color intensities in the red and green images. Each image has 256 possible color intensities for both the red and green images. Thus the maximum H(r) and the maximum H(g) is $\log_2(256) = 8$ bits which would occur if each of 256 color intensities were equally likely.

2.5.2. Joint Entropy

We use joint entropy to measure the uncertainty in the outcome of two variables:

$$H(r,g)=-\sum_{r}\sum_{g}p(r,g)\log_2 p(r,g), \tag{2}$$

where p(r, g) is the joint probability distribution function of r and g.

The two variables may be unrelated. For example, the joint entropy in the outcome of tossing a fair coin twice is calculated from the probabilities of four possible events [heads, heads], [heads, tails], [tails, heads], and [tails, tails]. The probability of each event is 1/4, resulting in a joint entropy of 2 bits. Since the events are independent, the joint entropy is equal to the sum of the entropies of each individual coin toss.

Alternatively, two variables could be related. In the extreme case, two variables could be completely correlated so that the value of one variable gives perfect information about the value of the other variable. For example, if the second coin toss occurred by picking up the coin and placing it back on the table with the same face up as before, then the probabilities of events [heads, heads] and [tails, tails] are both 1/2, and the probabilities of [heads, tails] and [tails, heads] are both 0. The joint entropy is 1, and equal to either of the individual entropies.

In our analysis of fluorescent images we are interested in the co-occurrence of red and green colors. That is, we wish to know whether knowing the color intensity of green pixels tells us anything about the color intensity of red ones in the same location. We calculate the probabilities of all possible color intensities (0 –255) in all corresponding locations of the red and green images. We define the joint probability p(r, g) as the probability of each pair of color intensities (0–255) occurring in the corresponding location in the red and green images. There are 256 × 256 = 65,536 possible combinations of color intensities. We calculate the number of times every intensity combination occurs in corresponding locations in an image. Then, we divide by the total number of locations in the images to turn those occurrences into probabilities. These probabilities are entered in equation (2) to calculate the joint entropy.

The joint entropy is low when color intensities repeatedly co-occur. Note that, joint entropy can be low when either the same color intensities repeatedly overlap, or when different color intensities overlap. For example, if red systematically has lower intensity than green, joint entropy would still be low if a green intensity of, say, 220 was frequently co-located with a red intensity of 180. Joint entropy only depends on the frequency of pairs of values co-occurring in the same locations. Joint entropy is high when there is no association in color intensities between the red and green images. Thus, in **Figure 2A** where red and green cells are uniformly randomly distributed, there is minimal co-occurrence of the intensities, and therefore all values in the probability table are low and uniformly distributed. By contrast, when red and green cells co-occur with the same intensities in the same locations (**Figure 2C**), the probabilities on the diagonal are high leading to the minimum possible joint entropy. We observe these scenarios in **Figures 2G,I** which are the corresponding joint probability tables for **Figures 2A,C**. For illustration purposes, the 256 color intensity values are binned into 4 color intensities.

2.5.3. Mutual Information

MI is calculated from the entropy of each image and the joint entropy of the two images using equation (3).

$$MI(r,g)=H(r)+H(g)-H(r,g). \tag{3}$$

Intuitively, this formula calculates MI by subtracting the joint entropy of r and g from the total entropy in both r and g, which leaves the overlap in entropy of r and g.

In **Figure 2**, we illustrate how MI is calculated from a set of 3 simulated images. The first case (**Figure 2A**) shows simulated red and green cells placed uniformly in random locations. In most cases, red and green do not overlap as shown in **Figure 2D** (although by random chance, there is some small co-occurrence of red and green cells that appear yellow). We calculate MI using equation (3). Because there is little or no co-occurrence of red and green pixels in **Figure 2A**, the joint entropy $H(r,g) \approx H(r)+H(g)$, so MI $\approx$ 0.

The second case, in **Figure 2B**, shows red cells placed within in a Gaussian distributed range of the green cells creating partial co-occurrence of red and green pixels. We can observe this region in **Figure 2E** (colored in yellow) which is the MI, calculated by summing the entropy of red and green images independently, and then subtracting the joint entropy (equation (2)). The process to calculate the joint entropy of the two images is described in Section 2.5.2 Joint Entropy.

The third case (**Figure 2C**) is a special case where the red and green pixels are of same intensity residing in the same location. When separated as two images, red and green cells completely overlap, shown in **Figure 2F**. In this case, information about the location of red cells provides all the information about the location of green cells. Because there is total correspondence between the intensity of red and intensity of green in the same location, the joint entropy $H(r, g) = H(r) = H(g)$, and the MI therefore equals $H(r)$ (and also equals $H(g)$).

2.6. Normalized Mutual Information

The MI analysis quantifies in bits the amount information shared by images showing the locations of two different cell types. However, the number of bits is influenced by the dimension of images and the numbers and sizes of cells. It does not provide us with a universal scale with which to compare the association of T cells with other cell types. For this, we define and calculate NMI as:

$$\mathrm{NMI} = \frac{\mathrm{MI}(r, g)}{\min(\mathrm{H}(r), \mathrm{H}(g))}. \tag{4}$$

We normalize MI by the minimum entropy image. MI depends on both the joint entropy and the internal (marginal) entropies of each color channel. The internal entropies vary across experiments, resulting in MI values that are not directly comparable. We normalize by dividing MI by the minimum of the internal entropies, since it provides an upper bound on MI, for a proof see Ref. (41).

The value of NMI is bounded between 0 and 1, where 0 indicates no occurrence of the red and green cells in the same location as in **Figure 2A**, and 1 indicates complete colocalization of the red and green cells as shown in **Figure 2C**. NMI allows us to directly compare spatial association of cells, regardless of the cell types, cell sizes, and image dimensions in our experiments.

We validated the NMI metric on simulated data generated as 512 × 512 RGB images shown in **Figure 3A**. Each cell is a square of 11 × 11 pixels with randomly chosen color intensities ranging from 0 to 255. In each image, 500 green cells are placed uniformly at random along with a number of red cells uniformly distributed between 100 and 500. We placed each red cell within a distance determined by a Gaussian distribution from each green cell with SDs (σ) ranging from 0 (generating complete correlation of the red and green pixels) to 10 (generating a low probability of overlap of red and green pixels). We treat the image as a torus to avoid edge effects when placing red cells. We also analyzed images in which both green and red cells are placed uniformly at random (u), and therefore with no spatial association and minimum MI.

NMI is designed to normalize for variations in cell numbers. To assess the potential effect of cell numbers on NMI, we simulated images in which we varied the cell numbers from 100 to 500 and calculated NMI for differing cell numbers with complete cell overlap ($\sigma = 0$, increasingly spatially separated $\sigma = 1$ or $\sigma = 3$ or cells placed in a uniform random distribution Figure S2 in Supplementary Material). We also calculated PCC as a comparison. We find that NMI is less sensitive to variations in cell numbers than PCC, particularly in cases in which there is spatial association.

2.7. Regionalization of Images

NMI is calculated from the intensity of pixels in corresponding locations. However, cells comprise multiple pixels. A naïve T cell has a diameter of approximately 5–7 μm whereas the approximate length of a pixel is 1.2 μm. Therefore, we created regions in the image and call this process "regionalization." In regionalization, for each pixel (p), we calculated a region around it with a specified length; for example in a 5 × 5 pixel (6 μm × 6 μm) region, p is the middle pixel. We replaced the value of p with the average color intensity of all cells in its region. We iterated over all pixels, discarding the regions along the image boundaries where complete regions could not be formed. This method produced new images where each pixel has the average intensity of its region. We calculated the MI, NMI, and PCC of these regionalized images. We used region sizes: 5 × 5 pixels (6 μm × 6 μm), 15 × 15 pixels (18 μm × 18 μm), and 25 × 25 pixels (30 μm × 30 μm). We are most interested in region sizes between 5 × 5 (6 μm × 6 μm) and 15 × 15 pixels (18 μm × 18 μm), since these scales are most relevant to our biological data.

We validated both NMI and PCC for regionalized images. For validation, we used 512 × 512 simulated images that are constructed using the same method mentioned in Section 2.6 Normalized Mutual Information. Analysis is performed on 500 green cells and 500 red cells. These simulated images are then divided into regions using the regionalization method. The size of the regions is consistent with the ones we used for experimental data. Results from NMI and PCC analysis on these images are shown in **Figure 4**. NMI and PCC decrease with decreasing spatial association, following a trend similar to that in the validation analysis shown in **Figure 3**, although region size influences PCC more than NMI.

3. RESULTS

3.1. PCC Shows T Cells Associate More With FRCs Than DCs in LN

To ask whether naïve T cells associate with DCs in the LN, we used PCC, a standard colocalization measure. As a comparison, we also calculated the PCC of T cells and FRCs because it has been suggested that T cells use FRCs as a network for migration through the LN (11). We transferred CMTMR-labeled T cells into CD11c-YFP mice, harvested LNs for 2PM imaging, and calculated PCC of T cells and DCs from multiple images of T cells and DCs. We imaged FRCs as previously described by Bajénoff et al. (11) by irradiating Ubiquitin-GFP animals, reconstituting with whole bone marrow from non-GFP animals for 4–8 weeks, and co-imaged GFP^+ FRCs with co-transferred CMTMR labeled T cells. We find the PCC of T:DC microscopy images was low (**Figure 1A**) (median = 0.1916, results given to four significant figures throughout). In fact, the PCC of T cells to DCs was significantly lower than PCC of T cell with FRCs (T:FRC PCC median = 0.3810). In **Figure 1**, we use interquartile-range notched box plots to visualize the statistical relationships between measurements (42). Non-overlapping notches indicate the measurements were drawn from different distributions at the 95% confidence level. While previous studies have determined

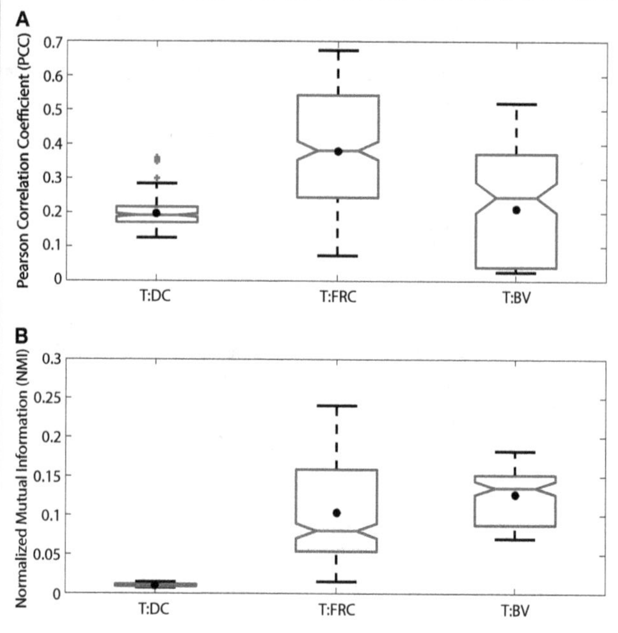

FIGURE 1 | Notched boxplots displaying PCC **(A)** and NMI **(B)** values for T:DC, T:FRC, and T:BV images. Data include 6 T:DC image z-stacks (2 experiments on 2 different days, 2 mice, 4 lymph nodes), 12 T:FRC image z-stacks (3 experiments on 3 different days, 6 lymph nodes), 4 T:BV image z-stacks (2 mice on 2 different days, 3 lymph nodes). Black dots indicate the mean. Median T:DC PCC value = 0.1922, median T:FRCs PCC value = 0.3810, median T:BV PCC value = 0.2447. Mann–Whitney p values for T:DC–T:FRCs < e–4, T:DC–T:BV = 0.0293, and T:FRC-T:BV < e–4. Median T:DC NMI value = 0.0101, median T:FRC NMI value = 0.0798, and median T:BV NMI value = 0.1355. Mann–Whitney p values for T:DC–T:FRC, T:DC–T:BV, and T:FRC-T:BV comparisons < e–4.

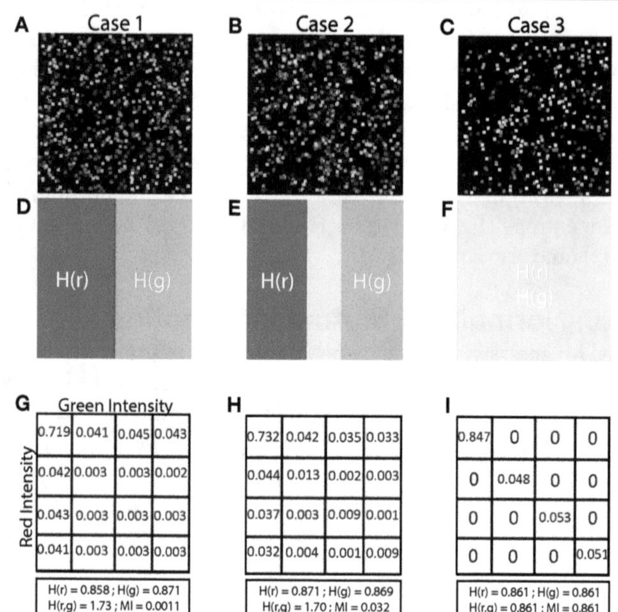

FIGURE 2 | Illustration of low, medium and high MI. Simulated images of 500 red and 500 green cells are shown in panels **(A–C)**. Each cell is a square of 11 × 11 pixels. The location and color intensity of each green cell is chosen from a uniform random distribution. A red cell is paired with each green cell. The red cell has the same color intensity as the green cell, but with a different spatial association in each case. In panel **(A)**, red cells are placed at random locations uncorrelated with green cell placements. In panel **(B)**, the placements of red and green cells are partially correlated. Red cell locations are chosen from a Gaussian distribution centered at the location of the paired green cell, but with a standard deviation ($\sigma = 5$). In panel **(C)**, the location of red and green cells is identical ($\sigma = 0$). **(D–F)** Set diagrams indicating the shared information between red and green channels. In panel **(D)**, the two color channels are independent since cell locations are uncorrelated with each other providing minimum MI. In panel **(E)**, the two images are partially correlated which increases the MI, shown by the yellow shaded region. In panel **(F)**, the two images are completely correlated maximizing the MI of the two color channels, resulting in complete intersection of the information in the red and green channels (yellow region). Panels **(G–I)** joint probability tables for images **(A–C)** where 256 color intensities are binned into 4 color intensities for purposes of illustration, resulting in a 4 × 4 probability table. In panel **(G)**, the probability values are low and evenly spread across the table, except for the upper left corner, indicating overlap in the space with no cells (MI = 0.0011 bits). In panel **(H)**, the probability values are higher along the diagonal than in other parts, indicating partial correlation in the placement of red and green cells (MI = 0.0320 bits). In panel **(I)**, there are probability values on the diagonal only and the probabilities off the diagonal are 0 since there is complete correlation in the placement of red and green cells (MI = 0.8610 bits). The calculation of entropy $H(r)$ and $H(g)$, joint entropy $H(r, g)$, and MI are shown for each case.

association of T cells with FRC and DC subsets separately, we quantitatively compare the effect of FRCs relative to DCs on T cell positioning. These results suggest that FRCs show much higher correlation with naïve T cell locations in the T cell zone of LNs than the presumed intended targets of DCs.

3.2. Application and Validation of NMI as a Novel Method to Assess T Cell Association With Cell Types in LN

While PCC provides a quantitative metric to assess the correlation among pixels in images, PCC assumes that these correlations are linear (22, 26, 43, 44). We use NMI (a normalized version of MI) to quantitatively assess spatial relationships between cell types without assuming linearity. The principles of MI are illustrated using simulated images in **Figure 2**.

We calculated the entropy of fluorescence signals using equation (1) and then calculated the joint entropy using equation (2) (for detail see Methods). We then calculated the MI of the signals using equation (3). To validate our MI calculations, we created simulated images with fields of green and red "cells" in which there is no association (**Figure 2A**), partial association (**Figure 2B**), and complete association (**Figure 2C**) of fluorescent objects with sizes similar to that of cells. The 3 cases can be simplified by observing the images in **Figure 2D** (no association), **Figure 2E** (partial association marked as yellow area), and **Figure 2F** (complete association marked as yellow area). The joint probability tables (simplified examples in 4 × 4 color intensities shown in **Figures 2G–I**) are used to calculate the joint entropy. If there is no spatial association, the joint probability table shows evenly distributed low values (**Figure 2G**). Given partial spatial association of cells, the joint probability table shows increased values across the diagonal (**Figure 2H**). Given completely overlapping signals, the joint probability table shows high values across the diagonal (**Figure 2I**). Because MI is calculated from fluorescent images in which different images possess different internal entropies, we normalized the MI values to provide a universal scale (between 0 and 1) with which to compare one image to another. We calculated NMI by normalizing MI with the minimum entropy of the two images, thus enabling quantitative comparisons across fields.

In **Figure 3A**, we show examples of simulated images created for validating NMI (described in Section 2.6 Normalized Mutual Information) in which red cells were placed with SD (σ) of 0 and 5 as well as red cells placed uniformly at random. We expect the MI and NMI values to decrease as the SD increases, as shown in **Figure 3B** (MI) and **Figure 3C** (NMI). As expected, MI and NMI are maximum in the special case 0* where the intensity, size and location of the cells are all identical; MI and NMI decrease as the spatial association between the cells decreases. While the MI can be greater than 1 bit (**Figure 3B**), the NMI metric is normalized to be between 0 and 1 (**Figure 3C**), demonstrating that NMI can provide comparisons to account for differing levels of fluorescence across multiple fields on a common scale.

As a further validation, we tested whether NMI calculations on our experimental data range between 0 and 1. Figure S1 in Supplementary Material shows that the NMI of an image with itself is 1 (Matched Red:Red and Matched Green:Green). We calculated NMI of two unrelated images from two different experimental fields (Unmatched Red:Green). For example, the red cell image may be taken from a T:DC experiment and the green cell image from a T:FRC experiment. As expected, NMI in these cases is very close to 0 (Figure S1 in Supplementary Material). We then calculated the NMI of T:DC and T:FRC interactions using the same images on which we calculated PCC (**Figure 1B**). We find that similar to PCC analyses, NMI shows significantly higher association for T:FRC than T:DC (T:FRC NMI median = 0.08; T:DC NMI median = 0.01).

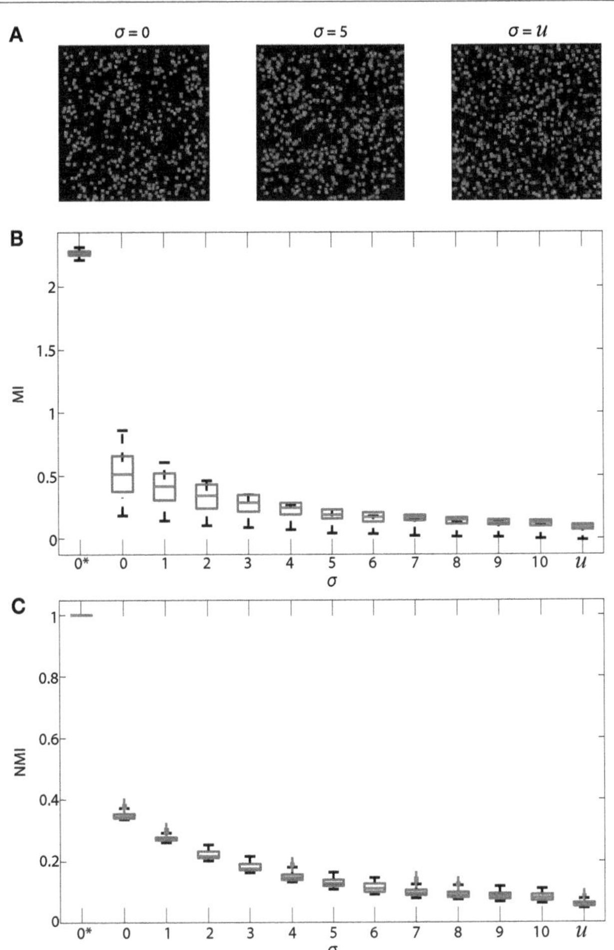

FIGURE 3 | Validation of MI and NMI. Panel **(A)** shows 3 samples of simulated 512 × 512 images that consist of 500 green cells and a number of red cells uniformly distributed between 100 and 500. Each pixel intensity of the red and green cells is randomly assigned, and each cell is a square of 11 × 11 pixels. The red cell locations are chosen from a Gaussian distribution centered at the location of green cells with SD (σ) 0 and 5 in the first and second images, and uniformly random in the third image. **(B)** shows boxplots of MI in bits and **(C)** shows boxplots of NMI (unitless) of simulated images where the SD (σ) ranges from 0 to 10. 2 additional special cases are shown: 0* and *u*. 0* indicates that red and green color intensities are identical in corresponding locations which maximizes both MI and NMI. *u* indicates that the cells are placed uniformly at random within the image and with uniform random color intensity, resulting in the lowest MI and NMI. Increasing σ decreases the spatial association of cells. As spatial association decreases, and both MI and NMI systematically decrease, demonstrating that they are useful metrics that indicate spatial association between cells.

3.3. Regional PCC and NMI Analyses

We first calculated both PCC and NMI using pixel-based comparisons (**Figure 1**). We find that PCC and NMI show a significantly higher association of T cells with FRCs than DCs. However, NMI and PCC pixel-based metrics can be problematic. Intercellular interactions in 2PM images are challenging to quantify by existing colocalization analyses because individual cells occupy discrete physical space, but pixel-based colocalization methods measure the amount of fluorescence signal overlap in individual pixels. In fact, any actual overlap in cell signal as measured by PCC and NMI is likely artifactual in that cells do not physically overlap in space. Also, it is possible that true intercellular contacts would be underestimated due to image resolution and the inability to resolve smaller protrusions such as dendrites of DCs. To account for cell-cell association rather than actual signal overlap based on pixels, we regionalized our images using sliding windows of multiple pixels, the size of which matched approximate sizes of T cells (estimated 5 μm diameter), DCs (estimated 10–15 μm diameter), and FRCs (estimated 5–7 μm diameter). The regionalized image has the same number of pixels as the original, but each pixel contains information drawn from the region surrounding it. Given that each pixel is approximately 1.2 μm in length, we created regions of 5 × 5 pixels (6 μm × 6 μm) and 15 × 15 pixels (18 μm × 18 μm) to account for potential extensions beyond the cell bodies. We also extended analysis to larger region sizes. Fluorescence in regions was determined by taking the average fluorescence of all the pixels within the region (for detail see

Section 2.7 Regionalization of Images). We used this method to generate new regionalized images and performed both PCC and NMI to take into account potential interactions of cells without directly overlapping fluorescent signals.

We first tested the "regionalization" effect by performing PCC and NMI on simulated images (as shown in **Figures 2A–C** and **3A**) to determine the effect of cell density, degree of pixel overlap, and regionalization on co-association (**Figure 4**). We created simulated images that approximate the amount of fluorescence in our experimental images. We varied the distance between the simulated cells to model different amounts of spatial association. We applied our regionalization method to these simulated images and calculated NMI and PCC values. We found that larger regions produce higher NMI and PCC values. Compared with NMI, PCC is less sensitive to changes in spatial association but more sensitive to region size (compare **Figures 4A,B**). Despite these differences, both NMI and PCC provide a quantitative measure that can be used to detect variation in spatial association among cell types.

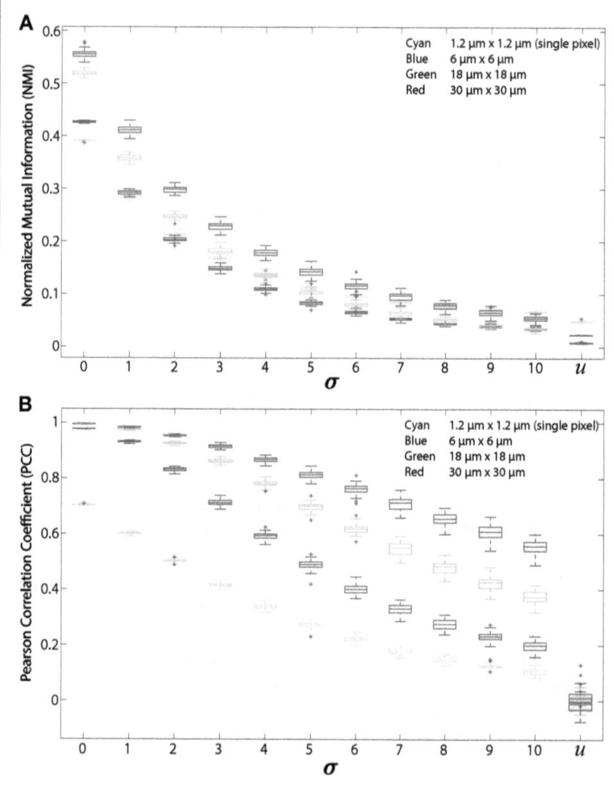

FIGURE 4 | Regionalized PCC and NMI on simulated data. Simulated images are 512 × 512 pixels with 500 red and 500 green 11 × 11 pixel square-shaped cells. The red cell locations are chosen from a Gaussian distribution centered at the location of green cells with SD (σ), which ranges from 0 to 10 and u. u indicates that the cells are placed uniformly at random within the images and with uniform random color intensity. **(A)** NMI calculated on simulated images with regions of sizes 6 μm × 6 μm (blue), 18 μm × 18 μm (green), 30 μm × 30 μm (red), and single pixels (1.2 μm × 1.2 μm, cyan). **(B)** PCC of simulated images using the same regions.

3.4. Regional Analyses Confirm That T Cells Are More Associated With FRCs Than With DCs

After validating both the NMI metric and the regionalization of images, we analyzed regionalized images to quantify spatial association of T cells with DCs and FRCs using both PCC and NMI (for sample images see **Figure 5A**). Both PCC and NMI show that T cells associate less with DCs than FRCs (**Figure 5B** for NMI and **Figure 5C** for PCC). T cells are more associated with FRCs across all region sizes. In pixel-based comparisons (without regionalizing), the T:DC association was very low (**Table 1**, NMI = 0.0101; PCC = 0.1916) while T:FRC association was significantly higher (NMI = 0.0798; PCC = 0.3810). Both NMI and PCC values for T:DC interactions increased with increasing region sizes, T:FRC association also increased at each region size. Regionalizing PCC into 18 μm × 18 μm region (15 × 15 pixels) resulted in the same trend among the compared cell types as NMI (**Figure 5B** NMI; T:DC median = 0.1427, T:FRC median = 0.3426; **Figure 5C** PCC T:DC median = 0.4396, T:FRC median = 0.7646, **Table 1**). **Figures 5D,E** compare physiologically relevant regions that approximate cell sizes and account for potential dendritic extensions with larger regions for DCs at 18 and 30 μm than FRCs at 6 μm. Again, T:FRC associations are greater than T:DC associations using both NMI and PCC. Thus, across region sizes, both NMI and PCC analyses show significantly higher T cell association with FRCs compared with DCs. These results suggest that despite the fact that DCs are considered the ultimate targets for T cell search, FRCs a greater determinant of naïve T cell positioning within the LN.

In addition to FRCs and DCs, structures such as blood vessels in the LN can be sources of chemokines (5, 45), and T cells may move along vessels in other tissues (21). Several studies suggest DCs are biased to localize near blood vessels and efficiently activate antigen-specific T cells (20, 46). We used NMI and PCC to ask whether vasculature can determine T cell localization in LN. We transferred GFP^+ T cells for 16 h as previously described, then just prior to imaging, we injected animals with DyLight 594-lectin which binds endothelial cells lining blood vessels. We then imaged T cells in conjunction with vasculature in LNs. With the pixel-based PCC (**Figure 1A**) and NMI analyses (**Figure 1B**), T cell association with blood vessels appears higher than T cell association with DCs, and NMI shows higher T cell association with blood vessels than even FRCs. However, with increasing region size, PCC and NMI analyses of T:BV values stayed consistent while T:DC values increased, for example, in the 18 μm length region, NMI of T:DC was 0.1427 and T:BV was 0.1036. The same trend was seen for PCC (T:DC = 0.4396, T:BV = 0.2603). The consistent value of NMI and PCC analyses of T:BV across regions likely reflects the sharp resolution of the blood vessel fluorescence compared with the more blurred extensions of FRCs and DCs. With increasing region size matching cellular scales, T cells show lower association with BVs (**Figures 5B,C**). These results suggest that T cells likely do not use crawling along vessels as a means to migrate within T cell zones of LNs.

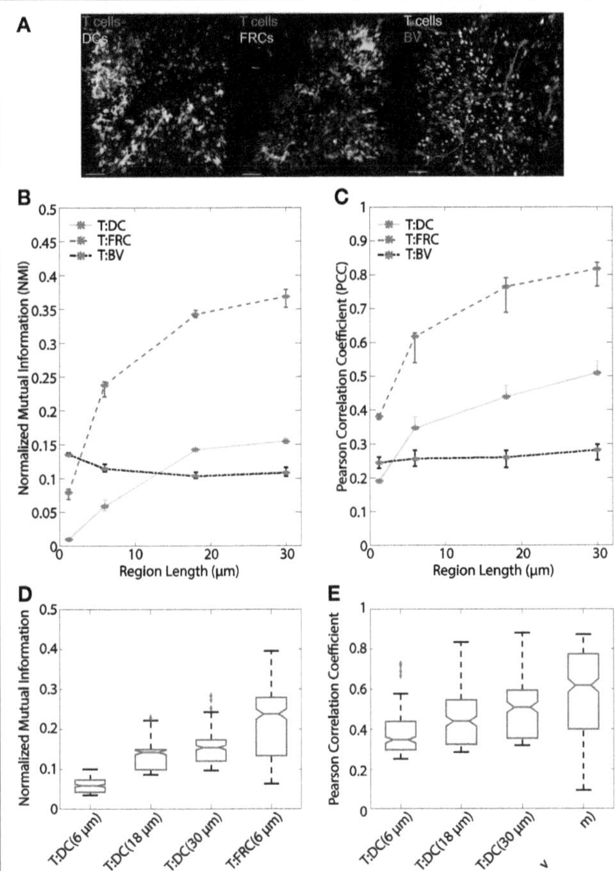

FIGURE 5 | **(A)** Sample images of T:DC (T cells labeled in red and DCs labeled in green), T:FRC (T cells labeled in red and FRCs labeled in green), and T:BV (T cells labeled in green and blood vessel labeled in red). **(B,C)** Line plots representing the NMI **(B)** and PCC **(C)** of T cells and DCs (T:DC, green line), T cells and FRCs (T:FRC, blue dashed line), and T cells and blood vessel (T:BV, black dotted line). NMI and PCC were calculated on pixels (region length = 1.2 μm), or regionalized images of increasing side length (6, 18, and 30 μm). Red stars indicate medians for the corresponding region size, and error bars indicate the 95% confidence interval around the median (40). For NMI, Mann–Whitney p values for T:DC–T:FRC, T:DC–T:BV, and T:FRC-T:BV comparisons < e−4 for all region lengths except T:DC–T:BV (region length = 18 μm) p value = 0.0012. For PCC, Mann–Whitney p values for T:DC–T:FRC, T:DC–T:BV, and T:FRC-T:BV comparisons < e−4 for all region lengths except T:DC–T:BV (region length = 1.2 μm) p value = 0.0293. **(D,E)** Notched box plots comparing the NMI **(D)** and PCC **(E)** of T cells and DCs with T cells and FRCs at physiologically relevant region lengths of (6, 18, and 30 μm) for T:DC associations and 6 μm for T:FRC associations. Note different scales on the y-axis. Both NMI and PCC are greater for the physiologically relevant region sizes for T:FRC than for T:DC (comparing T:DC at 30 μm to T:FRC at 6 μm p = 0.0022; for all other comparisons p < e−4). T:DC images were from 6 image z-stacks consisting of 4,089 frames from 2 mice and 4 lymph nodes. T:FRC images were from 12 image z-stacks consisting of 9,468 frames from 3 mice and 6 lymph nodes. T:BV images were from 4 image z-stacks consisting of 4,361 frames from 2 mice and 3 lymph nodes.

3.5. CCR7 Does Not Enhance T:DC Association

The chemokine CCL21 plays an important role in driving rapid motility of naïve T cells in LNs, and this rapid motility has been suggested to enhance T cell interactions with DCs (3). We tested whether signaling through CCR7 might provide information to T cells to enable closer T:DC associations. To do this, we transferred CMTMR-labeled $CCR7^{-/-}$ T cells into CD11c-YFP mice, harvested LNs for 2PM imaging, and calculated NMI and PCC of $CCR7^{-/-}$ T cells and DCs (**Figure 6A**). Contrary to our hypothesis, we found that in general, $CCR7^{-/-}$ T cells and DCs showed slightly higher NMI and PCC than WT T:DCs (**Figure 6B**, NMI WT: 0.0101; $CCR7^{-/-}$: 0.0158 and **Table 1**). WT T cells showed higher co-association with DCs compared with $CCR7^{-/-}$ T cells in only one case, pixel-based PCC analysis, while with increasing region size and in all NMI analyses, $CCR7^{-/-}$ T cells were slightly increased in DC association over WT T cells (**Figures 6B,C**; **Table 1**). Based on both NMI and PCC analyses, these data show that CCR7 does not promote increased T cell localization with DCs. Absence of CCR7 did not increase T:DC association to the level of T:FRC, as NMI and PCC values of T:FRC remained significantly higher than $CCR7^{-/-}$ T:DC association. These results suggest that high speed motility promoted by CCR7 signaling likely functions to promote T cell exploration of the LN paracortex rather than increase T cell localization close to DCs.

TABLE 1 | Median NMI and PCC values among cell types with 95% confidence interval.

Data type	Median NMI	95% Confidence interval	Median PCC	95% Confidence interval
Random control	0.0008	[0.0007, 0.0008]	0.0008	[0.0005, 0.0010]
Same image control	1	[1, 1]	1	[1, 1]
1.2 μm × 1.2 μm (single pixel)				
T:DC (WT)	0.0101	[0.0090, 0.0102]	0.1916	[0.1879, 0.1941]
T:DC ($CCR7^{-/-}$)	0.0158	[0.0156, 0.0161]	0.1527	[0.1338, 0.1589]
T:FRC	0.0798	[0.0691, 0.0846]	0.3810	[0.3729, 0.3886]
T:BV	0.1355	[0.1348, 0.1381]	0.2447	[0.2281, 0.2610]
6 μm × 6 μm				
T:DC (WT)	0.0588	[0.0524, 0.0685]	0.3467	[0.3427, 0.3808]
T:DC ($CCR7^{-/-}$)	0.0857	[0.0808, 0.0886]	0.4252	[0.3720, 0.4334]
T:FRC	0.2377	[0.2207, 0.2427]	0.6175	[0.5392, 0.6283]
T:BV	0.1144	[0.1101, 0.1214]	0.2565	[0.2342, 0.2815]
18 μm × 18 μm				
T:DC (WT)	0.1427	[0.1418, 0.1443]	0.4396	[0.4327, 0.4734]
T:DC ($CCR7^{-/-}$)	0.2633	[0.2576, 0.2679]	0.5866	[0.5794, 0.5957]
T:FRC	0.3426	[0.3384, 0.3487]	0.7646	[0.6893, 0.7913]
T:BV	0.1036	[0.1002, 0.1093]	0.2603	[0.2302,0.2805]
30 μm × 30 μm				
T:DC (WT)	0.1547	[0.1509, 0.1589]	0.5089	[0.5020, 0.5448]
T:DC ($CCR7^{-/-}$)	0.3075	[0.2980, 0.3165]	0.6590	[0.6527, 0.6673]
T:FRC	0.3685	[0.3525, 0.3789]	0.8169	[0.7659, 0.8352]
T:BV	0.1080	[0.1034, 0.1159]	0.2816	[0.2514,0.2984]

Both NMI and PCC values increase with region size except for T:BV.

4. DISCUSSION

In this work, we analyze 2PM z-stacks to quantitatively compare T cell association with different cell types and structures in the naïve lymph node using both PCC and NMI. To account for the limitations of 2PM to resolve cell structures, we create regions that correspond to physiologically relevant cell sizes. Both PCC and NMI across multiple region sizes show that T cells share

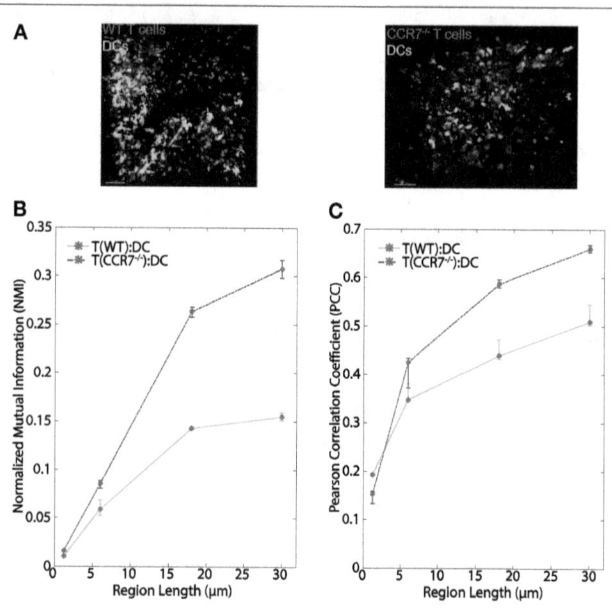

FIGURE 6 | (A) Sample images of WT T:DC and CCR7$^{-/-}$ T:DC. T cells are labeled in red and DCs are labeled in green. In WT T:DC, T cells are wild-type naïve T cells and in CCR7$^{-/-}$ T:DC, T cells are from CCR7-deficient animals. **(B,C)** Line plots representing the NMI **(B)** and PCC **(C)** of WT T cells and DCs (T(WT):DC, green line) and CCR7$^{-/-}$ T cells and DCs (T(CCR7$^{-/-}$):DC, blue dashed line). NMI and PCC were calculated on pixels (region length = 1.2 μm), or regionalized images of increasing side length (6, 18, and 30 μm). Red stars indicate medians for the corresponding region size, and error bars indicate the 95% confidence interval around the median (40). For NMI, Mann–Whitney p values for T(WT):DC–T(CCR7$^{-/-}$):DC comparisons < e–4 for all region lengths. For PCC Mann–Whitney p values for T(WT):DC–T(CCR7$^{-/-}$):DC comparisons for region lengths 1.2, 6, 18, and 30 μm: Region length 1.2 μm p < e–4, 6 μm p = 0.9152, 18 μm p = 0.0021, 30 μm p < e–4. WT T:DC images were from 6 image z-stacks consisting of 4,089 frames using 2 mice and 4 lymph nodes. CCR7$^{-/-}$ data are from 12 image z-stacks consisting of 11,294 frames using 4 mice and 8 lymph nodes.

more spatial association with FRCs than with DCs. Furthermore, CCR7$^{-/-}$ T cells do not associate less with DCs than WT T cells; in fact, our results suggest that CCR7$^{-/-}$ T cells may associate slightly more with DCs than WT T cells.

Many studies have investigated T cell search for DCs in the naïve LN since DCs are the key cell type that is required to present cognate antigen to T cells leading to the initiation of the adaptive immune response (3, 47). Westermann et al. suggest that cell positioning within the LN maximizes the likelihood of T cell interaction with DCs (48). Other studies hypothesize that DCs are situated atop the FRC network to facilitate T cell interactions with DCs as the T cells move along the FRCs (49) and that T cells enter the paracortex from HEVs at specific entry points contiguous with the FRCs network, enabling T cells to be "received" by a greeting line of DCs positioned on top of the FRCs near the HEV entry points (50). Furthermore, different subpopulations of DCs have been shown to localize to specific regions in the LN, suggesting that DC positioning relative to T cells may facilitate T cell activation (51). However, our quantitative analysis using NMI and PCC suggest that T cell association with FRCs does not necessarily lead to similarly high association with DCs. The lack of association between T cells and DCs suggests that T cells have no *a priori* knowledge of DC positions and that DCs are unlikely to attract T cells to DC locations prior to infection. While there is evidence that upon DC activation and infection, chemokines are important to mediate T cell repositioning to DCs (52–54), our data suggests that chemokines CCL19/21 that bind to CCR7 do not play a role in T cell positioning to DCs in the absence of infection. We previously demonstrated that T cells move with a lognormal correlated random walk (55), which aligns with several other studies in the LN (56, 57). Our results suggest that random movement, rather than guided movement, may be the strategy that naive T cells use to interact with DCs prior to infection.

Although T cells and DCs have low NMI and PCC, we find that unexpectedly, lack of CCR7 does not decrease association between T cells and DCs, in fact, CCR7-deficient T cells show slightly increased association with DCs. CCR7 mediates high speed motility in LNs (58). One possible explanation for our finding is that CCR7 deficiency in T cells results in slower T cells that cannot efficiently move away from DCs once they have made contact. Alternatively, CCR7 signaling might be important for T cells to move along FRCs where they receive chemokinetic and survival signals, including both CCL21 and other cytokines such as IL-7 so that in the absence of CCR7, T cells stay closer to DCs, which are not the primary source of CCL21 (59, 60). While it is known that CCR7-deficient T cells are less capable of activation, our quantitative analysis suggests that this may not be due to lack of T:DC contacts but rather may be due to CCR7 effects on overall motility or effects on cosignaling with T cell receptors.

We validated both NMI and PCC on simulated data where we directly manipulated the spatial association of cells and showed that both metrics decrease as spatial association decreases and as region size increases (**Figure 4**). We designed NMI to normalize for differences in fluorescence between fields, and NMI can quantify non-linear relationships between variables (27) while PCC is based on correlation coefficients (22, 26). In addition, information based measures are theoretically insensitive to coarse graining (34). Our regional NMI analyses in both simulated and experimental images is consistent with this theoretical prediction in that NMI is less sensitive to region size than PCC (**Figures 4** and **5**). We find that NMI is also less sensitive to variations in cell number than PCC, particularly in cases in which there is already spatial association (Figure S2 in Supplementary Material). Furthermore, NMI based on regions avoids problems associated with pixel-distance measures that arise from 2PM images containing transient single pixel noise (61). Cell-distance measures are also problematic because they require the boundaries of cells, or their centroids, to be well defined. That is usually not the case in 2PM images, especially in the case of DCs and FRCs.

While both NMI and PCC consistently show that T cells are more spatially associated with FRCs than with DCs, we note several caveats in interpreting these results. We considered that T cells may share the highest NMI or PCC with the most numerous cells or structures that occupy the most volume in the paracortex, simply because they cannot move away from the abundant cell type or structure without encountering another cell or structure of the same kind. However, our simulations (**Figure 3C**) validated that NMI is insensitive to variation in cell number, with fivefold variation in cell number causing much less effect on NMI than changes in spatial association. While the amount of background noise (low-level fluorescence of individual pixels) has some effect on NMI and PCC, that effect does not change the conclusion that NMI and PCC both indicate higher spatial association of T cells with FRCs than with DCs.

Similar to previous studies, our experimental method uses irradiation to image FRCs showing residual GFP$^+$ hematopoeitic cells (between 5 and 10%). Thus, it is possible that T:DC can contribute to the T:FRC NMI and PCC. However, because NMI and PCC of T cells with DCs are significantly lower, it is unlikely that the increase in T cell association seen with FRCs is due to residual DC signal. There may also be limitations in the use of two photon imaging as the primary mode of visualizing T cell interactions in the T cell zone as the T cell zone is usually deeper in the LN cortex. Thus, although many publications have used two photon imaging to understand T cell motion in LNs, T cell associations with FRCs and DCs may vary depending on the specific areas that are imaged. In addition, it is possible that staining specific subsets of T cells or DCs may reveal more or less spatial association than we see with total T cells and all CD11c$^+$ cells.

In summary, our results show that NMI and PCC both provide quantitative methods to analyze the relationship between two sets of objects, validated in simulations. NMI and PCC show significant differences for different cell populations labeled with two different fluorescent markers, providing quantitative comparisons of fluorescent microscopy images across multiple fields (62). Thus, both NMI and PCC of physiologically relevant regions are useful tools to quantify the relationship between fluorescent cell types. Since MI is a general method for measuring colocalization of fluorescence microscopy images including 2PM signals, the NMI and regional analyses may be broadly applied to any colocalization study of differentially fluorescent objects.

AUTHOR CONTRIBUTIONS

GMF and MEM conceived of MI as a measure of cell-type interactions. JRB, under JLC, conducted 2PM imaging of *ex vivo* lymph nodes. JRB, HT, JOS, and GMF wrote software to analyze the images. HT wrote a simulation to validate the MI approach. HT, GMF, JRB, MEM, and JLC wrote sections of the paper. HT and JRB created the figures. All authors contributed to manuscript revision and approved the submitted version.

ACKNOWLEDGMENTS

We would like to thank Nick Watkins and Sandra Chapman for useful discussion as well as the very helpful suggestions by reviewers to include analysis of regions of 2PM images, rather than just pixel-based comparisons.

FUNDING

This work was supported by funding from the following: DOD STTR Contract FA8650-18-C-6898 (JLC and MEM), NIH 1R01AI097202 (JLC), the Spatiotemporal Modeling Center (P50 GM085273), the Center for Evolution and Theoretical Immunology 5P20GM103452 (JLC), and a James S. McDonnell Foundation grant for the study of Complex Systems (MEM and GMF). Thanks to the UNM Cancer Center Fluorescence Microscopy Facility (P30-CA118100) as well as the BRAIN Imaging Center (P30GM103400) for help with two-photon microscopy. JRB was supported by T32 NIH 5 T32 AI007538-19 as well as the Ruby Predoctoral Travel Fellowship from the Molecular Genetics and Microbiology Department at UNM HSC. JLC is a member of the Center of Biomedical Research Excellence (CoBRE) Autophagy, Inflammation, and Metabolism (AIM) in Disease (P20GM121176). HT and MEM were supported by an LDRD grant from Sandia National Laboratories.

SUPPLEMENTARY MATERIAL

FIGURE S1 | Illustration of the highest and lowest NMI that can be generated from the experimental data. The NMI of an image with itself is the maximum value of 1, shown for an example image of red cells and an example image of green cells. To obtain a minimum value, we calculate NMI between two images, one red and one green from two different fields so that the images are unrelated. We calculated NMI from 5,036 pairs of frames (Unmatched Red:Green). For this unmatched scenario, the NMI is very close to 0 (median is 0.008).

FIGURE S2 | NMI is more robust than PCC to cell count. Simulated images were generated in which numbers of cells in the green and red channels are varied by number and positions varied as indicated. Apparent association of cell types based purely on the increased chance of two cells being near one another as the number of cells goes up is a concern. The normalization factor in NMI is intended to compensate for this artifact. Insensitivity to variation in cell number while preserving sensitivity to the underlying association between cell types distinguishes NMI from PCC. The number of cells in the green channel is kept constant at 500 while the number of cells in the red channel is varied. NMI results are shown in the left column and PCC in the right column. The spatial association between cell types in the model decreases from $\sigma = 0$ in the top row to uniform random placement in the bottom row.

REFERENCES

Mirsky HP, Miller MJ, Linderman JJ, Kirschner DE. Systems biology approaches for understanding cellular mechanisms of immunity in lymph nodes during infection. *J Theor Biol* (2011) 287:160–70. doi:10.1016/j.jtbi.2011.06.037

Brewitz A, Eickhoff S, Dähling S, Quast T, Bedoui S, Kroczek RA, et al. CD8+ T cells orchestrate pDC-XCR1+ dendritic cell spatial and functional cooperativity to optimize priming. *Immunity* (2017) 46(2):205–19. doi:10.1016/j.immuni.2017.01.003

Wong HS, Germain RN. Robust control of the adaptive immune system. *Semin Immunol* (2018) 36:17–27. doi:10.1016/j.smim.2017.12.009

Baekkevold ES, Yamanaka T, Palframan RT, Carlsen HS, Reinholt FP, von Andrian UH, et al. The CCR7 ligand elc (CCL19) is transcytosed in high endothelial venules and mediates T cell recruitment. *J Exp Med* (2001) 193(9):1105–12. doi:10.1084/jem.193.9.1105

Gretz JE, Norbury CC, Anderson AO, Proudfoot AEI, Shaw S. Lymph-borne chemokines and other low molecular weight molecules reach high endothelial venules via specialized conduits while a functional barrier limits access to the lymphocyte microenvironments in lymph node cortex. *J Exp Med* (2000) 192(10):1425–40. doi:10.1084/jem.192.10.1425

Palframan RT, Jung S, Cheng G, Weninger W, Luo Y, Dorf M, et al. Inflammatory chemokine transport and presentation in HEV. *J Exp Med* (2001) 194(9):1361–74. doi:10.1084/jem.194.9.1361

Sixt M, Kanazawa N, Selg M, Samson T, Roos G, Reinhardt DP, et al. The conduit system transports soluble antigens from the afferent lymph to resident dendritic cells in the T cell area of the lymph node. *Immunity* (2005) 22(1):19–29. doi:10.1016/j.immuni.2004.11.013

Stein JV, Nombela-Arrieta C. Chemokine control of lymphocyte trafficking: a general overview. *Immunology* (2005) 116(1):1–12. doi:10.1111/j.1365-2567.2005.02183.x

von Andrian UH, Mackay CR. T-cell function and migration—two sides of the same coin. *N Engl J Med* (2000) 343(14):1020–34. doi:10.1056/NEJM200010053431407

Novkovic M, Onder L, Cupovic J, Abe J, Bomze D, Cremasco V, et al. Topological small-world organization of the fibroblastic reticular cell network determines lymph node functionality. *PLoS Biol* (2016) 14(7):e1002515. doi:10.1371/journal.pbio.1002515

Bajénoff M, Egen JG, Koo LY, Laugier JP, Brau F, Glaichenhaus N, et al. Stromal cell networks regulate lymphocyte entry, migration, and territoriality in lymph nodes. *Immunity* (2006) 25(6):989–1001. doi:10.1016/j.immuni.2006.10.011

Girard J-P, Moussion C, Förster R. HEVs, lymphatics and homeostatic immune cell trafficking in lymph nodes. *Nat Rev Immunol* (2012) 12(11):762–73. doi:10.1038/nri3298

Donovan GM, Lythe G. T cell and reticular network co-dependence in HIV infection. *J Theor Biol* (2016) 395:211–20. doi:10.1016/j.jtbi.2016.01.040

Katakai T, Hara T, Lee J-H, Gonda H, Sugai M, Shimizu A. A novel reticular stromal structure in lymph node cortex: an immuno-platform for interactions among dendritic cells, T cells and B cells. *Int Immunol* (2004) 16(8):1133–42. doi:10.1093/intimm/dxh113

Textor J, Mandl JN, de Boer RJ. The reticular cell network: a robust backbone for immune responses. *PLoS Biol* (2016) 14(10):e2000827. doi:10.1371/ journal.pbio.2000827

Zeng M, Southern PJ, Reilly CS, Beilman GJ, Chipman JG, Schacker TW, et al. Lymphoid tissue damage in HIV-1 infection depletes naïve T cells and limits T cell reconstitution after antiretroviral therapy. *PLoS Pathog* (2012) 8(1):e1002437. doi:10.1371/journal.ppat.1002437

Takeda A, Kobayashi D, Aoi K, Sasaki N, Sugiura Y, Igarashi H, et al. Fibroblastic reticular cell-derived lysophosphatidic acid regulates confined intranodal T-cell motility. *Elife* (2016) 5:e10561. doi:10.7554/eLife.10561

Asperti-Boursin F, Real E, Bismuth G, Trautmann A, Donnadieu E. CCR7 ligands control basal T cell motility within lymph node slices in a phosphoinositide 3-kinase-independent manner. *J Exp Med* (2007) 204(5):1167–79. doi:10.1084/jem.20062079

Letendre K, Asperti-Boursin F, Donnadieu E, Moses ME, Cannon JL. Bringing statistics up to speed with data in analysis of lymphocyte motility. *PLoS One* (2015) 10(5):e0126333. doi:10.1371/journal.pone.0126333

Mempel TR, Henrickson SE, Von Andrian UH. T-cell priming by dendritic cells in lymph nodes occurs in three distinct phases. *Nature* (2004) 427(6970):154–9. doi:10.1038/nature02238

Mrass P, Oruganti SR, Fricke GM, Tafoya J, Byrum JR, Yang L, et al. ROCK regulates the intermittent mode of interstitial T cell migration in inflamed lungs. *Nat Commun* (2017) 8(1):1010. doi:10.1038/s41467-017-01032-2

Adler J, Parmryd I. Quantifying colocalization by correlation: the Pearson correlation coefficient is superior to the Mander's overlap coefficient. *Cyto metry A* (2010) 77(8):733–42. doi:10.1002/cyto.a.20896

Barlow AL, MacLeod A, Noppen S, Sanderson J, Guérin CJ. Colocalization analysis in fluorescence micrographs: verification of a more accurate calculation of Pearson's correlation coefficient. *Microsc Microanal* (2010) 16(6): 710–24. doi:10.1017/S143192761009389X

Shannon CE. A mathematical theory of communication. *Bell Syst Tech J* (1948) 27(3):379–423. doi:10.1002/j.1538-7305.1948.tb01338.x

Dinic J, Riehl A, Adler J, Parmryd I. The T cell receptor resides in ordered plasma membrane nanodomains that aggregate upon patching of the receptor. *Sci Rep* (2015) 5:10082. doi:10.1038/srep10082

Dunn KW, Kamocka MM, McDonald JH. A practical guide to evaluating colocalization in biological microscopy. *Am J Physiol Cell Physiol* (2011) 300(4):C723–42. doi:10.1152/ajpcell.00462.2010

Smith R. A mutual information approach to calculating nonlinearity. *Stat* (2015) 4(1):291–303. doi:10.1002/sta4.96

Kim J. Visual correspondence using energy minimization and mutual information. *Proceedings Ninth IEEE International Conference on Computer Vision, 2003*. New York: IEEE (2003). p. 1033–40.

Pluim JPW, Maintz JBA, Viergever MA. Mutual-information-based registration of medical images: a survey. *IEEE Trans Med Imaging* (2003) 22(8):986–1004. doi:10.1109/TMI.2003.815867

Studholme C, Hill DLG, Hawkes DJ. An overlap invariant entropy measure of 3D medical image alignment. *Pattern Recognit* (1999) 32(1):71–86. doi:10.1016/S0031-3203(98)00091-0

Viola P, Wells WM III. Alignment by maximization of mutual information. *Int J Comput Vis* (1997) 24(2):137–54. doi:10.1023/A:1007958904918

Lizier JT. JIDT: an information-theoretic toolkit for studying the dynamics of complex systems. *Front Robot AI* (2014) 1:11. doi:10.3389/frobt.2014.00011

Prokopenko M, Boschetti F, Ryan AJ. An information-theoretic primer on complexity, self-organization, and emergence. *Complexity* (2009) 15(1):11–28. doi:10.1002/cplx.20249

DeDeo S, Hawkins RXD, Klingenstein S, Hitchcock T. Bootstrap methods for the empirical study of decision-making and information flows in social systems. *Entropy* (2013) 15(6):2246–76. doi:10.3390/e15062246

Fricke GM. *Search in T cell and Robot Swarms: Balancing Extent and Intensity*. Albuquerque: University of New Mexico, PhD thesis (2017).

Coombs CH, Dawes RM, Tversky A. *Mathematical Psychology: An Elementary Introduction*. Oxford, England: Prentice-Hall (1970).

Press WH. *Numerical Recipes 3rd Edition: The Art of Scientific Computing*. Cambridge: Cambridge University Press (2007).

Vinh NX, Epps J, Bailey J. Information theoretic measures for clusterings comparison: variants, properties, normalization and correction for chance. *J Mach Learn Res* (2010) 11:2837–54.

Witten IH, Frank E, Hall MA, Pal CJ. *Data Mining: Practical Machine Learning Tools and Techniques*. Burlington, Massachusetts: Morgan Kaufmann (2016).

Altman D, Machin D, Bryant T, Gardner M, editors. *Statistics with Confidence: Confidence Intervals and Statistical Guidelines, BMJ*. 2nd ed. London: John Wiley & Sons (2000).

Gray RM. *Entropy and Information Theory*. New York: Springer Science & Business Media (2011).

McGill R, Tukey JW, Larsen WA. Variations of box plots. *Am Stat* (1978) 32(1):12–6. doi:10.1080/00031305.1978.10479236

Fletcher PA, Scriven DRL, Schulson MN, Moore EDW. Multi-image colocalization and its statistical significance. *Biophys J* (2010) 99(6):1996–2005. doi:10.1016/j.bpj.2010.07.006

Reshef DN, Reshef YA, Finucane HK, Grossman SR, McVean G, Turnbaugh PJ, et al. Detecting novel associations in large data sets. *Science* (2011) 334(6062):1518–24. doi:10.1126/science.1205438

Stein JV, Rot A, Luo Y, Narasimhaswamy M, Nakano H, Gunn MD, et al. The CC chemokine thymus-derived chemotactic agent 4 (TCA-4, secondary lymphoid tissue chemokine, 6Ckine, exodus-2) triggers lymphocyte function–associated antigen 1–mediated arrest of rolling T lymphocytes in peripheral lymph node high endothelial venules. *J Exp Med* (2000) 191(1):61–76. doi:10.1084/jem.191.1.61

Bajénoff M, Granjeaud S, Guerder S. The strategy of T cell antigen-presenting cell encounter in antigen-draining lymph nodes revealed by imaging of initial T cell activation. *J Exp Med* (2003) 198(5):715–24. doi:10.1084/jem.20030167

Krummel MF, Bartumeus F, Gérard A. T cell migration, search strategies and mechanisms. *Nat Rev Immunol* (2016) 16(3):193. doi:10.1038/nri.2015.16

Westermann J, Bode U, Sahle A, Speck U, Karin N, Bell EB, et al. Naive, effector, and memory T lymphocytes effi tly scan dendritic cells in vivo: contact frequency in T cell zones of secondary lymphoid organs does not depend on LFA-1 expression and facilitates survival of effector T cells. *J Immunol* (2005) 174(5):2517–24. doi:10.4049/jimmunol.174.5.2517

Gasteiger G, Ataide M, Kastenmüller W. Lymph node – an organ for T-cell activation and pathogen defense. *Immunol Rev* (2016) 271(1):200–20. doi:10.1111/imr.12399

Lindquist RL, Shakhar G, Dudziak D, Wardemann H, Eisenreich T, Dustin ML, et al. Visualizing dendritic cell networks in vivo. *Nat Immunol* (2004) 5(12):1243–50. doi:10.1038/ni1139

Gerner MY, Torabi-Parizi P, Germain RN. Strategically localized dendritic cells promote rapid T cell responses to lymph-borne particulate antigens. *Immunity* (2015) 42(1):172–85. doi:10.1016/j.immuni.2014.12.024

Castellino F, Huang AY, Altan-Bonnet G, Stoll S, Scheinecker C, Germain RN. Chemokines enhance immunity by guiding naive {CD}8+ {T} cells to sites of{CD}4+ {T} cell-dendritic cell interaction. *Nature* (2006) 440(7086):890–5. doi:10.1038/nature04651

Groom JR, Richmond J, Murooka TT, Sorensen EW, Sung JH, Bankert K, et al. CXCR3 chemokine receptor-ligand interactions in the lymph node optimize CD4+ T helper 1 cell differentiation. *Immunity* (2012) 37(6):1091–103. doi:10.1016/j.immuni.2012.08.016

Lian J, Luster AD. Chemokine-guided cell positioning in the lymph node orchestrates the generation of adaptive immune responses. *Curr Opin Cell Biol* (2015) 36:1–6. doi:10.1016/j.ceb.2015.05.003

Fricke GM, Letendre KA, Moses ME, Cannon JL. Persistence and adaptation in immunity: T cells balance the extent and thoroughness of search. *PLoS Comput Biol* (2016) 12(3):e1004818. doi:10.1371/journal.pcbi.1004818

Banigan EJ, Harris TH, Christian DA, Hunter CA, Liu AJ, Asquith B. Heterogeneous CD8+ T cell migration in the lymph node in the absence of inflammation revealed by quantitative migration analysis. *PLoS Comput Biol* (2015) 11(2):e1004058. doi:10.1371/journal.pcbi.1004058

Miller MJ, Wei SH, Cahalan MD, Parker I. Autonomous T cell trafficking examined in vivo with intravital two-photon microscopy. *Proc Natl Acad Sci U S A* (2003) 100(5):2604–9. doi:10.1073/pnas.2628040100

Katakai T, Kinashi T. Microenvironmental control of high-speed interstitial T cell migration in the lymph node. *Front Immunol* (2016) 7:194. doi:10.3389/fimmu.2016.00194

Katakai T, Suto H, Sugai M, Gonda H, Togawa A, Suematsu S, et al. Organizer-like reticular stromal cell layer common to adult secondary lym- phoid organs. *J Immunol* (2008) 181(9):6189–200. doi:10.4049/jimmunol.181.9.6189

Link A, Vogt TK, Favre S, Britschgi MR, Acha-Orbea H, Hinz B, et al. Fibroblastic reticular cells in lymph nodes regulate the homeostasis of naive T cells. *Nat Immunol* (2007) 8(11):1255. doi:10.1038/ni1513

Pawley JB, Masters BR. Handbook of biological confocal microscopy. *J Biomed Opt* (2008) 13(2):9902. doi:10.1117/1.2911629

Strehl A, Ghosh J. Cluster ensembles – a knowledge reuse framework for combining multiple partitions. *J Mach Learn Res* (2002) 3:583–617.

2

Variable Effect of HIV Superinfection on Clinical Status: Insights from Mathematical Modeling

*Ágnes Móréh [1], András Szilágyi [2,3], István Scheuring [2,3] and Viktor Müller [2,4]**

[1] MTA Centre for Ecological Research, Danube Research Institute, Budapest, Hungary, [2] Evolutionary Systems Research Group, MTA Centre for Ecological Research, Tihany, Hungary, [3] MTA-ELTE Theoretical Biology and Evolutionary Ecology Research Group, Institute of Biology, Eötvös Loránd University, Budapest, Hungary, [4] Department of Plant Systematics, Ecology and Theoretical Biology, Institute of Biology, Eötvös Loránd University, Budapest, Hungary

***Correspondence:**
Viktor Müller
mueller.viktor@ttk.elte.hu

HIV superinfection (infection of an HIV positive individual with another strain of the virus) has been shown to result in a deterioration of clinical status in multiple case studies. However, superinfection with no (or positive) clinical outcome might easily go unnoticed, and the typical effect of superinfection is unknown. We analyzed mathematical models of HIV dynamics to assess the effect of superinfection under various assumptions. We extended the basic model of virus dynamics to explore systematically a set of model variants incorporating various details of HIV infection (homeostatic target cell dynamics, bystander killing, interference competition between viral clones, multiple target cell types, virus-induced activation of target cells). In each model, we identified the conditions for superinfection, and investigated whether and how successful invasion by a second viral strain affects the level of uninfected target cells. In the basic model, and in some of its extensions, the criteria for invasion necessarily entail a decrease in the equilibrium abundance of uninfected target cells. However, we identified three novel scenarios where superinfection can substantially increase the uninfected cell count: (i) if the rate of new infections saturates at high infectious titers (due to interference competition or cell-autonomous innate immunity); or when the invading strain is more efficient at infecting activated target cells, but less efficient at (ii) activating quiescent cells or (iii) inducing bystander killing of these cells. In addition, multiple target cell types also allow for modest increases in the total target cell count. We thus conclude that the effect of HIV superinfection on clinical status might be variable, complicated by factors that are independent of the invasion fitness of the second viral strain.

Keywords: HIV superinfection, AIDS, mathematical model, virus dynamics, invasion analysis

1. INTRODUCTION

HIV superinfection occurs when a person already infected with HIV acquires a second (unrelated) strain of the virus. While estimates for the incidence of superinfection vary widely [from virtually zero (Gonzales et al., 2003; Tsui et al., 2004) to rates comparable to that of initial infection (Piantadosi et al., 2008; Redd et al., 2011; Kraft et al., 2012)], the ubiquitous imprint of recombination on the global evolution of HIV diversity (Rambaut et al., 2004; Vuilleumier and Bonhoeffer, 2015) indicates that superinfection cannot be very rare. At the population level, superinfection might affect the evolution of virulence (Nowak and May, 1994; van Baalen and Sabelis, 1995; Alizon and van Baalen, 2008), it might potentially contribute to the spread of drug resistance (Chakraborty et al., 2004; Smith et al., 2005), and, in the case of HIV, it also allows for recombination between distant lineages, which might facilitate adaptation and evolutionary innovation in the virus (Vuilleumier and Bonhoeffer, 2015).

Superinfection can also have an impact on the health status of the affected individual. A number of studies have reported either abrupt deterioration of clinical status (a drop in the CD4+ T cell count and/or increase in the virus load), or accelerated disease progression following superinfection (Altfeld et al., 2002; Jost et al., 2002; Gottlieb et al., 2004, 2007; Yerly et al., 2004; van der Kuyl et al., 2005; Clerc et al., 2010; Cornelissen et al., 2012; Brener et al., 2018). However, there are also counterexamples, where superinfection did not have a negative impact (Casado et al., 2007) or the effect was only transient (Rachinger et al., 2008). Furthermore, superinfection events with no (or, possibly, beneficial) effects might often go unnoticed, as the detection of superinfection requires the sequencing of the viral genome, which is rarely done in unproblematic infections. This led the authors of a comprehensive review on HIV superinfection to conclude that "the full extent and potency of the detrimental effects of superinfection remain unclear and might depend on several viral and host factors" (Redd et al., 2013).

Here, following up on Fung et al. (2010), we use simple mathematical models of HIV infection to analyze a set of biologically relevant scenarios with respect to the possible outcomes of superinfection. Mathematical modeling has been used to study various aspects of the complexity of HIV infection (Nowak and May, 2000; Perelson, 2002; Müller and Bonhoeffer, 2003), including within-host evolution (e.g., Iwasa et al., 2004, 2005) and some scenarios for superinfection (Fung et al., 2010). From an ecological perspective, both cases can be regarded as "invasion tests" (Chesson, 2000): is the second strain (the mutant or the "invader") able to spread in the steady state (chronic infection) established by the first strain? We use invasion analysis to determine under what conditions a second strain of the virus can establish superinfection, either coexisting with, or excluding the original strain. For the cases where superinfection is successful, we assess the range of possible effects on the uninfected target cell count, which serves as a proxy for the clinical status (health) of the patient. We find that, contrary to intuition, there are biologically plausible scenarios that allow superinfection not only to decrease, but also to increase the target cell count.

2. MODELS AND METHODS

The mathematical framework of virus dynamics describes the interactions between relevant cell and virus types within an infected individual (see e.g., Nowak and May, 2000). Models consist of differential equations that describe the rate of change of each cell and virus type (the variables of the model). We extended the basic model of virus dynamics to explore systematically a set of model variants incorporating various details of HIV infection.

Exposure to superinfection can be implemented by adding a low initial inoculum of a second viral strain to a chronic (steady-state) infection established by the first strain in the models (equivalent to modeling the outcome of within-host mutation events Iwasa et al., 2004). Three outcomes are possible: (i) successful invasion and exclusion of the resident strain; (ii) successful invasion, followed by stable coexistence of both strains; (iii) unsuccessful invasion, the system remains in the original equilibrium with only the resident strain. The invasion is successful (superinfection occurs) if the initial growth rate of the new strain is positive when introduced into the established steady state of the original strain. Exclusion of the original strain occurs if the steady-state cell count of the original strain is zero in the presence of the new strain. Finally, successful invasion results in coexistence if both strains can grow when introduced into a steady-state infection established by the other strain (mutual invasibility).

The impact of superinfection on clinical status can be approximated by comparing the steady-state level of uninfected cells (corresponding to functional CD4+ T cells) before and following the invasion of the superinfecting strain. The possible range of outcomes can be determined by analyzing whether and how the conditions for superinfection constrain the relation of prior and subsequent steady-state target cell levels. In particular, superinfection is strictly associated with the deterioration of clinical status when the (mathematical) conditions for superinfection unambiguously imply that the stable steady-state level of the uninfected cells will be lower in the presence of the invading strain. In this case, only strains that reduce the steady state and thus have negative clinical impact will be able to establish superinfection.

In some of the models, the steady states (equilibrium points) of the system, and the conditions for invasion (and superinfection) could be readily calculated and characterized analytically. In the cases where the analytical approach was impractical due to the complexity of the equations, we employed numerical simulations. We selected credible intervals for all parameter values (Table A5 in Appendix), and then sampled the parameters from their respective intervals independently for each simulation run. We integrated the set of equations corresponding to the uninfected system until equilibrium, then Strain 1 was added. After the system attained steady state (and stable infection with Strain 1 was verified), Strain 2 was added with a low concentration as an invader; the parameters for Strain 2 were selected with the same procedure (including the requirement to establish stable infection given its independently generated set of both viral and host parameters). In case of successful superinfection, we recorded the steady-state level of uninfected target cells both before and after superinfection, along with the corresponding parameter values. We repeated the simulations until we obtained 20000 independent runs with successful superinfection. Numerical integration was performed with the SUNDIALS/CVODE package (Hindmarsh et al., 2005) (C source code is available upon request). In each simulation, we verified the local asymptotic stability of the final steady states by computing the leading eigenvalue of the corresponding Jacobian matrix.

In the following we illustrate the analytical method on a slightly simplified version of the basic model of virus dynamics, then introduce the model variants that we have tested in our analyses.

2.1. Basic Model

As a starting point, we use a two-strain variant of the established model of virus dynamics, consisting of uninfected target cells (T) and two types of infected cells (I_1 and I_2) that harbor the resident and the invading strain of the virus, respectively. The dynamics has the form:

$$\dot{T} = \sigma - (\beta_1 I_1 + \beta_2 I_2)\, T - \delta_T T \tag{1}$$

$$\dot{I}_1 = \beta_1 T I_1 - \delta_1 I_1 \tag{2}$$

$$\dot{I}_2 = \beta_2 T I_2 - \delta_2 I_2, \tag{3}$$

where σ is the influx rate, δ_T is the death rate of uninfected cells, respectively. β_i denotes the infection efficiency of the ith viral strain, and δ_i is the death rate of cells infected with strain i. This is a slightly reduced form of the "basic model of virus dynamics" (Nowak and May, 2000), as it does not explicitly follow the levels of virus particles. This established simplification is justified by the faster turnover of free virions (compared with infected cells), which implies that the concentration of free virions follows (in a quasi steady state) the level of virus producing cells, and the rate of new infections can be made a function of the level of infected cells without loss of generality (Nowak and May, 2000).

The equilibrium values of the target cells can be determined analytically. If infected cells are not present, the system reduces to Equation (1), and the equilibrium value of uninfected cells is $\hat{T}^{()} = \frac{\sigma}{\delta_T}$, where empty brackets in the superscript denote the absence of infection.

If only Strain 1 is present, the corresponding system is Equations (1, 2), and the equilibrium values are: $\hat{T}^{(I_1)} = \frac{\delta_1}{\beta_1}$ and $\hat{I}_1^{(I_1)} = \frac{\sigma}{\delta_1} - \frac{\delta_T}{\beta_1}$. Substituting the uninfected steady state into Equation (2), it follows that infection can be established only if $\frac{\sigma}{\delta_T} > \frac{\delta_1}{\beta_1}$, implying

$$\hat{T}^{()} > \hat{T}^{(I_1)}. \tag{4}$$

That is, infection always decreases the uninfected target cell count. Because of the symmetry in the dynamics of infected cells, the same result is obtained for the situation when Strain 2 is present alone. Finally, because $\dot{I}_1 = 0$ and $\dot{I}_2 = 0$ are satisfied at different target cell levels (except for the special case when $\frac{\delta_1}{\beta_1} = \frac{\delta_2}{\beta_2}$), there is no generic equilibrium point with both strains present. The equilibrium values are listed in **Table 1**.

To illustrate the method, in the following we analyze the possibility and the possible outcomes of superinfection in this basic model. The criterion of successful invasion by Strain 2 is the positivity of the growth rate of I_2 ($\dot{I}_2 > 0$) in a chronic infection established by the first strain ($ES2$: $\hat{T}^{(I_1)}$, $\hat{I}_1^{(I_1)}$). By substituting $\hat{T}^{(I_1)}$ into Equation (3), it follows that the condition for successful

TABLE 1 | The equilibrium states (ES) of the basic model.

	$\hat{T}$	$\hat{I}_1$	$\hat{I}_2$
*ES*1 ()	$\frac{\sigma}{\delta_T}$	0	0
*ES*2 (I_1)	$\frac{\delta_1}{\beta_1}$	$\frac{\sigma}{\delta_1} - \frac{\delta_T}{\beta_1}$	0
*ES*3 (I_2)	$\frac{\delta_2}{\beta_2}$	0	$\frac{\sigma}{\delta_2} - \frac{\delta_T}{\beta_2}$

The viral strain present in each state is indicated in brackets; empty brackets in ES1 () denote the absence of infection.

invasion is $\frac{\delta_1}{\beta_1} > \frac{\delta_2}{\beta_2}$, which can be rewritten in terms of the equilibrium target cell counts as:

$$\hat{T}^{(I_1)} > \hat{T}^{(I_2)}, \tag{5}$$

implying that successful superinfection always decreases the uninfected target cell count at steady state, because only strains that lower the count can establish superinfection. The criterion for the stable coexistence of both types of infected cells is a positive growth rate of each type of infected cells in the established population of the other. However, mutual invasibility cannot be satisfied as Equation (5) and its reverse cannot be satisfied simultaneously. As a consequence, successful invasion results in the extinction of the resident strain, and the lower steady-state cell count associated with the superinfecting strain is attained.

In this simple system the coexistence of both strains in not possible, and the impact of superinfection is unequivocal. However, implementing some aspects of the complexity of HIV infection can open up the possibility of more complicated behavior in the models. In the following, we introduce extended models of HIV dynamics that incorporate homeostatic target cell dynamics, bystander killing (with or without inducible HIV-specific immunity), interference competition in the infection process, multiple target cell types, or the virus-induced activation of quiescent target cells. The analysis of these models, following the procedure described above, is presented in the Results.

2.2. Homeostatic Target Cell Dynamics

The basic model of virus dynamics assumes a constant rate of influx for the susceptible target cells. However, at least some of the new production is likely to arise from the division of existing target cells, and this process must then inevitably be regulated to maintain stable cell counts. Such homeostatic dynamics can be described by a logistic growth term that is a decreasing function of the current size of the cell pool, and we employed the following equation to describe such self-limiting dynamics for the target cells:

$$\dot{T} = rT\left(1 - \frac{T}{K}\right) - (\beta_1 I_1 + \beta_2 I_2)\, T - \delta_T T. \tag{6}$$

Here r defines the maximal per capita growth rate of the uninfected target cells, and K is the "carrying capacity" at which divisions stop entirely. Note that we have retained the simple exponential death term ($\delta_T T$) for consistence with the basic model, and the dynamics of the infected cells remain unchanged (cf. Equations 2, 3).

2.3. Models With Bystander Killing of Uninfected Cells

Accumulating evidence indicates that the killing of uninfected cells (induced, primarily, by pyroptosis (Doitsh et al., 2014; Ke et al., 2017) might be a major mechanism of HIV-associated loss of CD4+ T lymphocytes. Viral strains are likely to differ in their ability to induce bystander killing, which gives rise to the following model variant:

$$\dot{T} = \sigma - [(\beta_1 + \gamma_1)I_1 + (\beta_2 + \gamma_2)I_2]T - \delta_T T \quad (7)$$

$$\dot{I_1} = \beta_1 T I_1 - \delta_1 I_1 \quad (8)$$

$$\dot{I_2} = \beta_2 T I_2 - \delta_2 I_2. \quad (9)$$

where the loss of target cells depends not only on the infection efficiency of the strains (β_i, cf. section 2.1), but also on the strength of the bystander killing effect of the infected cells (γ_i).

In addition, inducible immunity that is activated proportional to the level of the antigen can have a profound effect on the equilibria and behavior of the models (De Boer and Perelson, 1998), and indeed on the competition of distinct viral strains (Iwasa et al., 2004). To investigate whether strain-specific immune responses can alter the invasion dynamics of viral strains with varying levels of bystander killing, we combined the earlier model of Iwasa et al. (2004) with bystander killing to obtain the following set of equations:

$$\dot{T} = \sigma - \sum_{i=1,2} (\beta_i + \gamma_i)I_i T - \delta_T T \quad (10)$$

$$\dot{I_i} = \beta_i T I_i - k_i E_i I_i - \delta_i I_i \quad (i = 1,2) \quad (11)$$

$$\dot{E_i} = \alpha_i I_i E_i - \delta_{E_i} E_i \quad (i = 1,2). \quad (12)$$

In this model, the two viral strains (i.e., the cells infected by them) activate, and are targeted by, two different populations of effector cells that are specific to the strains. The effector cells proliferate proportional to the level of infected cells with rate constants α_i, die at rates δ_{E_i}, and they kill infected cells in a concentration dependent manner, with rate constants k_i. The scheme of the models is shown in **Figure 1A**.

We also tested model variants with alternative immune effector mechanisms. Cytotoxic lymphocytes might be able to kill newly infected cells before they could start producing virus (Klenerman et al., 1996), which can be implemented by making the fraction of newly infected cells that enter the virus-producing cell population a decreasing function of the immune response:

$$\dot{I_i} = \frac{\beta_i T}{1 + f_i E_{(i)}} I_i - \delta_i I_i \quad (i = 1,2). \quad (13)$$

The same equation applies also if some effector cells exert a non-cytotoxic effect that reduces the rate of new infections (Levy et al., 1996); in this case the reduction in the infection terms involves also the loss of uninfected cells:

$$\dot{T} = \sigma - \sum_{i=1,2} \frac{\beta_i I_i}{1 + f_i E_{(i)}} T - \delta_T T \quad (14)$$

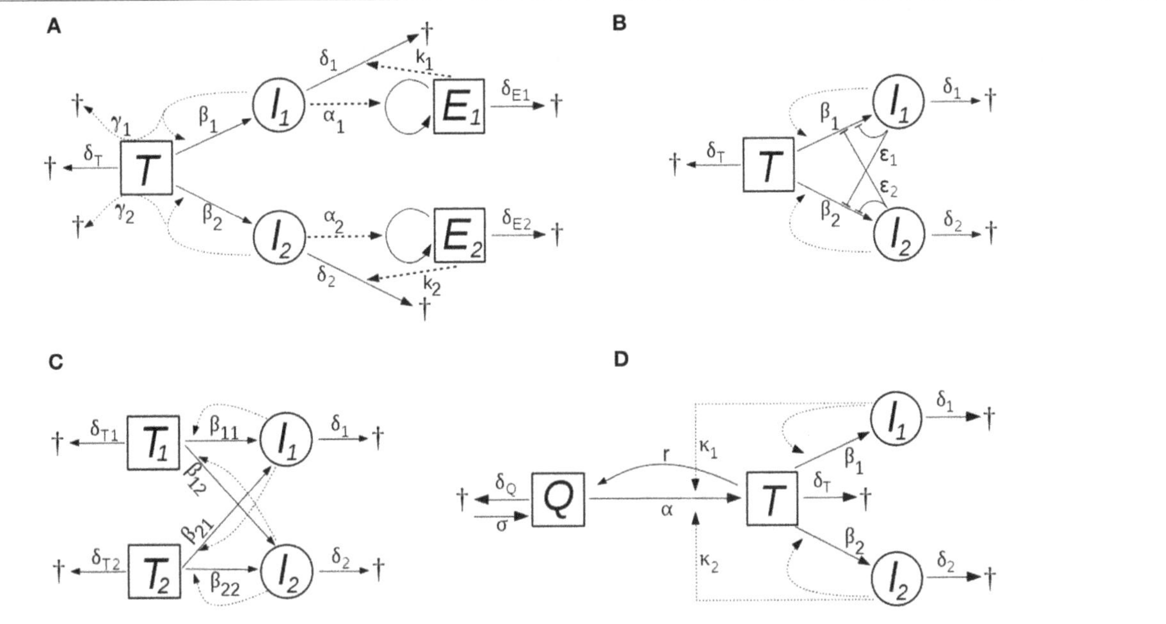

FIGURE 1 | The schemes of the models with **(A)** bystander killing and (optional) strain-specific cytotoxic immunity, **(B)** saturating dynamics of new infections, **(C)** multiple target cell types, and **(D)** HIV induced activation of target cells. New infections occur proportional to the level of infected cells in all models; the level of infectious virions is assumed to follow that of the infected cells, with a proportionality constant implicit in the infection parameter (β). The processes and parameters are explained in the text.

2.4. Saturating Dynamics of New Infections

Two biological scenarios can be implemented by the following formalism:

$$\dot{T} = \sigma - \left(\frac{\sum_{i=1,2} \beta_i I_i}{1 + \sum_{i=1,2} \epsilon_i I_i} \right) T - \delta_T T \quad (15)$$

$$\dot{I}_i = \frac{\beta_i T I_i}{1 + \sum_{i=1,2} \epsilon_i I_i} - \delta_i I_i \quad (i = 1,2), \quad (16)$$

in which the rate of new infections increases slower than linearly with increasing infectious titer, and saturates at high titers; ϵ_i parameters characterize the strength of the effect. First, this can be regarded as a "functional response" in the infection term, acknowledging that the linear proportionality between the rate of infections and the level of infected cells cannot be valid indefinitely as the level of the infected cells increases: at high levels, competitive saturation occurs due to interference (crowding) effects (Schoener, 1978). Alternatively, the same model structure applies also if the presence of the virus induces innate antiviral mechanisms in the target cells (e.g., in the context of abortive infections). HIV is known to be affected by several cell-autonomous innate immune mechanisms (Zheng et al., 2012), some of which are likely to be inducible. In this setting, the effective infection rate might decrease already at lower levels of the infected cells. **Figure 1B** illustrates the scheme of this model.

2.5. Multiple Target Cell Types

Strains of HIV can differ in their target cell tropism, which might also have an effect on their competition dynamics. With regard to the blood CD4+ T cell count (which we use as a proxy for clinical status), the major distinction lies between cells expressing either the CCR5 or the CXCR4 coreceptor (Bleul et al., 1997). Some viral strains are specific for the former, but dual-tropic viruses often evolve during the course of disease progression, with varying levels of affinity for the two coreceptors (Connor et al., 1997). For simplicity, we here investigate two target cell types that are produced independently of each other at rates σ_i, and can be infected by one or both viral strains with coefficients β_{ij}:

$$\dot{T}_i = \sigma_i - T_i \sum_{j=1,2} \beta_{ij} I_j - \delta_{T_i} T_i \quad (i = 1,2; j = 1,2) \quad (17)$$

$$\dot{I}_j = \sum_{i=1,2} \beta_{ij} T_i I_j - \delta_j I_j \quad (i = 1,2; j = 1,2) \quad (18)$$

The total target cell level comprises $\sum_i T_i$; the scheme of the model is shown in **Figure 1C**.

2.6. HIV-Induced T-Cell Activation

Our last scenario implements some of the complexity in the dynamics of the target cells of HIV infection. While the majority of CD4+ T cell cells in the body are in a quiescent state, HIV infects only activated cells efficiently (Bukrinsky et al., 1991; Chiu et al., 2005). In addition, the presence of the virus itself might increase the rate of activation, which complicates the dynamics and brings up the possibility that the impact of superinfection might also be affected. Building on earlier models (e.g., Bartha et al., 2008), we consider the following system of equations:

$$\dot{Q} = \sigma - \delta_q Q - (\alpha + \sum_{i=1,2} \kappa_i I_i) Q + rT \quad (19)$$

$$\dot{T} = \left(\alpha + \sum_{i=1,2} \kappa_i I_i \right) Q - (r + \delta_T) T - \sum_{i=1,2} \beta_i I_i T \quad (20)$$

$$\dot{I}_i = \beta_i I_i T - \delta_i I_i \quad (i = 1,2), \quad (21)$$

where T now denotes activated CD4+ T cells (corresponding, as before, to the susceptible target cells in the system), and Q indicates quiescent CD4+ T cells that are in a resting state. Quiescent cells are generated at a constant rate σ, and die at a rate $\delta_Q Q$. They become activated at a rate composed of an HIV-independent component, αQ, and an HIV-dependent component that is proportional to the level of infected cells, $\kappa_i I_i Q$, where κ_i denotes the efficiency of activation mediated by the ith viral strain. Activated target cells (T) revert to quiescent state at the rate rT; the death and infection of target cells, and the dynamics of infected cells are the same as in the basic model (see **Figure 1D**).

Because the dynamics of infected cells is unchanged from the basic model, here, too, coexistence of the two strains is not possible, and successful superinfection always decreases the count of susceptible target cells (T). However, in this model the total CD4+ T cell count includes also the quiescent cells, and for this total, the outcome can be different. For details, see section 3.4.

In each scenario we followed the method introduced above, i.e., we investigated the criteria for invasions (mutual invasibility) and the positivity of the steady-state cell levels. We distinguished the possible equilibrium states based on which cell types are present with nonzero steady-state levels at the equilibrium point; we present the distinct equilibrium states of all models in **Table 2** for easy reference.

3. RESULTS

In Models and Methods we showed that in the basic model of virus dynamics superinfection always entails a decrease in the uninfected target cells. This followed because the criteria for invasion in that model can be fulfilled only for strains that ultimately establish a new steady state of the target cells that is lower than the one set by the resident virus before the invasion. In the following, we use the same methodology of invasion analysis on multiple variants of the HIV dynamics model. The model variants are extensions to the basic model, incorporating various aspects of the complexity of HIV infection. The main results are presented here, while the details of the calculations and simulations are presented in the Appendix. We refer the non-mathematical reader to the beginning of the Discussion, where we summarize the main results in intuitive non-mathematical terms.

TABLE 2 | Summary of the possible equilibrium states in the analyzed models, showing the cell types that are present in each equilibrium point.

	Q	*T*	*I₁*	*I₂*	*E₁*	*E₂*	
ES1		*					Basic model; Homeostatic dynamics; Saturating dynamics
ES2		*	*				
ES3		*		*			
ES4		*	*		*		Bystander killing with strain-specific immunity
ES5		*		*		*	
ES6		*	*	*	*		
ES7		*	*	*		*	
ES8		*	*	*	*	*	
ES1		*					Multiple target cell types*
ES2		*	*				
ES3		*		*			
ES4		*	*	*			
ES1	*	*					HIV-induced T-cell activation
ES2	*	*	*				
ES3	*	*		*			

*For analytical forms see Appendix 1–4. Note, that "homeostatic dynamics" refers to the self-limiting dynamics of uninfected target cells, whereas "saturating dynamics" refers to the dynamics of new infections. In the case of multiple target cell types (denoted by *), T refers to the simultaneous presence of both target cell types T_1 and T_2.*

3.1. Models With Uniform Negative Effect of Superinfection

We first briefly discuss the scenarios (model variants) where superinfection either always decreases the uninfected target cell count (as in the basic model), or it might leave the count unchanged in some cases.

3.1.1. Homeostatic Target Cell Dynamics

The equilibrium points of the model are listed in (**Table 3**). The target cell count in the absence of infection, and the steady states of infected cells differ from those of the basic model of virus dynamics. However, the criteria for successful invasion by a second viral strain, and the steady-state target cell counts before and after superinfection, are derived from the dynamical equations of the infected cells, which are the same as in the basic model. As a consequence, this model variant also predicts a uniform negative impact of superinfection on the target cell level (cf. Equation 5).

We also tested models that combined homeostatic target cell dynamics with other extensions if the basic model, and found that the effect of superinfection was generally independent of the choice between homeostatic dynamics and constant influx of new cells. In the following we therefore present models employing the simpler approximation of constant influx for the uninfected cells, consistent with the basic model.

3.1.2. Bystander Killing of Uninfected Cells

We then studied models that allow for the bystander killing of uninfected cells, which appears to be a major factor in the loss of CD4+ T cells in HIV infection (Doitsh et al., 2014). We aimed to investigate whether differences in the rate of bystander killing can influence the impact of superinfection on clinical status.

TABLE 3 | The equilibrium states (*ES*) of the basic model with homeostatic target cell dynamics.

	$\hat{T}$	$\hat{I}_1$	$\hat{I}_2$
ES1 ()	$\frac{K(r-\delta_T)}{r}$	0	0
ES2 (I_1)	$\frac{\delta_1}{\beta_1}$	$(\hat{T}^{()} - \hat{T}^{(I_1)})\frac{r}{K\beta_1}$	0
ES3 (I_2)	$\frac{\delta_2}{\beta_2}$	0	$(\hat{T}^{()} - \hat{T}^{(I_2)})\frac{r}{K\beta_2}$

TABLE 4 | Equilibrium states in the case of bystander killing of uninfected cells without immune response.

	$\hat{T}$	$\hat{I}_1$	$\hat{I}_2$
ES1 ()	$\frac{\sigma}{\delta_T}$	0	0
ES2 (I_1)	$\frac{\delta_1}{\beta_1}$	$\frac{(\hat{T}^{()}-\hat{T}^{(I_1)})\delta_T}{\hat{T}^{(I_1)}(\beta_1+\gamma_1)}$	0
ES3 (I_2)	$\frac{\delta_2}{\beta_2}$	0	$\frac{(\hat{T}^{()}-\hat{T}^{(I_2)})\delta_T}{\hat{T}^{(I_2)}(\beta_2+\gamma_2)}$

Without immune response the dynamics of the system is described by Equations (7–9). The equilibrium points of the system are easily computed (**Table 4**), revealing that the steady-state counts of uninfected cells remain the same as in the basic model, and only the steady states of the infected cells are different. The relations determining the positivity of the infected cell counts, and the criteria for successful invasion (superinfection) are also unchanged: successful invasion always decreases the uninfected target cell count in this implementation of bystander killing of uninfected target cells.

3.1.3. Bystander Killing With Strain-Specific Cytotoxic Immunity

We next investigated whether an inducible immune response against the virus [which can change the equilibria and behavior of the models profoundly (De Boer and Perelson, 1998)] can affect the outcome of superinfection. Because cross-reactive immunity (that targets both strains) has already been shown to allow for both increasing and decreasing target cell counts after successful invasion (Iwasa et al., 2004), we combined strain-specific immunity with bystander killing. Strain-specific immunity, by itself, does not allow for increasing target cell counts (Iwasa et al., 2004); we aimed to investigate whether immune control by strain-specific immunity might allow for the invasion of a viral strain with reduced bystander killing, possibly increasing the target cell count.

In brief, we found that in models with bystander killing of uninfected cells and strain-specific immunity, superinfection imposed on a steady state with induced immunity always decreases the target cell count (for details see Appendix 1). In the case with an initial virus that is not able to elicit an immune response, superinfection with a fitter virus can result in a situation with stable coexistence, an immune response against the second strain, and no change in the target cell level. Finally, we also tested alternative action mechanisms for the immune response (early cytotoxicity, non-cytotoxic immunity); however, the results of the previous analyses remained robust irrespective of the effector mechanism.

3.2. Saturating Dynamics of New Infections

We next explored whether implementing interference competition between the viral strains can influence the outcome of superinfection. Such competition arises from a "crowding effect" that reduces the per capita rate of new infections at high virus load, acknowledging that the rate of new infections cannot increase indefinitely with the level of infected cells. Alternatively, the same model applies also if innate antiviral mechanisms are activated in the target cells proportional to the virus load they are exposed to.

In this model variant there is no immune control and infected cell originate from a single pool of target cells (see **Figure 1B**); the coexistence of both strains is therefore not possible. The dynamics of the system is described in Equations (15, 16), where the rate of new infections increases slower than linearly with increasing infectious titer, and saturates at high titers. The three possible equilibrium points are listed in Table A2 in Appendix 2.1. In the case of successful superinfection the new strain excludes the old one. The condition of successful invasion by the second strain has the same form as in the basic model (for details, see Appendix 2.2):

$$\frac{\delta_1}{\delta_2} > \frac{\beta_1}{\beta_2}. \tag{22}$$

However, in this model, the total target cell count can both decrease and increase after successful superinfection. The count increases if the following relation holds:

$$(\delta_1\beta_2 - \delta_2\beta_1) + \delta_T(\delta_1\epsilon_2 - \delta_2\epsilon_1) + \sigma(\epsilon_1\beta_2 - \epsilon_2\beta_1) < 0. \tag{23}$$

As the expression in the first pair of brackets must be positive for superinfection to occur (c.f. Equation 22), the relation can hold if the sum of the remaining two expressions is negative and of greater magnitude. If $\sigma \gg \delta_T$ (which is a realistic assumption) the condition is mainly affected by the ϵ_i coefficients of interference and the β_i coefficients of infection efficiency, yielding the following necessary (though not sufficient) condition for an increase in the target cell count after superinfection:

$$\frac{\epsilon_1}{\epsilon_2} < \frac{\beta_1}{\beta_2}. \tag{24}$$

If $\sigma \ll \delta_T$ the condition is mainly affected by the δ_i rates of infected cell turnover, in addition to the coefficients of interference, and an increase in the target cell count is possible only if

$$\frac{\epsilon_1}{\epsilon_2} < \frac{\delta_1}{\delta_2}. \tag{25}$$

In general, superinfection can increase the level of uninfected target cells, if the relative difference between the two strains is smaller with respect to the coefficients of interference than with respect to the relative difference in the infection efficiency and/or in the infected cell turnover. As interference by a "crowding effect" is likely to be relatively invariable, this condition might often be fulfilled under this scenario.

As the above calculations are only approximate, we also carried out a series of numerical simulations to investigate the effect of superinfection on the uninfected target cell count. We fixed the parameters of the uninfected cells such that $\sigma \gg \delta_T$, when the condition for increasing target cell count is expected to be approximated by $\frac{\epsilon_1}{\epsilon_2} < \frac{\beta_1}{\beta_2}$; all other parameters were chosen randomly from the intervals presented in Table A5 in Appendix. Overall about 50% of the invasion tests resulted in successful superinfection (from a random pair of strains, one can always exclude the other, except for the degenerate case when $\beta_1/\delta_1 = \beta_2/\delta_2$). In each run the increase/decrease of the uninfected target cell counts after the superinfection and the ratios of β_i and ϵ_i parameters were recorded. **Figure 2** shows the results from a randomly selected subset of simulations with successful superinfection (300 cases of both increasing and decreasing target cell counts), confirming the validity of the approximate criterion; the distribution of the relative change in the cell count is shown for the whole set of 20,000 simulation runs with successful superinfection.

3.3. Multiple Target Cell Types

This model variant was motivated by the observation that different virus strains can differ in their target cell tropism (e.g., Bleul et al., 1997), which might influence their competition dynamics by introducing multiple resources into the system. The scheme of the model is shown in **Figure 1C**. With two target cell types, exposure to a second strain can lead to three different outcomes: unsuccessful invasion; successful superinfection with exclusion of the original strain; and successful superinfection followed by the coexistence of both strains. There are four equilibrium states of the system, but the complexity of their form (c.f. Appendix 3.1) precludes an analytical investigation of the effect of superinfection. We therefore assessed the impact of superinfection with numerical simulations of the model, using

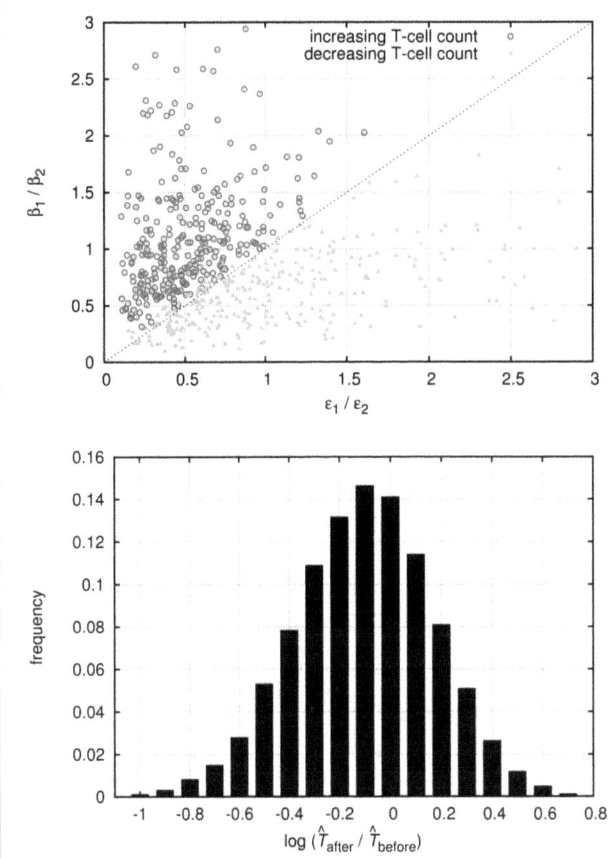

FIGURE 2 | The top panel shows the change in the uninfected target cell count after superinfection as a function of the relative differences in the interference (ϵ) and infection efficiency (β) parameters of both strains; results from 600 randomly selected simulation runs of the saturating infection dynamics model (300–300 runs with both increasing and decreasing cell counts) are shown. Red circles represent runs with increasing uninfected target cell count; green triangles represent runs with decreasing cell counts. The blue dashed line of the diagonal corresponds to $\frac{\epsilon_1}{\epsilon_2} = \frac{\beta_1}{\beta_2}$; Equation (24) is fulfilled above the diagonal. In all runs we set $\sigma = 10$ cells per day and $\delta_T = 0.1$ per day; all other parameters were drawn randomly with uniform distribution from the intervals presented in Table A5 (Appendix). The lower panel shows the histogram of the (log-transformed) ratios of the uninfected target cell counts after and before superinfection, from 20,000 simulation runs with successful superinfection.

parameters sampled randomly from credible intervals (see Table A5 in Appendix), and recording the total number of target cells ($T_1 + T_2$) before and after a successful superinfection (see Models and Methods for details). The ratio of simulations with successful superinfection was again, as expected, close to 50%. In 20,000 simulation runs with successful superinfection, the most frequent scenario was the exclusion of the first strain accompanied by a decrease in the total uninfected target cell count ($T_1 + T_2$); however, a modest increase in the total count was also observed in some of the cases (**Table 5**), and coexistence of the two strains was also possible with both increasing and decreasing total uninfected target cell counts. We found no parameters or simple parameter combinations that could predict the increase or decrease of total counts.

TABLE 5 | The observed frequencies of the possible outcomes of successful superinfection, and the median and interquartile range of the ratio of change in the uninfected target cell count for each case, calculated from 20,000 simulation runs with successful superinfection (50% of the total number of runs) in the multiple target cell types model.

Outcome	Frequency	Median ratio of change (Q1–Q3)
Exclusion–increasing total count	0.005	1.029 (1.010 – 1.062)
Exclusion–decreasing total count	0.815	0.467 (0.290 – 0.672)
Coexistence–increasing total count	0.020	1.010 (1.003 – 1.033)
Coexistence–decreasing total count	0.160	0.889 (0.759 – 0.965)

3.4. HIV-Induced Activation of Target Cells

Our final extension of the basic model takes into account that only activated CD4+ T cells are highly susceptible to HIV infection, while the majority of the CD4+ T cells are in a resting or quiescent state. By equating the susceptible target cells (T) with activated T cells, the model can preserve much of the basic architecture, while adding a new variable for the levels of quiescent cells (Q) allows it to track the total CD4+ T cell count with more realism. An important feature of the system is that HIV itself contributes to the activation of quiescent cells. The dynamics of the system is described by the set of differential equations introduced in Equations (19–21); the scheme of the model is shown in **Figure 1D**. The three equilibrium states (*ES*1, *ES*2, and *ES*3; see **Table 2**, but note that Q is also present) and the corresponding equilibrium values of different cell counts can be found in Appendix 4.1.

As there is no immune control, and both strains of the virus infect the same pool of (activated) target cells, coexistence of strains is not possible, analogous to the basic model (cf. section 2.1). In the case of successful invasion, the original strain is excluded, and the level of activated target cells decreases, in line with the results of the basic model: $\hat{T}^{(I_2)} < \hat{T}^{(I_1)}$, see Equation (5). In the equilibrium states with infection, the steady-state values of susceptible target cell levels, T, are the same in the basic model and this model; however, the addition of quiescent cells allows for a more complicated behavior of the total uninfected target cell count ($Q + T$) in this case. From Equation (19), the steady-state level of quiescent cells can be expressed in the following way:

$$\hat{Q}^{(I_i)} = \frac{r\hat{T}^{(I_i)} + \sigma}{\delta_q + \alpha + \kappa_i \hat{I}^{(I_i)}}. \tag{26}$$

While the complexity of the fully expanded formula of the steady state (see Appendix 4.1) precludes a fully analytical study of the possible consequences of superinfection, the possibility of increasing cell count can be gleaned by expressing the increase of the total CD4+ T cell count ($\hat{Q}^{(I_2)} + \hat{T}^{(I_2)} > \hat{Q}^{(I_1)} + \hat{T}^{(I_1)}$) in the following form:

$$\frac{\delta_2}{\beta_2} + \frac{r\frac{\delta_2}{\beta_2} + \sigma}{\delta_q + \alpha + \kappa_2 \hat{I}^{(I_2)}} > \frac{\delta_1}{\beta_1} + \frac{r\frac{\delta_1}{\beta_1} + \sigma}{\delta_q + \alpha + \kappa_1 \hat{I}^{(I_1)}}. \tag{27}$$

Although the level of activated target cells decreases, (i.e., $\delta_2/\beta_2 < \delta_1/\beta_1$), the inequality can be fulfilled if the invading Strain 2 exerts a (sufficiently) lower level of virus-mediated target cell activation ($\kappa_2\hat{I}_2 < \kappa_1\hat{I}_1$), which might be possible for some parameter combinations. We tested this by numerical integration of the set of differential equations Equations (19–21), following the method used in the previous two scenarios (for details see section 2). In about 10% of the cases, with single infection the system attained stable oscillations with large amplitude in all variables, which is biologically unrealistic; we have therefore excluded these cases from further analysis. We performed invasion tests with pairs of strains that both attained stable equilibria in single infections; of these tests, about 11% resulted in successful superinfection. This is considerably lower than the "neutral" expectation observed in the other models, and can be explained by the additional positive feedback of infected cell levels on the supply of susceptible (activated) cells. The second strain still has 50% probability to have higher replicative fitness (β/δ) than the resident strain; however, in some of these cases it has too low activation potential to sustain infection in the new host. The results of 20,000 successful invasions are presented in **Figure 3**.

In line with the qualitative predictions, the total target cell count increased for some cases of superinfection where the $(\kappa_1 I_1)/(\kappa_2 I_2)$ ratio was greater than 1. The κ_1/κ_2 ratio was also a good proxy: substantial increase in the total target cell count seems to be possible only if $\kappa_1/\kappa_2 > 1$, i.e., when the invading strain is less efficient at activating quiescent target cells. Based on these numerical results, we conclude that the total uninfected cell count can both decrease and increase after superinfection, if the dynamics of target cell activation and quiescence is taken into account.

Finally, we also tested a minor variant of this model, in which quiescent cells affected by the virus die instead of entering the pool of activated target cells [i.e., the $\kappa_i I_i$ terms appear only in the equation of quiescent cells (Equation 19) but not in the equation of activated cells (Equation 20)]. This formalism corresponds to a mechanism of bystander killing that affects resting uninfected cells, which might apply to the pyroptotic pathway in particular (Doitsh et al., 2014). The behavior of this model was analogous to the structurally similar case of HIV-induced T cell activation: superinfection with a strain that has higher replicative capacity but a lower rate of HIV-induced bystander killing of the quiescent cells, compared with the resident strain, can increase the total CD4+ T cell count.

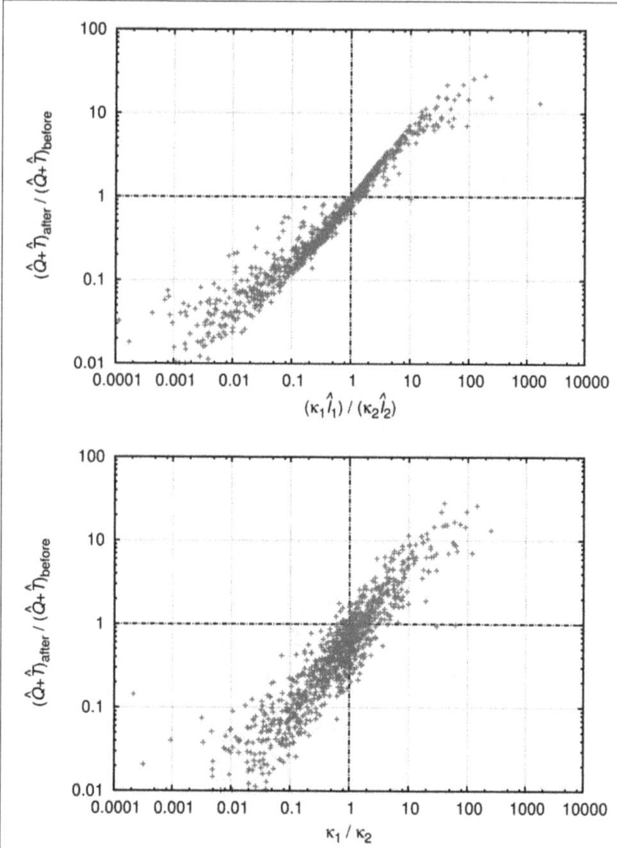

FIGURE 3 | Relative change of the total uninfected target cell count ($\hat{Q}+\hat{T}$) after and before successful superinfection, plotted against the total rates of activation $(\kappa_1\hat{I}_1)/(\kappa_2\hat{I}_2)$ (top) or the ratio of the activation parameters κ_1/κ_2 (bottom) of the two virus strains in the HIV-induced activation model. The results of 20,000 simulation runs with successful superinfection are shown. In each run, all parameters were drawn randomly with uniform distribution from the intervals presented in Table A5 (Appendix); the cases with healthy (uninfected) cell counts between 500 and 1,500 per μL were used for the analyses. Both axes are logarithmic.

4. DISCUSSION

Using simple models of HIV infections, we demonstrated that superinfection with a second strain of HIV can, under different assumptions, result in both a deterioration, but also an improvement of clinical status (approximated by uninfected target cell counts in the models). This runs counter to the widespread view that associates superinfection with a negative outcome. In our exploration of biologically motivated extensions to the basic model of HIV dynamics, we have identified four new scenarios in which superinfection can also have a positive impact on the level of uninfected target cells.

The first scenario assumed interference competition for the susceptible target cells between the competing viral clones. Such interference is almost inevitable at high densities of a predator or infectious agent (Schoener, 1978): the rate of new infections cannot grow indefinitely with increasing infectious titer. Furthermore, the same model structure is applicable also if inducible mechanisms of innate antiviral defense reduce the susceptibility of uninfected cells upon exposure to the virus that does not result in productive infection. Interference competition (saturating infection dynamics) can therefore be expected to occur, although the magnitude of the effect is unclear. In this model, the total uninfected target cell count increased upon superinfection when the relative difference between the two viral strains was smaller with respect to the coefficients of interference than with respect to the relative difference in the infection efficiency and/or in the infected cell turnover.

Variable tropism for multiple distinct cell types also allowed for increasing total uninfected cell counts, although in this case the increase was modest and it occurred in only a minority of the simulation runs with randomized parameters. Larger increases in the total count were possible in models that distinguished between activated (susceptible) and resting (non-permissive) target cells, and included an effect of the virus on the resting cell pool (activation to susceptible state or bystander killing). In these models, "invasion fitness" of a virus strain is independent of its effect on quiescent cells, allowing for superinfection with strains that induce less depletion of this cell pool, which constitutes the dominant component of the total CD4+ T cell count.

In all scenarios that allow for increasing target cell level after superinfection, this positive outcome is expected to arise (in some of the cases) when there are independent sources of variability in the relevant parameters, e.g., if the intensity of interference effects, or the potential for immune activation can vary, at least in part, independent of the components of replicative fitness (production and infectiousness of virions, turnover rates of infected cells and virus particles). Since a complete coupling is not expected between the parameters, the possibility of increasing target cell levels is likely if any of the relevant structural features of these scenarios is indeed important *in vivo*. This is a robust result, independent of the uncertainties in the parameters of both viral and host immune dynamics.

Our results add to the earlier modeling work of Fung et al. who found that HIV superinfection can occur with a less fit (and virulent) strain if target cells can be multiply infected (which reduces or eliminates competition for this resource) (Fung et al., 2010). Furthermore, since exposure to superinfection is fully analogous to the appearance of new virus strains by mutation, earlier modeling results pertaining to the within-host emergence and competition of new strains are also applicable in the context of superinfection (e.g., Iwasa et al., 2004, 2005; Ball et al., 2007), and vice versa. Altogether, there are now five mechanisms known to allow for a positive impact of HIV superinfection on clinical status (uninfected target cell count): in addition to the four cases identified in this paper, the earlier work of Iwasa et al. (2004) identified cross-reactive immunity as a mechanism that is also compatible with a positive outcome – all of these scenarios could, in principle, also allow for evolution toward decreasing HIV virulence within the host. We summarize the predictions of various mathematical models with regard to the impact of HIV superinfection on clinical status in **Table 6**.

While modeling suggests that HIV superinfection could have counterintuitive beneficial effects by several possible mechanisms, the data are not sufficient to predict how often this might occur. Elucidating the true distribution of outcomes might be elusive in the era of broadly accessible antiretroviral therapy, but it might be possible through the retrospective identification of superinfection events from stored samples. Finding cases where the CD4+ T cell count improved, at least temporarily, after superinfection, would indicate that at least one of the complicating factors that allow such an effect are indeed at work in the infection. Insights from the models and a detailed examination of these cases could narrow down the list of possible mechanisms, and improve our understanding of the within-host dynamics of HIV infection.

TABLE 6 | Possible outcomes of HIV superinfection on the total uninfected target cell count.

Scenario	After superinfection the target cell count	Source
Basic model	Always decreases	Iwasa et al., 2004
Homeostatic target cell dynamics	Always decreases	This paper
Strain-specific immunity	Decreases or unchanged	Iwasa et al., 2004
Cross-specific immunity	Can decrease or increase	Iwasa et al., 2004, 2005
Multiple infection of target cells	Decreases or unchanged*	Fung et al., 2010
Bystander killing		
of susceptible target cells	Always decreases	This paper
of non-permissive target cells	Can decrease or increase	This paper
Saturating infection dynamics	Can decrease or increase	This paper
Multiple target cell types	Can decrease or increase	This paper
HIV-induced T-cell activation	Can decrease or increase	This paper

**Fung et al. (2010) used a non-steady-state model of disease progression: when dual infection of the target cells was allowed to occur unhindered, the rate of disease progression was unaffected or slightly accelerated after superinfection.*

Finally, our results might also have some relevance with regard to the impact of superinfection on the evolution of HIV virulence at the population level. The possibility of ambiguous outcomes implies that superinfection might contribute to the spreading of not only virulent, but also of attenuated strains under some circumstances. We also note that even in the scenarios when superinfection could spread only strains with higher virulence, this predicted effect could be mitigated by factors that were not incorporated in our models. For example, the initial dissemination of the virus is likely to be aided considerably by the large susceptible population of CD4+CCR5+ T cells in the gut-associated lymphoid tissue (Mehandru et al., 2004). This pool is quickly and irreversibly depleted when an individual first becomes infected with HIV, and the absence of this readily infectable cell population might reduce the probability of successful superinfection upon subsequent exposure to other viral strains. This and other factors (e.g., cross-specific immunity) might inhibit superinfection, which would constrain the spreading of strains with higher within-host fitness also at the population level (Ferdinandy et al., 2015). Furthermore, the current broad application of antiretroviral therapy is likely to reduce also the incidence of superinfection, especially considering that therapeutic guidelines increasingly advise the treatment of all diagnosed individuals. In principle, superinfection by drug resistant viruses could still occur (Chakraborty et al., 2004; Smith et al., 2005), but currently available evidence suggests that such events are extremely rare (Bartha et al., 2013). Finally, the population-level dynamics and evolution of HIV is also influenced by factors that act on between-host transmission (Nowak and May, 1994; van Baalen and Sabelis, 1995; Alizon and van Baalen, 2008), and trade-offs between viral traits might also complicate the evolutionary dynamics (Ball et al., 2007).

In summary, we have shown that the effect of HIV superinfection on clinical status is not straightforward: while the simplest models predict that only a more virulent strain can successfully establish superinfection, adding biologically relevant details of HIV infection opens up the possibility that superinfection might also improve clinical status in some cases. The impact of superinfection at the population (epidemic) level is likely to be modulated by further factors.

AUTHOR CONTRIBUTIONS

VM conceived and supervised the study. ÁM, AS, IS, and VM developed the models. ÁM, AS, IS, and VM performed the analyses. ÁM, AS, IS, and VM wrote the paper.

FUNDING

This research was supported by the the Hungarian Scientific Research Fund (OTKA grants NF72791 and K124438) and by the grant GINOP-2.3.2-15-2016-00057 (Az evolúció fényében: elvek és megoldások). VM holds a Bolyai János Research Fellowship of the Hungarian Academy of Sciences.

REFERENCES

Alizon, S., and van Baalen, M. (2008). Multiple infections, immune dynamics, and the evolution of virulence. *Am. Nat.* 172, E150–E168. doi: 10.1086/590958

Altfeld, M., Allen, T. M., Yu, X. G., Johnston, M. N., Agrawal, D., Korber, B. T., et al. (2002). HIV-1 superinfection despite broad CD8+ T-cell responses containing replication of the primary virus. *Nature* 420, 434–439. doi: 10.1038/nature01200

Ball, C. L., Gilchrist, M. A., and Coombs, D. (2007). Modeling within-host evolution of HIV: mutation, competition and strain replacement. *Bull. Math. Biol.* 69, 2361–2385. doi: 10.1007/s11538-007-9223-z

Bartha, I., Assel, M., Sloot, P. M., Zazzi, M., Torti, C., Schülter, E., et al. (2013). Superinfection with drug-resistant HIV is rare and does not contribute substantially to therapy failure in a large European cohort. *BMC Infect. Dis.* 13:537. doi: 10.1186/1471-2334-13-537

Bartha, I., Simon, P., and Müller, V. (2008). Has HIV evolved to induce immune pathogenesis? *Trends Immunol.* 29, 322–328. doi: 10.1016/j.it.2008.04.005

Bleul, C. C., Wu, L., Hoxie, J. A., Springer, T. A., and Mackay, C. R. (1997). The HIV coreceptors CXCR4 and CCR5 are differentially expressed and regulated on human T lymphocytes. *Proc. Natl. Acad. Sci. U.S.A.* 94, 1925–1930. doi: 10.1073/pnas.94.5.1925

Brener, J., Gall, A., Hurst, J., Batorsky, R., Lavandier, N., Chen, F., et al. (2018). Rapid HIV disease progression following superinfection in an HLA-B*27:05/B*57:01-positive transmission recipient. *Retrovirology* 15:7. doi: 10.1186/s12977-018-0390-9

Bukrinsky, M., Stanwick, T., Dempsey, M., and Stevenson, M. (1991). Quiescent T lymphocytes as an inducible virus reservoir in HIV-1 infection. *Science* 254, 423–427. doi: 10.1126/science.1925601

Casado, C., Pernas, M., Alvaro, T., Sandonis, V., García, S., Rodríguez, C., et al. (2007). Coinfection and superinfection in patients with long-term, nonprogressive HIV-1 disease. *J. Infect. Dis.* 196, 895–899. doi: 10.1086/520885

Chakraborty, B., Kiser, P., Rangel, H., Weber, J., Mirza, M., Marotta, M., et al. (2004). Can HIV-1 superinfection compromise antiretroviral therapy? *AIDS* 18, 132–134. doi: 10.1097/00002030-200401020-00019

Chesson, P. (2000). Mechanisms of maintenance of species diversity. *Annu. Rev. Ecol. Syst.* 31, 343–366. doi: 10.1146/annurev.ecolsys.31.1.343

Chiu, Y., Soros, V., Kreisberg, J., Stopak, K., Yonemoto, W., and Greene, W. (2005). Cellular APOBEC3G restricts HIV-1 infection in resting CD4+ T cells. *Nature* 435, 108–114. doi: 10.1038/nature03493

Clerc, O., Colombo, S., Yerly, S., Telenti, A., and Cavassini, M. (2010). HIV-1 elite controllers: beware of super-infections. *J. Clin. Virol.* 47, 376–378. doi: 10.1016/j.jcv.2010.01.013

Connor, R. I., Sheridan, K. E., Ceradini, D., Choe, S., and Landau, N. R. (1997). Change in coreceptor use correlates with disease progression in HIV-1–infected individuals. *J. Exp. Med.* 185, 621–628. doi: 10.1084/jem.185.4.621

Cornelissen, M., Pasternak, A. O., Grijsen, M. L., Zorgdrager, F., Bakker, M., Blom, P., et al. (2012). HIV-1 dual infection is associated with faster CD4+ T-cell decline in a cohort of men with primary HIV infection. *Clin. Infect. Dis.* 54, 539–547. doi: 10.1093/cid/cir849

De Boer, R. J., and Perelson, A. S. (1998). Target cell limited and immune control models of HIV infection: a comparison. *J. Theor. Biol.* 190, 201–214. doi: 10.1006/jtbi.1997.0548

Doitsh, G., Galloway, N. L., Geng, X., Yang, Z., Monroe, K. M., Zepeda, O., et al. (2014). Cell death by pyroptosis drives CD4 T-cell depletion in HIV-1 infection. *Nature* 505, 509–514. doi: 10.1038/nature12940

Ferdinandy, B., Mones, E., Vicsek, T., and Müller, V. (2015). HIV competition dynamics over sexual networks: first comer advantage conserves founder effects. *PLoS Comput. Biol.* 11:e1004093. doi: 10.1371/journal.pcbi.1004093

Fung, I. C.-H., Gambhir, M., van Sighem, A., de Wolf, F., and Garnett, G. P. (2010). Superinfection with a heterologous HIV strain *per se* does not lead to faster progression. *Math. Biosci.* 224, 1–9. doi: 10.1016/j.mbs.2009.11.007

Gonzales, M., Delwart, E., Rhee, S., Tsui, R., Zolopa, A., Taylor, J., et al. (2003). Lack of detectable human immunodeficiency virus type 1 superinfection during 1072 person-years of observation. *J. Infect. Dis.* 188, 397–405. doi: 10.1086/376534

Gottlieb, G. S., Nickle, D. C., Jensen, M. A., Wong, K. G., Grobler, J., Li, F., et al. (2004). Dual HIV-1 infection associated with rapid disease progression. *Lancet* 363, 619–622. doi: 10.1016/S0140-6736(04)15596-7

Gottlieb, G. S., Nickle, D. C., Jensen, M. A., Wong, K. G., Kaslow, R. A., Shepherd, J. C., et al. (2007). HIV type 1 superinfection with a dual-tropic virus and rapid progression to AIDS: a case report. *Clin. Infect. Dis.* 45, 501–509. doi: 10.1086/520024

Hindmarsh, A. C., Brown, P. N., Grant, K. E., Lee, S. L., Serban, R., Shumaker, D. E., et al. (2005). SUNDIALS: suite of nonlinear and differential/algebraic equation solvers. *ACM Trans. Math. Softw.* 31, 363–396. doi: 10.1145/1089014.1089020

Iwasa, Y., Michor, F., and Nowak, M. (2004). Some basic properties of immune selection. *J. Theor. Biol.* 229, 179–188. doi: 10.1016/j.jtbi.2004.03.013

Iwasa, Y., Michor, F., and Nowak, M. A. (2005). Virus evolution within patients increases pathogenicity. *J. Theor. Biol.* 232, 17–26. doi: 10.1016/j.jtbi.2004.07.016

Jost, S., Bernard, M.-C., Kaiser, L., Yerly, S., Hirschel, B., Samri, A., et al. (2002). A patient with HIV-1 superinfection. *N. Engl. J. Med.* 347, 731–736. doi: 10.1056/NEJMoa020263

Ke, R., Cong, M.-E., Li, D., Garcia-Lerma, J. G., and Perelson, A. S. (2017). On the death rate of abortively infected cells: estimation from simian-human immunodeficiency virus infection. *J. Virol.* 91:e00352-17. doi: 10.1128/JVI.00352-17

Klenerman, P., Phillips, R., Rinaldo, C., Wahl, L., Ogg, G., May, R., et al. (1996). Cytotoxic T lymphocytes and viral turnover in HIV type 1 infection. *Proc. Natl. Acad. Sci. U.S.A.* 93, 15323–15328. doi: 10.1073/pnas.93.26.15323

Kraft, C. S., Basu, D., Hawkins, P. A., Hraber, P. T., Chomba, E., Mulenga, J., et al. (2012). Timing and source of subtype-C HIV-1 superinfection in the newly infected partner of Zambian couples with disparate viruses. *Retrovirology* 9:22. doi: 10.1186/1742-4690-9-22

Levy, J. A., Mackewicz, C. E., and Barker, E. (1996). Controlling HIV pathogenesis: the role of the noncytotoxic anti-HIV response of CD8+ T cells. *Immunol. Today* 17, 217–224. doi: 10.1016/0167-5699(96)10011-6

Mehandru, S., Poles, M. A., Tenner-Racz, K., Horowitz, A., Hurley, A., Hogan, C., et al. (2004). Primary HIV-1 infection is associated with preferential depletion of CD4+ T lymphocytes from effector sites in the gastrointestinal tract. *J. Exp. Med.* 200, 761–770. doi: 10.1084/jem.20041196

Müller, V., and Bonhoeffer, S. (2003). Mathematical approaches in the study of viral kinetics and drug resistance in HIV-1 infection. *Curr. Drug Targets Infect. Disord.* 3, 329–344. doi: 10.2174/1568005033481042

Nowak, M., and May, R. M. (2000). *Virus Dynamics: Mathematical Principles of Immunology and Virology.* Oxford: Oxford University Press.

Nowak, M. A., and May, R. M. (1994). Superinfection and the evolution of parasite virulence. *Proc. R. Soc. B* 255, 81–89. doi: 10.1098/rspb.1994.0012

Perelson, A. S. (2002). Modelling viral and immune system dynamics. *Nat. Rev. Immunol.* 2, 28–36. doi: 10.1038/nri700

Piantadosi, A., Ngayo, M., Chohan, B., and Overbaugh, J. (2008). Examination of a second region of the HIV type 1 genome reveals additional cases of superinfection. *AIDS Res. Hum. Retroviruses* 24:1221. doi: 10.1089/aid.2008.0100

Rachinger, A., Navis, M., van Assen, S., Groeneveld, P. H. P., and Schuitemaker, H. (2008). Recovery of viremic control after superinfection with pathogenic HIV type 1 in a long-term elite controller of HIV type 1 infection. *Clin. Infect. Dis.* 47:e86. doi: 10.1086/592978

Rambaut, A., Posada, D., Crandall, K., and Holmes, E. (2004). The causes and consequences of HIV evolution. *Nat. Rev. Genet.* 5, 52–61. doi: 10.1038/nrg1246

Redd, A., Collinson-Streng, A., Martens, C., Ricklefs, S., Mullis, C., Manucci, J., et al. (2011). Identification of HIV superinfection in seroconcordant couples in Rakai, Uganda, by use of next-generation deep sequencing. *J. Clin. Microbiol.* 49, 2859–2867. doi: 10.1128/JCM.00804-11

Redd, A., Quinn, T., and Tobian, A. (2013). Frequency and implications of HIV superinfection. *Lancet Infect. Dis.* 13, 622–628. doi: 10.1016/S1473-3099(13)70066-5

Schoener, T. W. (1978). Effects of density-restricted food encounter on some single-level competition models. *Theor. Population Biol.* 13, 365–381. doi: 10.1016/0040-5809(78)90052-7

Smith, D., Wong, J., Hightower, G., Ignacio, C., Koelsch, K., Petropoulos, C., et al. (2005). HIV drug resistance acquired through superinfection. *AIDS* 19, 1251–1256. doi: 10.1097/01.aids.0000180095.12276.ac

Tsui, R., Herring, B., Barbour, J., Grant, R., Bacchetti, P., Kral, A., et al. (2004). Human immunodeficiency virus type 1 superinfection was not detected following 215 years of injection drug user exposure. *J. Virol.* 78, 94–103. doi: 10.1128/JVI.78.1.94-103.2004

van Baalen, M., and Sabelis, M. W. (1995). The dynamics of multiple infection and the evolution of virulence. *Am. Nat.* 146, 881–910. doi: 10.1086/285830

van der Kuyl, A. C., Kozaczynska, K., van den Burg, R., Zorgdrager, F., Back, N., Jurriaans, S., et al. (2005). Triple HIV-1 infection. *New Engl. J. Med.* 352, 2557–2559. doi: 10.1056/NEJM200506163522420

Vuilleumier, S., and Bonhoeffer, S. (2015). Contribution of recombination to the evolutionary history of HIV. *Curr. Opin. HIV AIDS* 10, 84–89. doi: 10.1097/COH.0000000000000137

Yerly, S., Jost, S., Monnat, M., Telenti, A., Cavassini, M., Chave, J.-P., et al. (2004). HIV-1 co/super-infection in intravenous drug users. *AIDS* 18, 1413–1421. doi: 10.1097/01.aids.0000131330.28762.0c

Zheng, Y. H., Jeang, K. T., and Tokunaga, K. (2012). Host restriction factors in retroviral infection: promises in virus-host interaction. *Retrovirology* 9:112. doi: 10.1186/1742-4690-9-112

3

Noise is not Error: Detecting Parametric Heterogeneity between Epidemiologic Time Series

Ethan O. Romero-Severson[1], *Ruy M. Ribeiro*[1,2] *and Mario Castro*[3,4*]

[1] Theoretical Biology and Biophysics Group, Los Alamos National Laboratory, Los Alamos, NM, United States, [2] Laboratorio de Biomatematica, Faculdade de Medicina, Universidade de Lisboa, Lisbon, Portugal, [3] Grupo Interdisciplinar de Sistemas Complejos and DNL, Universidad Pontificia Comillas, Madrid, Spain, [4] Department of Applied Mathematics, School of Mathematics, University of Leeds, Leeds, United Kingdom

***Correspondence:**
Mario Castro
marioc@comillas.edu

Mathematical models play a central role in epidemiology. For example, models unify heterogeneous data into a single framework, suggest experimental designs, and generate hypotheses. Traditional methods based on deterministic assumptions, such as ordinary differential equations (ODE), have been successful in those scenarios. However, noise caused by random variations rather than true differences is an intrinsic feature of the cellular/molecular/social world. Time series data from patients (in the case of clinical science) or number of infections (in the case of epidemics) can vary due to both intrinsic differences or incidental fluctuations. The use of traditional fitting methods for ODEs applied to noisy problems implies that deviation from some trend can only be due to error or parametric heterogeneity, that is noise can be wrongly classified as parametric heterogeneity. This leads to unstable predictions and potentially misguided policies or research programs. In this paper, we quantify the ability of ODEs under different hypotheses (fixed or random effects) to capture individual differences in the underlying data. We explore a simple (exactly solvable) example displaying an initial exponential growth by comparing state-of-the-art stochastic fitting and traditional least squares approximations. We also provide a potential approach for determining the limitations and risks of traditional fitting methodologies. Finally, we discuss the implications of our results for the interpretation of data from the 2014-2015 Ebola epidemic in Africa.

Keywords: stochastic, deterministic, epidemiology, panel data, random effects, fixed effects

1. INTRODUCTION

Mathematical models play an increasingly central role in the analysis of infectious disease data at both the within-host and epidemiological levels (Perelson et al., 1996; Heesterbeek, 2000; Molina-París and Lythe, 2011). The traditional modeling approach involves formulating a set of structural assumptions about the processes involved, such as infection, recovery, death, etc. Often, these structural assumptions are then implemented in terms of differential equations, predominantly ordinary (ODE), but sometimes partial (PDE), or delayed (dODE) differential equations. The advantage of this approach is its amenability for both analytical treatment and powerful numerical and fitting algorithms even for non-linear problems. We will refer to those approaches collectively as *deterministic*.

However, stochasticity is an intrinsic feature of infections at multiple levels from the cellular/molecular world to the level of epidemics (Süel et al., 2006; Bressloff and Newby, 2013). The deterministic framework conceptualizes all deviation from the model prediction as **error**. For example, in a simple univariate linear regression we say that the data are equal to a linear predictor plus some error. Put another way, we can say that error is the density of the data conditional on the model. However, stochasticity generates intrinsic fluctuations in the underlying dynamics of a system (for instance, in the number of secondary cases an incident case generates), even when the process follows the structural model envisaged. That is, stochasticity generates **noise**, which we define as the set of outcomes that are consistent with a fixed set of assumptions (i.e., a model).

One of the central challenges of using the deterministic framework is to delineate its limitations (Roberts et al., 2015). If the world and its data truly are stochastic, then how much of a problem is it to conflate noise with error? Likewise, how much information in the data are we neglecting by treating all deviation as uninformative error? To what extent is the assumption of deterministic dynamics plus error providing misleading results?

This question is not gratuitous as some parameters estimated within the deterministic framework, such as the basic reproduction number (R_0), are often invoked to quantify the aggressiveness of a pathogen and to determine the conditions under which a pathogen will go extinct (Dietz, 1993; Heffernan et al., 2005) or to create public health information such as risk maps (Hartemink et al., 2011).

The potential problems in applying the deterministic framework can become even more pronounced when we have data that represent multiple realizations of a heterogeneous stochastic process. For example, a set of viral load profiles in different infected individuals (e.g., primary HIV infection; Ribeiro et al., 2010) or epidemic curves in different regions (e.g., cases of Ebola in multiple counties of the same country ; Krauer et al., 2016), that is, any data that can be represented as a panel over discrete units. In those scenarios, an important question is whether the variability seen between units can be attributed to a genuine difference in the process that generated the data (e.g., some parameters of the dynamics are different for each unit), simple stochastic fluctuation, or a mixture of the two, in addition to measurement error. Given a common error model across the units, the deterministic framework assumes that all deviation that cannot be explained by error must be due to parametric variability between units, that is the units are fundamentally different from one another. For this reason, the deterministic framework is ill-suited to tackle the question of stochastic effects.

We address in this paper two related questions regarding modeling of panel data: (i) can we use a stochastic modeling approach to partition variability into stochastic and parametric components? and (ii) can we quantify the bias induced by modeling the data by a deterministic approach with error? Put in other words, is there a best and a good-enough fitting method for the practitioner? In section 2.1, we consider two simple structural models that will help us emphasize the essence of the problem without having to invoke unnecessary complexities that may cloud our main arguments. In section 3.1, we present our approach to analyze those models, which will then be used to benchmark comparisons between traditional (deterministic) fitting methods and more sophisticated stochastic ones, that we explore in section 3.2. As a case study, in section 4, we compare deterministic and stochastic modeling approaches to data from the 2014-2015 Ebola epidemic in West Africa. We use epidemic data from multiple counties of those countries that were most heavily affected. If one thinks of each county as a realization of some epidemic generating process, then the relevant question is whether differences between the counties can be accounted for by stochastic variability or if it is possible to detect a signal for different growth rates of the epidemic in different counties. Finally, in section 5 we summarize our results and discuss the implications of our work.

2. METHODS

2.1. Simulated Data

The general framework we employ is to simulate data *in silico* from two structural models, birth-only or birth-death process (see Karlin, 2014), by a discrete-time stochastic simulation and then fit those data using both deterministic and stochastic methods under a variety of assumptions.

The code used to generate the data and fit the models is given in Appendix A. We simulate panel data according to the following process

$x_{1:U,1:O} \leftarrow 0$
$a \leftarrow \Gamma(\mu = \mu_A, \sigma = \sigma_A)$
$b \leftarrow \Gamma(\mu = \mu_B, \sigma = \sigma_B)$
$j, k \leftarrow 0$
for $j \leq U$ **do**
  $j \leftarrow j + 1$
  $I \leftarrow 1$
  for $k \leq O$ **do**
    $\phi_A \leftarrow \text{Poisson}(Ia)$
    $I \leftarrow I + \phi_A$
    $I \leftarrow I - \text{Poisson}(Ib)$
    $x_{j,k} \leftarrow \phi_A$
  end for
end for

where U is the number of units in the panel, O is the number of observations (time points) per unit, and $x_{j,k}$ is the number of new infected cases in each time period k for unit j—this is the output of the simulation used for the fits described below. If the number of deaths exceeds the infected population size, I, this variable is set to 0. These simple models capture both the initial exponential growth phase when infected population sizes are small and stochastic die out that is common in many epidemiological processes. For simplicity, we focus only on the early stages of the epidemic, i.e., the approximately exponential phase in the growth of infected individuals. Note that throughout we use arbitrary time units.

Each simulated data set is specified by 6 parameters: mean growth rate, μ_A; standard deviation of the growth rate, σ_A; mean death rate, μ_B; standard deviation of the death rate, σ_B; the number of units in the panel, U; and the number of observations per unit, O. From this we consider 4 possible scenarios: birth-only without parametric variability ($\mu_B = \sigma_B = \sigma_A = 0$), birth-only with parametric variability ($\mu_B = \sigma_B = 0$), birth-death without parametric variability ($\sigma_A = \sigma_B = 0$), and birth-death with parametric variability. In all cases with parametric variability, we assume a Gamma distribution for the respective parameter (where μ and σ are the corresponding mean and standard deviation). We chose the Gamma distribution because it can easily be re-parameterized into its mean and standard deviation, which makes interpreting the parameters straightforward.

We set up four sets of simulated experiments to explore the effects of (1) model misspecification, (2) the number of observations per unit, (3) the number of units in the panel, and (4) the heterogeneity in parameters (growth rates) between units (see **Table 1** for reference).

In the first set of experiments, we simulate data from a birth-only process without parametric variability ($\mu_A = 0.15$), birth-only with parametric variability ($\mu_A = 0.15, \sigma_A = 0.02$), birth-death without parametric variability ($\mu_A = 0.25$, $\mu_B = 0.1$), and birth-death with parametric variability ($\mu_A = 0.25$, $\sigma_A = 0.02$, $\mu_B = 0.1$, $\sigma_B = 0.01$). In each case, we assume ($U =$) 20 units per panel and ($O =$) 20 observations per unit, at equal time intervals. We then fit each of these four data sets using each of four possible models (birth or birth-death with and without random effects) with both stochastic and deterministic approaches for a total of 32 fits.

In the next three sets of experiments we use the birth-only model with parametric variability and the default parameters $\mu_A = 0.15$, $\sigma_A = 0.02$, $U = 20$, $O = 20$. In the second set of experiments, we vary the number of observations per unit ($O \in \{10, 20, 30, 40, 50\}$), in the third set of experiments we vary the number of units in the panel ($U \in \{10, 20, 30, 40, 50\}$), and in the fourth set of experiments we vary the heterogeneity in growth rates ($\sigma_A \in \{0.01, 0.02, 0.03, 0.04, 0.05\}$).

2.2. Parameter Inference

To infer the parameter values, we use a fitting scheme based on simulations that can account both for the intrinsic stochasticity of the process and the potential variation among individuals. Here all model formulations (both stochastic and deterministic versions) are fit using the iterated filtering method implemented in the R library `pomp` (King et al., 2016). This approach allows us to fit all the models to the data using the same framework and likelihood functions, such that the model fits are all comparable. We specifically use the iterated filtering for panel data (IFPD) formulation detailed in Romero-Severson et al. (2015). Code used to specify the `pomp` process are given in Appendix A.

Models were fit using 5,000 or 15,000 particles for the deterministic and stochastic models respectively. For stochastic fits, the density of the number of incident cases in the *kth* time period of the *jth* unit, $x_{j,k}$, is assumed to be Poisson($x_{j,k}|I_{j,k-1}\alpha$) were $I_{j,k}$ is the simulated number of extant infected cases in the *kth* time period of the *jth* unit and α is the growth rate, which itself may be sampled from a Gamma distribution. For the deterministic fits, $x_{j,k}$ is simply $x_{j,k} = \alpha I_{j,k-1}$.

To obtain confidence intervals (CIs) for the parameters, we used a profile likelihood method (Romero-Severson et al., 2014) where the parameter of interest was varied over a grid of values and the likelihood was calculated, by refitting the data allowing all other parameters to be free. We used the `mif2` method (King et al., 2016) in `pomp`. A local regression (loess) curve was fitted to the profile likelihood curve and both the MLE and CIs were calculated from the interpolated curve (King et al., 2015, 2016).

2.3. Ebola Data and Analysis

The Ebola case count data was compiled from publicly available datasets published by the World Health Organization (from the "Ebola Data and Statistics" section of the WHO website). Case counts were stratified by country and county of origin. All descriptive analyses were done on the full data. However, to fit the models to the data using the simulation-based method described, we restrcited the data in the following way.

(i) For every county, we define time $= 1$ as the first week where the total number of cases is larger or equal to 1.
(ii) We truncated the data at 10 weeks after that time, in order to have homogeneous sets (same number of points) during the approximately exponential initial growth of the epidemic. To emphasize this latter point, we re-plot the data in linear-log scale.
(iii) Finally, we removed those counties where the data does not include at least 10 data points.

Note that in the simulated data, we assumed no measurement error in time or in number of infected. However, this is not a good assumption for real epidemiological data. Thus, for the Ebola data, we fit a modified version of both the deterministic and stochastic birth-only model accounting for measurement error (e.g., missed cases and reporting delays) in a simple way, by assuming that the number of new cases is distributed according to a Negative Binomial, rather than a Poisson, conditional on the simulated state of the system at the previous time. We re-parameterize the typical NB(n, p) as NB($\delta, \frac{\mu}{\mu+\delta}$) where μ is the mean of new cases and δ is an overdispersion parameter such that $\lim_{\delta\to\infty}$ NB($\delta, \frac{\mu}{\mu+\delta}$) = Poisson($\mu$). Therefore, the mass of the data conditional on the simulated state of the system is NB$\left(y_{j,k}|\delta, \frac{x_{j-1,k}a}{x_{j-1,k}a+\delta}\right)$. The parameter δ controls the level of overdispersion (smaller values, more overdispersion) in the data

TABLE 1 | Summary of groups of numerical experiments, the aim of each experiment and the figure summarizing the main results for each case.

Experiment #	Description	Model	Results
1	Effect of model misspecification	Birth only and birth-death	**Figure 3**
2	Effect of number of observations	Birth only	**Figure 4**
3	Effect of number of units in the panel	Birth only	**Figure 5**
4	Effect of parametric variance	Birth only	**Figure 6**

In all cases (in particular in Experiment 4), we compare fitted parameters using the stochastic and deterministic methods described in section 3.1. In all cases, we made use of simulated data with and without random effects to account for the impact of parametric variance.

conditional on the simulated state and is free (estimated) for each point in the likelihood profiles. This formulation puts the stochastic and deterministic models on a level playing field in that the deterministic model can model variance between epidemic trajectories with increased overdispersion rather than increased population-level heterogeneity. The deterministic and stochastic models were fit with 5,000 and 15,000 particles, respectively, for each value in the profiles (**Figure 10**).

3. RESULTS

3.1. Motivation: Noise as Parametric Heterogeneity

Traditional inference is based on maximum likelihood estimates of some well-defined functions. For instance, for the cases considered here (pure birth and birth-death) an ODE-based deterministic approximation provides differential equations that, upon solving, can be fit to the data to determine the parameters ($\mu_A = \alpha$ and $\mu_B = \gamma$) that best describe the data (see **Table 2**, and Appendix B for a succinct derivation for the pure birth case). Similarly, the stochastic version of those models can be solved and in that case one could also fit the mean and variance of a given observable (last two rows in **Table 2**), and indeed higher moments.

In these cases, as the models are linear, both deterministic and stochastic predictions for the average are the same (because averaging and integrating the evolution equation are exchangeable operations). However, the latter has the benefit that it also allows to fit the variance of the data (thus, in principle, increasing the reliability of the inferred parameters).

The main point that we wish to address is how to interpret different trajectories of an intrinsic stochastic process. To illustrate this point, **Figure 1** shows 100 realizations of the simple stochastic pure birth model with rate parameter $\alpha = 0.1$ time-unit^{-1} measured without error at integer times. If we use a naive deterministic approach (top of **Table 2**), we fit $I(t) = e^{\alpha t}$ to each trajectory (data set) and estimate α independently, obtaining a distribution for this parameter (**Figure 1**, bottom panel). If this process were observed at time 25, it would be tempting to conclude that there is a high degree of heterogeneity in the growth rates of these epidemics. Even by time 75, when the expected population size is over 1,000, we still see a large heterogeneity in the estimated rates.

TABLE 2 | Number of infected, new cases and total cases for the birth and the birth-death processes as defined in the deterministic (top part of the table) and stochastic (bottom part) approaches.

	Birth process	Birth-death process
Differential equation	$\frac{dI}{dt} = \alpha I$	$\frac{dI}{dt} = (\alpha - \gamma)I$
Infected, I	$e^{\alpha t}$	$e^{(\alpha-\gamma)t}$
New cases per unit time, N	$\alpha e^{\alpha t}$	$\alpha e^{(\alpha-\gamma)t}$
New cases in Δt, N_t	$e^{\alpha t}(e^{\alpha \Delta t} - 1)$	$\frac{\alpha}{\alpha - \gamma} e^{(\alpha-\gamma)t}(e^{(\alpha-\gamma)\Delta t} - 1)$
Total cases, T	$e^{\alpha t}$	$\frac{\gamma}{\alpha - \gamma}(\frac{\alpha}{\gamma} e^{(\alpha-\gamma)t} - 1)$
Mean of infected, $\langle I \rangle$	$e^{\alpha t}$	$e^{(\alpha-\gamma)t}$
Variance of infected, σ_I^2	$e^{\alpha t}(e^{\alpha t} - 1)$	$\frac{\alpha^2 - \gamma^2}{(\alpha - \gamma)^2} e^{(\alpha-\gamma)t}(e^{(\alpha-\gamma)t} - 1)$

In all cases, the epidemic starts with one infected case, namely, $I(0) = 1$. Here we only consider models without parametric variability ($\sigma_A = \sigma_B = 0$).

If we used the stochastic version of the pure birth process (bottom of **Table 2**), by definition we would assume that there was just one value for the α parameter and could fit the mean and variance (and possibly other moments) of the trajectories to estimate that growth rate.

Another possible deterministic fitting approach is to allow for random effects, where we assume an underlying distribution (e.g., normal) for the growth rate parameter (α) and allow each trajectory to be the realization of a pure birth process with parameter drawn from that distribution (Gelman and Hill, 2007). In this case, the estimation method yields the parameters of the distribution (i.e., the mean and variance). This is a mixed effects approach, where we still assume no stochasticity and that all differences are due to parametric variability.

This approach of assuming parametric variability can also be used with the stochastic version of the model. In fact, it is instructive to analyze in more detail such situation by calculating analytically the distribution of the number of infected accounting both for the stochasticity of the process and the parameter distribution for the pure birth process.

If we assume that the growth rate, α, is distributed according to a normal, $\alpha \sim \mathcal{N}(\mu_A, \sigma_A)$, then the probability of having $I(t)$ total infected is the product of the geometric distribution for fixed α, which is the solution of the pure birth process, (see Allen, 2010), and the normal distribution for α, namely

$$P(I|\mu_A, \sigma_A, t) = P(I|\alpha, t)P(\alpha|\mu_A, \sigma_A) = [p(1-p)^{I-1}]\frac{e^{-(\alpha-\mu_A)^2/2\sigma_A^2}}{\sqrt{2\pi\sigma_A^2}}$$

where $p = e^{-\alpha t}$. Therefore,

$$P(I|\mu_A, \sigma_A, t) = \frac{\left(1 - e^{-\alpha t}\right)^{I-1} e^{-\frac{(\alpha - \mu_A)^2}{2\sigma_A^2} - \alpha t}}{\sqrt{2\pi\sigma_A^2}}, \quad I = 1, 2, \ldots \tag{1}$$

From this expression, we can obtain the mean and variance of I, including the contributions of both stochasticity and parametric variability (see also Appendix C)

$$\langle I \rangle = e^{\mu_A t + \frac{\sigma_A^2 t^2}{2}} \tag{2}$$

and

$$\sigma_I^2 = e^{\mu_A t + \frac{\sigma_A^2 t^2}{2}} \left(e^{\mu_A t + \frac{\sigma_A^2 t^2}{2}} \left(2e^{\sigma_A^2 t^2} - 1 \right) - 1 \right) \tag{3}$$

(These expressions reduce to the forms in **Table 2**, when $\sigma_A = 0$). It is worth noting that both the mean and the variance of I depend

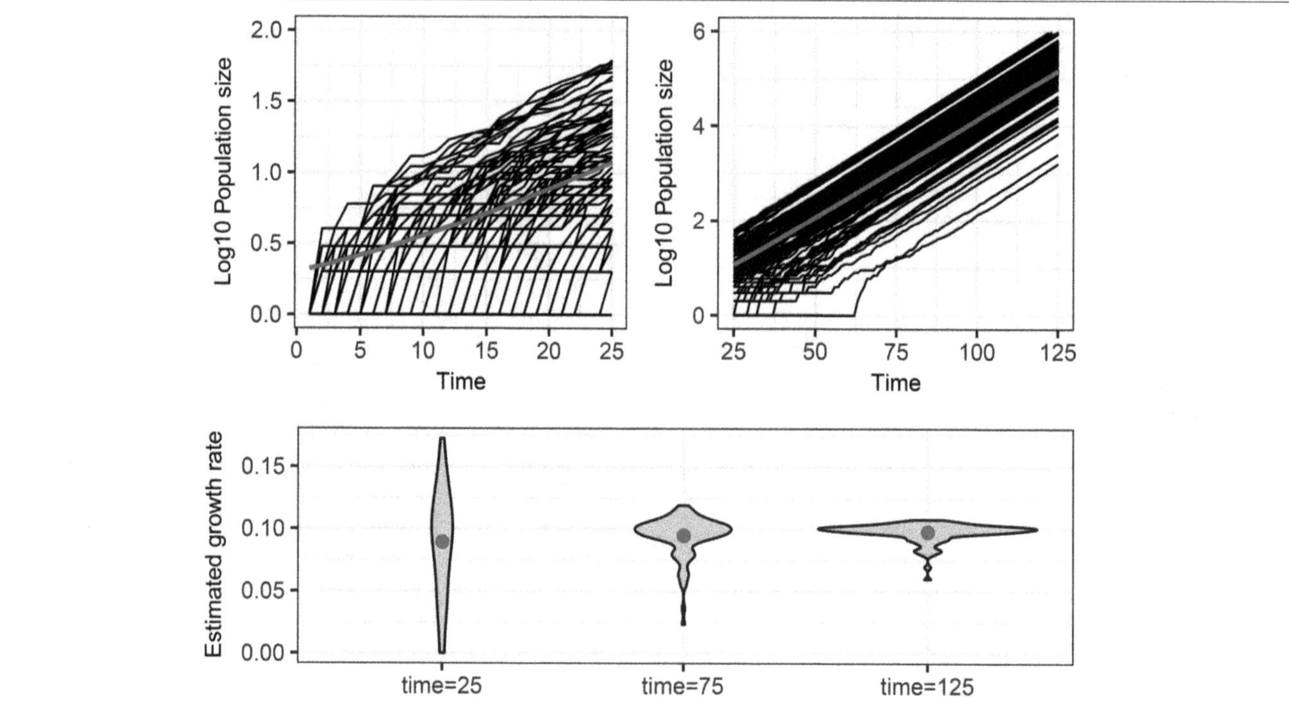

FIGURE 1 | Stochastic realizations of a pure birth process and distributions of deterministic estimation of the growth rate at different times. Top figures show 100 trajectories from a continuous time pure-birthh process with parameter $\alpha = 0.1$ over two time scales. The only difference between each trajectory is intrinsic stochastic variability. The red line shows the expected population size assuming a deterministic process, which is also the mean number of infected of the stochastic process if there is no parametric variability. The bottom plot shows the distribution of estimated growth rates obtained by fitting a linear model to the $\log_{10}$ of the population size for each of the 100 trajectories from time 0 to times 25, 75, and 125. The red dots indicate the mean of the estimated growth rates, which are all close to the true value of 0.1.

on μ_A and σ_A, suggesting that an ODE or stochastic fit to the mean ignoring parametric variability would estimate the growth rate incorrectly.

These four different ways to fit the same data set (e.g., **Figure 1**) beg the question of which one is the best approach and whether that depends on the data containing actual parametric variability or not. On the other hand, the explicit knowledge of the stochastic form of σ_I, both in the presence of parametric variability (expression 3) and pure stochastic variability (**Table 2**), suggests the definition of a quantity, R^2 (analogous to a coefficient of determination) as

$$R^2 = \frac{\sigma^2_{\text{param}}}{\sigma^2_{\text{param}} + \sigma^2_{\text{noise}}} = 1 - \frac{\sigma^2_{\text{noise}}}{\sigma^2_I} \tag{4}$$

For the pure birth process (see Appendix C for details):

$$R^2 = \frac{\frac{1}{2}\sigma_A^2 t^2 e^{\mu_A t}\left(6e^{\mu_A t} - 1\right)}{e^{\mu_A t}\left(e^{\mu_A t} - 1\right) + \frac{1}{2}\sigma_A^2 t^2 e^{\mu_A t}\left(6e^{\mu_A t} - 1\right)} \left(\simeq \frac{3\sigma_A^2 t^2}{1 + 3\sigma_A^2 t^2}\right) \tag{5}$$

This expression helps us to determine (in a prescriptive way) whether the process is governed by stochasticity ($R^2 \rightarrow 0$) or by parametric variability ($R^2 \rightarrow 1$). Also, as it can be expected, the variance at shorter times is governed by pure random fluctuations but as time proceeds, parametric variance, if present, is increasingly more relevant. We plot R^2 as a function of time in **Figure 2**

To analyze these issues in more detail, we now use *in silico* generated data fitted in multiple ways, with and without stochastic effects and with and without assuming parametric variability, to assess the quality of the parameter estimation.

3.2. Comparison of Fitting Methods With Simulated Data

In Appendix D (Tables I to IV) we summarize the fitted parameters discussed in the Sections 3.2.1 to 3.2.4.

3.2.1. Experiment 1: Model Misspecification

We fit 4 models (birth-only and birth-death, with and without random effects) using both deterministic and stochastic model formulations allowing us to consider the effect of both model structure misspecification and other model assumptions. Parameter estimates for each data set are given in Table I in Appendix. Also, in **Figure 3** we summarize succinctly the main conclusions of this section.

3.2.1.1. Correct model

When the data are generated without population heterogeneity (i.e., $\sigma_A = \sigma_B = 0$) and fit with the correct structural model, both the deterministic and the stochastic fits have reasonable point

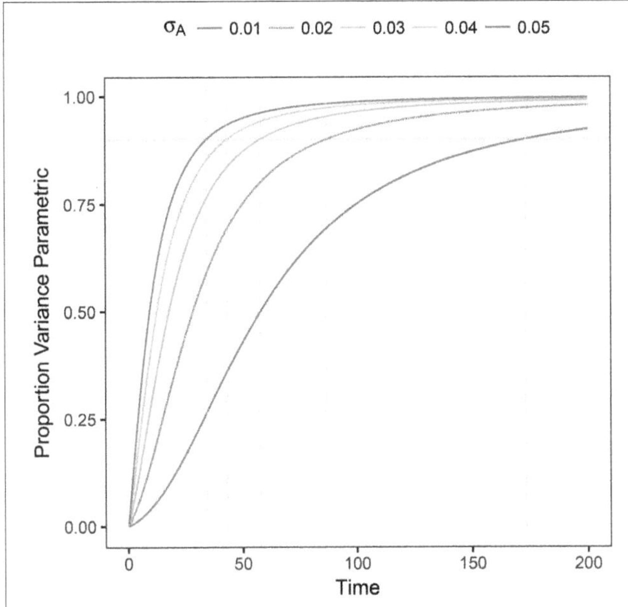

FIGURE 2 | Plot of R^2 as a function of time for heterogeneous stochastic exponential growth. Each line shows R^2 for the specified level of σ_A assuming $\mu_A = 0.1$. The horizontal gray line indicates 90% of the variance being due to parametric heterogeneity; the dashed vertical gray lines indicate the time at which each line reaches 90%.

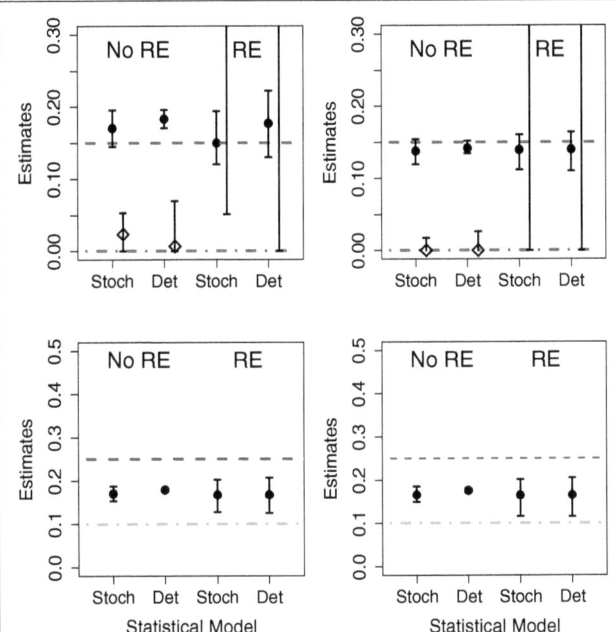

FIGURE 3 | Results of fits when using mismatched structural models. The symbols correspond to the estimates of the growth rate (circles) and death rates (diamonds) under different scenarios. In the **(Left)**, the data was generated without parametric variability and in the **(Right)** the data was generated with parametric variability. Top row: results of fits with a birth-death model to data generated by a pure birth process. In each case, we used stochastic or deterministic fits, without ("No RE") or with ("RE") random effects. The horizontal dashed blue lines indicate the value μ_A (birth rate) and the dot-dashed red line the value of σ_A used in the data generation. Bottom row: results of fits with a pure birth model to data generated by a birth-death process. The horizontal dashed blue lines stand for μ_A and the dot-dashed green lines for μ_B. In all cases, the vertical whiskers are the 95% CI obtained in the fits. Note that the estimates of the death rate for the random effects fits (in the top panel) are off the plot, and only the bottom segments of the whiskers are visible).

estimates and their confidence intervals (CIs) contain the true parameter value (shown in Table I in Appendix). However, CIs on the death rates are very broad suggesting that the incidence data are only weakly informative. When we introduce population heterogeneity into both the data and fits, the stochastic fit still contains the true parameter values in its CIs; although fitting all 4 parameters leads to very broad estimates for the mean and standard deviation of the death rate. The deterministic model, however, is unable to estimate either the mean or standard deviation of the growth rates correctly.

3.2.1.2. Random effects in the model but not the data

When the fit attempts to estimate random effects when no parametric variability is actually present, the CIs for the estimated standard deviation of the parameters in the stochastic fits contain 0, while the deterministic CIs do not. That is, the deterministic model finds evidence for population-level heterogeneity when none actually exists.

3.2.1.3. Random effects in the data but not the model

When there is population-level heterogeneity in the data but the model assumes that there is none, the stochastic fit still obtains correct point estimates and CIs of the mean effects for both the birth-only and birth-death models. However, in the deterministic fits the CIs for the mean effects did not contain the true values of the growth rates.

3.2.1.4. Death in the data but not in the model

When fitting the birth-death data with a birth-only model, we found that, in both the stochastic and deterministic fits, the estimate of the growth rate is close to the net growth rate (i.e., birth rate minus death rate). However, if we allow random effects on the growth rate, the deterministic fits finds a very high level of heterogeneity in the growth rate when none actually exists. The CI for the standard deviation of the parameter in the stochastic fit correctly contains 0, suggesting limited evidence for heterogeneity in growth rates.

3.2.1.5. Death in the model but not in the data

Conversely, if there is death in the model, but not in the data, both the fixed effects stochastic and deterministic fits the CIs for the death rate correctly contained 0. However the deterministic fit overestimated the growth rate while the stochastic fit did not.

3.2.2. Experiment 2: Number of Units in the Panel

Results for data generated by a pure birth process, with different number of units in the panel, are shown in **Figure 4**. Using the stochastic or the deterministic fits resulted in point estimates for the mean growth rates that were very close to the mean value and the CIs contain the true value for all cases. Increasing the

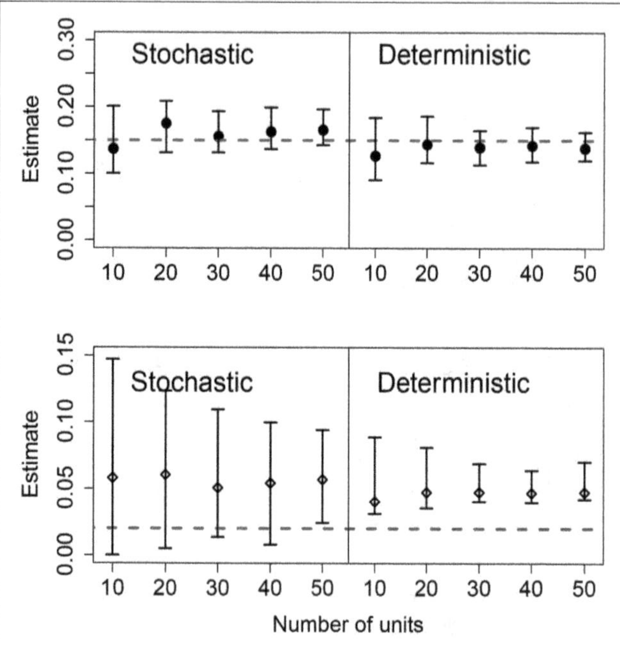

FIGURE 4 | Results of fits when there is a variable number of units. The data in all cases was generated by a pure birth process with parametric variability and fit with a birth-only model. The top row shows the estimates for the mean growth rate with stochastic or deterministic fits, and the bottom row the estimate of the standard deviation of the growth rate. The horizontal dashed blue lines indicate the parameter values used in the data generation. The vertical whiskers are the 95% CI obtained in the fits. In each case, the number of observations per unit was $O = 20$, the growth rate was $\alpha = 0.15$ and the standard deviation of the growth rate was $\sigma = 0.02$.

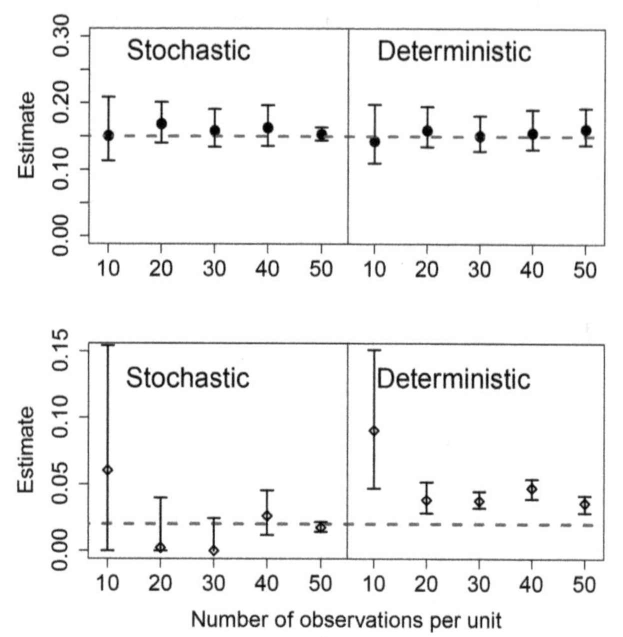

FIGURE 5 | Results of fits when there is a variable number of observations in each unit. The data in all cases was generated by a pure birth process with parametric variability. The top row shows the estimates for the mean growth rate with stochastic or deterministic fits, and the bottom row the estimate of the standard deviation of the growth rate. The horizontal dashed blue lines indicate the parameter values used in the data generation. The vertical whiskers are the 95% CI obtained in the fits. In each case, the number of units was $U = 20$, the growth rate was $\alpha = 0.15$ and the standard deviation of the growth rate was $\sigma = 0.02$.

number of units in the panel causes slightly narrower CIs for the mean growth rate as well. The standard deviation of the growth rates was correctly estimated in the stochastic model for all but one case; however, the deterministic model overestimated the population-level heterogeneity in all cases. Also, as the number of units in the panel increases, the CIs narrow suggesting a higher degree of certainty in an incorrect conclusion.

3.2.3. Experiment 3: Number of Observations Per Unit

The effects of increasing the number of observations per units was similar to increasing the number of units in the panel. For both the stochastic and deterministic fits, the mean growth rates where correctly estimated. As before, the deterministic fit consistently overestimated the standard deviation in the growth rates and increasing the number of observations per unit led to narrower but wrong CIs. Increasing the number of observations per unit is more efficient at improving the accuracy of the estimation compared to increasing the number of units in the panel for the stochastic model. Results are shown in **Figure 5**.

3.2.4. Experiment 4: Increasing Heterogeneity Between Units

We also analyzed the effect of different values for the heterogeneity of the parametric variability. As before, the deterministic fit consistently overestimated the level of heterogeneity regardless of the actual value of the standard deviation of the growth rate, however, these estimates became closer to the true value with increasing heterogeneity in the data. In the stochastic fits, when the heterogeneity was less than 0.04, the estimated CIs included the true parameter and increasing heterogeneity led to a narrower CI. At the highest heterogeneity levels the CI did not contain the true value; we found that using a stochastic fit to data with high levels of parametric heterogeneity leads to numerical instability making estimation of the CIs difficult. Results are shown in **Figure 6**.

3.3. Quantifying Parametric Variability With R^2

As shown in **Figure 6**, the deterministic CIs do not include the real value of σ_A, albeit the estimate of μ_A is accurate enough. To test the ability of different methods to quantify the relevance of parametric variance vs. noise (through R^2), we use the estimation of σ_A from the different methods with Equation (5), at the final observation, $t = 20$. The results are shown in **Figure 7**. Note that the stochastic prediction, at least, is able to include the real R^2 inside the whisker, especially at low values of parametric variability. This means

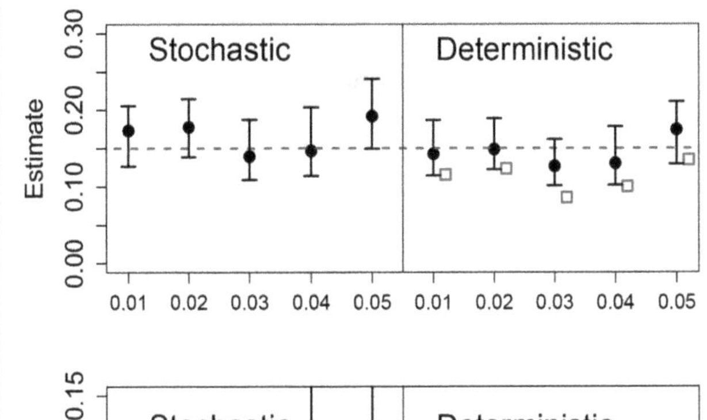

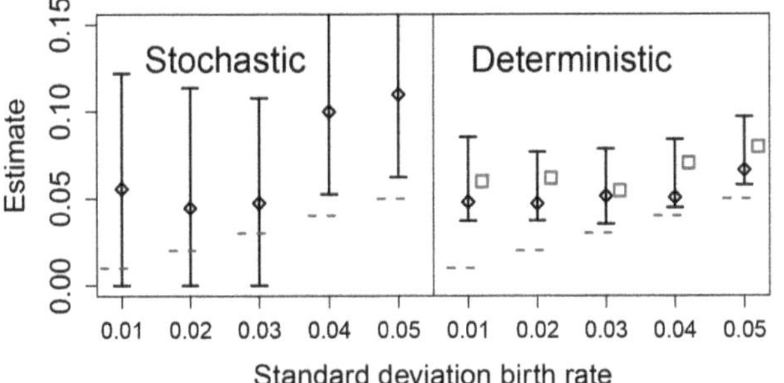

FIGURE 6 | Results of fits with increasing standard deviation for the growth rate. The data in all cases was generated by a pure birth process with parametric variability. The top row shows the estimates for the mean growth rate with stochastic or deterministic fits, and the bottom row the estimate of the standard deviation of the growth rate. The horizontal dashed blue lines indicate the parameter values used in the data generation. The vertical whiskers are the 95% CI obtained in the fits. In the right panels, the red empty squares are the estimated values obtained from standard linear mixed-effect models (regression). In each case, the number of observations per unit was $O = 20$ and the numbers of units was $U = 20$.

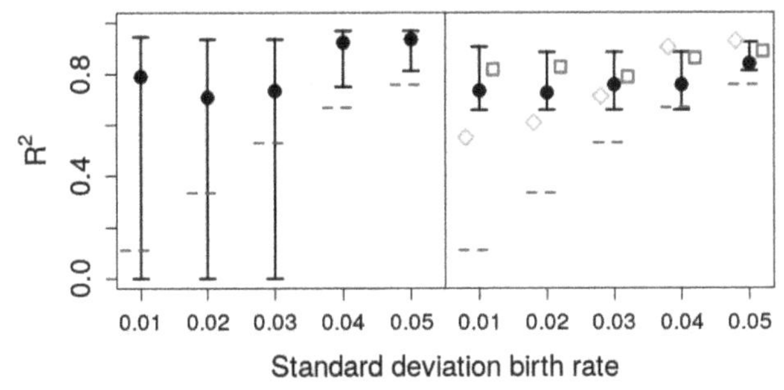

FIGURE 7 | Estimated R^2 with increasing standard deviation for the growth rate. The data in all cases was generated by a pure birth process with parametric variability. The horizontal short dashed lines indicate the parameter values used in the data generation. The left panel corresponds to the stochastic fits and the right panel to the deterministic fits, where the vertical whiskers are the 95% CI obtained in the fits. The red empty squares in the right panel stand for the value of R^2 calculated with Equation (5) at time $t = 20$ with parameters estimated using standard linear mixed-effect models (regression). The empty green diamonds are an alternative way to estimate R^2 using the empirical data variance and the theoretical (stochastic) noise variance, Equation (8). In each case, the number of observations per unit was $O = 20$.

that this fitting method is able to capture (in a probabilistic way) the cases where parametric variance is not as relevant as fluctuations.

We have used throughout simulation-based inference, because it allows us to compare directly likelihood profiles between stochastic and deterministic implementations of the models. Nevertheless, it is worth remembering that traditional methods (based, loosely speaking, on regression) are usually the preferred way to estimate parameters from the data. This is not a matter of taste but of computational efficiency. Even for the simple models in the present work, simulation-based inference is computationally expensive (and, as such, not suitable as of writing for models with many parameters). Thus, for the sake of completeness we discuss briefly the role of regression-based methods in our framework and fit the data in Experiment 4 using a standard linear mixed-effect model (Gelman and Hill, 2007). We find that this fit results in a systematic underestimation of the mean, μ_A (red squares in **Figure 6** top), and in an overestimation of the standard deviation σ_A (red squares in **Figure 6** bottom).

While Equation (5) was derived under the assumption of an unerlying stochastic process, and traditional methods ignore the stochasticity of the underlying process, we can still use hybrid information to obtain a *rough* estimate the relative weight between noise and parametric variance. We can mix both approaches (linear mixed-effect models and stochatic predictions) in two ways: In the first one (corresponding to the red empty squares in **Figure 7**) we use μ_A and σ_A from the linear mixed-effects model fit to the data in Equation (5). The second method, consists in calculating the empirical variance of the data and the expected value of the noise variance from Equation (8) and calculate R^2 using Equation (4). Remarkably, inspection of **Figure 7** (green empty diamonds) suggest that using this second method, the estimated value of R^2 is sometimes closer to the original one.

In summary, combining standard methods with analytical results coming from the exact solution of the stochastic process might be useful to estimate the level of noise in the data. Notwithstanding, in all cases, this hybrid method used to calculate R^2 also overestimates the true value.

4. CASE STUDY: THE 2014-15 EBOLA EPIDEMIC

4.1. Heterogeneity of Epidemic Spread of Ebola

In **Figure 8** we show the total number of cases reported for the 2014-15 Ebola epidemic in Guinea, Liberia and Sierra Leone. In each case, the solid line is the fit of an exponential function to the data for the first 29 weeks. Despite the fluctuations (specially in the first days) the fit provides an (apparently) accurate account for the growth during those early weeks. Note that the estimated slopes are highly variable among countries. Since for simple models, the slope in the exponential fit (α) is proportional to the basic reproductive number minus one ($R_0 - 1$) (Heffernan et al., 2005), with this approach one would conclude that the severity of Ebola in different countries is highly variable. Indeed, this variability has been reported for the 2014-15 epidemic (with R_0 ranging between 1.51 and 2.53), see (Althaus, 2014; Kucharski

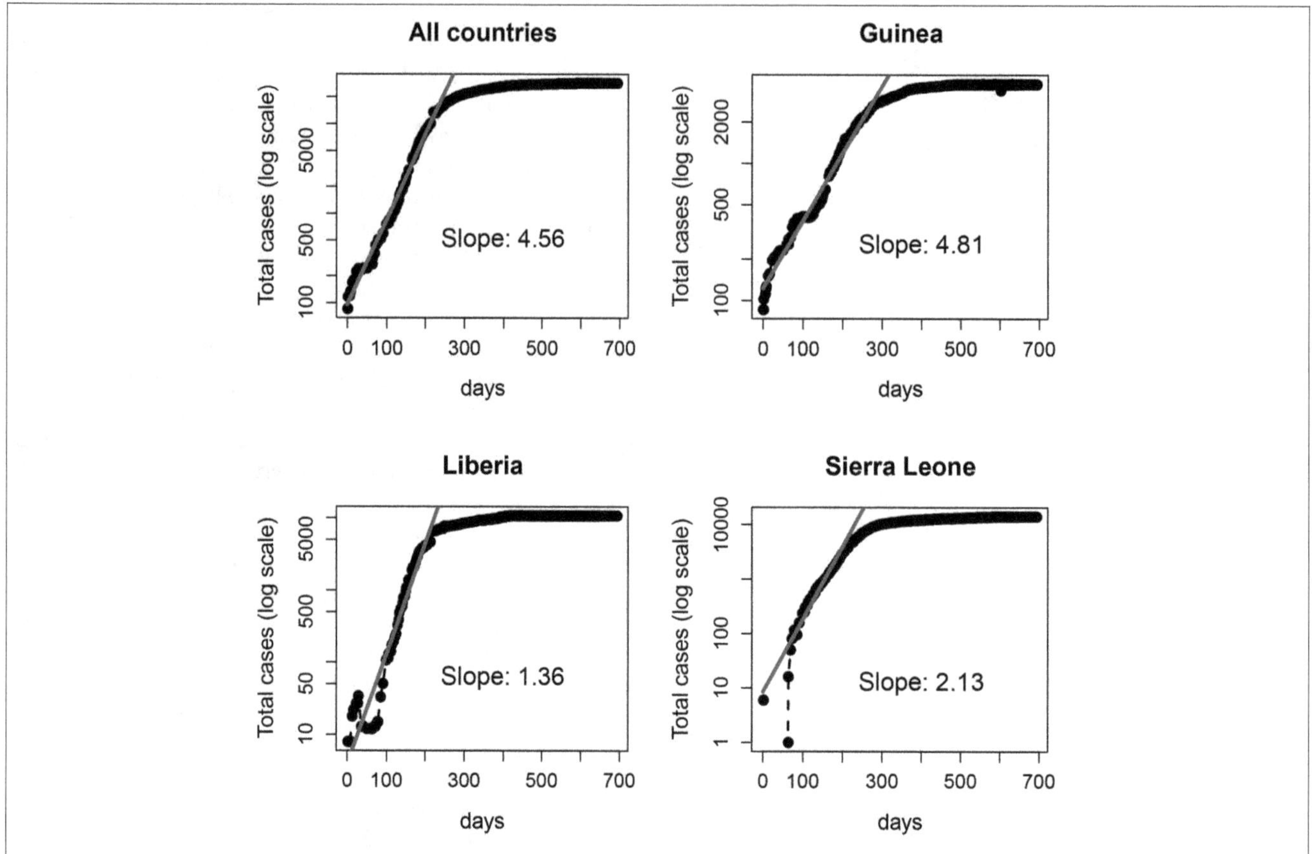

FIGURE 8 | Number of Ebola cases (logarithmic scale) of the 2014-15 Ebola epidemic. **(Top left)** total number of cases in the three countries: Guinea **(Top right)**, Liberia **(Bottom left)**, and Sierra Leone **(Bottom right)**. The solid line represents the fit of an exponential function to the data in each panel over the first 200 days (~ 29 weeks).

et al., 2015; Krauer et al., 2016) , as well as for earlier outbreaks (Chowell et al., 2004).

From a traditional deterministic approach we might come to two conclusions: (1) The Ebola epidemic is well described by a deterministic model that predicts accurately the initial exponential growth and (2) the epidemic was more aggressive in Guinea, followed by Sierra Leone and Liberia. However, a closer inspection of the data (collected by counties) before the aggregation shows a different picture. In **Figure 9**, we plot the same dataset (for Liberia and Sierra Leone) but separately for the different counties.

Now, the conclusions that can be drawn are more nuanced and perhaps contrary to the picture of uniform growth suggested by **Figure 8**. On the one hand, the starting dates of the epidemic in different counties are highly variable, and the initial slopes (the plot is in logarithmic scale) also display a large variability. This suggests that assigning a simple value per country (and, consequently a single R_0) can be misleading and lead to erroneous interpretations and, more importantly, interventions or policies. On the other hand, and this is what we are interested in, this fine grained view of the data begs for a stochastic approach to fitting. Even when the data is aggregated (which tends to smooth the underlying stochasticity), the initial part of the curves are reminiscent of the trajectories in **Figure 1** (left panel).

4.2. Ebola Model Fits

We fitted both deterministic and stochastic versions of a birth-only model with random effects to the Ebola data, allowing for negative binomial measurement error (see section 2.3 for details). The stochastic model was, in terms of the likelihood values, objectively better than the deterministic model (−556.4 vs. −565.0) despite being identical in all respects except stochasticity. The estimate of the mean growth rate was nearly identical in both models, 0.62, with CI (0.53, 0.73) deterministic and 0.59, with CI (0.52, 0.67) stochastic (**Figure 10**). However, the deterministic model found a very high level of heterogeneity, 0.16 CI (0.11, 0.25), while the stochastic model found low levels of heterogeneity, 0.03 CI(0, 0.15). In the stochastic model, the profile likelihood for the standard deviation in growth rates, σ_A, suggests that the likelihood surface is virtually flat around very small values of σ_A (see **Figure 10** right). However, in the deterministic model—even when we allow variable levels of overdispersion—the likelihood rapidly drops off as the heterogeneity decreases from the MLE.

Overall, these results show that, while deterministic fitting is as good as stochastic fitting to estimate the mean growth rates, it performs poorly as a predictor of the parametric variability. Specifically, using our definition of R^2, and the MLE of σ_A = 0.03, obtained with the stochastic method, we can estimate the

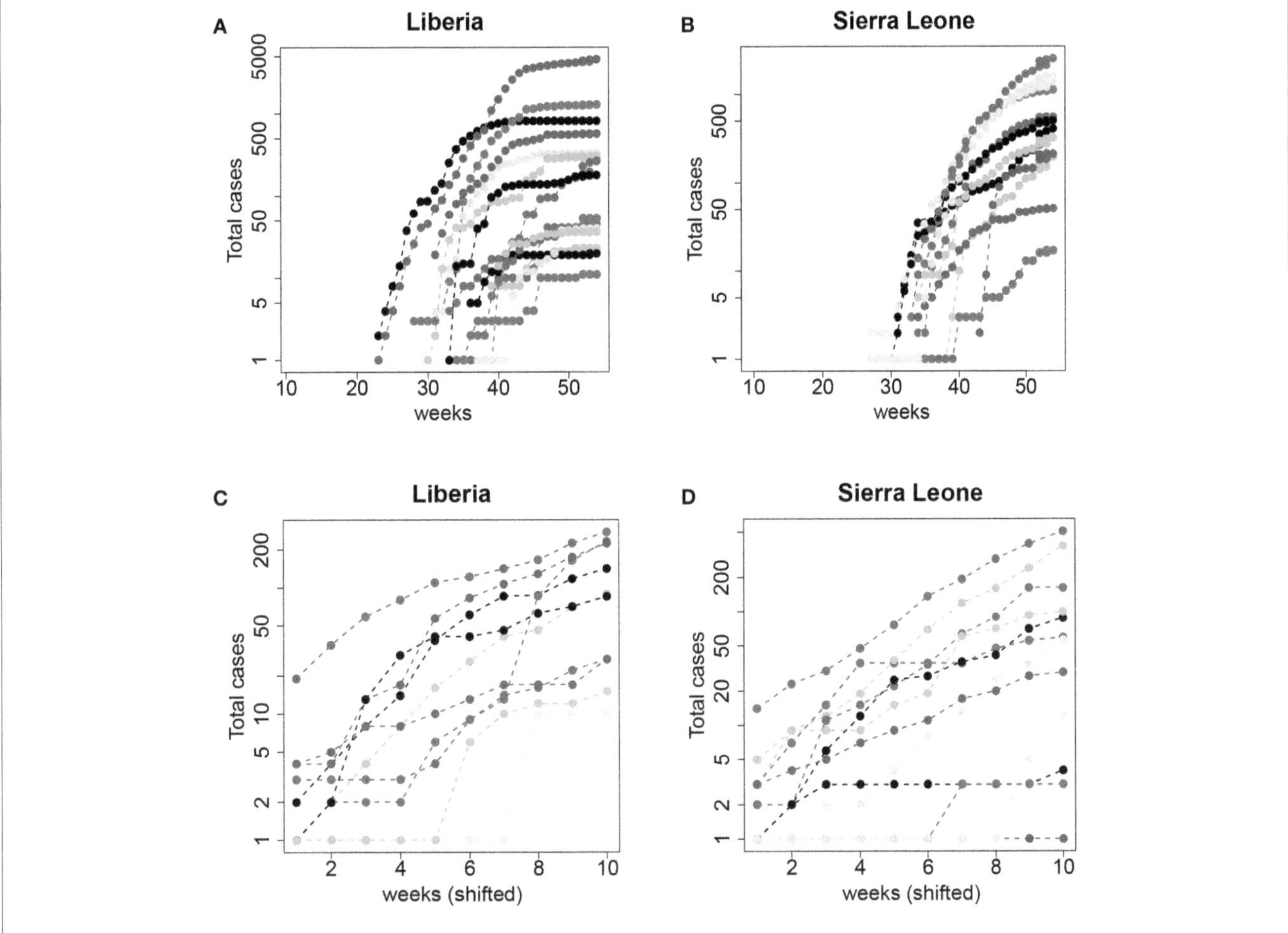

FIGURE 9 | Top: Total number of cases (logarithmic scale) per county in **(A)** Liberia and **(B)** Sierra Leone. Bottom: The same but aligning week 1 to the date of the first event with $I \geq 1$ and restricting to the first 10 observations (see text for details); **(C)** Liberia and **(D)** Sierra Leone.

contribution of parametric variability to overall variability in the data. Using Equation (5) results in $R^2 \simeq 0.21$. This analysis would suggest that, in the case of Ebola, 10 weeks after the start of the epidemic, around 79% of the measured variability could be attributed to noise rather than to inter-county differences. Taking into account that, as we showed in **Figure 7**, this empirical way to calculate R^2 overestimates the true coefficient, the conclusion is even more substantiated. Doing the same calculation with the value obtained in the deterministic fitting, $\sigma_A = 0.16$, we get $R^2 \simeq 0.88$, so we would conclude that 88% of the variability is due to true differences among counties.

5. DISCUSSION AND CONCLUSIONS

The aim of modeling is not to capture every specific feature of the system under consideration but, rather, to describe succinctly the main mechanisms of the process and, ideally, to be able to differentiate among competing hypotheses (Ganusov, 2016). The art of modeling involves balancing multiple levels of complexity to achieve predictability, accuracy, and tractability. In this context, here we have added another concern: is the methodological approach suitable? Following an approach of keeping things simple, we have shown that even for the most basic cases, deterministic fitting methods, which assume that all variability is either error or parametric, provide misleading results. Although, not all aspects of the models were sensitive to the assumption of determinism, since for example the mean of a parameter was usually reasonably estimated.

This study is not a purely academic exercise on the role of fluctuations for small populations because our results point to important practical implications. A case in point is our example of the initial spread of the Ebola epidemic. Although different counties seem to have different growth rates, our fitting indicates that the variability is also well explained by stochastic (i.e., non-systematic) differences among the counties. This does not mean that there are no differences in epidemic spread among the counties, only that stochasticity alone is a statistically better and more parsimonious explanation. That is, when stochasticity is taken into account the evidence for differences in early growth rates is negligible.

The ability to accurately detect and measure heterogeneity is an important topic with practical implications. Take, for example, the expanding field of personalized medicine, where individual

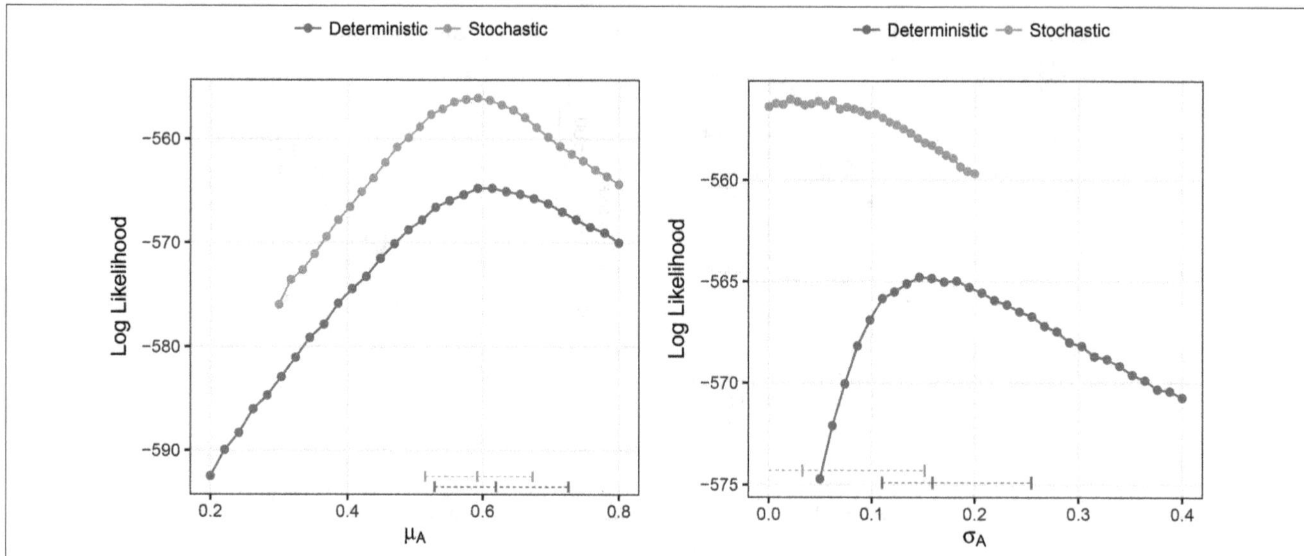

FIGURE 10 | Profile likelihood plots for the parameter estimates for the Ebola data. The plot on the left shows the profile likelihood for the mean growth rate, μ_A, while the plot on the right shows the profile likelihood for the standard deviation of growth rates over counties, σ_A. Horizontal dashed lines indicate the MLE and 95% CIs for the parameter estimates. The overdispersion parameter was free to vary in the calculation of each point along the profile.

treatment plans may be designed under the potentially faulty assumption that there is heterogeneity in response to treatment regimes. Likewise, scientific resources may be wasted in a quest to search for individual-level correlates of heterogeneity that may not exist. Our results suggest that measuring heterogeneity in panel data time series is prone to bias and misinterpretation and that including more data in terms of additional observations per unit or increasing the number of units will not alleviate this bias caused by methodological misspecification.

In this regard, it is important to note that the simulation-based stochastic fits, generally speaking, appropriately partitioned variability into stochastic and parametric components even with relatively short time series. This means that such methods should be preferred for fitting data. However, there are practical issues with implementing stochastic fitting methods when the models are complex (e.g., multiple populations or many parameters) or the populations involved are large. This is because the computational resources needed and the time to fit a given model would be, in most cases, prohibitive. As an alternative, if a fully stochastic model is not possible, one could explore the possibility of using stochastic models for a limited time window (for instance, early on). Although, this will need the development of hybrid fitting methodologies. Generally, one should be cautious when interpreting the fit of deterministic models to panel data, since the observation of parametric heterogeneity or even structural heterogeneity in terms of model selection may be the result of overfitting stochastic fluctuation. Also, the term R^2 can be estimated numerically for a given model to provide a warning of potential problems based on deterministic model fits.

In summary, here we analyzed the effect of neglecting stochastic noise (i.e., in addition to the error term) in panel data of biological time series. We found that deterministic approaches usually overestimate the parametric variability, although (at least in our simple models) the parameter average is less difficult to estimate. On the other hand, stochastic fitting, in general, did a good job of dividing variability between stochastic and parametric.

AUTHOR CONTRIBUTIONS

All authors listed have made a substantial, direct and intellectual contribution to the work, and approved it for publication.

FUNDING

This work was funded by NIH grants R01-AI087520 and R01-AI104373; grants FIS2013-47949-C2-2-P and FIS2016-78883-C2-2-P and PRX 16/00287 (Spain); and PIRSES-GA-2012-317893 (7th FP, EU). The funders had no responsibility in devising the study, developing it or writing it up.

ACKNOWLEDGMENTS

MC thanks the hospitality of Los Alamos National Laboratory (LANL) where this work was conceived. We would like to thank James (Mac) Hyman and Nicholas Hengartner for helpful discussions early on.

REFERENCES

Allen, L. J. (2010). *An Introduction to Stochastic Processes With Applications to Biology*. CRC Press.

Althaus, C. L. (2014). Estimating the reproduction number of ebola virus (ebov) during the 2014 outbreak in west africa. *PLoS Curr.* 6:ecurrents.outbreaks.91afb5e0f279e7f29e7056095255b288. doi: 10.1371/currents.outbreaks.91afb5e0f279e7f29e7056095255b288

Bressloff, P. C., and Newby, J. M. (2013). Stochastic models of intracellular transport. *Rev. Mod. Phys.* 85:135. doi: 10.1103/RevModPhys.85.135

Chowell, G., Hengartner, N. W., Castillo-Chavez, C., Fenimore, P. W., and Hyman, J. M. (2004). The basic reproductive number of ebola and the effects of public health measures: the cases of congo and uganda. *J. Theor. Biol.* 229, 119–126. doi: 10.1016/j.jtbi.2004.03.006

Dietz, K. (1993). The estimation of the basic reproduction number for infectious diseases. *Stat. Methods Med. Res.* 2, 23–41.

Ganusov, V. V. (2016). Strong inference in mathematical modeling: a method for robust science in the twenty- first century. *Front. Microbiol.* 7:1131. doi: 10.3389/fmicb.2016.01131

Gelman, A., and Hill, J. (2007). *Data Analysis Using Regression and Multilevel/Hierarchical Models.* New York, NY: Cambridge University Press.

Hartemink, N., Vanwambeke, S. O., Heesterbeek, H., Rogers, D., Morley, D., Pesson, B., et al. (2011). Integrated mapping of establishment risk for emerging vector-borne infections: a case study of canine leishmaniasis in southwest france. *PLoS ONE* 6:e20817. doi: 10.1371/journal.pone.0020817

Heffernan, J. M., Smith, R. J., and Wahl, L. M. (2005). Perspectives on the basic reproductive ratio. *J. R. Soc. Interface* 2, 281–293. doi: 10.1098/rsif.2005.0042

Heesterbeek, J. (2000). *Mathematical Epidemiology of Infectious Diseases: Model Building, Analysis and Interpretation, Vol. 5.* Sussex: John Wiley & Sons.

Krauer, F., Gsteiger, S., Low, N., Hansen, C. H., and Althaus, C. L. (2016). Heterogeneity in district-level transmission of ebola virus disease during the 2013-2015 epidemic in west africa. *PLoS Negl. Trop. Dis.* 10:e0004867. doi: 10.1371/journal.pntd.0004867

Karlin, S. (2014). *A first Course in Stochastic Processes.* New York, NY: Academic press.

King, A. A., Nguyen, D., Ionides, E. L. (2016). Statistical inference for partially observed markov processes via the r package pomp. *J. Stat. Softw.* 69, 1–43. doi: 10.18637/jss.v069.i12

King, A. A., Domenech de Cellès M, Magpantay, F. M., and Rohani, P. (2015). Avoidable errors in the modelling of outbreaks of emerging pathogens, with special reference to ebola. *Proc. R. Soc. B* . 282:20150347. doi: 10.1098/rspb.2015.0347

Kucharski, A. J., Camacho, A., Flasche, S., Glover, R. E., Edmunds, W. J., and Funk, S. (2015). Measuring the impact of ebola control measures in sierra leone. *Proc. Natl. Acad. Sci. U.S.A.* 112, 14366–14371. doi: 10.1073/pnas.1508814112

Molina-París, C., and Lythe, G. (2011). *Mathematical Models and Immune Cell Biology.* New York, NY: Springer Science & Business Media.

Perelson, A. S., Neumann, A. U., Markowitz, M., Leonard, J. M., and Ho, D. D. (1996). Hiv-1 dynamics in vivo: virion clearance rate, infected cell life-span, and viral generation time. *Science* 271, 1582.

Roberts, M., Andreasen, V., Lloyd, A., and Pellis, L. (2015). Nine challenges for deterministic epidemic models. *Epidemics* 10 49–53. doi: 10.1016/j.epidem.2014.09.006

Ribeiro, R. M., Qin, L., Chavez, L. L., Li, D., Self, S. G., and Perelson, A. S. (2010). Estimation of the initial viral growth rate and basic reproductive number during acute hiv-1 infection. *J. Virol.* 84, 6096–6102. doi: 10.1128/JVI.00127-10

Romero-Severson, E. O., Volz, E., Koopman, J. S., Leitner, T., and onides, E. L. (2015). Dynamic Variation in Sexual Contact Rates in a Cohort of HIV-Negative Gay Men. *Am. J. Epidemiol.* 182, 255–262. doi: 10.1093/aje/kwv044

Romero-Severson, E., Skar, H., Bulla, I., Albert, J., and Leitner, T. (2014). Timing and order of transmission events is not directly reflected in a pathogen phylogeny. *Mol. Biol. Evol.* 31, 2472-2482. doi: 10.1093/molbev/msu179

Süel, G. M., Garcia-Ojalvo, J., Liberman, L. M., and Elowitz, M. B. (2006). An excitable gene regulatory circuit induces transient cellular differentiation. *Nature* 440, 545-550. doi: 10.1038/nature04588

4

Correlation between Anti-gp41 Antibodies and Virus Infectivity Decay During Primary HIV-1 Infection

Naveen K. Vaidya[1*], *Ruy M. Ribeiro*[2,3], *Pinghuang Liu*[4], *Barton F. Haynes*[5], *Georgia D. Tomaras*[5] *and Alan S. Perelson*[2]

[1] Department of Mathematics and Statistics, San Diego State University, San Diego, CA, United States, [2] Theoretical Biology and Biophysics Group, MS K710, Los Alamos National Laboratory, Los Alamos, NM, United States, [3] Laboratório de Biomatemática, Faculdade de Medicina, Universidade de Lisboa, Lisboa, Portugal, [4] Harbin Veterinary Research Institute, Chinese Academy of Agricultural Sciences, Harbin, China, [5] Duke University School of Medicine, Durham, NC, United States

***Correspondence:**
Naveen K. Vaidya
nvaidya@sdsu.edu

Recent experiments have suggested that the infectivity of simian immunodeficiency virus (SIV) and human immunodeficiency virus type-1 (HIV-1) in plasma decreases over time during primary infection. Because anti-gp41 antibodies are produced early during HIV-1 infection and form antibody-virion complexes, we studied if such early HIV-1 specific antibodies are correlated with the decay in HIV-1 infectivity. Using a viral dynamic model that allows viral infectivity to decay and frequent early viral load data obtained from 6 plasma donors we estimate that HIV-1 infectivity begins to decay after about 2 weeks of infection. The length of this delay is consistent with the time before antibody-virion complexes were detected in the plasma of these donors and is correlated ($p = 0.023$, $r = 0.87$) with the time for antibodies to be first detected in plasma. Importantly, we identify that the rate of infectivity decay is significantly correlated with the rate of increase in plasma anti-gp41 IgG concentration ($p = 0.046$, $r = 0.82$) and the increase in IgM+IgG anti-gp41 concentration ($p = 8.37 \times 10^{-4}$, $r = 0.98$). Furthermore, we found that the viral load decay after the peak did not have any significant correlation with the rate of anti-gp41 IgM or IgG increase. These results indicate that early anti-gp41 antibodies may cause viral infectivity decay, but may not contribute significantly to controlling post-peak viral load, likely due to insufficient quantity or affinity. Our findings may be helpful to devise strategies, including antibody-based vaccines, to control acute HIV-1 infection.

Keywords: antibodies, primary HIV-1 infection, viral dynamics model, viral load, virus infectivity

INTRODUCTION

Primary human immunodeficiency virus type 1 (HIV-1) infection is associated with an initial eclipse phase, during which the viral load remains below the limit of detection of conventional assays, followed by a rapid viral load increase (Daar et al., 1991; Schacker et al., 1996; Fiebig et al., 2003; Ribeiro et al., 2010; Cohen et al., 2011). After the viral load reaches its peak, it declines and reaches a set-point level (i.e., a quasi-steady state). The early events during primary HIV-1 infection not only have particular relevance for vaccine, microbicide and pre/post-exposure prophylaxis (Chun et al., 1998; Pope and Haase, 2003; Shattock and Moore, 2003; Haase, 2005), they are also important in defining the set-point viral load later in infection (Lifson et al., 1997) and the time period over which a successful vaccine needs to induce a protective response prior to establishment of the latent pool of HIV-1 infected CD4$^+$ T cells (Wong and Siliciano, 2003; Johnston and Fauci, 2007).

Based on a previous experiment involving simian immunodeficiency virus (SIV) infection of macaques that revealed a difference in infectivity between virus in plasma obtained 7 days after infection and set-point virus (Ma et al., 2009), we introduced an SIV dynamic model with time-dependent viral infectivity (Vaidya et al., 2010). Also, preliminary data comparing the ratio of the 50% tissue culture infectious dose ($TCID_{50}$) with HIV-1 RNA copy number suggests a decrease in virus infectivity over time during primary infection in HIV-1 infected patients, although the magnitude of this effect varies among subjects (Genevieve Fouda and David Montefiori, Duke University School of Medicine, unpublished data). Although the mechanisms responsible for the decay in viral infectivity have not been established, it has been speculated that binding of antibodies to HIV-1 might be in part responsible (Ma et al., 2009). Consistent with this, during early HIV-1 infection it has been shown that anti-gp41 antibodies are produced and form virion-antibody complexes (Tomaras et al., 2008; Liu et al., 2011).

Here we sought to determine whether these early anti-gp41 antibodies influence HIV infectivity by fitting a mathematical model to frequently measured plasma viral loads obtained from 6 plasma donors. The model, which incorporates a time-dependent infectivity rate, fits the acute infection HIV-1 data well. We show the infectivity decay predicted by our model significantly correlates with the anti-gp41 antibody response observed in these plasma donors.

MATERIALS AND METHODS

Experimental Data

Sequential HIV-1 viral load data from 6 plasma donors was obtained as previously described (Gasper-Smith et al., 2008; Tomaras et al., 2008; Stacey et al., 2009). The study was approved by the Duke Health Institutional Review Board, protocol number Pro00006579. Each individual donated 600–800 ml of plasma which was frozen within 8 h to −20°C or less. The plasma samples were stored up to 2 months then sent in pools to be serologically screened for HIV. Donors who were HIV-1 positive were notified and deferred from subsequent donation. HIV-1 positive samples were aliquoted, and refrozen at −20°C. Aliquoted samples of plasma donors were quantified with the Roche Amplicore HIV-1 RT PCR Ultra assay by Quest Diagnostics (Lyndhurst, NY), with a lower limit of quantification of 50 HIV-1 RNA copies/ml (Tomaras et al., 2008). There was a median of 9 data points per donor with a median of 4 data points before the viral peak. The median peak viral load was 6.0 (range 4.5–6.8) $\log_{10}$ viral RNA (vRNA) copies/ml. In these plasma donors, the anti-gp41 IgG and IgM responses were also measured and recorded as optical density (O.D.) (Tomaras et al., 2008). In addition, circulating antibody-virion immune complexes were measured (Tomaras et al., 2008; Liu et al., 2011). The data analyzed below is provided in Table S1.

Viral Dynamic Model

To study the effect of antibody responses in decreasing viral infectivity early during infection, we use the standard model of viral infection (Phillips, 1996; Nowak et al., 1997; Little et al., 1999; Perelson and Nelson, 1999; Stafford et al., 2000), but allow the virus infectiousness to decay in time after a certain delay τ, which accounts for the time needed to generate an anti-HIV-1 response. The model is

$$\begin{aligned}\frac{dT}{dt} &= \lambda - dT - \beta(t)\,TV, \quad T(0) = T_0,\\ \frac{dI}{dt} &= \beta(t)\,TV - \delta I, \quad I(0) = I_0,\\ \frac{dV}{dt} &= pI - cV, \quad V(0) = V_0,\end{aligned} \tag{1}$$

where

$$\beta(t) = \begin{cases} \beta_0, & t \le \tau,\\ \beta_\infty + (\beta_0 - \beta_\infty)\, e^{-k(t-\tau)}, & t > \tau. \end{cases} \tag{2}$$

The model consists of target cells (CD4$^+$ T cells), T, productively infected CD4$^+$ T cells, I, and free virus, V. We assume that target cells are generated at a constant rate λ, have a per capita net loss rate d, which is the difference between loss from cell death and gain due to cell division, and become infected at a rate proportional to the product of target cell density and virus concentration with a time-dependent rate $\beta(t)$. The parameters δ, p, and c are the rate constants of infected cell loss, virus production by infected cells and virus clearance, respectively. As in Vaidya et al. (2010), we assume a simple exponential decay in infectivity over time from the initial rate β_0 to the final rate β_∞ with a decay rate k, but for a more general formulation here we include a time-delay τ before infectivity decay begins.

Data Fits and Parameter Estimation

We fit the model, Equations (1) and (2), to plasma viral load data obtained from 6 HIV-1-infected plasma donors during the acute phase of infection. Earlier studies have shown that the percentage of proliferating CD4$^+$ T cells in the peripheral blood of healthy individuals, as measured by Ki-67 antigen expression, is ~1% (Sachsenberg et al., 1998). We use Ki-67$^+$ CD4$^+$ cells as a surrogate for target cells and thus take the initial number of target cells, T_0, as 10^4 per ml (1% of 10^6/ml CD4$^+$ T cell count). We note that, as in Stafford et al. (2000), the model system (1) becomes independent of T_0 if the scaling $p \to p/T_0$ is performed. This shows that taking the value of T_0 different from 10^4 per ml affects the estimates of only p, not the infectivity rate, $\beta(t)$, and thus, our conclusions will remain unaffected if one uses other values of T_0. Assuming CD4$^+$ T cells were at equilibrium before infection, we set $\lambda = dT_0$. Because the route of infection of the plasma donors is not known, we first assumed infection was initiated by free virus particles rather than infected cells, and thus we set $I_0 = 0$ (Pearson et al., 2011). Then we also analyzed the data assuming infection was initiated by an infected cell. Recent estimates show that the virion clearance rate constant, c, varies between 9.1 day^{-1} and 36.0 day^{-1}, with an average of 23 day^{-1}

(Ramratnam et al., 1999). Thus, we take $c = 23$ day^{-1}, although other values in this range were also considered in a sensitivity analysis.

It is difficult to obtain information about the initial virus concentration that established infection. At least one virion, i.e., 2 viral RNA (vRNA) copies, is needed to establish infection. A 70-kg person has about 15 L of extracellular body water and about 3 L of plasma. Thus, the initial plasma viral load needed to establish systemic infection is >2 vRNA copies per 3,000 ml or >2 vRNA copies per 15,000 ml depending upon whether the virus distributes throughout only the plasma or the total extracellular body water before initiating infection. Here, we present results with $V_0 = 10^{-3}$ vRNA copies per ml assuming that the virus distributes in the plasma and then study the sensitivity of parameter estimates on the initial viral load (V_0) by varying V_0 from 10-fold lower considering the possibility of virus being distributed through extracellular body water to 1,000-fold higher corresponding to the possibility of much higher levels of virus initially entering the circulation.

The exact time of initial infection is not available for this data set. However, the initial viral expansion rates for these subjects have been estimated in a previous study (Ribeiro et al., 2010). Using the slope of viral increase estimated in Ribeiro et al. (2010) and the base value of V_0, we calculated the time of infection and then the time to the first measured viral load above the detection limit for each of these subjects. This allowed us to associate a time since infection with each data point. To estimate τ, we varied τ in 1 day increments, and chose the one which provided the best fit for each plasma donor. The other 6 parameters, β_∞, β_0, k, δ, d, and p, were kept free and estimated by fitting the model to the data from each plasma donor. We also performed fitting by making τ a free parameter and obtained approximately the same value as the best estimate from 1-day increment fitting. Since the fit was not improved with τ as an extra free parameter, we fixed τ as the best estimate obtained from the 1-day increment fitting.

Parameter identifiability in HIV models, including those with time-varying parameters, was discussed in Wu et al. (2008) and Miao et al. (2011). As shown in Miao et al. (2011) and Wu et al. (2008), with λ fixed as in our case, all the constant parameters are structurally identifiable. Miao et al. (2011) showed that the time-varying parameter ($\beta(t)$ in our case) is also identifiable if all the constant parameters are identifiable. Therefore, we expect that the parameters of our model are identifiable for the number of data points available in this study.

The data fitting protocol used to estimate parameters was as described previously in Vaidya et al. (2010). We solved the system of ordinary differential equations (ODEs) numerically using a fourth-order Runge-Kutta in Berkeley Madonna. Using Madonna's "curve fitter" option, we obtain a set of initial parameter estimates. The curve fitting method uses nonlinear least-squares regression that minimizes the following sum of the squared residuals:

$$J(\beta_0, \beta_\infty, k, \delta, p, d) = \frac{1}{N}\sum_{i=1}^{N}\left[\log_{10} V(t_i) - \log_{10} \overline{V}(t_i)\right]^2. \quad (3)$$

Here, V and $\overline{V}$ are virus concentrations predicted by the model and those given by the experimental data, respectively. N is the total number of data points.

Using the set of parameters obtained from Madonna as initial guesses, we refined the fits by using "fmincon.m" and/or "fminsearch.m" functions in MATLAB. For each best fit parameter estimate, we provide a 95% confidence interval (CI), which was computed from 500 bootstrap replicates (Efron and Toibshirani, 1986). Since we analyze only 6 subjects, we present results as medians and ranges, unless otherwise indicated.

Sensitivity Analysis

The viral load establishing systemic infection, V_0, is not known. To study the sensitivity of our results to the choice of V_0, we randomly selected 200 different V_0 from 10-fold lower (i.e., 10^{-4} vRNA copies/ml) to 1,000-fold higher (i.e., 1 vRNA copies/ml) and estimated parameters for each of the 6 donors.

Statistical Analysis

We performed linear regression to obtain the slope of the IgG increase, the IgM increase and the IgG+IgM increase. We then carried out correlation analyses using Pearson's correlation between these slopes and the decay slope of infectivity estimated by our model. We also calculated the slope of the viral load decay after the peak and performed correlation analyses of the viral decay rate with the antibody response.

To evaluate the statistical significance of models comparisons, we performed an F-test (Bates and Watts, 2007) as the models considered in this study without and with infectivity decay are nested.

RESULTS

Model Fitting to Data

We fitted Equations (1) and (2) to the HIV-1 data. We estimated six parameters β_∞, β_0, k, δ, d, and p from the data fitting. The estimated parameters along with their 95% confidence intervals are summarized in **Table 1**. Using these estimated parameters, we plotted the viral load dynamics predicted by the model along with the data for each of the 6 HIV-1 infected plasma donors in **Figure 1**. The predictions of our time-varying infectivity delay model (solid curve) agree well with the data (filled circles).

For comparison, we also fitted these viral load data using a constant infectivity (i.e., $\beta(t)$ constant) model (Stafford et al., 2000), and found that the delay model with time-dependent infectivity provides statistically significant better fits ($p = 0.001$, F-test with all the subjects combined as in Vaidya et al., 2010). Moreover, we compared the data fitting using a time-dependent model without delay (Vaidya et al., 2010) (i.e., $\tau = 0$), and found that including a delay in the model significantly improved the fits ($p = 0.008$, F-test, Vaidya et al., 2010).

Virus Infectivity Decay

We estimated the median initial and late viral infection rate constants to be $\beta_0 = 4.20 \times 10^{-7}$ ml RNA^{-1} day^{-1} and $\beta_\infty = 0.76 \times 10^{-7}$ ml RNA^{-1} day^{-1}, respectively (**Table 1**). This suggests that infectivity decays during acute HIV-1 infection

TABLE 1 | Estimated parameter values β_0, β_∞, k, δ, p, d, τ, and time t_h to reach the mid-value $(\beta_0 + \beta_\infty)/2$.

Patient	β_0 (10^{-6}ml/RNA/day)	β_∞ (10^{-6}ml/RNA/day)	k (1/day)	δ (1/day)	p (10^3 RNAs/day)	d (1/day)	τ (day)	t_h (day)
CHID46	0.409 (0.376–0.441)	0.233 (0.169–0.297)	0.249 (0.234–0.250)	0.775 (0.737–0.814)	14.500 (14.499–14.501)	0.030 (0.023–0.038)	7	2.8
CHID77	0.431 (0.417–0.444)	0.140 (0.129–0.151)	0.077 (0.067–0.093)	0.420 (0.417–0.433)	10.000 (9.999–10.001)	0.021 (0.019–0.025)	24	9.0
CHID79	0.201 (0.195–0.208)	0.001 (0.000–0.027)	0.013 (0.012–0.015)	1.048 (0.992–1.064)	30.172 (30.166–30.178)	0.036 (0.033–0.041)	10	53.3
CHID32	9.203 (4.320–11.011)	0.011 (0.000–0.112)	0.013 (0.011–0.020)	0.851 (0.325–1.360)	0.548 (0.391–0.901)	0.055 (0.048–0.156)	12	53.3
CHID40	0.485 (0.457–0.513)	0.291 (0.161–0.339)	0.096 (0.062–0.103)	0.803 (0.623–0.910)	11.425 (11.422–11.428)	0.033 (0.022–0.037)	5	7.2
CHID08	0.057 (0.050–0.112)	0.004 (0.000–0.019)	0.021 (0.019–0.031)	0.821 (0.491–1.170)	89.892 (48.541–130.952)	0.003 (0.000–0.028)	22	33.0
Median	0.420	0.076	0.049	0.812	12.962	0.032	11	21.0

Numbers in parentheses indicate 95% confidence intervals (see Materials and Methods).

($p = 0.031$, paired Wilcoxon Test). Such infectivity decay over time was also observed previously in SIV infection (Ma et al., 2009; Vaidya et al., 2010). Assuming that the decay of $\beta(t)$ occurs exponentially with rate k, we found that HIV-1 infectivity decays with a median rate of $k = 0.049$ day^{-1} (**Table 1**) (range: $k = 0.013$ day^{-1} to $k = 0.249$ day^{-1}). Also, the time, t_h, to reduce the virus infectivity to its mid-value, $(\beta_0 + \beta_\infty)/2$, given by $\ln(2)/k$, was found to be 21 days (**Table 1**).

Correlation of Infectivity With Antibody Response

It is known that antibodies bind to virions and form antibody-virion complexes (Dianzani et al., 2002; Tomaras et al., 2008; Liu et al., 2011). Such antibodies bound to virions might interfere with the infection process (Ma et al., 2009). Therefore, we examined if there is any correlation between the infectivity decay and the earliest antibody responses detected during acute infection, i.e., the anti-gp41 IgM and/or IgG response (Tomaras et al., 2008; Liu et al., 2011).

While we acknowledge some uncertainty due to sparsity in early Ab data, in general, as shown in **Figure 2**, the anti-gp41 IgM concentration (measured in optical density. i.e., O.D. units) increases approximately linearly up to a maximum value and then decays, whereas the anti-gp41 IgG concentration increases monotonically over the time period studied. This pattern of IgM increasing and then decreasing is consistent with the known features of the IgM-IgG isotype switch (Murphy et al., 2008). We performed a linear regression analysis to find the slope of the IgM increase, of the IgG increase and of the IgM+IgG increase using the antibody data to the time point where antibody levels saturate or start to decay. The IgM and IgG concentrations increase by a median rate of 0.19 day^{-1} and 0.09 day^{-1}, respectively, while the median rate of increase in the IgM + IgG concentration is 0.27 day^{-1} (Table S2).

While there was a positive association between the rate of infectivity decay estimated by our model (k) and the slope of IgM increase (**Figure 3**), this correlation was not statistically significant ($p = 0.33$, $r = 0.48$). However, we found that the rate of infectivity decay has a statistically significant positive correlation with the slope of IgG increase ($p = 0.046$, $r = 0.82$) and a very significant positive correlation with the IgM+IgG anti-gp41 concentration with p-value $= 8.37 \times 10^{-4}$ and r-value $= 0.98$ (**Figure 3**). This suggests that the antibody response might contribute to the loss of virus infectivity. To check the robustness of this finding, we performed correlation analysis by iteratively excluding each donor one at a time, and found that the correlation of infectivity decay with slope of increase of IgM+IgG remained statistically significant ($p < 0.01$ in each case, Table S3).

The Delay Before the Start of Infectivity Decay Correlates With the Time Until the Antibody Response Is Detected

Our model predicts that the virus infectivity begins to decay after a median time of 11 days (range: 5–24 days) of infection. The exact delay from the time of infection to the initiation of antibody increase is not known. However, from the experimental

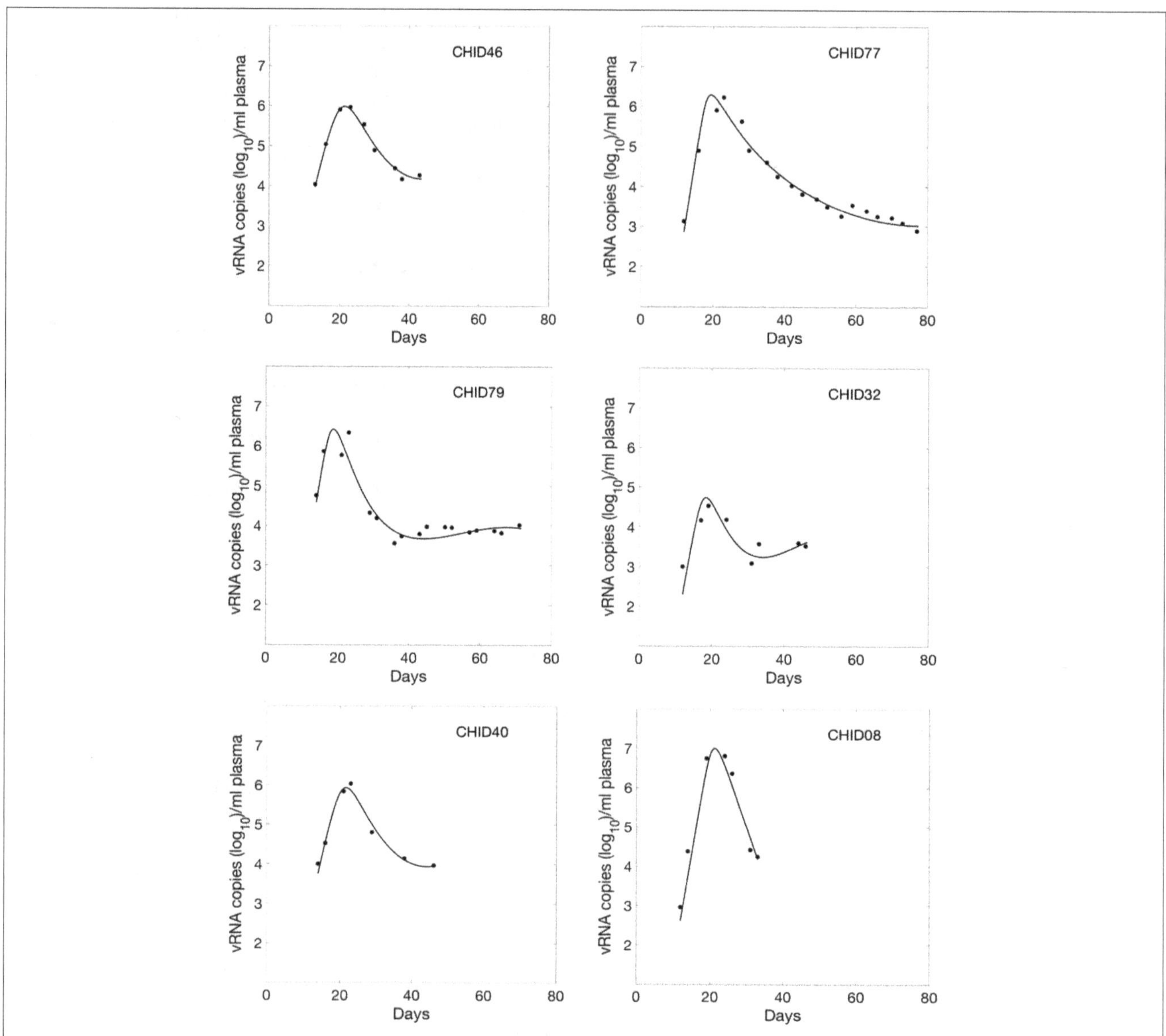

FIGURE 1 | Fitted viral dynamics curve using the delay model with time-varying infectivity to the observed viral load data (filled circle) during primary infection of 6 HIV-1 infected plasma donors.

data we estimated the time from infection (as estimated by our calculation) to the time when the free IgM+IgG level begin to increase in plasma. In the donated plasma, antibodies were measured and, in every case, O.D. readings of both IgM and IgG began to increase on the same day. Since the antibodies were assayed in every sample, we defined the time when antibody becomes detectable as the first time point for which the O.D. of IgM+IgG level was above the limit of detection (i.e., O.D. > 0.5). We found a statistically significant correlation ($p = 0.0233$, $r = 0.87$) between the time that antibody became detectable in plasma and the delay before infectivity decay began predicted by our model (**Figure 4**). Furthermore, for three donors (CHID77, CHID08, CHID79), the times for antibody-virion complexes to be experimentally detectable in plasma were reported previously as 13, 9, and 6 days, respectively, where this was measured relative to the time at which the plasma viral load first reached 100 copies/ml (Tomaras et al., 2008). Using the eclipse phase of acute infection in these plasma donors, calculated from the slope of viral increase estimated in Ribeiro et al. (2010), these times translate to 24, 18, and 14 days from the time of infection. These values and their rank-order are consistent with the delay for infectivity decay predicted by our model (24, 22, 10 days, respectively, **Table 1**).

Correlation of Post-peak Viral Load Drop With Antibody Response

To observe if antibodies have any significant impact on viral load decay after the viral load peak, we performed a correlation analysis between the slope of IgM increase, IgG increase, IgM+IgG increase and the slope of the viral load drop after the

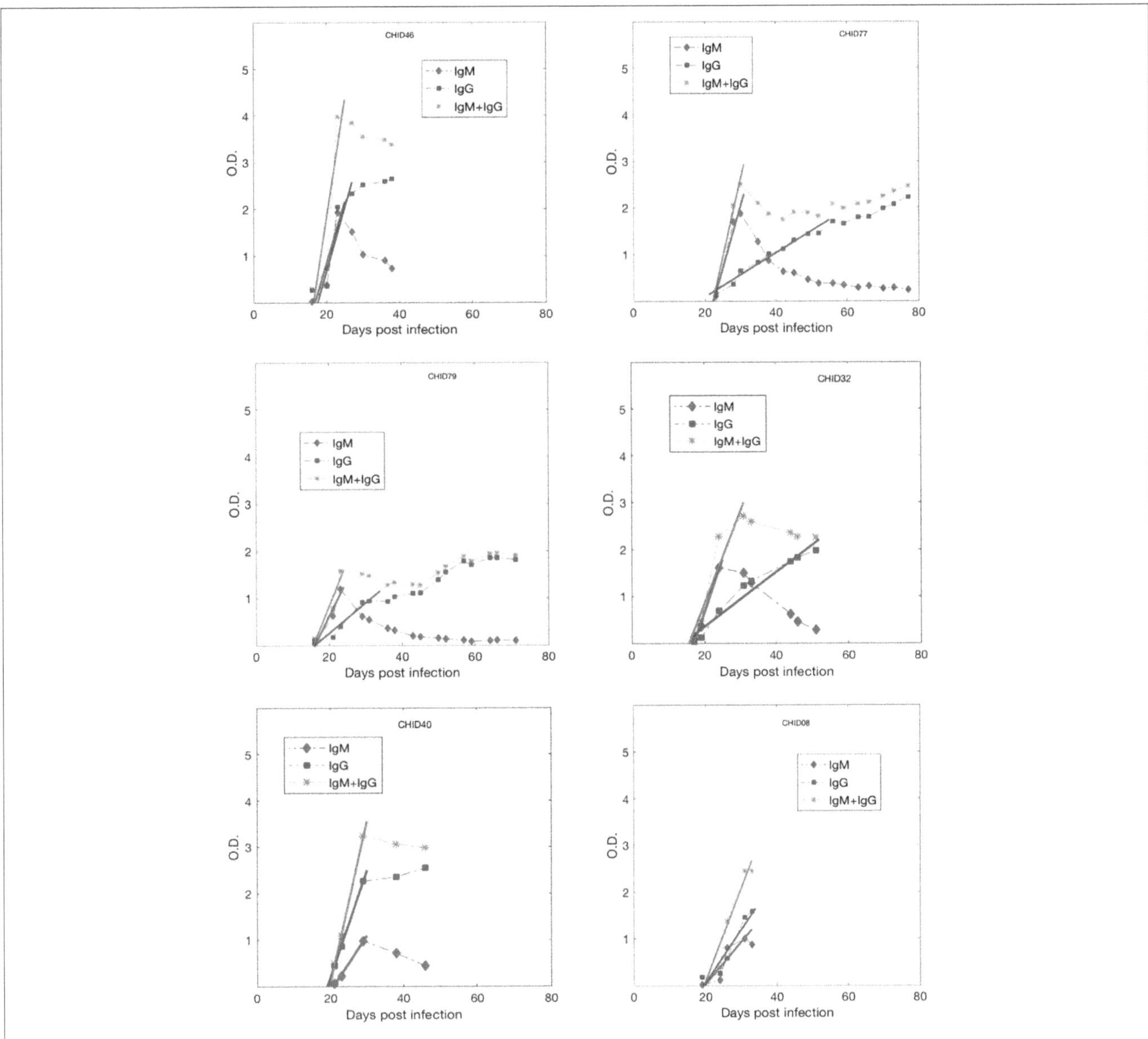

FIGURE 2 | Anti-gp41 IgM, IgG and (IgM+IgG) antibody response data during primary infection from 6 HIV-1 infected plasma donors. The lines represent the best fits used to estimate the upward slope of the antibody increase.

peak (Table S2). We did not find any significant correlation with IgM, IgG or IgM+IgG indicating that this antibody response might not be the primary cause for the drop of viral load after the peak, consistent with previous findings (Tomaras et al., 2008). In our viral dynamic model, Equation (1), viral load drop after the peak is due to target cell limitation and death of productively infected cells.

Sensitivity Analysis

Above we analyzed the correlation of two parameters, k and τ, with the antibody response. We estimated these parameters by fitting our model to viral load data. Due to lack of information about the actual number of virions initiating infection, V_0, we assumed $V_0 = 10^{-3}$ vRNA copies/ml. To ensure that the choice of V_0 did not bias our results, we re-fit the data taking 200 different values of V_0 selected randomly from 10-fold lower to 1,000-fold higher (i.e., 10^{-4} to 1) than the base-case. We find that the estimate of τ is not affected at all, and that the median change in the estimates of k is below 5% (Figure S1). Therefore, our results are not sensitive to the choice of V_0.

We assumed that the infection was initiated with free virus particles. To study how the estimates are affected if the infection was initiated with infected cells, we compared the estimates between an infection with one virus particle distributed in 15 L body water (i.e., $V_0 = 2/15000$ vRNA copies/ml) and an infection with one infected cell distributed in 15 L body water (i.e., $I_0 = 1/15000$ cells/ml). We found that the estimates of k are essentially the same in these two cases (Figure S2).

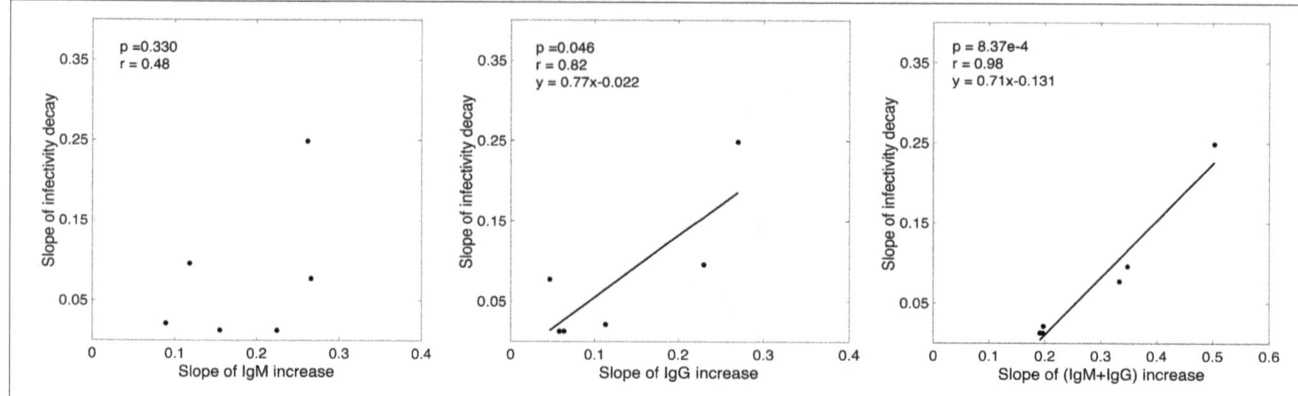

FIGURE 3 | Correlation analysis of the slope of experimentally measured IgM, IgG and (IgM+IgG) antibody increase with the rate of infectivity decay predicted by our model.

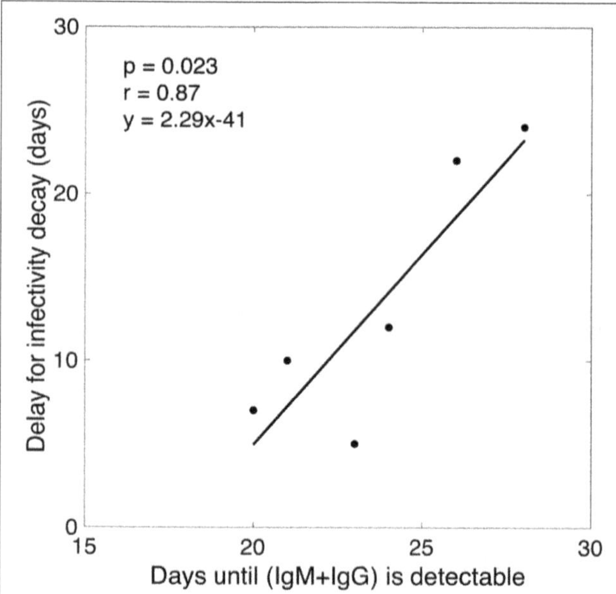

FIGURE 4 | Correlation analysis between the time for total antibody (IgM+IgG) response to be experimentally detectable in plasma and the delay for the start of infectivity decay predicted by our model.

We chose $c = 23\ d^{-1}$ based on the average of the experimentally estimated range between 9 and 36 d^{-1}. To test the robustness of our results to this assumption, we refitted the data with different values of c within this range. The only parameters that is mainly affected is the viral production rate. Therefore, our results regarding k and τ are not affected by the specific value of c.

DISCUSSION

During primary HIV-1 infection, a decay of virus infectivity over time has been suggested by comparing the ratio of tissue culture infectious dose ($TCID_{50}$) with HIV RNA copy number in sequential early viral load samples from a limited number of subjects (Genevieve Fouda and David Montefiori, unpublished data). In addition, HIV-1-specific anti-gp41 antibodies have been detected in plasma a median of 13 days after the viral load reaches 100 vRNA copies/ml (Tomaras et al., 2008). Moreover, anti-gp41 IgM-virion or IgG-virion complexes were found as early as 5 days after the viral load became detectable (Tomaras et al., 2008; Liu et al., 2011). The presence of such antibodies might affect the infectivity of HIV-1 (Tomaras et al., 2008; Ma et al., 2009). Therefore, one of the main objectives of this study was to ask if there is a correlation between the infectivity decay of plasma virus and the anti-gp41 antibody response in HIV-1 infected individuals.

Since there are delays before antibodies and antibody-virion complexes become detectable in plasma (Tomaras et al., 2008), we extended a previous infection model (Vaidya et al., 2010) used to study acute SIV infection by incorporating a time-delay before infectivity decay begins. We then used this delay model to quantify the time-variation of HIV-1 infectivity during primary infection. Our data fitting procedure reveals that both time-dependent nature and delay of infectivity decay are necessary to better describe the viral load data from primary HIV-1 infection.

According to our model estimates, plasma HIV-1 infectivity decays exponentially with a median rate of 0.049 day^{-1} (**Table 1**), and there is a time delay of about 2 weeks (range 5–24 days) before virus infectivity begins to decay. The length of this delay is consistent with the period from infection to the time when the virion-antibody complexes were detected in plasma (Tomaras et al., 2008), and is significantly correlated ($p = 0.0233$, $r = 0.87$) with the time post-infection for anti-gp41 antibody (IgG+IgM) to be detectable in plasma (**Figure 4**).

Our analyses also showed a statistically significant and strong correlation between the rate of increase of the IgM+IgG anti-gp41 antibody concentration and the rate of infectivity decay estimated by the model ($p = 0.0008$, $r = 0.98$) (**Figure 3**). On the other hand, we did not observe a significant correlation between the slope of the IgM, IgG or IgM+IgG increase and the slope of viral load drop after the viral load peak. Taken together, these results indicate that the anti-gp41 (IgM+IgG) response might contribute to the reduction of virus infectivity, but that these anti gp41 antibodies have minimal effect on controlling post peak viral load as seen in Tomaras et al. (2008). Thus other factors, such as target cell limitation (Stafford et al., 2000) and cytotoxic T cell responses (Goonetilleke et al., 2009) may be playing a role in determining the post-peak viral decline. Because cells are not collected from plasma donors quantifying the change in target cell levels and the magnitude of the CTL response was not possible in this study.

A contribution of antibodies to reducing viral infectivity was suggested by Ma et al. (2009), and supported by their observation that mixing plasma obtained at set-point with plasma obtained 7 days after SIV infection reduced the infectivity of the 7-day plasma. However, our inference that antibody affects the infectivity of HIV-1 during early infection is derived from a correlation based on limited viral load and antibody data from only 6 individuals. We cannot rule out other possible causes of infectivity decay such as the production of non-infectious viral genomes that reduce infectivity, as the virus that founds the infection diversifies due to mutation during early infection, or other plasma proteins binding to virions and mediating infectivity decay. Also, the correlation between the slope of the infectivity decay and the up-slope of antibody responses obtained in this study is for the early stages post-infection. Once a plasma donor was identified as being HIV+ donations were stopped and hence no long-term data were collected. Later in the infection antibody responses saturate or decay. To capture the long-term effect, the model needs to be extended to incorporate such behavior and longer-term data is needed to validate such extended models.

While this study supports the hypothesis that antibodies reduce viral infectivity, we acknowledge that antibodies might have other anti-HIV effects, such as enhanced virion clearance and/or antibody-dependent cellular cytotoxicity (Tomaras and Haynes, 2009, 2010). However, these effects were found to have negligible contribution to HIV-1 viral dynamics (Tomaras et al., 2008). In our previous study, we (Tomaras et al., 2008) also investigated the effects of antibody in neutralizing virus by reducing the infectivity rate in a mathematical model including antibody data, but we did not find a significant antibody effect in most patients. The difference with the current results could be due to differences in the two modeling approaches: the delay in the antibody effect in Tomaras et al. (2008) was entirely given by the free antibody data, i.e., the delay corresponded to the time delay for antibody to become detectable in plasma, while the delay in our model (estimated to be much shorter, **Figure 4**) corresponds to the delay for the formation of antibody-virion complexes. Note that antibody-virion complexes are detectable earlier than free antibodies in plasma (Tomaras et al., 2008). The second difference in the two modeling approaches is the functional form of the infectivity decay introduced into the models (see Text S1). A study with more antibody data may help to accurately and explicitly incorporate antibody effects into viral dynamic models. While direct comparison between these two models might not be appropriate as our model does not have explicit dynamics for antibodies, clarifying these issues might be important for future development of models that take explicit antibody responses into account. We also acknowledge uncertainty in the route of infection and the actual time of infection; if the time of initial infection is different, then this may imply a different dose of infecting virus, or even differences in host immune response to the virus infection. However, we note that it is very difficult to find HIV infected individuals so early in infection. This complexity makes this data set unique and highlights the importance of this study.

Although our model cannot conclusively address the causes of decay in HIV-1 infectivity, the quantitative agreement between our model's predictions and the measured viral load curves in all 6 subjects, and the correlation of the rate of infectivity decay with the measured increase in anti-gp41 antibody concentrations strongly suggest the early anti-HIV-1 response, even though non-neutralizing may still provide benefit. More data, especially on early antibody responses (including IgA responses), the formation of antibody-virion complexes, and the ratio of infectious virus to total HIV-1 RNA are needed to provide a more accurate picture of virus infectivity during primary HIV-1 infection.

AUTHOR CONTRIBUTIONS

NV and AP designed the study. NV performed mathematical analysis and numerical experiments. NV, RR, and AP analyzed the data. PL, BH, and GT provided the experimental data. All authors contributed to writing the paper.

ACKNOWLEDGMENTS

This work was funded by NSF grant DMS-1616299 (NV), DMS-1836647(NV) and the start-up fund from San Diego State University (NV). Portions of this work were done under the auspices of the US Department of Energy under contract DE-AC52-06NA25396 and supported by NIH grants R01-AI028433 and R01-OD011095 (AP), R01-AI104373 (RR), and the NIH CHAVI grant U01-AI067854.

REFERENCES

Bates, D. M., and Watts, D. G. (2007). *Nonlinear Regression Analysis and its Applications*. Hoboken, NJ: John Wiley & Sons, Inc.

Chun, T. W., Engel, D., Berrey, M. M., Shea, T., Corey, L., and Fauci, A. S. (1998). Early establishment of a pool of latently infected, resting CD4(+) T cells during primary HIV-1 infection. *Proc. Natl. Acad. Sci. U.S.A.* 95, 8869–8873. doi: 10.1073/pnas.95.15.8869

Cohen, M. S., Shaw, G. M., McMichael, A. J., and Haynes, B. F. (2011). Acute HIV-1 infection. *N. Engl. J. Med.* 364, 1943–1954. doi: 10.1056/NEJMra1011874

Daar, E. S., Moudgil, T., Meyer, R. D., and Ho, D. D. (1991). Transient high levels of viremia in patients with primary human immunodeficiency virus type 1 infection. *N. Engl. J. Med.* 324, 961–964. doi: 10.1056/NEJM199104043241405

Dianzani, F., Antonelli, G., Riva, E., Turriziani, O., Antonelli, L., Tyring, S., et al. (2002). Is human immunodeficiency virus RNA load composed of neutralized immune complexes? *J. Infect. Dis.* 185, 1051–1054. doi: 10.1086/340043

Efron, B., and Toibshirani, R. (1986). Bootstrap methods for standard errors, confidence intervals, and other measures of statistical accuracy. *Stat. Sci.* 1, 54–75. doi: 10.1214/ss/1177013815

Fiebig, E. W., Wright, D. J., Rawal, B. D., Garrett, P. E., Schumacher, R. T., Peddada, L., et al. (2003). Dynamics of HIV viremia and antibody seroconversion in plasma donors: implications for diagnosis and staging of primary HIV infection. *AIDS* 17, 1871–1879. doi: 10.1097/00002030-200309050-00005

Gasper-Smith, N., Crossman, D. M., Whitesides, J. F., Mensali, N., Ottinger, J. S., Plonk, S. G., et al. (2008). Induction of plasma (TRAIL), TNFR-2, Fas ligand, and plasma microparticles after human immunodeficiency virus type 1 (HIV-1) transmission: implications for HIV-1 vaccine design. *J. Virol.* 82, 7700–7710. doi: 10.1128/JVI.00605-08

Goonetilleke, N., Liu, M. K., Salazar-Gonzalez, J. F., Ferrari, G., Giorgi, E., Ganusov V. V., et al. (2009). The first T cell response to transmitted/founder virus contributes to the control of acute viremia in HIV-1 infection. *J. Exp. Med.* 206, 1253–1272. doi: 10.1084/jem.20090365

Haase, A. T. (2005). Perils at mucosal front lines for HIV and SIV and their hosts. *Nat. Rev. Immunol.* 5, 783–792. doi: 10.1038/nri1706

Johnston, M. I., and Fauci, A. S. (2007). An HIV vaccine–evolving concepts. *N. Engl. J. Med.* 356, 2073–2081. doi: 10.1056/NEJMra066267

Lifson, J. D., Nowak, M. A., Goldstein, S., Rossio, J. L., Kinter, A., Vasquez, G., et al. (1997). The extent of early viral replication is a critical determinant of the natural history of simian immunodeficiency virus infection. *J. Virol.* 71, 9508–9514.

Little, S. J., McLean, A. R., Spina, C. A., Richman, D. D., and Havlir, D. V. (1999). Viral dynamics of acute HIV-1 infection. *J. Exp. Med.* 190, 841–850. doi: 10.1084/jem.190.6.841

Liu, P., Overman, R. G., Yates, N. L., Alam, S. M., Vandergrift, N., Chen, Y., et al. (2011). Dynamic antibody specificities and virion concentrations in circulating immune complexes in acute to chronic HIV-1 infection. *J. Virol.* 85, 11196–11207. doi: 10.1128/JVI.05601-11

Ma, Z. M., Stone, M., Piatak, M. Jr., Schweighardt, B., Haigwood, N. L., Montefiori, D., et al. (2009). High specific infectivity of plasma virus from the pre-ramp-up and ramp-up stages of acute simian immunodeficiency virus infection. *J. Virol.* 83, 3288–3297. doi: 10.1128/JVI.02423-08

Miao, H., Xia, X., Perelson, A. S., and Wu, H. (2011). On identifiability of nonlinear ode models and applications in viral dynamics. *SIAM Rev.* 53, 3–39. doi: 10.1137/090757009

Murphy, K., Travers, P., and Walport, M. (2008). *Janeway's Immunobiology*. New York, NY: Garland Science.

Nowak, M. A., Lloyd, A. L., Vasquez, G. M., Wiltrout, T. A., Wahl, L. M., Bischofberger, N., et al. (1997). Viral dynamics of primary viremia and antiretroviral therapy in simian immunodeficiency virus infection. *J. Virol.* 71, 7518–7525.

Pearson, J. E., Krapivsky, P., and Perelson, A. S. (2011). Stochastic theory of early viral infection: continuous versus burst production of virions. *PLoS Comput. Biol.* 7:e1001058. doi: 10.1371/journal.pcbi.1001058

Perelson, A. S., and Nelson, P. W. (1999). Mathematical analysis of HIV-1 dynamics of *vivo*. *SIAM Rev.* 41, 3–44. doi: 10.1137/S0036144598335107

Phillips, A. N. (1996). Reduction of HIV concentration during acute infection: independence from a specific immune response. *Science* 271, 497–499. doi: 10.1126/science.271.5248.497

Pope, M., and Haase, A. T. (2003). Transmission, acute HIV-1 infection and the quest for strategies to prevent infection. *Nat. Med.* 9, 847–852. doi: 10.1038/nm07 03-847

Ramratnam, B., Bonhoeffer, S., Binley, J., Hurley, A., Zhang, L., Mittler, J. E., et al. (1999). Rapid production and clearance of HIV-1 and hepatitis C virus assessed by large volume plasma apheresis. *Lancet* 354, 1782–1785. doi: 10.1016/S0140-6736(99)02035-8

Ribeiro, R. M., Qin, L., Chavez, L. L., Li, D., Self, S. G., and Perelson, A. S. (2010). Estimation of the initial viral growth rate and basic reproductive number during acute HIV-1 infection. *J. Virol.* 84, 6096–6102. doi: 10.1128/JVI.00127-10

Sachsenberg, N., Perelson, A. S., Yerly, S., Schockmel, G. A., Leduc, D., Hirschel, B., et al. (1998). Turnover of CD4+ and CD8+ T lymphocytes in HIV-1 infection as measured by Ki-67 antigen. *J. Exp. Med.* 187, 1295–1303. doi: 10.1084/jem.187.8.1295

Schacker, T., Collier, A. C., Hughes, J., Shea, T., and Corey, L. (1996). Clinical and epidemiologic features of primary HIV infection. *Ann. Intern. Med.* 125, 257–264. doi: 10.7326/0003-4819-125-4-199608150-00001

Shattock, R. J., and Moore, J. P. (2003). Inhibiting sexual transmission of HIV-1 infection. *Nat. Rev. Microbiol.* 1, 25–34. doi: 10.1038/nrmicro729

Stacey, A. R., Norris, P. J., Qin, L., Haygreen, E. A., Taylor, E., Heitman, J., et al. (2009). Induction of a striking systemic cytokine cascade prior to peak viremia in acute human immunodeficiency virus type 1 infection, in contrast to more modest and delayed responses in acute hepatitis B and C virus infections. *J. Virol.* 83, 3719–3733. doi: 10.1128/JVI.01844-08

Stafford, M. A., Corey, L., Cao, Y., Daar, E. S., Ho, D. D., and Perelson, A. S. (2000). Modeling plasma virus concentration during primary HIV infection. *J. Theor. Biol.* 203, 285–301. doi: 10.1006/jtbi.2000.1076

Tomaras, G. D., and Haynes, B. F. (2009). HIV-1-specific antibody responses during acute and chronic HIV-1 infection. *Curr. Opin. HIV AIDS* 4, 373–379. doi: 10.1097/COH.0b013e32832f00c0

Tomaras, G. D., and Haynes, B. F. (2010). Strategies for eliciting HIV-1 inhibitory antibodies. *Curr Opin HIV AIDS* 5, 421–427. doi: 10.1097/COH.0b013e32833d2d45

Tomaras, G. D., Yates, N. L., Liu, P., Qin, L., Fouda, G. G., Chavez, L. L., et al. (2008). Initial B-cell responses to transmitted human immunodeficiency virus type 1: virion-binding immunoglobulin M (IgM) and IgG antibodies followed by plasma anti-gp41 antibodies with ineffective control of initial viremia. *J. Virol.* 82, 12449–12463. doi: 10.1128/JVI.01708-08

Vaidya, N. K., Ribeiro, R. M., Miller, C. J., and Perelson, A. S. (2010). Viral dynamics during primary simian immunodeficiency virus infection: effect of time-dependent virus infectivity. *J. Virol.* 84, 4302–4310. doi: 10.1128/JVI.02284-09

Wong, S. B. J., and Siliciano, R. F. (2003). "Biology of early infection and impact on vaccine design," in *AIDS Vaccine Development: Challenges and Opportunities*, eds P. K. Wayne, C. Koff, and I. D. Gust (Norfold: Caister Academic Press), 17–22.

Wu, H., Zhu, H., Miao, H., and Perelson, A. S. (2008). Parameter identifiability and estimation of HIV/AIDS dynamic models. *Bull. Math. Biol.* 70, 785–799. doi: 10.1007/s11538-007-9279-9

5

A Bistable Switch in Virus Dynamics can Explain the Differences in Disease Outcome Following SIV Infections in Rhesus Macaques

Stanca M. Ciupe[1], Christopher J. Miller[2] and Jonathan E. Forde[3]*

[1] Department of Mathematics, Virginia Tech, Blacksburg, VA, United States, [2] Department of Pathology, Microbiology, and Immunology, School of Veterinary Medicine, Center for Comparative Medicine and California National Primate Research Center, University of California, Davis, Davis, CA, United States, [3] Department of Mathematics and Computer Science, Hobart and Williams Smith Colleges, Geneva, NY, United States

***Correspondence:**
Stanca M. Ciupe
stanca@vt.edu

Experimental studies have shown that the size and infectious-stage of viral inoculum influence disease outcomes in rhesus macaques infected with simian immunodeficiency virus. The possible contribution to disease outcome of antibody developed after transmission and/or present in the inoculum in free or bound form is not understood. In this study, we develop a mathematical model of virus-antibody immune complex formation and use it to predict their role in transmission and protection. The model exhibits a bistable switch between clearance and persistence states. We fitted it to temporal virus data and estimated the parameter values for free virus infectivity rate and antibody carrying capacity for which the model transitions between virus clearance and persistence when the initial conditions (in particular the ratio of immune complexes to free virus) vary. We used these results to quantify the minimum virus amount in the inoculum needed to establish persistent infections in the presence and absence of protective antibodies.

Keywords: SIV, immune complexes, mathematical model, bistable dynamics, stochastic model

INTRODUCTION

The humoral immune response is one of the first barriers against infecting pathogens and forms the basis for most vaccines that are currently in use (Plotkin, 2008; Deal and Balazs, 2015). The rapidly mutating human immunodeficiency virus (HIV), however, evades humoral immune responses in most human infections due to difficulties in eliciting neutralizing antibodies that are effective against the enormous diversity of virus strains (Haynes, 2015). In a few cases broadly neutralizing antibodies (bnAbs) are produced, but they appear 2–4 years following infection (Gray et al., 2011; Tomaras et al., 2011), are ineffective against co-circulating virus strains, and have unusual traits such as autoreactivity and high levels of somatic hypermutations (Mascola and Haynes, 2013). Inducing protective antibodies *in vivo* is challenging (Mascola and Haynes, 2013; Haynes, 2015), with the partially successful RV144 vaccine clinical trial offering a 31.2% decrease in transmission through non-neutralizing antibody dependent cellular toxicity-mediated responses (ADCC) (Rerks-Ngarm et al., 2009; Tomaras et al., 2013; Pollara et al., 2014).

Animal models have proven useful in examining the mechanisms of virus-antibody interactions that lead to protection against HIV infections. Studies using the chimeric simian-human rhesus macaque model (SHIV) have shown that passive transfer of broadly neutralizing monoclonal antibodies (bnMAbs) can induce protection against mucosal challenge (Moldt et al., 2012). The protection is dependent on the ratio between the challenge dose and the concentration of broadly neutralizing antibodies in the serum (Mascola et al., 1999), the breadth and potency of bnMAbs (Walker et al., 2011; Moldt et al., 2012), as well as the timing of antibody infusion (Nishimura et al., 2003). The potential for inducing neutralizing antibodies that correlate with protection *in vivo* has been shown during simian immunodeficiency virus (SIV) infections of ENV-vaccinated rhesus macaques (Letvin et al., 2011), suggesting that it may be possible to elicit antibody-mediated protection through vaccination. Understanding the properties of antibodies, such as concentration and avidity needed for protection based on known virus count in the inoculum, is important information that can guide vaccine design.

In 2009, Ma et al. used SIV infection in rhesus macaques to examine the connection between infection outcome, the size of the challenge inoculum and the disease stage in the SIV infected animals used as donors (Ma et al., 2009). They found that ~20 viral RNA (vRNA) copies titrated from a plasma pool containing virus collected during the ramp-up-stage of infection in donor animals are needed to successfully infect recipient animals. By contrast, ~1,500 vRNA copies titrated from a plasma pool containing virus collected during the set-point-stage of infection in donor animals are needed to establish infection in recipient animals. This led to the conclusion that the virus infectivity decreases over time due to a combination of virological and immunological factors. In Vaidya et al. (2010) used mathematical models to quantify the decrease in infectivity during the ramp-up and set-point infection and found that the decrease happens during both acute and chronic stages with a sharper decrease during acute infections. They did not, however, examine the mechanisms underlying the decrease.

In this study we investigate whether antiviral factors can explain the change in virus infectivity observed in experiments. Briefly, we hypothesize that donor's ramp-up-stage plasma transferred into the recipient animal contains mostly free virus. By contrast, donor's set-point-stage plasma transferred into the recipient animal contain a large amount of antibody-virus immune complexes in addition to free virus. If such immune complexes can still infect, then their infectivity rate is reduced compared to that of the free virus. To test this hypothesis, we develop a mathematical model of antibody-virus dynamics that assumes interaction between virus, recipient and donor antibody, and the corresponding immune complexes. We fit the model to viral load data from two recipient animals challenged with donor's ramp-up-stage plasma, three challenged with donor's set-point-stage plasma, and one infused with donor's set-point antibody and challenged with donor's ramp-up-stage plasma. The fits give us parameter estimates for long-run antibody concentration, free virus infectivity rates, and the relation between protection and free virus - immune complex ratio in the inoculum.

METHODS

Data

We are using published data from the Ma et al. (2009) (all information regarding approvals by IRB can be found in the original study). Briefly, plasma samples from seven SIV infected rhesus macaques were collected during the ramp-up and set-point-stages of infections. Various amounts of vRNA were titrated from the two plasma pools and used for intravenous infection of SIV naive rhesus macaques (see Ma et al., 2009 for additional details). Animals 35036, 33815, and 3297 were challenged with virus from ramp-up-stage plasma and animals 33952, 34846, and 34373 were challenged virus from set-point-stage plasma. Lastly, animals 33681, 32350, 32970, and 36068 were challenged with virus from an aliquot of ramp-up-stage plasma containing heat inactivated set-point-stage plasma. Longitudinal virus load data (vRNA copies per ml) was collected for all recipient animals that became viremic.

Model of Recipient-Virus Interaction

We develop a mathematical model of virus-antibody interaction that investigates the connection between inoculum size and disease outcome. We start with the basic SIV model (Perelson et al., 1996; Bonhoeffer et al., 1997) which considers the interaction between activated uninfected CD4 T cells T, infected CD4 T cells I, and free virus V, as follows

$$\begin{aligned} \frac{dT}{dt} &= s - dT - \beta TV, \\ \frac{dI}{dt} &= \beta TV - \delta I, \\ \frac{dV}{dt} &= N\delta I - cV. \end{aligned} \tag{1}$$

Uninfected cells are produced at rate s, die at per capita rate d, and become infected upon encountering virus at rate β. Infected cells die at per capita rate δ and produce N virions throughout their average lifespan. Free virus is eliminated at per capita rate c.

During challenge with donor's plasma, we assume that donor's antibody A_D and donor's virus-antibody immune complexes X_D are transferred into the recipient animals. A_D decays exponentially at rate d_A. We assume that donor's immune complexes X_D can still infect target cells at rate β_1. Their infectivity rate, however, is smaller than that of free virus, $\beta_1 < \beta$. X_D unbind to give rise to free virus

$$X_D \underset{k_p}{\overset{k_m}{\rightleftharpoons}} V + A_D, \tag{2}$$

where k_p and k_m are binding and unbinding rates. Lastly, X_D are cleared faster than free virus. We model this in a density dependent manner, with c_{AV} being the maximum removal rate and M the complexes at which the removal is half-maximal.

We next assume that a *de novo* antibody response to the SIV infection occurs in recipients. Recipient antibody, A_R, binds free virus, V, and forms antibody-virus immune complexes, X_R

$$A_R + V \underset{k_p}{\overset{k_m}{\rightleftharpoons}} X_R, \tag{3}$$

with the same binding and unbinding rates as the those of the donor antibody. Recipient antibody expands in an antigen dependent manner at rate α. We account for immunological memory by assuming that recipient antibodies persist in an antigen independent manner with maximum proliferation r and carrying capacity K. Recipient immune complexes have the same infectivity rate, $\beta_1 < \beta$, and the same removal rate, $c_{AV} > c$, as the donor's immune complexes.

The model becomes

$$\begin{aligned}
\frac{dT}{dt} &= s - dT - \beta TV - \beta_1 T(X_D + X_R),\\
\frac{dI}{dt} &= \beta TV + \beta_1 T(X_D + X_R) - \delta I,\\
\frac{dV}{dt} &= N\delta I - cV - k_p(A_R + A_D)V + k_m(X_R + X_D),\\
\frac{dA_R}{dt} &= \alpha A_R V + rA_R\left(1 - \frac{A_R}{K}\right) - k_p A_R V + k_m X_R, \qquad (4)\\
\frac{dX_R}{dt} &= k_p A_R V - k_m X_R - c_{AV}\frac{X_R}{X_R + M},\\
\frac{dA_D}{dt} &= -d_A A_D - k_p A_D V + k_m X_D,\\
\frac{dX_D}{dt} &= k_p A_D V - k_m X_D - c_{AV}\frac{X_D}{X_D + M},
\end{aligned}$$

with initial values $T(0) = s/d$, $I(0) = 0$, $V(0) = V_0 > 0$, $A_R(0) = A_0, X_R(0) = 0, A_D(0) \geq A_0$ and $X_D(0) \geq 0$.

Parameter Values and Initial Conditions

We assume that we have $T(0) = 10^6$ per ml and $I(0) = 0$ per ml at the beginning of infection. Uninfected CD4 T cells are produced at rate $s = 10^4$ per ml per day (Sachsenberg et al., 1998) and die at rate $d = 0.01$ per day (Stafford et al., 2000). We use previous estimates for the infected cells death rate, $\delta = 0.39$ per day (Markowitz et al., 2003), virus clearance rate, $c = 23$ per day (Ramratnam et al., 1999), and virus production by an infected cells, $N = 2{,}000$ per day (Ciupe, 2015). We fix the immune complexes infectivity rate $\beta_1 = 10^{-8}$ ml per day per virion.

Since all donor and recipient animals were negative for anti-SIV antibodies, we assume the antibodies are below their limit of detection of 3.8×10^8 molecules per ml (0.1 ng/ml[1]). Without loss of generality, $A_D(0) = A_R(0) = 3.5 \times 10^8$ molecules per ml. The recipient immune complexes are absent at the time of infection, $X_R(0) = 0$ molecules per ml. Donor antibodies decay at rate $d_A = 0.07$ per day (Zalevsky et al., 2010). Once infection occurs, recipient antibodies are produced and expand in both virus-dependent and virus-independent manners, at rates α and r, respectively. Since α and r have complementary functions (see Supplementary Material), we can ignore one of them. For simplicity, we set $\alpha = 0$. Immune complexes dissociate at rate $k_m = 100$ per day (Schwesinger et al., 2000; Zhou et al., 2007; Tabei et al., 2012). The IgG affinity $K_A = k_p/k_m$ in a humoral response frequently starts at 10^5 M^{-1} (Gopalakrishnan and Karush, 1975). For SIV, each virion can have ten to hundreds of potential antibody binding sites and affinity maturation may occur. Taking both effects into account can increase the functional affinity K_A to 10^8 M^{-1}. Therefore, we consider a binding rate $k_p = K_A \times k_m = 10^{10} M^{-1}$/day= 1.6×10^{-11} ml per molecule per day, higher than in Tabei et al. (2012), Ciupe (2015) and a carrying capacity $K = 5 \times 10^{13}$ molecules per ml. We assume that a maximum of $c_{AV} = 10^6$ immune complexes are removed per day, and that the removal rate is half-maximal for $M = 500$ immune complexes.

When an animal is challenged with SIV, the inoculum plasma may contain both free virus or donor's immune complexes. As in Vaidya et al. (2010), we assume that the initial virus distributes throughout the entire plasma volume of a 7 kg macaque, approximately 300 ml. Therefore, our initial conditions are $X_D(0) + V(0) = D(0)/300$ copies per ml, where $D(0)$ is the inoculum vRNA (Ma et al., 2009), and $V(0)$ and $X_D(0)$ vary.

We assume that the free virus infectivity rate $\beta(> \beta_1)$ ml per day per virion, antibody carrying capacity K molecules per ml, and antibody independent expansion rate r per day are unknown and we estimate them through data fitting. All fixed parameters and initial conditions are presented in **Table 1**.

Data Fitting

We estimate parameters β and r by simultaneously fitting $V_T(t) = V(t) + X_D(t) + X_R(t)$ given by model (4) with known total virus initial conditions to both chronic and no-infection virus data. Two monkeys (35036 and 33815) were protected when challenged with 2 ramp-up vRNA and chronically infected when challenged with 20 ramp-up vRNA. We use these to get initial concentrations of $V_T(0) = 2/300$ and $V_T(0) = 20/300$ copies per ml, respectively. When a monkey is protected, no vRNA data is collected. We create an artificial data set $VTiter_{low} = \{2/300, 1/300\}$ copies per ml at times $\tau_j \in \{0, 30\}$ days in each animal that did not get infected. When a monkey gets infected, total virus concentrations $VTiter_{high}(t_i)$ above the limit of detection were collected at $t_i \in \{2, 5, 7, 9, 12, 14, 21, 28\}$ days post infection for each subject.

Similarly, three monkeys (33952, 34846, and 34373) were protected when challenged with 1.5, 15, and 150 set-point vRNA and chronically infected when challenged with 1500 set-point vRNA. We therefore use initial concentrations $V_T(0) = 150/300$ and $V_T(0) = 1{,}500/300$ copies per ml for $V_T(0)$ in model (4). When a monkey is protected, no vRNA data is collected. We create an artificial data set $VTiter_{low} = \{150/300, 1/300\}$ copies per ml at times $\tau_j \in \{0, 30\}$ days in each animal that did not get infected. When a monkey gets infected, total virus concentrations $VTiter_{high}(t_i)$ above the limit of detection were collected at $t_i \in \{5, 7, 9, 12, 14, 21, 28\}$ days post infection for subjects 33952 and 34373, and $t_i \in \bar{t} = \{14, 21, 28\}$ days post infection for subject 34846.

[1] IgG Human ELISA Kit ab100547. http://www.abcam.com/IgG-Human-ELISA-Kit-ab100547.html.

TABLE 1 | Parameter values and initial conditions used in model (4).

Variables	Description	Initial values
T	Target cells (cells ml^{-1})	$T(0) = 10^6$
I	Infected cells (cells ml^{-1})	$I(0) = 0$
V	Free virus (virion ml^{-1})	$V(0)$ varies
A_D	Donor antibody (molecules ml^{-1})	$A_D(0)$ varies
A_R	Recipient antibody (molecules ml^{-1})	$A_H(0) = 3.5 \times 10^8$
X_D	Donor immune complexes (complexes ml^{-1})	$H_D(0)$ varies
X_R	Recipient immune complexes (complexes ml^{-1})	$H_X(0) = 0$
Parameters	**Description**	**Values**
s	CD4 T cell production rate (cells ml-day^{-1})	10^4
d	Target CD4 T cells death rate (day^{-1})	0.01
β	Free virus infectivity rate (ml day-virion^{-1})	estimated
β_1	Immune complexes infectivity rate (ml day-virion^{-1})	10^{-8}
δ	Infected cells death rate (day^{-1})	0.39
N	Burst size (virion)	2000
c	Virus clearance rate (day^{-1})	23
α	Antigen dependent expansion of antibodies (ml day-virion^{-1})	10^{-9}
r	Antibody division rate (day^{-1})	estimated
d_A	Antibody degradation rate(day^{-1})	0.07
K	Antibody carrying capacity (molecules ml^{-1})	5×10^{13}
k_p	Binding rate (ml day-virion^{-1})	1.6×10^{-11}
k_m	Unbinding rate (day^{-1})	100
c_{AV}	Immune complexes clearance rate (complexes day^{-1})	10^6
M	Immune complexes where clearance is half maximal (ml^{-1})	500

We use the "fminsearch" algorithm in MATLAB R2016b [The MathWorks Inc., Natick, MA] to minimize the functional

$$J(\beta, K, r) = \left(\sum_{i=1}^{n} \left(\log V_T(t_i) - \log VTiter_{high}(t_i)\right)^2 + \sum_{j=1}^{2} \left(\log V_T(\tau_j) - \log VTiter_{low}(\tau_j)\right)^2 \right)^{1/2}, \quad (5)$$

where n is the number of data points. Finally, $V_T(t_i)$ and $V_T(\tau_j)$ are the theoretical predictions for the total viral concentration as given by model (4) at times t_i and τ_j.

RESULTS

Antibody-Dependent Basic Reproduction Number

The model exhibits bistable switch between a clearance state $S_0 = (s/d, 0, 0, K, 0, 0, 0)$ and a positive chronic state $S_1 = (T_1, I_1, V_1, A_{R1}, X_{R1}, 0, 0)$. We can show analytically that steady state S_0 is locally asymptotically stable when $R_0^a < 1$ (see Supplementary Material), where

$$R_0^a = R_0 \frac{k_m + \frac{c_{AV}}{M} + \frac{\beta_1}{\beta} k_p K}{k_m + \frac{c_{AV}}{M} + \frac{c_{AV}}{cM} k_p K} < 1. \quad (6)$$

Inequality (6) shows that even if viremia occurs in the absence of antibodies, $R_0 = \frac{N\beta s}{dc} > 1$, viral clearance can be reached when the combined contribution of the protective and/or infused antibodies make $R_0^a < 1$. We name R_0^a, the antibody-dependent basic reproduction number, which represents the number of virion produced in average by an infected cell in an otherwise infection-free population throughout its lifetime when antibodies are present.

$R_0^a < 1$ is a necessary but not sufficient condition for virus clearance. Indeed, numerical results show that for $R_0^a < 1$, the chronic state S_1 is asymptotically stable as well. That means that given $R_0^a < 1$ and appropriate initial conditions the chronic steady state S_1 can be reached. We numerically investigate the relationship between the model's initial conditions, animal data and the model's long-term behavior.

Infection With Ramp-Up-Stage Virus

Animals 35036 and 33815 were challenged with 20 vRNA copies that were titrated from a plasma pool containing virus collected from seven monkeys during the ramp-up-stage of infection (defined as approximately 7 days after challenge). Following challenge they became viremic. In contrast, animal 32970, who was challenged 2 vRNA copies from the same plasma pool, did not develop a persistent infection (Ma et al., 2009). Since immune complexes are detected around 21 days post infection (Tomaras et al., 2008; Liu et al., 2011), we assume that the ramp-up inoculum contains only free virus. Therefore, our initial concentrations are $X_D(0) = 0$ and $V(0) = 20/300$ copies per ml in animals 35036 and 33815; $V(0) = 2/300$ copies per ml in animal 32970. The best estimates for β and r were obtained by minimizing J given by (5) for the above initial conditions (see **Table 2**).

Our model predicts a bistable switch in the virus dynamics between persistence and clearance when the free virus initial concentration changes from 20/300 to 2/300 copies per ml (see **Figure 1**, left panels). For median estimates among the two animals, we predict that for $V(0) = 20/300$ copies per ml, the total virus load increases to a maximum of 2×10^8 copies per ml, before decreasing to equilibrium levels of 9×10^6 copies per ml, three months after infection. By contrast, when $V(0) = 2/300$ copies per ml, the total virus concentration grows to 850 copies per ml four days following infection, before it decays below the limit of detection of 50 vRNA copies per ml.

The antibody populations do not depend of the initial viral inoculum (see **Figure 1**, right panels). They reach maximum carrying capacity 5×10^{13} molecules per ml (0.0125 mg per ml) seven days after infection. When $V(0) = 20/300$ vRNA copies per ml, free virions bind recipient antibodies to form recipient immune complexes which, at equilibrium, exceed the free virus concentration 7.8 times. When $V(0) = 2/300$ copies per ml, immune complexes are formed, but they decay below limit of

TABLE 2 | Parameter estimates and 95% confidence intervals from minimizing the likelihood function J given by (5) for the ramp-up data.

Animal	β (ml day-virion^{-1})	95% CI	r(day^{-1})	95% CI	R_0^a
35036	1.58×10^{-7}	$[1.57 \times 10^{-7}, 1.59 \times 10^{-7}]$	2.32	[2.3, 2.33]	0.42
33815	1.34×10^{-7}	$[1.33 \times 10^{-7}, 1.35 \times 10^{-7}]$	1.95	[1.945, 1.952]	0.35
Median	1.46×10^{-7}	–	2.14	–	–

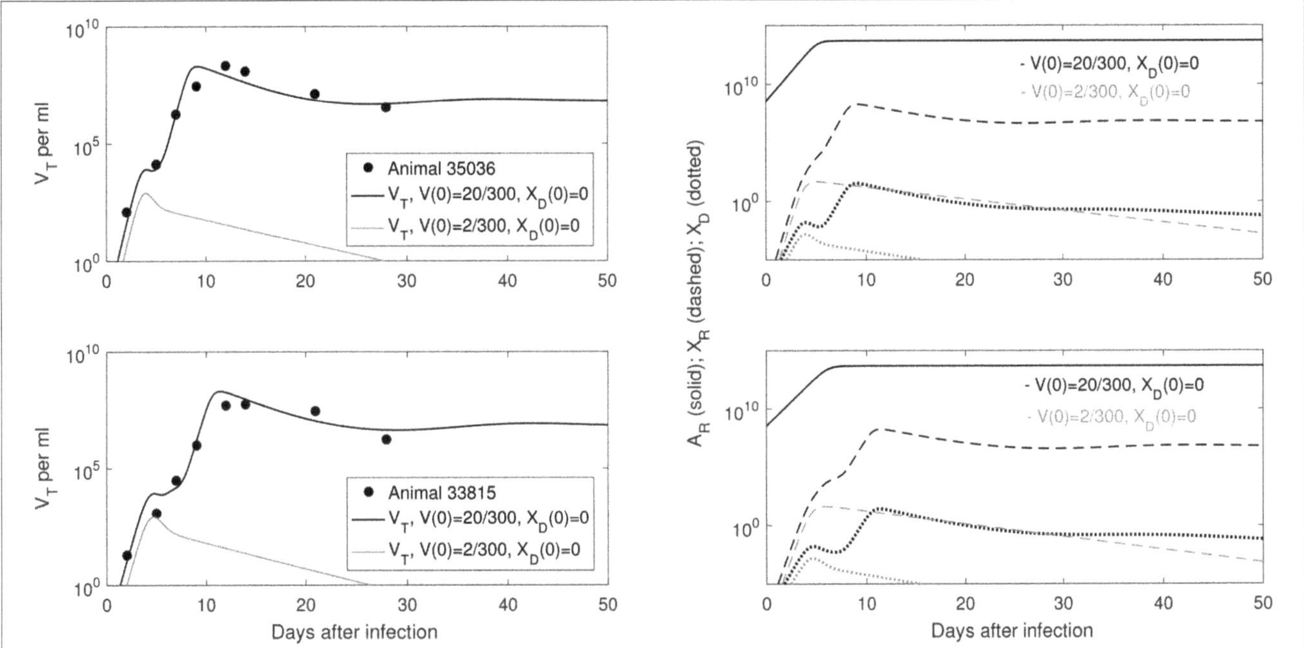

FIGURE 1 | **(Left)** Basin of attraction for V_T given by (4) vs. data; **(Right)** Free antibody (solid lines); recipient immune complexes (dashed lines) and donor immune complexes (dotted lines) for $V(0) = 20/300$ vRNA copies per ml, $X_D(0) = 0$ vRNA copies per ml (black) and $V(0) = 2/300$ vRNA copies per ml, $X_D(0) = 0$ vRNA copies per ml (gray). Note that antibody populations are identical regardless of initial conditions (solid black and gray lines overlap).

detection 7 days after inoculation. Model (4) assumed that B-cell priming by the virus is followed by an antigen-independent antibody expansion with a maximum per capita growth rate r. We estimated a median per capita growth rate $r = 2.14$ per day, corresponding to the doubling time of antibody population of 7.8 h.

We are interested in determining the largest initial virus inoculum that allows for viral clearance under the ramp-up-stage modeling assumptions. For the median r parameter in **Table 2** we derived a bifurcation diagram showing the asymptotic free virus concentrations three months following infection when the infectivity rate β is varied (see Figure S1). The system is displaying hysteresis. For the median infectivity rate β in **Table 2**, we plotted the basins of attractions for the total virus concentration V_T when the inoculum concentration varies (see **Figure 2**, left panel). We predict that V_T is cleared for $V(0) < 17.5/300$ copies per ml and persists otherwise.

Infection With Set-Point-Stage Virus

Animals 33952, 34846, and 34373, were challenged with vRNA copies titrated from a plasma pool containing virus collected during the set-point-stage of infection (defined as the time several months after the peak when plasma vRNA levels were relatively stable, and antibody responses were well developed) of the seven donor monkeys (Ma et al., 2009). The animals were protected when challenged with set-point-stage plasma titrated to contain 1.5, 15, and 150 vRNA and became viremic when challenged with set-point-stage plasma containing 1500 vRNA. We aim to determine the parameter sets for which model (4) predicts a switch between viral persistence for $V(0) + X_D(0) = 1500/300$ copies per ml and clearance for $V(0) + X_D(0) = 150/300$ copies per ml (and consequently for 1.5/300 and 15/300 vRNA copies per ml).

As before, we assume that the donor's antibody concentration is below the limit of detection. However, there are 7.8 times more immune complexes than free virus in the inoculum plasma, $X_D(0)/V(0) = 7.8$, as predicted by the model (4) fitted to ramp-up data and run to equilibrium values. We minimize functional J given by (5) with $X_D(0)/V(0) = 7.8$. The estimated parameters are presented in **Table 3**.

We predict a bistable switch between persistent and cleared virus populations based on initial conditions (see **Figure 3**,

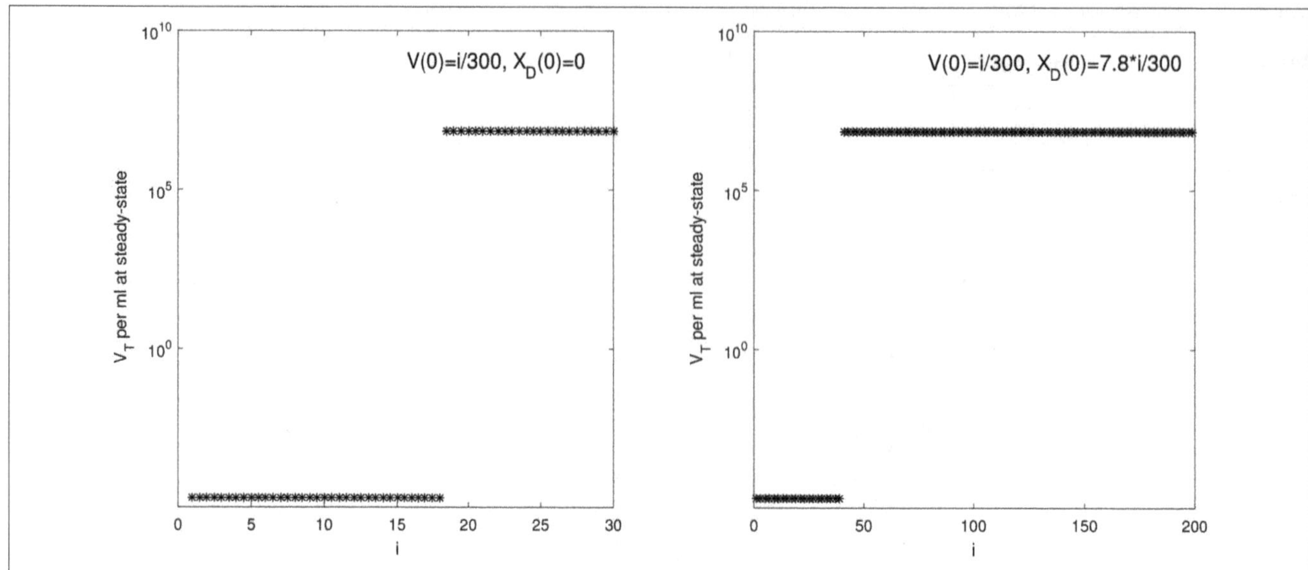

FIGURE 2 | V_T given by (4) at steady state vs. i for: **(Left)** $V(0) = i/300$ vRNA copies per ml, $X_D(0) = 0$ vRNA copies per ml and median parameters in **Table 2**; **(Right)** $V(0) = i/300$ vRNA copies per ml, $X_D(0) = 7.8 \times i/300$ vRNA copies per ml and median parameters in **Table 3**.

TABLE 3 | Parameter estimates and 95% confidence intervals from minimizing the likelihood function J given by (5) for the set-point data.

Animal	β (ml day-virion^{-1})	95% CI	r(day^{-1})	95% CI	R_0^a
33952	9.3×10^{-8}	$[9.23 \times 10^{-8}, 9.33 \times 10^{-8}]$	1.37	[1.369, 1.375], 0.25	
34846	4.09×10^{-8}	$[4.07 \times 10^{-8}, 4.1 \times 10^{-8}]$	0.515	[0.512, 0.518]	0.108
34373	1.07×10^{-7}	$[9.51 \times 10^{-8}, 1.07 \times 10^{-7}]$	1.66	[1.5, 1.8]	0.2673
Median	9.3×10^{-8}	–	1.37	–	–

left panels). The median set-point virus infectivity rate is 1.5 times smaller than the median infectivity rate of the animals infected with the ramp-up-stage plasma. Moreover, the median set-point antibody antigen-dependent growth rate, r is 1.55 times smaller, corresponding to a median antibody population's doubling time of 12 h. We decided to compare median values, rather than averages, since the set-point plasma results are biased by the estimates in animal 34846 whose virus growth is delayed.

We next quantified the largest initial virus inoculum that allows for viral clearance when the initial inoculum is comprised of 7.8 times more immune complexes than free virion. We set all parameters at the median values in **Table 3** and plotted the basins of attractions for the total virus concentration three months following infection as the inoculum concentration varies (see **Figure 2**, right panel). We predict that V_T is cleared when $V_T(0) \leq 42/300$ vRNA copies per ml, $X_D(0)/V(0) = 7.8$ and persists otherwise. We also investigated the relation between viral clearance, $V_T(0)$ and the ratio $X_D(0)/V(0)$. We note that when the ratio between the immune complexes and free virus in the initial plasma is low, even a small inoculum size can create virus persistence. Conversely, when the immune complexes dominate the initial plasma, a large initial virus inoculum is needed to establish an infection (see **Figure 4**).

Infection With a Mix of Heat Inactivated Set-Point-Stage Plasma Mixed With Ramp-Up-Stage Virions

To determine whether antibodies play a role in reducing virus infectivity, Ma et al. designed an aliquot of ramp-up stage plasma containing 20 vRNA/0.5 ml mixed with 0.5 ml of heat inactivated set-point-stage plasma (Ma et al., 2009). The set-point-stage plasma contained antibodies capable of *in vitro* neutralization. They used the aliquot on four animals: 33681, 32350, 32970, and 36068, with the first three animals being protected and the last animal developing persistent infection.

To address this experimental setting we assume the model follows the dynamics given by median parameter values in the ramp-up case with $V(0) = 20/300$ copies per ml and $X_D(0) = 0$ copies per ml (see **Tables 1, 2**). However, we vary $A_D(0)$ to account for donor's antibody being present in the inoculum. We find that a minimum of $A_D(0) = 7.4 \times 10^9$ donor antibody molecules per ml (1.8×10^{-6} mg per ml) are needed for clearance. This value is above the antibody's limit of detection, but more than three orders of magnitude below the antibody's equilibrium values. This suggests that even low antibody levels may help protect the host.

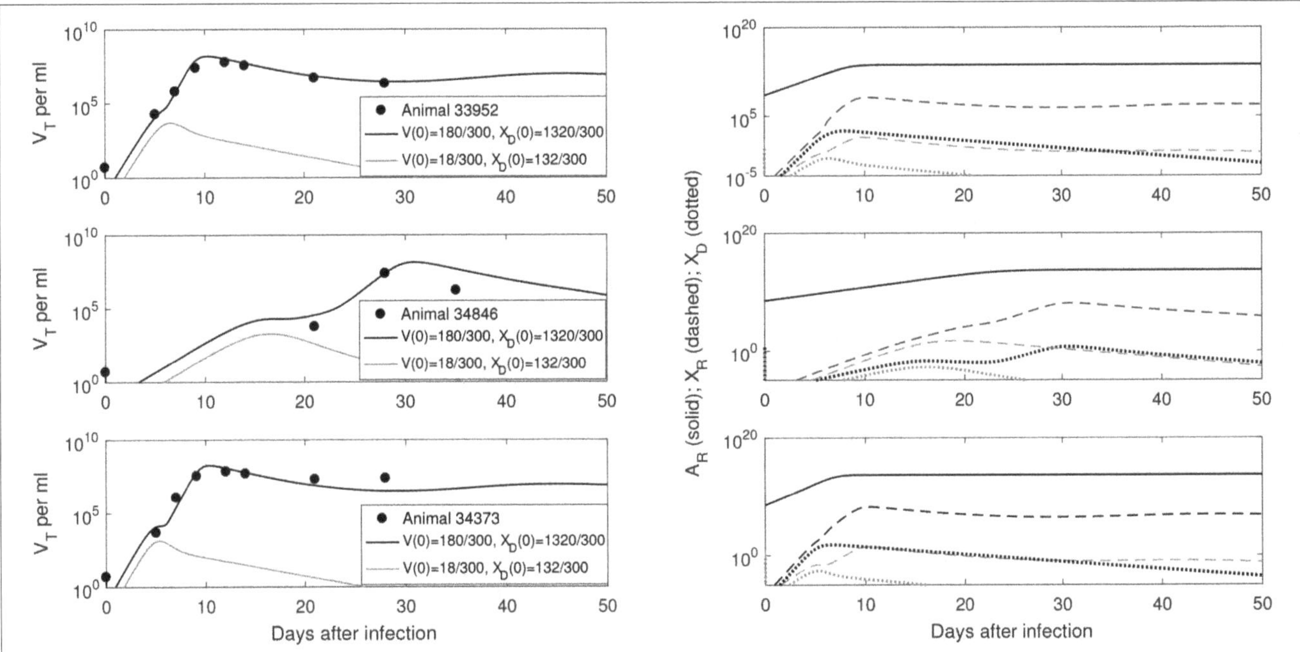

FIGURE 3 | (**Left**) V_T given by (4) vs. data; (**Right**) Free antibody (solid lines), recipient immune complexes (dashed lines) and donor immune complexes (dotted lines): for $V(0) + X_D(0) = 1500/300$ vRNA copies per ml, $X_D(0)/V(0) = 7.8$ (black) and $V(0) + X_D(0) = 150/300$ vRNA copies per ml, $X_D(0)/V(0) = 7.8$ (gray). Note that antibody populations are identical regardless of initial conditions (solid black and gray lines overlap) but the immune complexes differ.

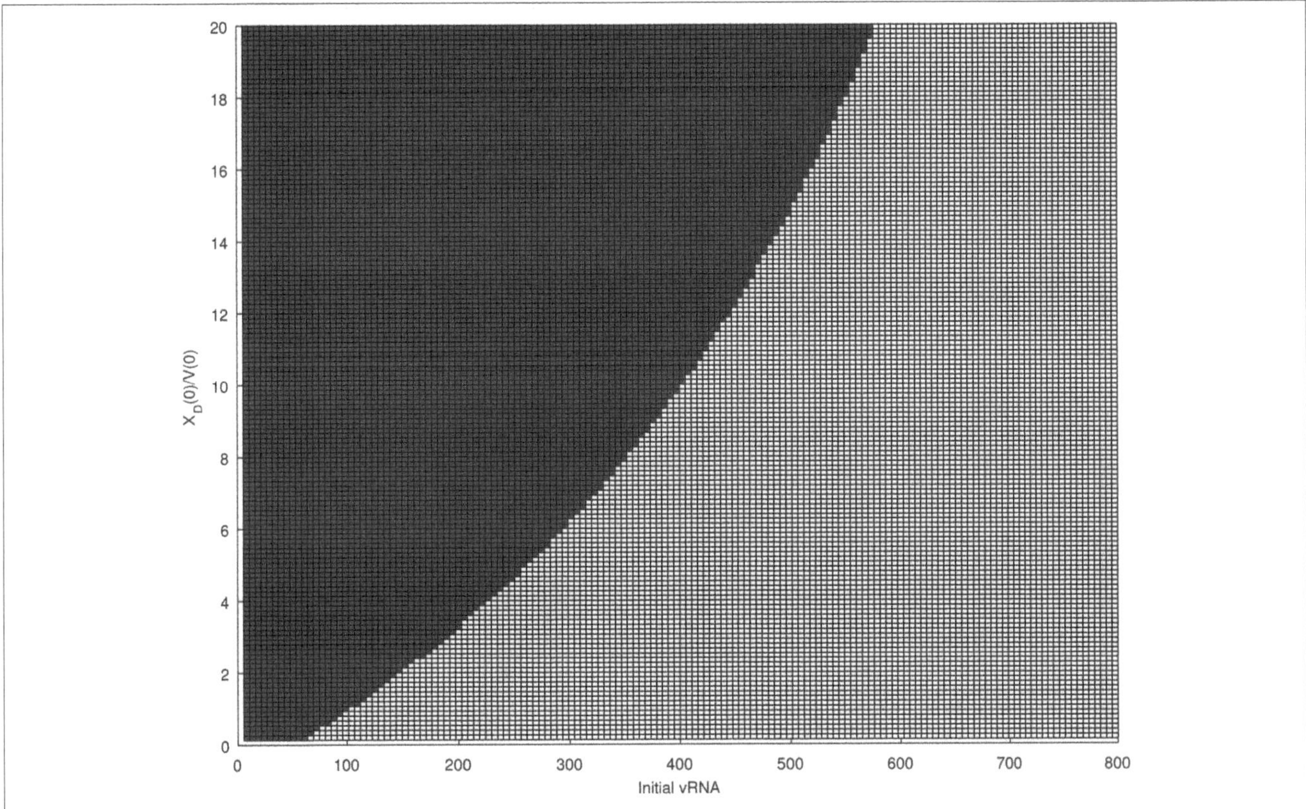

FIGURE 4 | Asymptotic behavior for the V_T solutions of (4) for median parameters in **Table 3** as the initial vRNA and $X_D(0)/V(0)$ are varied. The blue region (left of the curve) corresponds to extinction asymptotic concentrations $V_T = 0$ copies per ml. The yellow region (right of the curve) corresponds to persistence asymptotic concentrations $V_T = 6.9 \times 10^6$ copies per ml.

We want to determine the additional recipient-virus dynamics that lead to infection in animal 36068. We fit V_T given by model (4) with $V(0) = 20/300$ vRNA copies per ml, $X_D(0) = 0$ vRNA copies per ml and $A_D(0) = 7.4 \times 10^9$ molecules per ml to animal 36068's virus data and found that virus persistence is due to the recipient antibody dynamics (see **Figure 5**, right panel). Indeed, for a good fit we need to decrease the recipient's antibody carrying capacity to $K = 5 \times 10^{12}$ molecules per ml, 10 times lower than the previous carrying capacity in ramp-up infected animals. The antigen-independent expansion rate $r = 1.62$ per day is 1.3 times smaller than the median per capita antibody expansion rate in the ramp-up infected animals, but similar to that of set-point infected animals (see **Table 4**). This implies that animal's 36068 immune response is not strong enough to prevent persistent viremia. Moreover, for these antibody parameters bistability does not occur ($R_0^a = 2.26 > 1$), and the virus reaches a positive steady state level regardless of the size and structure of the initial inoculum.

Can Random Infection and Clearance Events Explain the Data?

To address whether the switch in virus dynamics is due to random effects, we use the stochastic model of virus infection and clearance developed in Pearson et al. (2011). Under the parametrization of model (1), the *burst stochastic model* in Pearson et al. (2011), is given by

$$\begin{aligned} V &\xrightarrow{\beta T} I, \\ I &\xrightarrow{\delta} NV, \\ V &\xrightarrow{c} \emptyset. \end{aligned} \tag{7}$$

Let $n = (n_V, n_I)$ be the number of viruses and infected cells starting the SIV infection,

$$\begin{aligned} \rho_V &= \Pr\{\text{Extinction}|n = (1,0)\} \text{ and} \\ \rho_I &= \Pr\{\text{Extinction}|n = (0,1)\}, \end{aligned} \tag{8}$$

be the probabilities of extinction given an infection that is started by one virus or one infected cell. Then the probability of virus persistence given n_V virion and n_I infected cells, $\epsilon = 1 - \rho_V^{nV} \rho_I^{n_I}$, can be computed analytically. Namely

$$\begin{aligned} \rho_V &= \min\{1, \rho_V^*\}, \\ \rho_I &= \min\{1, (\rho_V^*)^N\}, \end{aligned} \tag{9}$$

where ρ_V^* is the positive solution of the equation

$$\gamma(\rho_V)^N - \rho_V + 1 - \gamma = 0. \tag{10}$$

Note that the probability of persistence ϵ is dependent on the burst size N and on the probability that a virus infects a cell, $\gamma = \frac{\beta T}{\beta T + c}$ (see Pearson et al., 2011 for a full derivation). For fixed $N = 300$ virions per infected cell, $T = 10^6$ cells per ml, and $c = 23$ per day, we determine the infectivity values β that can explain the relationship between extinction/persistence and the inoculum size in ramp-up/set-point vRNA cases when free virus establishes the infection, i.e., $n_I = 0$ (see **Figure 6**).

We find that a 99% probability of persistence for a ramp-up-stage inoculum of 20 vRNA occurs when the infectivity rate $\beta > 8 \times 10^{-6}$, while the same persistence probability for a set-point inoculum of 1500 vRNA occurs for $\beta > 1.15 \times 10^{-7}$ (see **Figure 6**, red circles). For these choices of β, the probability of extinction for the lower 2 ramp-up stage and 150 set-point-stage vRNA inoculum are 64% and 65%, respectively (see **Figure 6**,

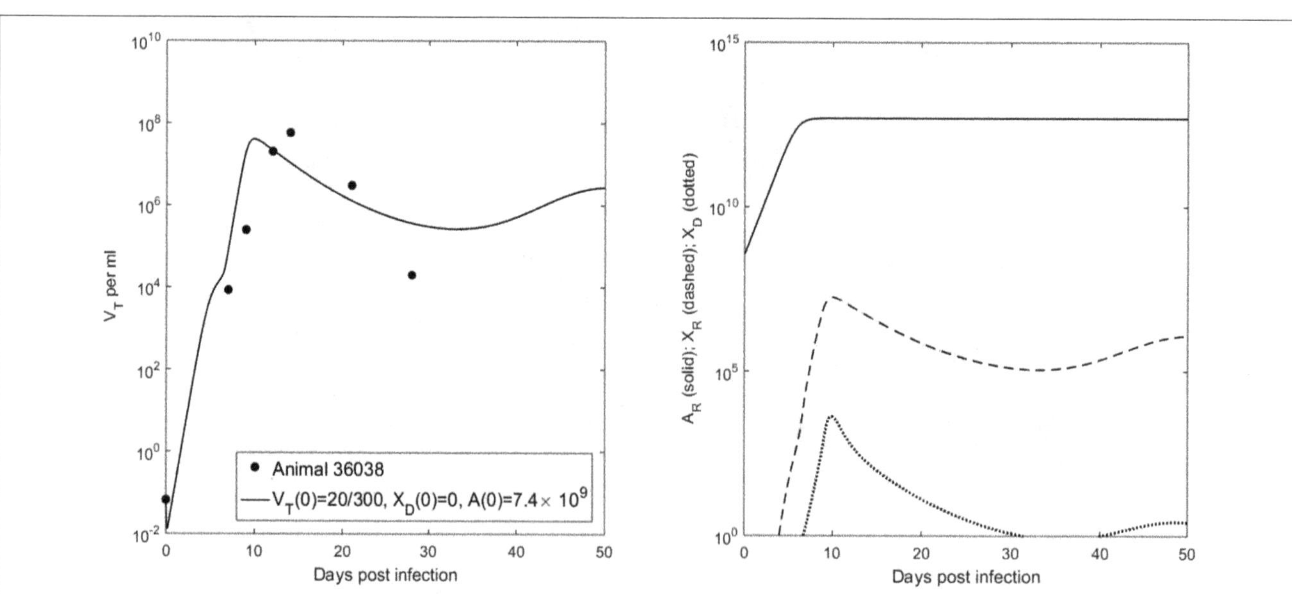

FIGURE 5 | (Left) V_T given by (4) vs. data; **(Right)** Free antibody (solid lines), recipient immune complexes (dashed lines) and donor immune complexes (dotted lines) for $V(0) = 20/300$ vRNA copies per ml, $X_D(0) = 0$ vRNA copies per ml and $A_D(0) = 7.4 \times 10^9$ molecules per ml.

TABLE 4 | Parameter estimates and 95% confidence intervals from fitting V_T to animal data for $V(0) = 20/300$ vRNA copies per ml, $X_D(0) = 0$ vRNA copies per ml and $A_D(0) = 7.4 \times 10^9$ molecules per ml.

Animal	β (ml day-virion^{-1})	95% CI	r(day^{-1})	95% CI	R_0^a
363068	1.11×10^{-7}	$[1.06 \times 10^{-7}, 1.17 \times 10^{-7}]$	1.62	[1.5, 1.74]	2.26

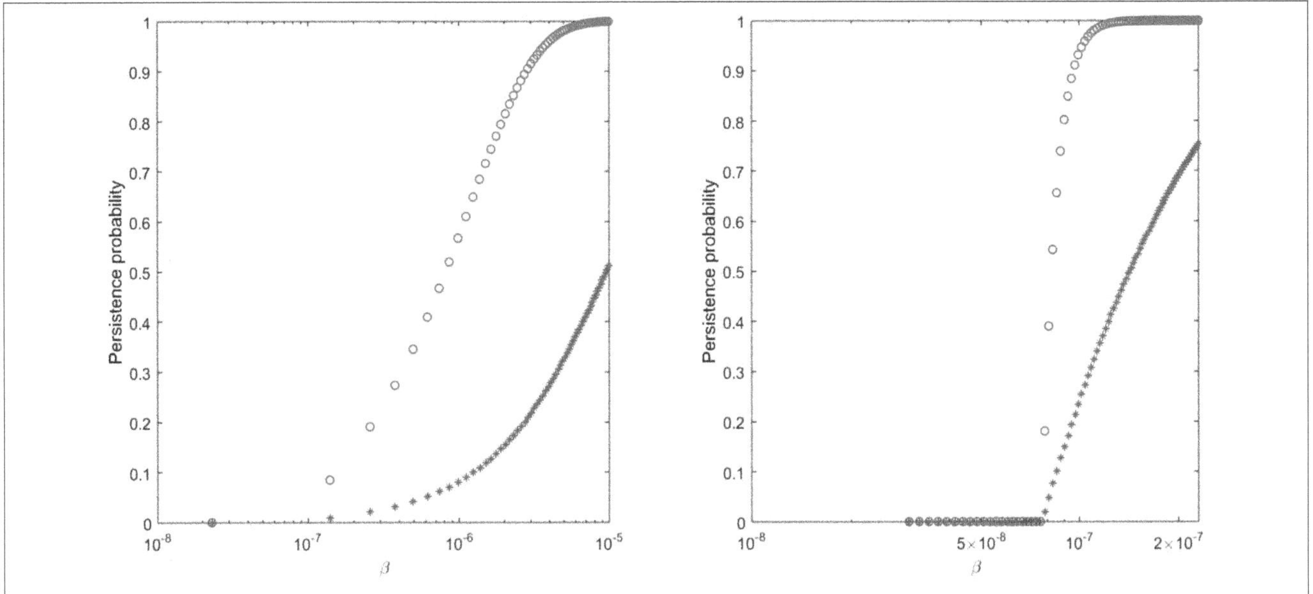

FIGURE 6 | The probability of virus persistence for (**Left**) ramp-up-stage and (**Right**) set-point-stage vRNA data under the assumption of the *burst stochastic model* (7). The red circles account for the probability of persistence for high inocula, while the blue stars account for the probability of persistence for low inocula.

blue stars). In order for the proposed stochastic process to explain the experimental observations, there must be a 70-fold reduction in the infectivity rate β between ramp-up and set-point virus (8.75 times higher than estimated in Vaidya et al., 2010). Moreover, the extinction probability for the lower inocula is lower than ideal. While the stochastic explanation is still conceivable, we conclude that the presence of immune complexes in the inoculum is a compelling alternative explanation for the experimental outcomes.

DISCUSSION

We developed a mathematical model of antibody responses to SIV infection that shows a bistable switch between persistent infection and virus clearance based on the composition of the plasma used for intravenous inoculation.

We made several interesting observations. When the plasma does not contain any free donor antibody, our model predicts that the difference between infection with high inoculum containing set-point-stage virus and infection with low inoculum containing ramp-up-stage virus can be explained by the presence of immune complexes in the inoculum that exceed free virus by a factor of 7.8. Such immune complexes can still infect target CD4 T cells, but have a 10-fold decrease in infectivity. Under these assumptions, the model fits the data when the infectivity of free virus is constant over time. There is a 1.5-fold decrease in the set-point-stage free virus infectivity compared to ramp-up-stage free virus infectivity, as reported in earlier studies (Ma et al., 2009; Vaidya et al., 2010). Such decrease may be due to temporal accumulation of non-infectious particles and to the emergence of other immune factors such as CD8 T cell responses.

When the inoculum plasma contains neutralizing antibody, our model predicts that infection is blocked even when free virus infectivity rates are as high as in the ramp-up stage. In order for virus to invade, antibody responses need to be 10 times lower at equilibrium. Moreover, their growth needs 1.3-fold reduction.

We assumed that the recipient and donor antibody have high avidity of 10^8 M^{-1} (as with infusion of broadly neutralizing antibody), a high antibody carrying capacity $K = 5 \times 10^{13}$ molecules per ml and estimated the recipient antibody expansion rate needed for protection. With our model, however, it is difficult to separate out the effects of changing the avidity rate $K_A = k_p/k_m$ and changing the antibody carrying capacity K. For example we can preserve the results by decreasing avidity and increasing the carrying capacity. Similarly, the antibody antigen-dependent and antigen-independent growth factors, r and α, have synergistic effects. If we decrease r we can maintain the overall virus-antibody dynamics by increasing α (as detailed in the sensitivity Figure S2).

We have also assumed that the immune complexes infect at rate $\beta_1 = 0.1 \times \beta$ ml per day per virion. This was an arbitrary choice, and the estimated infectivity rate β may change when the β to β_1 ratio is varied.

An important variable in our study is the basic reproduction number R_0^a, which has to remain below one for viral clearance. However, even when $R_0^a < 1$, a persistent infection can still occur when either inoculum is composed of mostly free virion, free virus infectivity rate is high, and/or equilibrium antibody levels are low. The presence of bistable switch allows us to alter the infection outcome in the model by changing the initial antibody levels. Knowing the minimum antibody concentration needed to prevent viremia under fixed parameter setting is important for guiding vaccine design.

To address whether stochastic effects alone can explain the data, we computed the probability of virus persistence under the assumption of a *burst stochastic* model developed in Pearson et al. (2011). We find that a 70-fold decrease in virus infectivity rate β is needed between the ramp-up and set-point-inoculum in order to obtain a 99% probability of persistence for a ramp-up inoculum of 20 vRNA and a set-point inoculum of 1500 vRNA occurs. This is higher than the 8-fold decrease reported in Vaidya et al. (2010). Furthermore, the extinction probabilities for the lower ramp-up inoculum of 2 vRNA and a set-point inoculum of 150 vRNA, 64% and 65%, are lower than ideal. While the stochastic explanation is still conceivable, we conclude that the presence of immune complexes in the inoculum is a possible alternative explanation for the experimental outcome.

Our study uses data from an intravenous inoculation experiment. It is not clear if a similar relationship exist with mucosal virus inoculation or with non-neutralizing antibody responses. In fact, some antibody responses were associated with enhanced risk of heterosexual HIV acquisition in RV144. Further, immune-complexed virus may be preferentially transported across epithelial surfaces by the neonatal Fc receptor (Haynes, 2012; Gorlani and Forthal, 2013; Gupta et al., 2013, 2015). Our analysis focused only on the role of antibody in infectivity after any epithelial barriers had been crossed.

In summary, we have developed a model of virus-host dynamics during SIV infection that gives insight into the relation between the structure of infecting inoculum, virus infectivity and disease outcomes. In particular, we showed that a large set-point-stage inoculum is needed for persistent infection due to the excess of immune complexes over the free virus. Moreover, we have estimated the antibody levels and the free virus infectivity and their relation to the disease outcome when the inoculum size and structure are well understood. Such predictions are important for vaccine design.

AUTHOR SUMMARY

We investigate whether antiviral factors can explain the change in virus infectivity during acute and chronic stages of simian immunodeficiency virus infections. Our hypothesis is that acute plasma contains mostly free virus while chronic plasma contains antibody-virus immune complexes in addition to free virus. If such immune complexes can still infect, then their infectivity rate is reduced compared to that of the free virus. We test this hypothesis by developing a mathematical model of antibody-virus dynamics that assumes interactions between virus, recipient and donor antibodies, and the corresponding immune complexes. We fit the model to published viral load data from recipient rhesus macaques challenged intravenously with different virus loads collected during donor's acute and chronic stages of SIV infection. The fits give us parameter estimates for long-run antibody concentration, free virus infectivity rate, and the relation between protection and the free virus—immune complexes ratio in the inoculum.

AUTHOR CONTRIBUTIONS

SC and JF designed the study and performed numerical experiments. CM provided the data. SC, CM, and JF wrote the paper.

ACKNOWLEDGMENTS

SC acknowledges support from NSF grants DMS-1214582, DMS-1813011, Simons Foundation grant 427115 and VT's OASF. CM was supported by Public Health Services grants U51RR00169, from the National Center for Research Resources; and P01 AI066314 from the National Institute of Allergy and Infectious Diseases. We are grateful to Dr Honghu Li for valuable discussions.

REFERENCES

Bonhoeffer, S., May, R., Shaw, G., and Nowak, M. (1997). Virus dynamics and drug therapy. *Proc. Natl. Acad. Sci. U.S.A.* 94, 6971–6976. doi: 10.1073/pnas.94.13.6971

Ciupe, S. (2015). Mathematical model of multivalent virus-antibody complex formation in humans following acute and chronic HIV infections. *J. Math. Biol.* 71, 513–532. doi: 10.1007/s00285-014-0826-3

Deal, C., and Balazs, A. (2015). Engineering humoral immunity as prophylaxis or therapy. *Curr. Opin. Immunol.* 35, 113–122. doi: 10.1016/j.coi.2015.06.014

Gopalakrishnan, P., and Karush, F. (1975). Antibody affinity. VIII. measurement of affinity of anti-lactose antibody by fluorescence quenching with a DNP-containing ligand. *J. Immunol.* 114, 1359–1362.

Gorlani, A., and Forthal, D. (2013). Antibody-dependent enhancement and the risk of HIV infection. *Curr. HIV Res.* 11, 421–426. doi: 10.2174/1570162X113116660062

Gray, E., Madiga, M., Hermanus, T., Moore, P., Wibmer, C., Tumba, N., et al. (2011). The neutralization breadth of HIV-1 develops incrementally over four years and is associated with CD4+ T cell decline and high viral load during acute infection. *J. Virol.* 85, 4828–4840. doi: 10.1128/JVI.00198-11

Gupta, S., Gach, J., Becerra, J., Phan, T., Pudney, J., Moldoveanu, Z., et al. (2013). The Neonatal Fc receptor (FcRn) enhances human immunodeficiency virus type 1 (HIV-1) trancytosis across epithelial cells. *PLoS Pathog.* 9:e1003776. doi: 10.1371/journal.ppat.1003776

Gupta, S., Pegu, P., Venzon, D., Gach, J., Ma, Z., Landucci, G., et al. (2015). Enhanced *in vitro* transcytosis of simian immunodeficiency virus mediated by vaccine-induced antibody predicts transmitted/founder strain number after rectal challenge. *J. Infect Dis.* 211, 45–52. doi: 10.1093/infdis/jiu300

Haynes, B. (2012). Immune-correlates analysis of an HIV-1 vaccine efficacy trial. *N. Engl. J. Med.* 366, 1275–1286. doi: 10.1056/NEJMoa1113425

Haynes, B. (2015). New approaches to HIV vaccine development. *Curr. Opin. Immunol.* 35, 39–47. doi: 10.1016/j.coi.2015.05.007

Letvin, N., Rao, S., Montefiori, D., Seaman, M., Sun, Y., Lim, S.-Y., et al. (2011). Immune and genetic correlates of vaccine protection against mucosal infection by SIV in monkeys. *Sci. Transl. Med.* 3:81ra36. doi: 10.1126/scitranslmed.3002351

Liu, P., Overman, R., Yates, N., Alam, S., Vandergrift, N., Chen, Y., et al. (2011). Dynamic antibody specificities and virion concentrations in circulating immune complexes in acute to chronic HIV-1 infection. *J. Virol.* 85, 11196–11207. doi: 10.1128/JVI.05601-11

Ma, Z., Stone, M., Piatak, M., Schweighardt, B., Haigwood, N., Montefiori, D., et al. (2009). High specific infectivity of plasma virus from the pre-ramp-up and ramp-up stages of acute simian immunodeficiency virus infection. *J. Virol.* 83, 3288–3297. doi: 10.1128/JVI.02423-08

Markowitz, M., Louie, M., Hurley, A., Sun, E., Di Mascio, M., Perelson, A., et al. (2003). A novel antiviral intervention results in more accurate assessment of human immunodeficiency virus type 1 replication dynamics and T-cell decay *in vivo*. *J. Virol.* 77, 5037–5038. doi: 10.1128/JVI.77.8.5037-5038.2003

Mascola, J., and Haynes, B. (2013). HIV-1 neutralizing antibodies: understanding nature's pathways. *Immunol. Rev.* 254, 225–244. doi: 10.1111/imr.12075

Mascola, J., Lewis, M., Stiegler, G., Harris, D., VanCott, T., Hayes, D., et al. (1999). Protection of macaques against pathogenic simian/human immunodeficiency virus 89.6PD by passive transfer of neutralizing antibodies. *J. Virol.* 73, 4009–4018.

Moldt, B., Rakasz, E., Schultz, N., Chan-Hui, P.-Y., Swiderek, K., Weisgrau, K., et al. (2012). Highly potent HIV-specific antibody neutralization *in vitro* translates into effective protection against mucosal SHIV challenge *in vivo*. *Proc. Natl. Acad. Sci. U.S.A.* 109, 18921–18925. doi: 10.1073/pnas.1214785109

Nishimura, Y., Igarashi, T., Haigwood, N., Sadjadpour, R., Donau, O., Buckler, C., et al. (2003). Transfer of neutralizing IgG to macaques 6 h but not 24 h after SHIV infection confers sterilizing protection: Implications for HIV-1 vaccine development. *Proc. Natl. Acad. Sci. U.S.A.* 100, 15131–15136. doi: 10.1073/pnas.2436476100

Pearson, J., Krapivsky, P., and Perelson, A. (2011). Stochastic theory of early viral infection: continuous versus burst production of virions. *PLoS Comput. Biol.* 7, 1–17. doi: 10.1371/journal.pcbi.1001058

Perelson, A., Neumann, A., Markowitz, M., Leonard, J., and Ho, D. (1996). HIV-1 dynamics *in vivo*: Virion clearance rate, infected cell life-span, and viral generation time. *Science* 271, 1582–1586. doi: 10.1126/science.271.5255.1582

Plotkin, S. (2008). Vaccines: correlates of vaccine-induced immunity. *Clin. Infect. Dis.* 47, 401–409. doi: 10.1086/589862

Pollara, J., Bonsignori, M., Moody, M., Liu, P., Alam, S., Hwang, K.-K., et al. (2014). HIV-1 vaccine-induced C1 and V2 env-specific antibodies synergize for increased antiviral activities. *J. Virol.* 88, 7715–7726. doi: 10.1128/JVI.00156-14

Ramratnam, B., Bonhoeffer, S., Binley, J., Hurley, A., Zhang, L., Mittler, J., et al. (1999). Rapid production and clearance of HIV-1 and hepatitis C virus assessed by large volume plasma apheresis. *Lancet* 354, 1782–1785. doi: 10.1016/S0140-6736(99)02035-8

Rerks-Ngarm, S., Pitisuttithum, P., Nitayaphan, S., Kaewkungwal, J., Chiu, J., Paris, R., et al. (2009). Vaccination with ALVAC and AIDSVAX to prevent HIV-1 infection in Thailand. *New Eng. J. Med.* 361, 2209–2220. doi: 10.1056/NEJMoa0908492

Sachsenberg, N., Perelson, A., Yerly, S., Schockmel, G., Leduc, D., Hirschel, B., and Perrin, L. (1998). Turnover of CD4 and CD8 T lymphocytes in HIV-1 infection as measured by Ki-67 antigen. *J. Exp. Med.* 187, 1295–1303. doi: 10.1084/jem.187.8.1295

Schwesinger, F., Ros, R., Strunz, T., Anselmetti, D., Guntherodt, H.-J., Honegger, A., et al. (2000). Unbinding forces of single antibody-antigen complexes correlate with their thermal dissociation rates. *Proc. Natl. Acad. Sci. U.S.A.* 97, 9972–9977. doi: 10.1073/pnas.97.18.9972

Stafford, M., Corey, L., Cap, Y., Daar, E., Ho, D., and Perelson, A. (2000). Modeling plasma virus concentration during primary HIV infection. *J. Theor. Biol.* 203, 285–301. doi: 10.1006/jtbi.2000.1076

Tabei, S., Li, Y., Weigert, M., and Dinner, A. (2012). Model for competition from self during passive immunization, with application to broadly neutralizing antibodies for HIV. *Vaccine* 30, 607–613. doi: 10.1016/j.vaccine.2011.11.048

Tomaras, G., Binley, J., Gray, E., Crooks, E., Osawa, K., Moore, P., et al. (2011). Polyclonal B cell responses to conserved neutralization epitopes in a subset of HIV-1-infected individuals. *J. Virol.* 85, 11502–11519. doi: 10.1128/JVI.05363-11

Tomaras, G., Ferrari, G., Shen, X., Alam, S., Liao, H.-X., Pollara, J., et al. (2013). Vaccine-induced plasma IgA specific for the C1 region of the HIV-1 envelope blocks binding and effector function of IgG. *Proc. Natl. Acad. Sci. U.S.A.* 110, 9019–9024. doi: 10.1073/pnas.1301456110

Tomaras, G., Yates, N., Liu, P., Qin, L., Fouda, G., Chavez, L., et al. (2008). Initial B-cell responses to transmitted human immunodeficiency virus type 1: virion-binding immunoglobulin IgM and IgG antibodies followed by plasma anti-gp41 antibodies with ineffective control of initial viremia. *J. Virol.* 82, 12449–12463. doi: 10.1128/JVI.01708-08

Vaidya, N., Ribeiro, R., Miller, C., and Perelson, A. (2010). Viral dynamics during primary simian immunodeficiency virus infection: effect of time-dependent virus infectivity. *J. Virol.* 84, 4302–4310. doi: 10.1128/JVI.02284-09

Walker, L., Huber, M., Doores, K., Falkowska, E., Pejchal, R., Julien, J.-P., et al. (2011). Broad neutralization coverage of HIV by multiple highly potent antibodies. *Nature* 477, 466–470. doi: 10.1038/nature10373

Zalevsky, J., Chamberlain, A., Horton, H., Karki, S., Leung, I., Sproule, T., et al. (2010). Enhanced antibody half-life improves *in vivo* activity. *Nat. Biotechnol.* 28, 157–159. doi: 10.1038/nbt.1601

Zhou, T., Xu, L., Dey, B., Hessell, A., Van Ryk, D., Xiang, S.-H., et al. (2007). Structural definition of a conserved neutralization epitope on HIV-1 gp120. *Nature* 445, 732–737. doi: 10.1038/nature05580

6

Examining the Reticulocyte Preference of Two *Plasmodium berghei* Strains During Blood-Stage Malaria Infection

Neha Thakre [1‡], ***Priyanka Fernandes*** [2†‡], ***Ann-Kristin Mueller*** [2,3*] ***and Frederik Graw*** [1*]

[1] Centre for Modeling and Simulation in the Biosciences, BioQuant-Center, Heidelberg University, Heidelberg, Germany, [2] Parasitology Unit, Centre for Infectious Diseases, University Hospital, Heidelberg, Germany, [3] German Center for Infectious Diseases (DZIF), Heidelberg, Germany

***Correspondence:**
Ann-Kristin Mueller
ann-kristin.mueller@uni-heidelberg.de
Frederik Graw
frederik.graw@bioquant.uni-heidelberg.de

† Present Address:
Priyanka Fernandes, CIMI-Paris, National Institute for Health and Medical Research U1135, Faculté de Médecine Pierre et Marie Curie, Site Pitié Salpêtrière 5éme ètage, Paris, France

‡ These authors have contributed equally to this work.

The blood-stage of the *Plasmodium* parasite is one of the key phases within its life cycle that influences disease progression during a malaria infection. The efficiency of the parasite in infecting red blood cells (RBC) determines parasite load and parasite-induced hemolysis that is responsible for the development of anemia and potentially drives severe disease progression. However, the molecular factors defining the infectivity of *Plasmodium* parasites have not been completely identified so far. Using the *Plasmodium berghei* mouse model for malaria, we characterized and compared the blood-stage infection dynamics of *Pb*ANKA WT and a mutant parasite strain lacking a novel *Plasmodium* antigen, *Pb*maLS_05, that is well conserved in both human and animal *Plasmodium* parasite strains. Infection of mice with parasites lacking *PbmaLS_05* leads to lower parasitemia levels and less severe disease progression in contrast to mice infected with the wildtype *Pb*ANKA strain. To specifically determine the effect of deleting *PbmaLS_05* on parasite infectivity we developed a mathematical model describing erythropoiesis and malarial infection of RBC. By applying our model to experimental data studying infection dynamics under normal and drug-induced altered erythropoietic conditions, we found that both *Pb*ANKA and *PbmaLS_05* (-) parasite strains differed in their infectivity potential during the early intra-erythrocytic stage of infection. Parasites lacking *PbmaLS_05* showed a decreased ability to infect RBC, and immature reticulocytes in particular that are usually a preferential target of the parasite. These altered infectivity characteristics limit parasite burden and affect disease progression. Our integrative analysis combining mathematical models and experimental data suggests that deletion of *PbmaLS_05* affects productive infection of reticulocytes, which makes this antigen a useful target to analyze the actual processes relating RBC preferences to the development of severe disease outcomes in malaria.

Keywords: Malaria, *Plasmodium*, mathematical modeling, infection dynamics, parasite infectivity, erythropoiesis

INTRODUCTION

Malaria caused by the *Plasmodium* parasite is one of the most serious tropical diseases with a major impact on global health. In 2015, malaria was responsible for 212 million clinical cases and an estimated number of 429,000 deaths worldwide (World Health Organization, 2016).

Within the host, *Plasmodium* parasites follow a complex life cycle involving parasite replication and differentiation in liver and blood (Portugal et al., 2011). Disease progression is mainly associated with the blood-stage of the parasite, as parasite-induced infection and lysis of red blood cells (RBC) leads to the development of anemia (Dondorp et al., 1999), one of the main symptoms characterizing a malaria infection.

Many *Plasmodium* parasite strains have been found to differ in their infectivity during the blood-stage infection phase by targeting RBC of different ages (McQueen and McKenzie, 2004). Several parasite species express a preference for immature RBC (reticulocytes) compared to mature RBC (erythrocytes/normocytes). Estimates indicate a 34- to 180-fold higher preference in *Plasmodium vivax* (Mons et al., 1988; Mons, 1990) and a 1.6- to 14-fold preference in *Plasmodium falciparum* in humans (Wilson et al., 1977; Pasvol et al., 1980; Clough et al., 1998), with the latter one being responsible for cerebral malaria, a severe neuropathy resulting in death or severe neurological sequelae in survivors (Seydel et al., 2015; Gupta et al., 2017). In rodents, strains of *Plasmodium chabaudi* show such age-specific targeting of RBC during the acute infection phase (Antia et al., 2008), while *Plasmodium berghei* (Singer et al., 1955; McNally et al., 1992; Sexton et al., 2004; Cromer et al., 2006, 2009) has an estimated $\sim$150-fold preference for reticulocytes during the late stages of infection (Cromer et al., 2006). It has been suggested that high reticulocyte preference is responsible for the highest parasite densities which in turn induce severe anemia (McQueen and McKenzie, 2004), i.e., with anemia-induced production of novel reticulocytes conversely fueling parasite replication. However, which factors govern and influence the infectivity of parasites and to which extent elevated parasite densities might also influence faster disease progression have not been determined so far (Beeson et al., 2016).

In this context, *Pb*maLS_05 was identified as a novel *Plasmodium* antigen that plays an important role in the development of experimental cerebral malaria (ECM) (Fernandes et al., submitted manuscript), a neuropathology that is characteristically similar to human cerebral malaria (de Souza et al., 2010; Hoffmann et al., 2016). The gene is well conserved in human and rodent *Plasmodium* strains and as it is expressed during both late intra-hepatic and intra-erythrocytic stages of the parasite, this cross-stage antigen represents a potential vaccine target. The protein localizes to the apicoplast organelle—an endosymbiotic relict of the parasite that is important for intra-erythrocytic survival. Deletion of *PbmaLS_05* was suggested to influence parasite replication or viability in the blood (Fernandes et al., submitted manuscript), but the effects on infectivity and potential cell preferences are not known.

Determining a parasite's infectivity potential during the intra-erythrocytic stage requires the disentangling of parasite replication dynamics and infection-induced changes to erythropoiesis. Mathematical modeling has been an essential tool to analyze these processes. In addition to detecting target cell preferences and differences in infection profiles of various pathogens, mathematical models allow us to specifically account for the processes of erythropoiesis, parasite infection and turnover, as well as disease-induced anemia (McQueen and McKenzie, 2004; Cromer et al., 2006, 2009; Antia et al., 2008; Fonseca and Voit, 2015). There have been various modeling approaches describing the blood-stage infection dynamics of different *Plasmodium* parasite strains in various levels of detail (Antia et al., 2008; Mideo et al., 2008; Cromer et al., 2009; Li et al., 2011).

In this study, we used a combination of different experimental protocols and mathematical models to investigate parasite blood-stage infection dynamics under physiological and drug-induced altered erythropoietic conditions to elucidate the effects of deletion of *PbmaLS_05* (KO) on parasite infectivity. We concentrated on the acute phase of infection, analyzing the first 4 days after infection with parasitized RBC until the time when mice infected by the *Pb*ANKA (WT) strain showed first signs of ECM. Our age-structured model explicitly accounts for RBC development and erythropoiesis and is thereby able to determine possible target cell preferences for both parasite strains. Our results indicate dynamic malaria-induced changes to erythropoiesis during disease progression and suggest that deletion of *Pb*maLS_05 has an effect on the productive infection of reticulocytes.

MATERIALS AND METHODS

Ethics Statement

All animal experiments were performed according to European regulations concerning FELASA category B and GV-SOLAS standard guidelines. Animal experiments were approved by German authorities (Regierungspräsidium Karlsruhe, Germany), § 8 Abs. 1 Tierschutzgesetz (TierSchG) under the license G-260/12 and were performed according to National and European regulations. For all experiments, female C57BL/6 mice (6- to 8-week-old) were purchased from Janvier laboratories, France. All mice were kept under specified pathogen-free (SPF) conditions within the animal facility at Heidelberg University (IBF).

Experimental Protocol and Data

In the first set of experiments, C57BL/6 mice were intravenously infected with 10^6 infected red blood cells (iRBC) taken from mice infected either with wild-type *Pb*GFP Luc_{con} (*P. berghei* line 676m1cl1) (WT), a GFP-luciferase transgenic derivative of *P. berghei* ANKA (Franke-Fayard et al., 2005), or the mutant *PbmaLS_05* (–) parasites (KO) generated in the wild-type *Pb*GFP Luc_{con} strain (Fernandes et al., submitted manuscript). An additional group of age-matched mice was left uninfected and treated as naïve controls. Daily blood samples of 10 μl were taken from all mice from the day of infection until day 4 post infection (p.i.). The total red blood cell count and reticulocyte percentage were measured using a Coulter counter and FACS analysis of CD71 (CD71-PE, eBioscience, Clone R17217) labeled reticulocytes, respectively. Parasitemia was determined by FACS analysis of GFP positive infected red blood cells. A sketch of the experimental protocol is shown in **Figure 1A**. Mice were sacrificed at day 5 p.i., when mice infected with WT parasites showed first symptoms of ECM.

A second set of mice were pretreated with two doses of phenylhydrazine (PHZ, 40 mg/kg), on two consecutive days prior to infection with 10^6 iRBC using the same groups of mice as before. Again, daily blood samples of 10 μl were taken from each mouse and analyzed up to day 5 p.i. before sacrificing the mice on day 6 p.i..

Mathematical Model for Erythropoiesis and Blood-Stage Infection Dynamics

To describe the blood stage-infection dynamics of the murine malaria parasite accounting for RBC age, we used a mathematical model for erythropoiesis as described before (Mackey, 1997). The age-structured model follows the population density of RBCs of age τ at time t based on a system of coupled ordinary differential equations that breaks the age ranges of RBC into $n = \tau_{RBC}/h$ different compartments with h being the compartment size and τ_{RBC} the maximal lifespan of RBCs. The concentration of RBCs within each compartment is denoted by $x_i(t)$, $i = 1, \ldots n$. New RBCs are constantly produced by the bone marrow that enter the population of RBCs after a delay T, with the actual influx at each time point determined by a Hill-function dependent on the maximal production rate of RBCs in the bone marrow, F_0, and the concentration of RBCs at time t-T, $X(t$-$T)$. Mathematically, the model is then described by the following system of ordinary differential equations:

$$\frac{dx_1}{dt} = F_0 \frac{\theta^k}{\theta^k + (X(t-T))^k} - \frac{1}{h} x_1(t) - \frac{1}{\tau_{RBC}} x_1(t) \quad (1)$$

$$\frac{dx_i}{dt} = \frac{1}{h}(x_{i-1}(t) - x_i(t)) - \frac{1}{\tau_{RBC}} x_i(t), \; i = 2, \ldots, n \quad (2)$$

$$X(t) = \sum_{i=1}^{n} x_i(t) \quad (3)$$

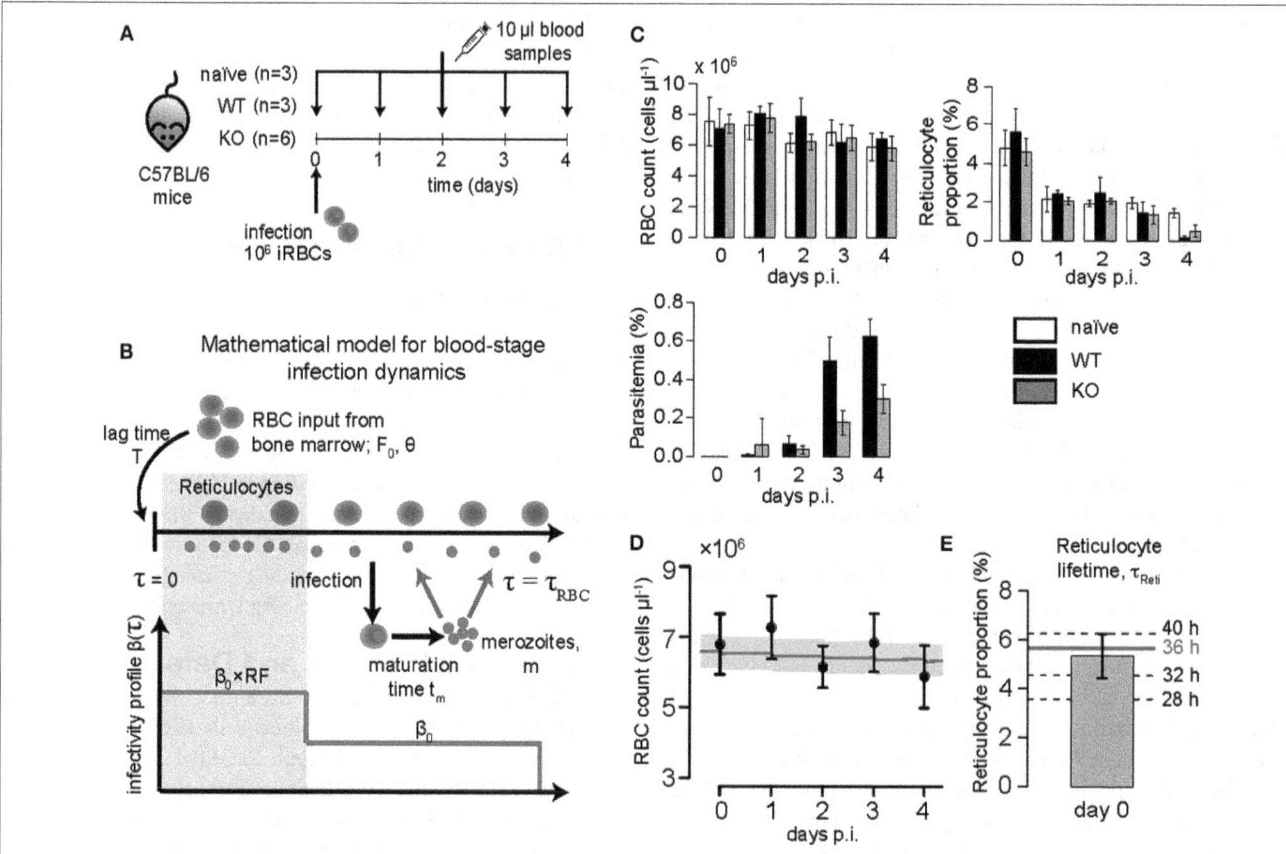

FIGURE 1 | (A) Experimental protocol: C57BL/6 mice were infected with 10^6 iRBC of *PbANKA* (WT), *PbmaLS_05* (-) (KO) or left uninfected. Daily samples of 10 μl blood were drawn to measure the concentration of RBC (cells/μl), reticulocyte proportion and parasitemia (in % of RBC). **(B)** Sketch of the mathematical model describing erythropoiesis and blood-stage infection dynamics of the parasite. For a detailed description of the model see section Materials and Methods.
(C) Measured concentration of RBC (cells/μl), reticulocyte proportion (in % of RBC) and parasitemia (in % of RBC) for each of the different groups analyzed. **(D)** The plot shows the measured concentration of red blood cells for naïve mice (mean + SD, $n = 3$), as well as the dynamics predicted by our model (best fit-red solid line, 95%-confidence interval- shaded area) using parameter estimates for RBC turnover and reticulocyte production as given in **Table 1**. **(E)** Based on model predictions and the measured proportion of reticulocytes on day 0, we consider a maturation time for reticulocytes of $\tau_{Reti} = 36$ h.

Hereby, the parameter θ describes the concentration of RBC where the production rate is half of the maximum and k the Hill-coefficient (Mackey, 1997). In addition, we also assumed that in each compartment x_i RBCs are lost by an age-independent loss-rate $1/\tau_{RBC}$ to have at least 85% of RBC lost until their assumed maximal lifespan τ_{RBC}. Equations (1–3) represent a mean-field approximation of the originally developed system relying on partial differential equations, thereby transforming assumed fixed, constant lifespans of RBC into gamma-distributed lifetimes (Mackey, 1997; Antia et al., 2008).

This basic model for erythropoiesis is then extended to account for malaria blood-stage infection as done previously (McQueen and McKenzie, 2004; Antia et al., 2008; **Figure 1B**). Uninfected RBCs can get infected by free merozoites, z, at a rate $\beta(\tau)$, which is dependent on the age-preference of the infecting parasite strain. Each infected RBC releases a number of merozoites, m, by bursting after having reached an infection maturation time, t_m. In addition, free merozoites are assumed to have an average lifetime of $1/d_m$. As for uninfected RBC, the concentration of infected cells, $Y(t)$, is broken down into $g = t_m/h$ different age compartments, $y_i(t), i = 1,\ldots,g$ leading to a system of coupled ordinary differential equations with a gamma-distributed maturation time with mean t_m. The basic model for erythropoiesis (Equations 1–3) is then extended to:

$$\frac{dx_1}{dt} = F_0\frac{\theta^k}{\theta^k + (X(t-T))^k} - \frac{1}{h}x_1(t) - \frac{1}{\tau_{RBC}}x_1(t) - \beta_1 z(t)\, x_1(t) \quad (4)$$

$$\frac{dx_i}{dt} = \frac{1}{h}(x_{i-1}(t) - x_i(t)) - \frac{1}{\tau_{RBC}}x_i(t) - \beta_i z(t)\, x_i(t),\ i = 2, \ldots, n \quad (5)$$

$$\frac{dy_1}{dt} = \sum_{i=1}^{n}\beta_i z(t) x_i(t) - \frac{1}{h}y_1(t) \quad (6)$$

$$\frac{dy_i}{dt} = \frac{1}{h}\left(y_{i-1}(t) - y_i(t)\right),\ i = 2,\ldots, g \quad (7)$$

$$\frac{dz}{dt} = \frac{m}{h}y_g(t) - \sum_{i=1}^{n}\beta_i z(t)\, x_i(t) - d_m z(t) \quad (8)$$

$$\beta_i = \begin{cases}\beta_0 RF, & i \le \tau_{Reti}/h \\ \beta_0, & i > \tau_{Reti}/h\end{cases} \quad (9)$$

Hereby, $z(t)$ describes the concentration of merozoites at time t and RF the so called reticulocyte factor, i.e., the fold-change in infectivity of the parasite for reticulocytes compared to the general infection rate assumed for normocytes, β_0 (see Cromer et al., 2006). The parameter τ_{Reti} defines the maturation time of reticulocytes into normocytes.

Calculating the Average Infectivity and Reticulocyte Preference

In order to compare parasite strains with possible different values for the infection rate, β_0, and the reticulocyte factor RF, we calculated an average infectivity β, which is defined as the infection rate of a single merozoite when placed into the erythropoietic system at the initiation of infection. In a naïve mouse, on average 5.8% of the RBC are reticulocytes, thus the average infectivity is calculated by $\beta = \beta_0(0.058RF + 0.942)$.

Besides the reticulocyte factor, RF, the reticulocyte preference, RP, is calculated based on the ratio between the percentage of infected reticulocytes (relative to all reticulocytes) and the percentage of infected normocytes (relative to all normocytes). Thus, if R and I_R define the concentration of reticulocytes and infected reticulocytes, respectively, and N and I_N the corresponding concentrations for normocytes, the reticulocyte preference is calculated by $RP = (I_R/R)/(I_N/N)$. In contrast to the reticulocyte factor, the reticulocyte preference can be directly calculated from experimental measurements.

Modeling the Effect of Phenylhydrazine Treatment on Erythropoiesis

Treatment with Phenylhydrazine (PHZ) is used for experimental induction of anemia in animal models to study hemolytic anemia or anemia caused by destruction or removal of RBCs from the bloodstream (Berger, 2007). Previous studies developed mathematical models to determine and quantify the effect of PHZ on the RBC age distribution and altered erythropoiesis (Savill et al., 2009). However, these models were inadequate to describe our experimental data suggesting that they incompletely addressed the effects of PHZ. To this end, we tested several different known hypotheses for the effect of PHZ on erythropoiesis (Jain and Hochstein, 1980; Berger, 2007; Savill et al., 2009; Moreau et al., 2012) by fitting them to the data of the PHZ-control group (see Supplementary Material Text S3). The models best explaining the experimental data included the following drug effects: (i) Treatment by PHZ leads to instantaneous lyses of a fraction $\rho(\tau)$ of RBCs at the time of treatment, t_p. Hereby, the effect of lysis depends on the age of the RBC, τ, with normocytes being more strongly affected than reticulocytes (Jain and Hochstein, 1980). (ii) An additional influx of reticulocytes from extra medullary sites is considered at a constant rate N_p with a time-delay T_p after the initiation of treatment to account for stress-induced erythropoiesis. Under severe anemia, such as that induced by PHZ-treatment, extra-medullary sites of erythropoiesis such as the spleen and liver are observed to show an increased contribution of RBCs to circulation (Spivak et al., 1973; Ploemacher et al., 1977; Kim, 2010). Thus, under PHZ-treatment, Equations (1, 2) describing RBC turnover are changed as follows:

$$\frac{dx_1}{dt} = F(t) - \left(\frac{1}{h} - \frac{1}{\tau_{RBC}}\right)x_1(t) - \rho_1 I(t = T_p)\, x_1(t) \quad (10)$$

$$\frac{dx_i}{dt} = \frac{1}{h}(x_{i-1}(t) - x_i(t)) - \frac{1}{\tau_{RBC}}x_i(t) - \rho_i I(t = T_p)\, x_i(t),\ i = 2, \ldots, n \quad (11)$$

$$\rho_i = \begin{cases}\rho_0\gamma, & i \le \tau_{Reti}/h \\ \rho_0, & i > \tau_{Reti}/h\end{cases} \quad (12)$$

$$F(t) = \begin{cases}F_0\frac{\theta_k}{\theta_k + (X(t-T))^k}, & t \le t_p + T_p \\ F_0\frac{\theta_k}{\theta_k + (X(t-T))^k} + N_p, & t > t_p + T_p\end{cases} \quad (13)$$

Hereby, ρ_0 defines the fraction of normocytes lysed by PHZ and γ represents the relative comparison of this fraction for reticulocytes. In addition, $I(t = T_p)$ defines the Indicator function, i.e., with $I(t = T_p) = 1$ if $t = T_p$ and 0 otherwise. A sketch of the effects of PHZ treatment on erythropoiesis is shown in **Figure 4A**. A detailed derivation of the model can be found in the Supplementary Material. During infection, we assume that malaria induced changes to RBC production affects both sources of novel reticulocytes, i.e., bone marrow and extra medullary sites alike.

Model Evaluation and Fitting Procedures

The mathematical models described above were implemented and analyzed using the **R** language of statistical computing (R Development Core Team, 2017). As indicated, the age of uninfected and infected RBC was compartmentalized leading to a tractable system of coupled ordinary differential equations with gamma-distributed lifetimes and maturation times for RBC and infected cells, respectively (Antia et al., 2008). In the following we used a compartment size of 4 h.

The differential equations were solved using the **deSolve** package and models were fitted to the experimental data using the *optim*-fitting routine in **R**. In cases where a strong correlation between parameters hindered convergence of fitting algorithms, a parameter sweep was performed to find combinations of parameters that fit the data. Proportion data (parasitemia levels and proportion of reticulocytes) were *logit*- transformed to allow for normally distributed residuals. Model performance was assessed based on simultaneous fitting for all obtained measurements including RBC concentration, reticulocyte proportion and, where applicable, parasitemia. Blood stage infection dynamics of parasites were determined in a stepwise approach: Parameters describing erythropoiesis were fixed to the indicated values obtained from the naïve control group before analyzing infection dynamics (**Table 1**). Therefore, measurements for the infection groups, i.e., reticulocyte proportion and RBC count, were scaled relative to the naïve group data when estimating parasite infectivity. To evaluate model performance, the average residual sum of squares (aRSS) was used which is the residual sum of squares divided by the number of data points.

The 95%-confidence intervals, as well as identifiability of parameter estimates were assessed by profile likelihood analysis (Raue et al., 2009). For the measured data, we report mean and standard error.

RESULTS

Characterizing the Dynamics of Erythropoiesis and Determining Reticulocyte Maturation Times in the Blood

To determine the dynamics of erythropoiesis in our experimental system, we fitted a mathematical model describing RBC production and subsequent aging (see Equations 1–3 in Materials and Methods; Mary et al., 1980; Mackey, 1997) to the observed progression of RBC concentration in uninfected mice that were sampled daily for 10 μl of blood (see Materials and Methods and **Figures 1A–C**). In general, bleeding leads to a decrease in the RBC concentration triggering the production of novel RBCs in the bone marrow that will enter the blood circulation after a time delay *T*. Thereby, the magnitude of the feedback depends on the severity of the anemia, i.e., the larger the loss of blood the larger the subsequent RBC production, which is accounted for in our model by a Hill-type function (Mackey, 1997). Assuming a maximal lifespan for RBC of $\tau_{RBC} = 40$ days (Bannerman, 1983) and a Hill-coefficient of $k = 7.6$ (Mackey, 1997), we estimated a maximal RBC production rate in the bone marrow of $F_0 = 5.95 \times 10^4$ cells μl^{-1} h^{-1} [4.02, 6.82] with half of the maximal production rate reached at a RBC concentration of $\theta = 6.65 \times 10^6$ cells μl^{-1}[5.28, 6.84], which is approximately 95% of the RBC concentration at steady state. Newly produced red blood cells are estimated to appear in the circulation after a lag-time of $T = 2$ days, testing different possible lag-times including $T = 0$, 1, 2, and 2.5 days. All our estimates are in agreement to parameters that have been determined previously for erythropoiesis in mice (Mary et al., 1980; Mackey, 1997; **Figure 1D** and **Table 1**).

As we were especially interested in the dynamics of reticulocytes, i.e., immature red blood cells, we compared model predictions for the proportion of different RBC age classes to the measured proportion of reticulocytes in order to determine the time these cells spend in the blood. We found that a maturation time for reticulocytes into normocytes in the blood of $\tau_{Reti} = 36$ h best described our measured proportion of reticulocytes (**Figure 1E**), which is in agreement to previous calculations determining a maturation time for reticulocytes between 1 and 3 days (Ganzoni et al., 1969; Gronowicz et al., 1984; Wiczling and Krzyzanski, 2008). Thus, for the following analyses we assume that after appearance in the blood, a reticulocyte will take on average 1.5 days to develop into a normocyte.

Parasite-Induced Cell Death Cannot Explain the Observed Loss in Reticulocyte Proportion

In order to compare the blood-stage infection dynamics of the two *Plasmodium berghei* strains investigated, mice were either infected with *Pb*ANKA (WT) or *PbmaLS_05* (-) (KO) infected red blood cells and sampled daily for 10 μl of blood. For both strains, we observe a substantial loss in the proportion of reticulocytes around day 3 post infection (p.i.) coinciding with an increase in parasitemia (**Figure 1C**). At day 4 p.i., when mice infected with WT show first signs of ECM, the parasitemia was approximately twice as high as the one measured for mice infected with the KO (0.63 ±0.05% WT compared to 0.29 ±0.03% KO) (**Figure 1C**).

To determine systematic differences in the infection dynamics between the two parasite strains, we extended our mathematical model describing erythropoiesis to include malaria blood-stage infection dynamics (see Equations 4–9). Hereby, RBCs get infected by merozoites at an infection rate β and infected RBC (iRBC) will release new merozoites m after a certain maturation

TABLE 1 | Estimated parameter values describing erythropoiesis in mice based on the model as described in Equations (1–3) in section Materials and Methods.

Parameter	Description	Unit	Value	References/Comparison
ERYTHROPOIESIS				
F_0	RBC production rate in Bone marrow	$(\times 10^4)$ cells μl^{-1} h^{-1}	5.95 (4.02, 6.82)	Mackey, 1997
θ	RBC concentration at which half of max. RBC production is reached	$(\times 10^6)$ cells μl^{-1}	6.65 (5.28, 6.84)	Mackey, 1997
T	Delay in RBC production feedback	days	2	Mackey, 1997
τ_{Reti}	Maturation time of reticulocytes in the blood	hours	36	Gronowicz et al., 1984; Wiczling and Krzyzanski, 2008
τ_{RBC}	Lifetime of RBC	days	40	Bannerman, 1983
k	Hill-coefficient for RBC feedback		7.6	Mackey, 1997
DISEASE-INDUCED FEEDBACK MODULATION				
λ	Loss-rate of gene-expression	day^{-1}	2.22 (1.31, 3.05)	
t_0	Time at which half of the max. gene expression is reached	days	3.70 (3.28, 4.23)	
PARASITE INFECTION				
t_m	Maturation time of iRBC	days	1	Cox, 1988; De Roode, 2004
m	Average number of merozoites released per burst		9	Cox, 1988; De Roode, 2004
d_m	Clearance rate of merozoites	day^{-1}	48	Garnham, 1966

Numbers in brackets represent 95%-confidence intervals of estimates obtained based on the profile likelihood method. In addition, the table contains the parameter estimates for the disease-induced modulation of the RBC feedback dynamics (see ***Figure 2A****), as well as the parameters that were fixed when analyzing the infectivity of the two different parasite strains.*

time t_m (see **Figure 1B** and Materials and Methods for a detailed explanation of the extended model). Assuming the average lifespan of a merozoite of $1/d_m = 30$ min (Garnham, 1966), a maturation time of an iRBC of $t_m = 24$ h (Cox, 1988; De Roode, 2004) and that an infected RBC releases on average $m = 9$ merozoites after bursting (Cox, 1988; De Roode, 2004; Reilly et al., 2007) we find that the observed loss in the proportion of reticulocytes around day 3 p.i. cannot be explained by the increased parasitemia when using the standard parameterization for erythropoiesis (**Table 1**). This observation is independent of the assumed infectivity of the parasite strain (Supplementary Figure S1) and is also the case if we assume that the infectivity for reticulocytes is substantially higher than for normocytes. This indicates that the reason for the observed decrease in reticulocyte proportion is not mainly due to reticulocytes being parasitized.

It is known that malarial-induced anemia causes erythropoietic suppression, starting during the early stages of infection (Villeval et al., 1990; Sexton et al., 2004; Thawani et al., 2014). By analyzing the expression levels of previously studied genes (Sexton et al., 2004), we found that the fold change in the expression of the genes most strongly associated with erythropoiesis, i.e., α-globin, β-globin major and β-1-globin, can be described by a logistic-loss function given by

$$F(t) = \frac{1+e^{-\lambda t_0}}{1+e^{-\lambda(t_0-t)}} \tag{14}$$

where λ defines the loss-rate of gene-expression, i.e., the loss of RBC production and t_0 the time point at which half of the maximal gene expression is reached. We estimate $\lambda = 2.22$ d^{-1} (95%-CI [1.31, 3.05]) and $t_0 = 3.70$ d [3.28, 4.23] (**Figure 2A**, **Table 1**). This parameterization is then used to account for malaria-induced modulation of RBC production during the analyses of blood stage infection dynamics in WT and KO infected mice.

*PbmaLS*_05 (-) Merozoites Express a Reduced Infectivity Compared to *Pb*ANKA WT

To analyze the infectivity of both parasite strains, we fitted our extended mathematical model (Equations 4–9 with Equation 14) to the experimental data on RBC count, reticulocyte proportion and parasitemia. Additionally accounting for a modulation of RBC production due to infection (i.e., replacing F_0 by $F_0F(t)$ with $\lambda = 2.22$ d^{-1} and $t_0 = 3.70$ d in Equation 3) improves model predictions, especially regarding the substantial loss in the proportion of reticulocytes starting 3 days p.i. (compare **Figure 2B** and Supplementary Figure S1A).

By estimating the infectivity for each parasite strain characterized by the rate of infection (β_0) and the reticulocyte factor (RF), our analysis indicates that the WT parasites have a higher preference for infecting reticulocytes than normocytes (**Figure 2B** and **Table 2**). During this early infection phase, we estimate a more than 22-fold higher infectivity for reticulocytes than for normocytes i.e., $RF > 22$ (**Table 2**). In contrast, a similar preference for reticulocytes could not be found explicitly for the KO parasite. Here, a model assuming equal infectivities for reticulocytes and normocytes, i.e., $RF = 1$, performs equally well as a model that assumes a reticulocyte preference (AIC 40.7 vs. AIC 42.7). However, our time courses are too short to clearly identify such a reticulocyte preference for both parasite strains. As a high infection rate β_0 can be compensated by a small value of RF and vice versa, several combinations of β_0 and RF can explain the observed dynamics (Supplementary Figure S2).

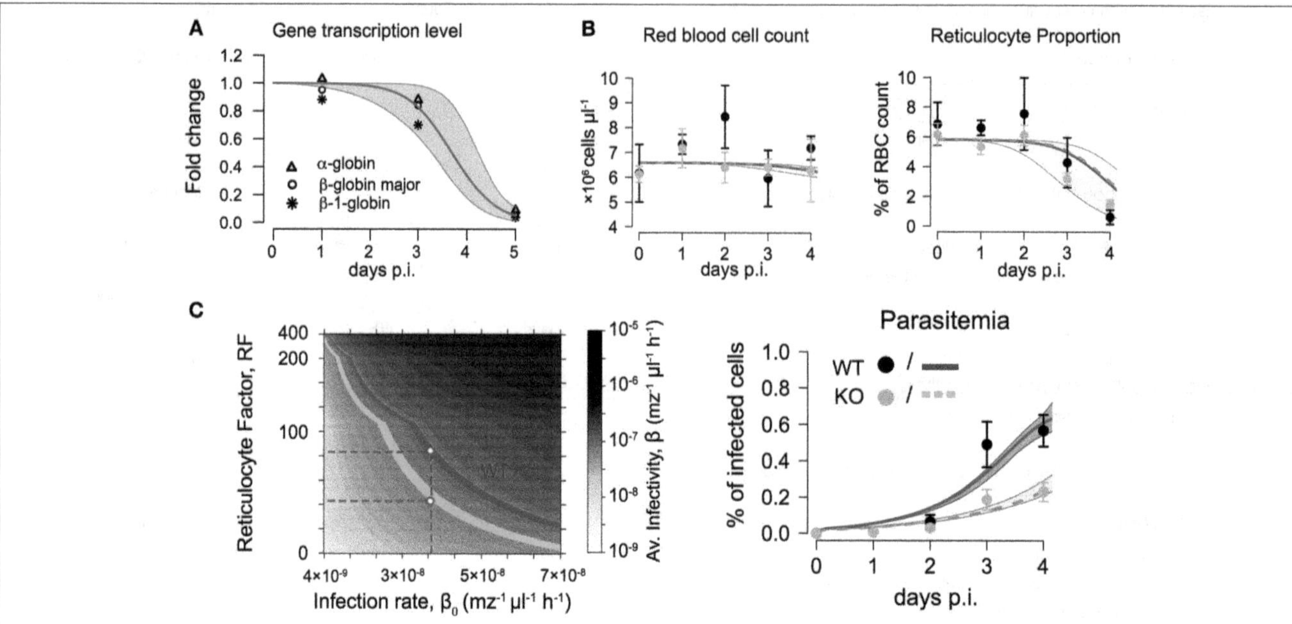

FIGURE 2 | (A) Fold change in expression levels of genes associated with erythropoiesis during malaria infection. Symbols represent gene-expression levels of α-globin (Δ), β-globin major ($\circ$) and β−1-globin ($\cdot$) as measured in Sexton et al. (2004). Dynamics can be described by a logistic-loss function with $F(t) = (1\text{-}exp(\text{-}\lambda t_0))/(1+exp(\text{-}\lambda(t\text{-}t_0)))$ (see main text). Red solid line indicates best fit with $\lambda = 2.22$ d^{-1} and $t_0 = 3.70$ days based on 10^4 bootstrap replicates simulated from the distribution given by the gene expression levels at each time point (shaded area – 95% confidence interval). **(B)** Dynamics of red blood cell concentration, reticulocyte proportion and parasitemia for mice infected by either WT, $n = 3$ or KO, $n = 6$. The mean and standard deviation for each group (WT-black, KO- gray) are shown. Model results simultaneously predicting the dynamics of all 3 measurements indicate a lower average infectivity for the WT (blue line) compared to KO (green line). Shaded areas indicate 95%-confidence intervals. Corresponding parameter estimates are shown in **Table 2**. **(C)** Obtained parameter combinations for reticulocyte factor *RF* and infection rate β_0 indicate a lower average infectivity β per merozoite per hour for the KO parasite compared to the WT. KO parasites have lower reticulocyte factors than the WT if similar infection rates β_0 for both parasites are assumed (red dashed lines).

TABLE 2 | Parameter estimates for parasite infectivity comparing *Pb*ANKA (WT) and *PbmaLS*_05(-) (KO).

Parameter	Unit	***Pb*ANKA (WT)**	***PbmaLS*_05(-) (KO)**
Infection rate, β_0	$\times 10^{-8}$ mz^{-1} µl^{-1} h^{-1}	(0, 4.84)	7.82 (7.36, 8.31)
Reticulocyte Factor, *RF*		(22.5, ∞)	1
Average Infectivity, β	$\times 10^{-7}$ mz^{-1} µl^{-1} h^{-1}	1.13 (1.08, 1.16)	0.78 (0.74, 0.83)

Because for PbANKA (WT) only combinations of β_0 and RF could be determined (structural non-identifiability), only the ranges of the parameters are given. For PbmaLS_05(-), there was no evidence for a reticulocyte preference, i.e., RF = 1. Numbers in brackets represent 95%-confidence intervals of estimates obtained by the profile likelihood method if boundaries could be determined.

To compare the infectivity of WT and KO parasites, we calculated an average infectivity β based on the estimates of β_0 and *RF*, which is defined as the infection rate of a single merozoite when placed into the erythropoietic system at the start of infection (see Materials and Methods for a detailed calculation). We find that KO parasites have a reduced average infectivity compared to WT parasites leading to less productive infections ($\beta = 1.13 \times 10^{-7}$ mz^{-1}µl^{-1} h^{-1} [1.08, 1.16] for WT vs. $\beta = 0.78 \times 10^{-7}$ mz^{-1}µl^{-1} h^{-1} [0.74, 0.83] for KO, numbers in brackets represent 95%-confidence intervals; **Table 2**). This reduced average infectivity can explain the slower increase in the parasitemia observed for the KO strain (**Figure 2B**).

If we assume that the infection rate β_0 does not differ between the two parasite strains, we find a consistently lower reticulocyte factor for the KO compared to the WT (**Figure 2C** and Supplementary Figure S2). Thus, our analysis indicates that KO parasites might have a particularly impaired ability to productively infect reticulocytes in comparison to the WT during the early erythrocytic stage of infection.

Parasite Infection Dynamics under Altered Erythropoietic Conditions

To elicit possible differences in reticulocyte preferences between the two parasite strains we pre-treated mice with the drug Phenylhydrazine (PHZ) before infecting them with either WT or KO parasites (**Figure 3A**). PHZ artificially induces anemia in mice causing peroxidation of RBC lipids leading to hemolysis and a change in RBC age distributions (Savill et al., 2009). In uninfected mice that were pre-treated with two doses of 40 mg/kg of PHZ on two consecutive days, we observe a substantial loss in the concentration of red blood cells to roughly ~1/3 of the concentration under homeostatic conditions 2 days after the last treatment with PHZ (2.5×10^6 cells/µl vs. 7.6×10^6 cells/µl, mean values; **Figure 3B**). There was a corresponding increase in

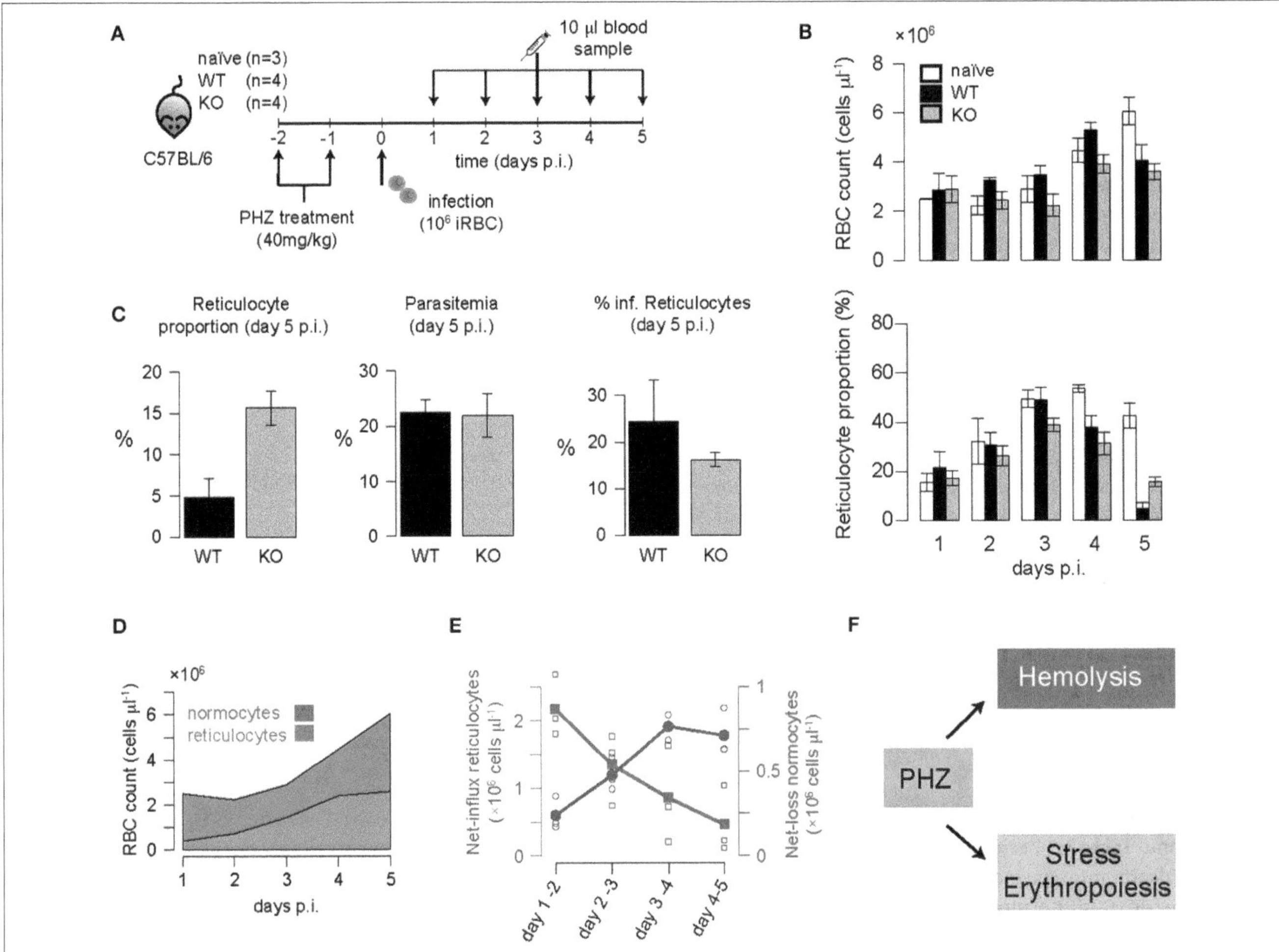

FIGURE 3 | (A) Experimental protocol: Mice were pre-treated with two doses of 40 mg/kg PHZ on two consecutive days before infection with 10^6 iRBC of WT or KO parasites on the following day. Blood samples (10 μl) were taken daily and analyzed. **(B)** Measured concentration of RBC (cells/μl) and reticulocyte proportion for each of the different groups. **(C)** Parasitemia (in % of RBC) above background was detected at day 5 post infection indicating equal levels between WT and KO-infected mice despite a roughly 3-fold higher reticulocyte proportion in KO- compared to WT-infected mice. The percentage of infected reticulocytes was determined as well. **(D)** The measured progression of normocytes and reticulocytes in PHZ-treated but uninfected animals (naïve) indicated an increasing net-influx of reticulocytes (blue line) and a decreasing net-loss of normocytes (red line) up to 5 days post PHZ treatment **(E)**. This corresponds to the assumed effects of PHZ leading to hemolysis and stress-induced erythropoiesis **(F)**.

the proportion of reticulocytes to up to 50% of the total RBC count at 5–6 days after the last treatment with PHZ (**Figure 3B**). Changes in RBC count and reticulocyte proportion of WT or KO infected mice that were pre-treated with PHZ are visible on day 5 p.i. with RBC counts reaching 4.0 ± 0.32 and $3.6 \pm 0.15 \times 10^6$ cells/μl for WT and KO, respectively, compared to $6.0 \pm 0.29 \times 10^6$ cells/μl in uninfected animals (**Figure 3C**). In addition, the proportion of reticulocytes in infected animals is substantially reduced compared to naïve mice; with KO infected mice still having ~3-fold higher levels than WT infected mice [42.6 ± 2.6% (naïve), 4.8 ± 1.2% (WT), 15.6 ± 1.0% (KO); **Figures 3B,C**]. While parasitemia levels are comparable between both infection groups (22.5 ± 1.2% vs. 21.0 ± 2.0%), the percentage of infected reticulocytes is slightly higher for WT compared to KO (24.3 ± 4.6% vs. 16.3 ± 0.8%; **Figure 3C**). Given these measurements, the average reticulocyte preference *RP*, calculated by the proportion of infected reticulocytes among reticulocytes divided by the proportion of infected normocytes among normocytes, is determined by $RP_{WT} = 1.46$ and $RP_{KO} = 0.76$, respectively. In accordance with our previous results (**Figure 2C**), these observations suggest that deletion of *PbmaLS_05* has a potential effect on the parasite's ability to productively infect reticulocytes.

Modeling the Effects of PHZ on Erythropoiesis and Predicting Infection Dynamics

To determine if the calculated infection characteristics for WT and KO during normal erythropoietic conditions also apply after PHZ treatment, we extended our previous model to account for drug-induced changes to erythropoiesis. The exact mechanisms by which PHZ induces hemolysis and changes in the RBC age distribution have not been determined so far. Several hypotheses including faster aging of RBCs or direct lysis have been suggested and corresponding mathematical models have been proposed (Savill et al., 2009). However, these models fail to fit our experimental data, partly because they are limited to a particular PHZ treatment protocol (Savill et al., 2009). Therefore, we performed a rigorous analysis, testing several different assumptions for the effect of PHZ on erythropoiesis and their ability to explain the observed changes in total RBC count and reticulocyte dynamics in our data (see Materials and Methods and Supplementary Material Text S3 for a detailed description of the different models tested).

Our data indicate an increasing influx of reticulocytes, as well as a decreasing net-loss in normocytes after the last PHZ-treatment (**Figures 3D,E**). Thereby, the increased production of reticulocytes cannot solely be explained by the anemia-induced production from the bone marrow. We found that the best models explaining the effect of PHZ treatment on erythropoiesis assume (i) instantaneous hemolysis with ~35–50% of the RBC being lysed upon PHZ administration, and (ii) stress-induced erythropoiesis with an additional production of reticulocytes from different sources than the bone marrow (**Figure 3F**). Thereby, this additional production starts around 4.5 days after the last PHZ-treatment has been given (**Table 3** and Text S3). In addition, our analysis indicates that PHZ leads to an increased death rate of RBC, reducing the average lifetime of RBC from τ_{RBC}~40 days to τ_{RBC}~8 days (see **Figure 3E** and **Table 3**). Besides a constant death rate, a linear decreasing death rate, as indicated by our calculation of the observed net-loss in normocytes (**Figure 3E**), could also be possible as it shows similar explanatory power for the data (**Table 3**). By incorporating these effects within our model, we are able to provide a modeling framework that describes PHZ-induced changes on erythropoiesis in our experimental system (**Figures 4A,B**).

We then simulated the pre-treatment of mice with PHZ and subsequent infection using different assumptions for parasite infectivity, β_0, and reticulocyte preference, *RF*, and predicted the expected levels of parasitemia and reticulocyte proportion on day 5 post infection (**Figure 4C**). For the KO strain, relevant parameter combinations as determined previously (**Table 2**) lead to reticulocyte proportions (~13%) comparable to the ones observed in the experimental data, but result in parasitemia levels of less than 1%. In contrast, combinations of *RF* and β_0 within the determined ranges for the WT parasite predict reticulocyte proportions that are twice as high as seen in the data (**Figure 3C**), and parasitemia levels that are only one-tenth of the observed level. However, neglecting previous knowledge and directly estimating *RF* and β_0 based on the observed parasitemia and reticulocyte proportion under PHZ treatment, both groups expect that nearly all reticulocytes are infected (80–100%), which does not agree with our data (**Figure 3C**). These findings indicate that there could be disease-induced changes to PHZ treatment effects that cannot be explained by a simple combination of separately determined processes of blood-stage infection kinetics, erythropoiesis and PHZ dynamics.

TABLE 3 | Parameters describing the effect of PHZ treatment on erythropoiesis.

Model	Parameter	Unit	Value
With extra-medullary production of RBC	ρ_0	–	0.52 (0.50, 0.54)
	γ	–	0.007 (0, 0.01)
	T_p	h	84.5 (83.2, 85.6)
	N_p	$\times 10^4$ cells μl^{-1} h^{-1}	7.8 (7.5, 8)
	r	–	0.97 (0.92, 0.99)
With extra-medullary production of RBC and constant change in RBC death rate	ρ_0	–	0.38 (0.37, 0.39)
	γ	–	0.006 (0, 0.04)
	T_p	h	82.8 (80.2, 84.1)
	N_p	$\times 10^4$ cells μl^{-1} h^{-1}	7.7 (7.2, 8.1)
	r	–	0.92 (0.90, 0.94)
	η	–	4.18 (3.91, 4.46)

For a detailed explanation of the different models tested to evaluate the different hypotheses for the effect of PHZ see Supplementary Material Text S3. The parameters describe PHZ induced hemolysis (ρ_0, fraction of RBC lysed; γ, reduction in lysis of reticulocytes) and stress-induced erythropoiesis (T_p, time delay after PHZ treatment before onset of extra-medullary RBC production; N_p, rate of RBC influx from extra-medullary sites; r, fraction of N_p being reticulocytes). The parameter "η" defines a factor at which the lifespan of RBC produced after treatment is permanently reduced.

DISCUSSION

Parasite replication and invasion of red blood cells during the pathological blood-stage of the *Plasmodium* life cycle is a critical determinant of the severity of disease progression in a malaria infection (Beeson et al., 2016). Determining the precise processes and host factors regulating parasite's infectivity is essential for the identification of appropriate therapeutic targets. Mathematical models have been widely used to understand within-host infection dynamics of the *Plasmodium* parasite through analysis of the complex life cycle and host-parasite interactions in various levels of details (Cromer et al., 2006; Mideo et al., 2008; Li et al., 2011; Kerlin and Gatton, 2013). In this study, we used an age-structured model based on partial differential equations similar to previous approaches (Antia et al., 2008) to specifically determine differences between *Pb*ANKA (WT) and *PbmaLS_05* (-) (KO) parasite strains in terms of age-preferences for RBC, and in particular reticulocytes.

We focused our analysis on the early erythrocytic stage of the parasite, i.e., studying the first 4 days post infection of mice with iRBC. We found that malarial-induced changes to erythropoiesis already play a role at this stage of infection. The observed decrease in reticulocyte proportions could not be explained solely by parasite-induced lysis of RBC (Supplementary Figure S1; Chang et al., 2004), similar to observations for *Plasmodium berghei* at later erythrocytic stages (Cromer et al., 2006). Several factors, including bystander destruction of uninfected RBC during infection (Cromer et al., 2006; Evans et al., 2006; Fonseca et al., 2016) might contribute to the substantial loss in reticulocytes. However, as total RBC counts are rather stable (**Figure 2**), an age-independent loss of RBC seemed to be insufficient to explain the observed decrease in reticulocyte proportion. Therefore, the mathematical model by Antia et al. (2008) used to describe blood-stage infection dynamics of *Plasmodium* parasites was extended in order to account for

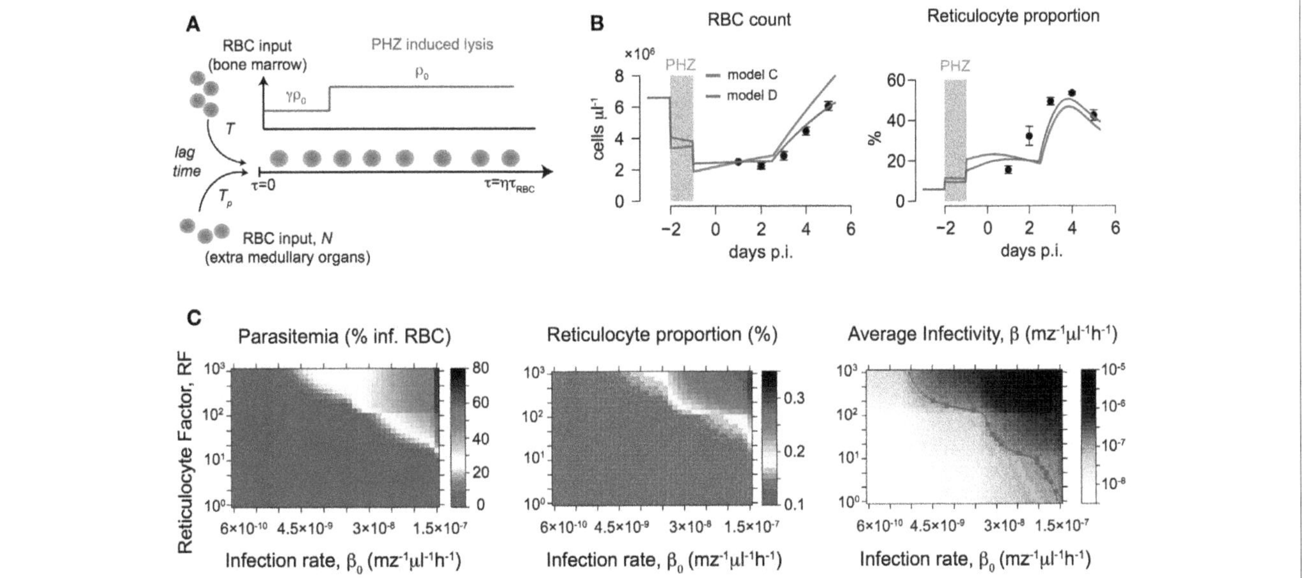

FIGURE 4 | (A) Sketch of the mathematical model describing the main effects of PHZ treatment on erythropoiesis. For a detailed description see section Materials and Methods. **(B)** Predictions of the best fit-mathematical model for the dynamics of RBC count and reticulocyte proportion under PHZ-induced changes to erythropoiesis. Gray areas indicate time of PHZ treatment. A model assuming an increased death rate of RBC, $1/\tau = 0.125\ d^{-1}$, i.e., due to hemolysis, (blue line) performs better than a model with unchanged RBC lifetimes, $1/\tau = 0.025\ d^{-1}$ (red line). **(C)** Predicted parasitemia and reticulocyte proportions after PHZ treatment on day 5 post infection for different combinations of reticulocyte factors, *RF*, and parasite infectivity, β_0. The right heat-map shows the relevant combinations for WT (blue) and KO (green) leading to the average infectivity as determined during untreated infection (see **Figure 2B** and **Table 1**). While for the KO-group relevant parameter combinations lead to matching reticulocyte proportions (~13%) as in the experimental data (compare to **Figure 3C**), combinations of *RF* and β_0 for the WT-group predict reticulocyte proportions roughly twice as high as seen in the data.

altered RBC production dynamics during infection (Sexton et al., 2004; Thawani et al., 2014).

By applying our extended model that disentangles erythropoietic and parasite infection dynamics to the experimental data, we found that *Pb*ANKA prefers to infect reticulocytes. This preference has been observed for various *Plasmodium* strains to different extents (Wilson et al., 1977; Mons et al., 1988; Mons, 1990; Cromer et al., 2006; Antia et al., 2008). We estimate a minimum 22-fold higher preference for reticulocytes compared to normocytes in *Pb*ANKA parasites relying on the early blood-stage of the parasite (**Table 2**). However, a maximal limit for the *RF* could not be determined (**Table 2**). As large values of *RF* can be compensated by lower values of the infection rate β_0, we can only identify combinations of both parameters that would lead to similar levels of parasitemia and reticulocyte proportion (*structural non-identifiability*) (Raue et al., 2009). Thus, even substantially higher values of *RF* could be possible for the WT if the age-independent infection rate β_0 is accordingly lower (**Figure 2C**). Cromer et al. (2006) estimated a value of $RF \sim 150$ based on data from later stages of infection with *Plasmodium berghei*, for which a particular reticulocyte preference was found at later times (Singer et al., 1955). With a $RF \sim 150$ as estimated by Cromer et al. (Cromer et al., 2006) our model would predict that infected reticulocytes account for ~65% of the parasitemia at day 4 p.i. (**Figure 5**). Although this is a slightly larger value than for previous observations in rats infected with *Plasmodium berghei* (Singer et al., 1955), which showed that reticulocytes represent ~50% of the infected RBC on day 4 p.i., such a high reticulocyte factor cannot be excluded based on our analysis.

We also find different combinations of the infection rate β_0 and the reticulocyte factor *RF* that could explain the observed dynamics for the KO-parasite (**Figure 2C**). However, we estimate that *Pb*ANKA parasites have a roughly 1.5-fold higher average infectivity than parasites lacking the *PbmaLS_05* gene (**Table 2**). Although quite small, this difference is sufficient to explain the observed reduced peripheral parasite load of KO compared to WT infected mice on day 4 p.i.. Moreover, the differences between both parasite strains might even be larger than currently estimated. Since WT-infected mice were sacrificed after showing signs of ECM, we were restricted in our analysis to the early exponential growth phase of the parasite in the blood. This could affect the identification of differing parasite infectivities for several reasons: Firstly, parasite levels are still low during this early phase (**Figure 1B**) and, hence, more prone to measurement noise. Therefore, differences between strains could be masked by the variation in the measurements. Secondly, by using our model to simulate blood-stage infection dynamics assuming various infectivity profiles, we find that differences between infectivity profiles only start to become visible in the measured parasitemia and reticulocyte proportion after 4–5 days p.i. (Supplementary Figure S2). However, comparison of long-term infection dynamics between both strains is hampered as mice infected by *Pb*ANKA WT develop ECM around day 5 p.i..

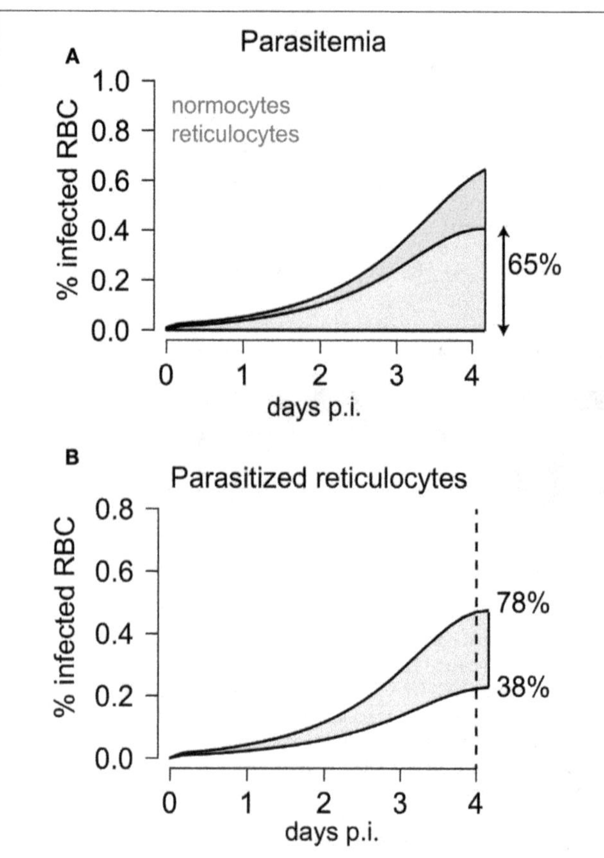

FIGURE 5 | (A) Development of infected normocytes and reticulocytes during infection with WT parasites as predicted by the model using a reticulocyte factor of $RF = 150$ as estimated by Cromer et al. (2006). The model predicts that 4 days after infection around 65% of the infected red blood cells are reticulocytes. **(B)** Using the estimated parameter combinations of the infection rate β_0 and RF for *Pb*ANKA (**Table 2**), the model predicts that 4 days after infection in between 38 and 78% of the infected red blood cells are reticulocytes.

Based on our analysis, the lower average infectivity for KO compared to *Pb*ANKA WT can be explained by two alternative hypotheses. On the one hand, KO-parasites could have a comparable or larger reticulocyte factor *RF* than the WT, but substantially lower infection rates β_0 (**Figure 2C** and Supplementary Figure S2). This would argue for a restriction of the parasite's infectivity to reticulocytes due to deletion of *PbmaLS*_05 (Hopp et al., 2017). In this case, we would expect that such a reticulocyte restriction is particularly visible in mice pre-treated with PHZ, a drug that artificially induces anemia and leads to an increased proportion of reticulocytes. However, we observe a 3-fold higher proportion of reticulocytes in KO- than WT-infected mice 5 days p.i. (**Figure 3C**). Given comparable levels of parasitemia and total RBC counts, this indicates enhanced reticulocyte survival during infection with the KO-parasite.

Therefore, our analysis rather suggests that deletion of *PbmaLS*_05 impairs the ability of the parasite to productively infect reticulocytes during the early infection phase. The estimated reticulocyte factor *RF* for the WT is around ~1.4 times higher than the one estimated for the KO when assuming similar infection rates (**Figure 2C**). Furthermore, the calculated reticulocyte preference for KO-infected mice after treatment with PHZ is roughly half the size of the one determined for WT-infected mice. As reticulocytes are usually the preferential targets of parasites (Mons et al., 1988; Mons, 1990), this impaired ability to infect reticulocytes would explain the observed slower increase in parasite burden in mice infected by the KO parasite. In fact, several studies have characterized the need for parasites to infect reticulocytes in order to spread infection. As shown through metabolomic analysis of RBC, reticulocytes possess a higher content of carbon sources and essential nutrients, both of which have been proposed to contribute to the higher reticulocyte preference of WT parasites during the early intra-erythrocytic stages of development (Srivastava et al., 2015). Furthermore, increased expression of CD47 on reticulocytes was shown to prevent phagocytosis and clearance of infected cells (Banerjee et al., 2015), thus allowing unchecked multiplication and infection of new red blood cells. It is therefore plausible that the reduced infectivity of *PbmaLS_05* (-) parasites reflected by the parasite's inability to develop within reticulocytes is a major contributing factor to the slower multiplication rates in the blood. Moreover, *PbmaLS_05* (-) infected mice do not develop experimental cerebral malaria but only late stage anemia (Fernandes et al., submitted manuscript), which is in line with previous studies that have proposed a link between severe disease progression and cell preference (McQueen and McKenzie, 2004; Iyer et al., 2007).

In addition to parasite infectivity, we also investigated if the reduced parasitemia in KO infected mice can be explained by impaired merozoite production or altered maturation times for infected RBCs. Assuming similar parasite infectivity for both strains, we do not find evidence for a reduced production of merozoites in KO infection compared to WT (Supplementary Figure S4). However, a roughly 2-fold longer maturation time for iRBC infected by the KO could provide an alternative explanation for the observed differing dynamics (Supplementary Figure S4). This supports the conclusion that deletion of *PbmaLS_05* particularly leads to impaired parasite development and less successful infections in reticulocytes during the initial blood-stage phase.

To fully determine the impact of *PbmaLS_05* deletion on parasite infectivity during the intra-erythrocytic stage and, thus, on disease progression, it remains to be investigated how infection affects erythropoiesis during later phases. Since mice infected with the KO-parasite do not develop ECM, they can be observed for longer time periods. During progression of infection, we observed a substantial increase in the proportion of reticulocytes before mice develop severe anemia and die ~21 days p.i., (Supplementary Figure S5). However, assuming continuous malarial-induced reduction of RBC production, our model is not able to explain the observed dynamics in reticulocytes and parasitemia (Supplementary Figure S5). These observations point toward a recovery of erythropoiesis at later time points, and potentially altered infectivity profiles of the parasite as has been observed for other *Plasmodium* strains. In fact, for the *Plasmodium chabaudi* strain it has been shown that reticulocyte production increases quickly after reaching a minimal production around 9 days after infection with 10^6 iRBC (Chang and Stevenson, 2004; Chang et al., 2004). In addition, *Plasmodium berghei* has been observed to alter its targeted age range during the progression of infection (Singer et al., 1955; Sexton et al., 2004). Understanding the changes in the erythropoietic processes in the time course of malaria infection remains critical to analyze long-term infection data and to further elucidate the effect of deleting maLS_05 on parasite infectivity and its importance for reticulocyte invasion. This also includes the understanding of the dynamics of infection and reticulocyte development under PHZ treatment. Our analysis revealed that these dynamics are more complex than a simple combination of altered erythropoiesis and infection processes that were parameterized independently.

In summary, our analysis based on a combination of mathematical modeling and experimental data suggests that deletion of *PbmaLS_05* affects productive infection of reticulocytes during the early blood-stage of the parasite's asexual development. Furthermore, our analysis supports previous findings on malarial-induced changes to erythropoiesis that also affect early blood-stage infection dynamics. Given the suggested outcome of *PbmaLS_05* on the productive infection of reticulocytes, we propose that the *PbmaLS_05* (-) mutant parasite strain can serve as a tool to study how the preference of parasites to infect particular RBC influences both disease progression and the development of experimental cerebral malaria. This will ultimately aid in revealing the factors that influence the activation of immune responses and that might enable efficient parasite control.

AUTHOR CONTRIBUTIONS

Conceived and designed the study: A-KM and FG; Performed the experiments: PF; Developed the mathematical models and analysis methods: NT and FG; Analyzed the experimental data: NT, PF, A-KM, and FG; Wrote the manuscript: NT, PF, A-KM, and FG.

FUNDING

This work was supported by a grant from the FRONTIER-program of Heidelberg University (ZUK 49/2 5.2.107) and by a grant from the Ministry of Science, Research and the Arts of Baden-Württemberg (Az: 0077.3.5.2.107) to FG and A-KM. NT and FG were additionally funded by the Center for Modeling and Simulation in the Biosciences (BIOMS). A-KM is a recipient of a maternity leave stipend through the Deutsche Zentrum für Infektionsforschung (DZIF). We acknowledge financial support by Deutsche Forschungsgemeinschaft within the funding programme Open Access Publishing, by the Baden-Württemberg Ministry of Science, Research and the Arts and by Ruprecht-Karls-Universität Heidelberg.

ACKNOWLEDGMENTS

We thank Annika Schneider and Sophia Eijkman for helpful contributions to the data analysis.

REFERENCES

Antia, R., Yates, A., and de Roode, J. C. (2008). The dynamics of acute malaria infections. I. Effect of the parasite's red blood cell preference. *Proc. Biol. Sci.* 275, 1449–1458. doi: 10.1098/rspb.2008.0198

Banerjee, R., Khandelwal, S., Kozakai, Y., Sahu, B., and Kumar, S. (2015). CD47 regulates the phagocytic clearance and replication of the *Plasmodium yoelii* malaria parasite. *Proc. Natl. Acad. Sci. U.S.A.* 112, 3062–3067. doi: 10.1073/pnas.1418144112

Bannerman, R. M. (1983). *Hematology.* London: Academic Press.

Beeson, J. G., Drew, D. R., Boyle, M. J., Feng, G., Fowkes, F. J., and Richards, J. S. (2016). Merozoite surface proteins in red blood cell invasion, immunity and vaccines against malaria. *FEMS Microbiol. Rev.* 40, 343–372. doi: 10.1093/femsre/fuw001

Berger, J. (2007). Phenylhydrazine haematotoxicity. *J. Appl. Biomed.* 5, 125–130.

Chang, K. H., and Stevenson, M. M. (2004). Malarial anaemia: mechanisms and implications of insufficient erythropoiesis during blood-stage malaria. *Int. J. Parasitol.* 34, 1501–1516. doi: 10.1016/j.ijpara.2004.10.008

Chang, K. H., Tam, M., and Stevenson, M. M. (2004). Modulation of the course and outcome of blood-stage malaria by erythropoietin-induced reticulocytosis. *J. Infect. Dis.* 189, 735–743. doi: 10.1086/381458

Clough, B., Atilola, F. A., Black, J., and Pasvol, G. (1998). *Plasmodium falciparum*: the importance of IgM in the rosetting of parasite-infected erythrocytes. *Exp. Parasitol.* 89, 129–132. doi: 10.1006/expr.1998.4275

Cox, F. E. G. (1988). *Major Animal Models in Malaria Research: Rodents.* New York, NY: Churchill Livingstone.

Cromer, D., Evans, K. J., Schofield, L., and Davenport, M. P. (2006). Preferential invasion of reticulocytes during late-stage *Plasmodium berghei* infection accounts for reduced circulating reticulocyte levels. *Int. J. Parasitol.* 36, 1389–1397. doi: 10.1016/j.ijpara.2006.07.009

Cromer, D., Stark, J., and Davenport, M. P. (2009). Low red cell production may protect against severe anemia during a malaria infection–insights from modeling. *J. Theor. Biol.* 257, 533–542. doi: 10.1016/j.jtbi.2008.12.019

De Roode, J. C. (2004). *Within-Host Competition and the Evolution of Malaria Parasites.* Ph.D. thesis, University of Edinburgh.

de Souza, J. B., Hafalla, J. C., Riley, E. M., and Couper, K. N. (2010). Cerebral malaria: why experimental murine models are required to understand the pathogenesis of disease. *Parasitology* 137, 755–772. doi: 10.1017/S0031182009991715

Dondorp, A. M., Angus, B. J., Chotivanich, K., Silamut, K., Ruangveerayuth, R., Hardeman, M. R., et al. (1999). Red blood cell deformability as a predictor of anemia in severe falciparum malaria. *Am. J. Trop. Med. Hyg.* 60, 733–737. doi: 10.4269/ajtmh.1999.60.733

Evans, K. J., Hansen, D. S., van Rooijen, N., Buckingham, L. A., and Schofield, L. (2006). Severe malarial anemia of low parasite burden in rodent models results from accelerated clearance of uninfected erythrocytes. *Blood* 107, 1192–1199. doi: 10.1182/blood-2005-08-3460

Fonseca, L. L., Alezi, H. S., Moreno, A., Barnwell, J. W., Galinski, M. R., and Voit, E. O. (2016). Quantifying the removal of red blood cells in *Macaca mulatta* during a Plasmodium coatneyi infection. *Malar. J.* 15:410. doi: 10.1186/s12936-016-1465-5

Fonseca, L. L., and Voit, E. O. (2015). Comparison of mathematical frameworks for modeling erythropoiesis in the context of malaria infection. *Math. Biosci.* 270(Pt B), 224-236. doi: 10.1016/j.mbs.2015.08.020

Franke-Fayard, B., Janse, C. J., Cunha-Rodrigues, M., Ramesar, J., Büscher, P., Que, I., et al. (2005). Murine malaria parasite sequestration: CD36 is the major receptor, but cerebral pathology is unlinked to sequestration. *Proc. Natl. Acad. Sci. U.S.A.* 102, 11468–11473. doi: 10.1073/pnas.0503386102

Ganzoni, A., Hillman, R. S., and Finch, C. A. (1969). Maturation of the macroreticulocyte. *Br. J. Haematol.* 16, 119–135. doi: 10.1111/j.1365-2141.1969.tb00384.x

Garnham, P. C. C. (1966). *Malaria Parasites and other Haemosporidia.* London: Blackwell Scientific Publishers.

Gronowicz, G., Swift, H., and Steck, T. L. (1984). Maturation of the reticulocyte *in vitro*. *J. Cell Sci.* 71, 177–197.

Gupta, S., Seydel, K., Miranda-Roman, M. A., Feintuch, C. M., Saidi, A., Kim, R. S., et al. (2017). Extensive alterations of blood metabolites in pediatric cerebral malaria. *PLoS ONE* 12:e0175686. doi: 10.1371/journal.pone.0175686

Hoffmann, A., Pfeil, J., Alfonso, J., Kurz, F. T., Sahm, F., Heiland, S., et al. (2016). Experimental cerebral malaria spreads along the rostral migratory stream. *PLoS Pathog.* 12:e1005470. doi: 10.1371/journal.ppat.1005470

Hopp, C. S., Bennett, B. L., Mishra, S., Lehmann, C., Hanson, K. K., Lin, J. W., et al. (2017). Deletion of the rodent malaria ortholog for falcipain-1 highlights differences between hepatic and blood stage merozoites. *PLoS Pathog.* 13:e1006586. doi: 10.1371/journal.ppat.1006586

Iyer, J., Grüner, A. C., Rénia, L., Snounou, G., and Preiser, P. R. (2007). Invasion of host cells by malaria parasites: a tale of two protein families. *Mol. Microbiol.* 65, 231–249. doi: 10.1111/j.1365-2958.2007.05791.x

Jain, S. K., and Hochstein, P. (1980). Membrane alterations in phenylhydrazine-induced reticulocytes. *Arch. Biochem. Biophys.* 201, 683–687. doi: 10.1016/0003-9861(80)90560-3

Kerlin, D. H., and Gatton, M. L. (2013). Preferential invasion by Plasmodium merozoites and the self-regulation of parasite burden. *PLoS ONE* 8:e57434. doi: 10.1371/journal.pone.0057434

Kim, C. H. (2010). Homeostatic and pathogenic extramedullary hematopoiesis. *J. Blood Med.* 1, 13–19. doi: 10.2147/JBM.S7224

Li, Y., Ruan, S., and Xiao, D. (2011). The within-host dynamics of malaria infection with immune response. *Math. Biosci. Eng.* 8, 999–1018. doi: 10.3934/mbe.2011.8.999

Mackey, M. C. (1997). "Mathematical models of hematopoietic cell replication and control," in *Case Studies in Mathematical Modeling - Ecology, Physiology, and Cell Biology*, eds H. G. Othmer, F. R. Adler, M. A. Lewis, and J. C. Dallon (New York, NY: Prentice-Hall), 151–181.

Mary, J. Y., Valleron, A. J., Croizat, H., and Frindel, E. (1980). Mathematical analysis of bone marrow erythropoiesis: application to C3H mouse data. *Blood Cells* 6, 241–262.

McNally, J., O'Donovan, S. M., and Dalton, J. P. (1992). Plasmodium berghei and *Plasmodium chabaudi* chabaudi: development of simple *in vitro* erythrocyte invasion assays. *Parasitology* 105(Pt 3), 355–362. doi: 10.1017/S0031182000074527

McQueen, P. G., and McKenzie, F. E. (2004). Age-structured red blood cell susceptibility and the dynamics of malaria infections. *Proc. Natl. Acad. Sci. U.S.A.* 101, 9161–9166. doi: 10.1073/pnas.0308256101

Mideo, N., Barclay, V. C., Chan, B. H., Savill, N. J., Read, A. F., and Day, T. (2008). Understanding and predicting strain-specific patterns of pathogenesis in the rodent malaria *Plasmodium chabaudi*. *Am. Nat.* 172, 214–238. doi: 10.1086/591684

Mons, B. (1990). Preferential invasion of malarial merozoites into young red blood cells. *Blood Cells* 16, 299–312.

Mons, B., Croon, J. J., van der Star, W., and van der Kaay, H. J. (1988). Erythrocytic schizogony and invasion of Plasmodium vivax *in vitro*. *Int. J. Parasitol.* 18, 307–311. doi: 10.1016/0020-7519(88)90138-5

Moreau, R., Tshikudi Malu, D., Dumais, M., Dalko, E., Gaudreault, V., Roméro, H., et al. (2012). Alterations in bone and erythropoiesis in hemolytic anemia: comparative study in bled, phenylhydrazine-treated and Plasmodium-infected mice. *PLoS ONE* 7:e46101. doi: 10.1371/journal.pone.0046101

Pasvol, G., Weatherall, D. J., and Wilson, R. J. (1980). The increased susceptibility of young red cells to invasion by the malarial parasite *Plasmodium falciparum*. *Br. J. Haematol.* 45, 285–295. doi: 10.1111/j.1365-2141.1980.tb07148.x

Ploemacher, R. E., van Soest, P. L., and Vos, O. (1977). Kinetics of erythropoiesis in the liver induced in adult mice by phenylhydrazine. *Scand. J. Haematol.* 19, 424–434. doi: 10.1111/j.1600-0609.1977.tb01497.x

Portugal, S., Drakesmith, H., and Mota, M. M. (2011). Superinfection in malaria: Plasmodium shows its iron will. *EMBO Rep.* 12, 1233–1242. doi: 10.1038/embor.2011.213

Raue, A., Kreutz, C., Maiwald, T., Bachmann, J., Schilling, M., Klingmüller, U., et al. (2009). Structural and practical identifiability analysis of partially observed dynamical models by exploiting the profile likelihood. *Bioinformatics* 25, 1923–1929. doi: 10.1093/bioinformatics/btp358

R Development Core Team (2017). *R: A Language and Environment for Statistical Computing and Graphics*. R-Project for Statistical Computing. Available online at: http://www.r-project.org

Reilly, H. B., Wang, H., Steuter, J. A., Marx, A. M., and Ferdig, M. T. (2007). Quantitative dissection of clone-specific growth rates in cultured malaria parasites. *Int. J. Parasitol.* 37, 1599–1607. doi: 10.1016/j.ijpara.2007.05.003

Savill, N. J., Chadwick, W., and Reece, S. E. (2009). Quantitative analysis of mechanisms that govern red blood cell age structure and dynamics during anaemia. *PLoS Comput. Biol.* 5:e1000416. doi: 10.1371/journal.pcbi.1000416

Sexton, A. C., Good, R. T., Hansen, D. S., D'Ombrain, M. C., Buckingham, L., Simpson, K., et al. (2004). Transcriptional profiling reveals suppressed erythropoiesis, up-regulated glycolysis, and interferon-associated responses in murine malaria. *J. Infect. Dis.* 189, 1245–1256. doi: 10.1086/382596

Seydel, K. B., Kampondeni, S. D., Valim, C., Potchen, M. J., Milner, D. A., Muwalo, F. W., et al. (2015). Brain swelling and death in children with cerebral malaria. *N. Engl. J. Med.* 372, 1126–1137. doi: 10.1056/NEJMoa1400116

Singer, I., Hadfield, R., and Lakonen, M. (1955). The influence of age on the intensity of infection with Plasmodium berghei in the rat. *J. Infect. Dis.* 97, 15–21. doi: 10.1093/infdis/97.1.15

Spivak, J. L., Toretti, D., and Dickerman, H. W. (1973). Effect of phenylhydrazine-induced hemolytic anemia on nuclear RNA polymerase activity of the mouse spleen. *Blood* 42, 257–266.

Srivastava, A., Creek, D. J., Evans, K. J., De Souza, D., Schofield, L., Müller, S., et al. (2015). Host reticulocytes provide metabolic reservoirs that can be exploited by malaria parasites. *PLoS Pathog.* 11:e1004882. doi: 10.1371/journal.ppat.1004882

Thawani, N., Tam, M., Bellemare, M. J., Bohle, D. S., Olivier, M., de Souza, J. B., et al. (2014). Plasmodium products contribute to severe malarial anemia by inhibiting erythropoietin-induced proliferation of erythroid precursors. *J. Infect. Dis.* 209, 140–149. doi: 10.1093/infdis/jit417

Villeval, J. L., Lew, A., and Metcalf, D. (1990). Changes in hemopoietic and regulator levels in mice during fatal or nonfatal malarial infections. I. Erythropoietic populations. *Exp. Parasitol.* 71, 364–374. doi: 10.1016/0014-4894(90)90062-H

Wiczling, P., and Krzyzanski, W. (2008). Flow cytometric assessment of homeostatic aging of reticulocytes in rats. *Exp. Hematol.* 36, 119–127. doi: 10.1016/j.exphem.2007.09.002

Wilson, R. J., Pasvol, G., and Weatherall, D. J. (1977). Invasion and growth of *Plasmodium falciparum* in different types of human erythrocyte. *Bull. World Health Organ.* 55, 179–186.

World Health Organization (2016). *WHO: World Malaria Report 2016*. Geneva.

7

Mathematical Analysis of Viral Replication Dynamics and Antiviral Treatment Strategies: From Basic Models to Age-Based Multi-Scale Modeling

Carolin Zitzmann and Lars Kaderali*

Institute of Bioinformatics and Center for Functional Genomics of Microbes, University Medicine Greifswald, Greifswald, Germany

Correspondence:
Carolin Zitzmann
carolin.zitzmann@uni-greifswald.de

Viral infectious diseases are a global health concern, as is evident by recent outbreaks of the middle east respiratory syndrome, Ebola virus disease, and re-emerging zika, dengue, and chikungunya fevers. Viral epidemics are a socio-economic burden that causes short- and long-term costs for disease diagnosis and treatment as well as a loss in productivity by absenteeism. These outbreaks and their socio-economic costs underline the necessity for a precise analysis of virus-host interactions, which would help to understand disease mechanisms and to develop therapeutic interventions. The combination of quantitative measurements and dynamic mathematical modeling has increased our understanding of the within-host infection dynamics and has led to important insights into viral pathogenesis, transmission, and disease progression. Furthermore, virus-host models helped to identify drug targets, to predict the treatment duration to achieve cure, and to reduce treatment costs. In this article, we review important achievements made by mathematical modeling of viral kinetics on the extracellular, intracellular, and multi-scale level for Human Immunodeficiency Virus, Hepatitis C Virus, Influenza A Virus, Ebola Virus, Dengue Virus, and Zika Virus. Herein, we focus on basic mathematical models on the population scale (so-called target cell-limited models), detailed models regarding the most important steps in the viral life cycle, and the combination of both. For this purpose, we review how mathematical modeling of viral dynamics helped to understand the virus-host interactions and disease progression or clearance. Additionally, we review different types and effects of therapeutic strategies and how mathematical modeling has been used to predict new treatment regimens.

Keywords: mathematical modeling, viral kinetics, viral replication, human immunodeficiency virus, Hepatitis C virus, Influenza A virus, antiviral therapy, immune response

INTRODUCTION

Viruses are small obligate intracellular parasites that are unable to reproduce independent of their host. Outbreaks of infectious viral diseases are a major global health concern, a circumstance that is evident by recent large epidemics of influenza, zika fever, Ebola virus disease, and the Middle East Respiratory Syndrome (MERS). According to the United Nations, the recent zika outbreak caused socio-economic costs of approximately US$7-18 billion in Latin America and the Caribbean from 2015 to 2017 (United Nations, 2017). A recent study estimated the socio-economic costs for symptomatic dengue cases (58.40 million) with US$8.9 billion in 141 countries in 2013 (Shepard et al., 2016). This number is expected to rise further in the coming years. Factors such as climate change and increasing air travel are furthermore increasing the risk of global pandemic infections; examples are recent global influenza outbreaks as much as the emergence of tropical infections such as Dengue Virus infections in previously unaffected regions in the United States and Europe (Mackey et al., 2014). To control this global threat, novel therapeutic and antiviral treatment approaches are urgently needed. To amplify the development of such novel drugs and to optimize treatment strategies, a comprehensive understanding of the viral infection dynamics, their parasitic interaction with their host, as well as host defense strategies against the invader are of major importance. In recent years, targeting viral agents that are essential for the viral replication has proven highly effective (Asselah et al., 2016). However, the emergence of resistance against these direct acting antiviral compounds leads more and more to treatment failure and multi-drug resistant viral strains (Poveda et al., 2014). In order to circumvent drug-resistance, novel antiviral strategies focus on the host by supporting the immune response or targeting host factors required for the viral life cycle. The advantage of these methods are higher barriers for the development of resistance and novel opportunity of broad-spectrum antivirals (Zeisel et al., 2013).

Mathematical modeling has proven to be a powerful tool to study viral pathogenesis and has yielded insights into the intracellular viral infection dynamics, the effect of the immune system, the evaluation of treatment strategies, and the development of drug resistance (Bonhoeffer et al., 1997; Perelson, 2002; Rong and Perelson, 2009; Perelson and Ribeiro, 2013; Boianelli et al., 2015; Perelson and Guedj, 2015; Ciupe and Heffernan, 2017). Modeling can deepen our understanding on different scales: From the molecular scale of intracellular virus-host interactions, extracellular cell-to-cell infection at the population scale, to virus spread within organs or whole organisms (Kumberger et al., 2016). In order to quantitatively study the viral growth at a molecular level and to investigate host requirements and limitations, first intracellular models have been developed for bacteriophages (Buchholtz and Schneider, 1987; Eigen et al., 1991; Endy et al., 1997), Baculovirus (Dee and Shuler, 1997), and Semliki Forest Virus (Dee et al., 1995). By studying cell-to-cell infection, early models for Human Immunodeficiency Virus (HIV) (Ho et al., 1995; Wei et al., 1995; Perelson et al., 1996, 1997; Stafford et al., 2000) provided insights into the pathogenesis, treatment strategies, and virus control by the immune system.

On the population scale, the target cell-limited model (Nowak and Bangham, 1996; Nowak et al., 1996; Bonhoeffer et al., 1997; Perelson, 2002; Wodarz and Nowak, 2002) has been extensively used to investigate the virus-host interaction of HIV, Hepatitis C Virus (HCV), and Influenza A Virus (IAV), which will be explained in this review in more detail. Furthermore, we describe the latest achievements made by modeling the dynamics of Ebola Virus (EBOV), Dengue Virus (DENV), and Zika Virus (ZIKV) that caused the most recent viral outbreaks. In addition, we give an introduction into the target cell-limited model with its extensions and applications to investigate the effects of direct antiviral therapy and immune response and highlight the most important achievements made by viral modeling of the intracellular, extracellular and the integration of both, the multi-scale level.

THE TARGET CELL-LIMITED MODEL AND ITS EXTENSIONS

Target Cell-Limited Model

The first mathematical models described the HIV progression by neglecting intracellular processes and taking only the key players of the virus-host interaction into account (Perelson et al., 1993, 1996, 1997; Ho et al., 1995; Bonhoeffer et al., 1997). The target cell-limited model (**Figure 1A**) includes three species: uninfected susceptible target cells (T), infected virus-producing cells (I), and the virus load (V) and is formulated by the following system of nonlinear ordinary differential equations (ODEs):

$$\begin{aligned} \frac{dT}{dt} &= \lambda - dT - kVT, \\ \frac{dI}{dt} &= kVT - \delta I, \\ \frac{dV}{dt} &= pI - cV. \end{aligned} \tag{1}$$

Uninfected target cells (T) are produced at a constant rate λ and die at rate d, corresponding to a target cell half-life of $t_{T_{1/2}} = \frac{\ln(2)}{d}$. By the interaction of virus (V) with uninfected target cells (T) at a constant infectivity rate k, the target cells become infected cells (I), which in turn produce infectious virus (V) with production rate p. Due to viral cytopathicity, immune elimination and/or apoptosis, infected cells (I) die at a rate δ [resulting in an infected cell half-life $t_{I_{1/2}} = \frac{\ln(2)}{\delta}$]. Virus is cleared at rate c from the cells [virion half-life $t_{V_{1/2}} = \frac{\ln(2)}{c}$] per virion by mechanisms such as immune elimination (Nowak and Bangham, 1996; Nowak et al., 1996; Bonhoeffer et al., 1997; Perelson, 2002; Wodarz and Nowak, 2002).

With average lifetimes of $1/d$, $1/\delta$, and $1/c$ for uninfected target cells, infected cells, and virus, respectively, the total number of virus particles N produced by one infected cell during

Abbreviations: AIR, Adaptive Immune Response; ART, Antiretroviral Therapy; CTL, Cytotoxic T lymphocytes; DAA, Direct-Acting Antiviral; DENV, Dengue Virus; EBOV, Ebola Virus; HAART, Highly Active Antiretroviral Therapy; HCV, Hepatitis C Virus; HIV, Human Immunodeficiency Virus; IAV, Influenza A Virus; IFN, Interferon; IIR, Innate Immune Response; NS, Nonstructural Protein; ODE, Ordinary Differential Equation; SVR, Sustained Virologic Response; WHO, World Health Organization; ZIKV, Zika Virus.

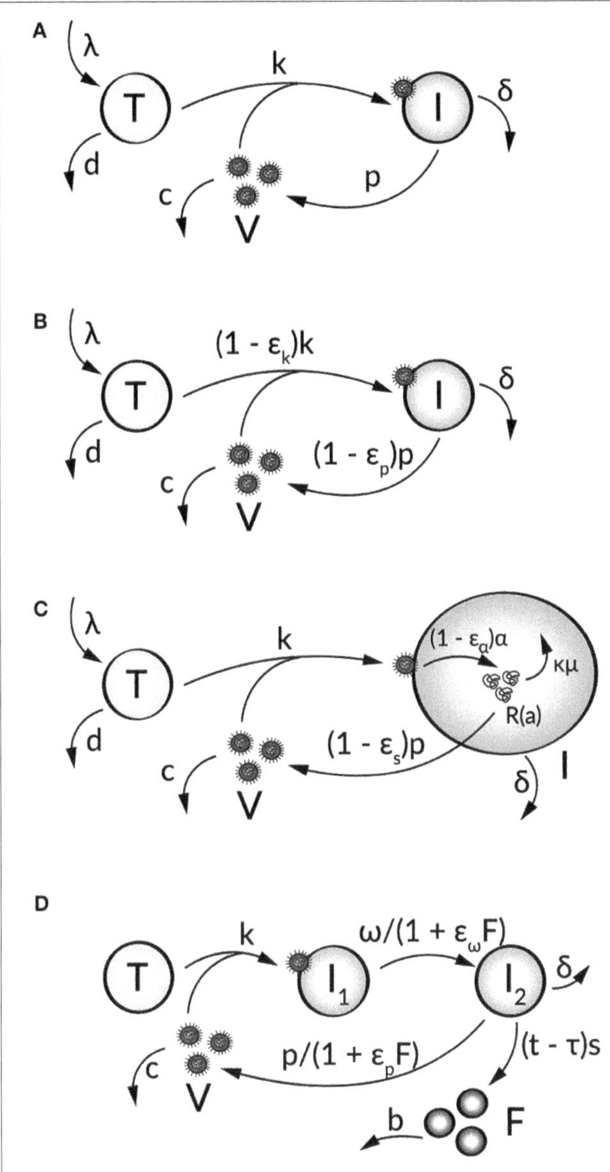

FIGURE 1 | Schematic illustration of **(A)** the target cell-limited model, **(B)** the target cell-limited model extended by antiviral inhibition, **(C)** the age-based multi-scale model, and **(D)** the target cell-limited model extended by the innate immune response.

its lifetime is calculated by p/δ. Therefore, the production rate p of one infected cell is $p = N\delta$. Without a viral infection ($I = 0$ and $V = 0$), target cells are in equilibrium with λ/d (Nowak and May, 2001; Perelson, 2002; Wodarz and Nowak, 2002).

The ability of a virus to develop an infection or to be cleared is given by the basic reproductive ratio $R_0 = \frac{\lambda kp}{d\delta c}$. R_0 represents the number of productively infected cells newly generated by one productively infected cell. With $R_0 > 1$ the infection grows due to an increase in virus-producing infected cells while $R_0 < 1$ refers to a decrease in productively infected cells and viral clearance (Nowak and May, 2001).

Target Cell-Limited Model and Antiviral Therapy

To analyze the effect of antiviral drugs that either block infection (ε_k) and/or production of viral particles (ε_p), the target cell-limited model is modified as follows (**Figure 1B**):

$$\begin{aligned}\frac{dT}{dt} &= \lambda - dT - (1 - \varepsilon_k)\, kVT,\\ \frac{dI}{dt} &= (1 - \varepsilon_k)\, kVT - \delta I,\\ \frac{dV}{dt} &= \left(1 - \varepsilon_p\right) pI - cV,\end{aligned} \tag{2}$$

with $0 \leq \varepsilon_{k,p} \leq 1$ (Neumann, 1998). Here, $\varepsilon_{k,p} = 0$ describes no drug effect while $\varepsilon_{k,p} = 1$ refers to the case of a 100% effective treatment—a perfect drug. Note that before treatment $\varepsilon_{k,p} = 0$. In simulating treatment, one assumes that the system is in steady state at treatment initiation, at which point the infection and/or production rates are modified depending on the type of antiviral drug used ($\varepsilon_k > 0$ and/or $\varepsilon_p > 0$). The overall drug efficacy ε_{tot} may be calculated as $\varepsilon_{tot} = 1-(1 - \varepsilon_k)\left(1 - \varepsilon_p\right)$, while the critical drug efficacy ε_c is given by $\varepsilon_c = 1 - \frac{d\delta c}{\lambda kp}$ and determines the transition from viral eradication to viral persistence. A successful drug therapy would clear the virus with $\varepsilon_{tot} > \varepsilon_c$ while the infection becomes chronic when $\varepsilon_{tot} < \varepsilon_c$ (Dahari et al., 2007a).

The relationship between a certain drug dose and the resulting response can be integrated into the target cell-limited model by the simple time-dependent pharmacodynamic equation

$$\varepsilon\,(t) = \frac{\varepsilon_{max} \cdot C\,(t)^n}{{EC_{50}}^n + C\,(t)^n}, \tag{3}$$

where ε_{max} describes the maximum of the drug effect, EC_{50} the drug concentration with 50% efficacy, and $C(t)$ the drug concentration or dose applied (Holford and Sheiner, 1982). Depending on the shape and steepness of the underlying drug effect, the Hill coefficient n describes either a sigmoidal curve for $n > 1$ or a hyperbolic curve otherwise. By substituting $C\,(t)$ by $C\,(t - \tau)$, a pharmacodynamic delay τ for the drug effect can be taken into account for $t > \tau$ (Holford and Sheiner, 1982; Guedj et al., 2010; Canini and Perelson, 2014).

Age-Based Multi-Scale Model for Direct Acting Antivirals

Age-based multi-scale models have been used in order to study the modes of action of antivirals within a virus-infected cell (Nelson et al., 2004; Guedj et al., 2013; Heldt et al., 2013; Clausznitzer et al., 2015). To include the effect of direct acting antivirals (DAAs), the target cell-limited model can be further extended by more detailed intracellular processes of the viral life cycle (**Figure 1C**). These multi-scale models that take the age of infected cells into account allow a biologically more realistic representation of intracellular processes with age-dependent reaction rates (Quintela et al., 2017). The target cell-limited model coupled to intracellular processes and an age-dependency is formulated as follows:

$$\frac{dT}{dt} = \lambda - dT - kTV,$$
$$\frac{\partial I}{\partial a} + \frac{\partial I}{\partial t} = \delta I(a,t), \tag{4}$$
$$\frac{\partial R}{\partial a} + \frac{\partial R}{\partial t} = (1-\varepsilon_\alpha)\alpha - \kappa\mu R - (1-\varepsilon_s)\rho R,$$
$$\frac{dV}{dt} = (1-\varepsilon_s)\rho \int_0^\infty R(a,t)I(a,t)\,da - cV,$$

with boundary and initial conditions $I(0,t) = kVT$, $I(a,0) = I_0(a)$, $R(0,a) = 1$, and $R(a,0) = R_0(a)$ (Guedj et al., 2013). Here, the intracellular viral genome (R) is produced at constant rate α and degraded at constant rate μ. The progeny virions are assembled and secreted at constant rate ρ. The drug effects regard intracellular processes or the viral genome replication: blocking viral RNA production ε_α and virion assembly/secretion ε_s, as well as increasing viral RNA degradation κ for $\kappa > 1$. Note that the intracellular viral genome [$R(a)$] and infected cells [$I(a)$] are dependent on the age a of the cell, measured as time elapsed since infection, and viral RNA levels increase with the age of the infected cell (Guedj et al., 2013; Canini and Perelson, 2014; Perelson and Guedj, 2015).

Extended Target Cell-Limited Model by the Immune Response

The innate and adaptive immune response provide various mechanisms in fighting a viral infection. The innate immune response (IIR) represents the first line of defense that recognizes the virus and triggers the adaptive immune response (AIR) (Braciale et al., 2013; Iwasaki and Medzhitov, 2013). In order to study the effect of the immune response on the viral dynamics, mathematical models incorporate key players of the immune response which inhibit processes in the viral life cycle. A further modification of the target cell-limited model has been developed to take the effect of the cell's IIR into account (**Figure 1D**). This is done by including the effect of interferon (IFN) into the model:

$$\frac{dT}{dt} = -kTV,$$
$$\frac{dI_1}{dt} = kTV - \frac{\omega}{1+\varepsilon_\omega F}I_1,$$
$$\frac{dI_2}{dt} = \frac{\omega}{1+\varepsilon_\omega F}I_1 - \delta I_2 - sI_2(t-\tau)F, \tag{5}$$
$$\frac{dV}{dt} = \frac{p}{1+\varepsilon_p F}I_2 - cV,$$
$$\frac{dF}{dt} = sI_2(t-\tau) - bF.$$

Herein, two populations of infected cells I_1 and I_2 describe a time delay. Infected but not yet virus producing cells (I_1) in the eclipse phase become productively virus producing cells (I_2) with average transition time $1/\frac{\omega}{1+\varepsilon_\omega F}$. Note that I_1 are not dying before the transition into I_2. Following a time delay τ for the IIR, IFN (F) is secreted by I_2 at constant rate s and degrades at constant rate b.

The effect of IFN has been modeled by decreasing the transition rate ω and/or the virus production rate p and effectiveness ε_ω and ε_p (Baccam et al., 2006).

Moreover, the effect of the IIR and the AIR can be coupled with the target cell-limited model by simple assumptions:

$$\frac{dT}{dt} = rD - kTV,$$
$$\frac{dI_1}{dt} = kTV - \omega I_1,$$
$$\frac{dI_2}{dt} = \omega I_1 - \delta I_2,$$
$$\frac{dD}{dt} = \delta I_2 - rD,$$
$$\frac{dV}{dt} = \frac{p}{1+\varepsilon_p R_{IIR}}I_2 - cV - \gamma kTV - hVR_{AIR}, \tag{6}$$
$$\frac{dR_{IIR}}{dt} = \psi V - bR_{IIR},$$
$$\frac{dR_{AIR}}{dt} = fV + \beta R_{AIR}.$$

In this model, the IIR (R_{IIR}) represent cytokines and recruited cells of the IIR, e.g., neutrophils and macrophages while the AIR (R_{AIR}) is represented as humoral immune response via B-cells and antibodies. With the free virus, the R_{IIR} expands at constant rate ψ and dies at constant rate b. Herein, the effect of the IIR is modeled by blocking the virus production rate p. The R_{AIR} is triggered by the virus and recruited at constant rate f. By clonal expansion at rate constant β, the R_{AIR} is activated and neutralizes the virus with constant rate h. Note that in this coupled model the dead cells D are replaced by new target cells at constant rate r that represents the regeneration of susceptible cells (Handel et al., 2010).

MODELING HIV INFECTIONS

HIV infects cells of the immune system and causes AIDS within 2–15 years post infection. In 2016, the World Health Organization (WHO) estimated that globally 36.7 million people were living with HIV with 1.8 million new infections in 2016. More than 19.5 million of these were treated with a lifelong antiretroviral therapy (ART), the current standard of care. Nowadays, the replication of HIV can be controlled and suppressed by the combination of at least three antiretroviral drugs, e.g., by reverse transcriptase inhibitors and protease inhibitors (World Health Organization, 2017b). These drugs have to be taken live-long and treatment regimens need to be adapted regularly to keep the infection under control. To date, no curative drugs and no vaccine against HIV are available.

Viral Dynamics

In the majority of cases, the infection with HIV follows a typical pattern of three different phases (**Figure 2**) (Simon and Ho, 2003; Munier and Kelleher, 2007). The first weeks post infection, the acute phase, are characterized by an exponential increase in viral load accompanied by a rapid depletion of CD4+ T cells,

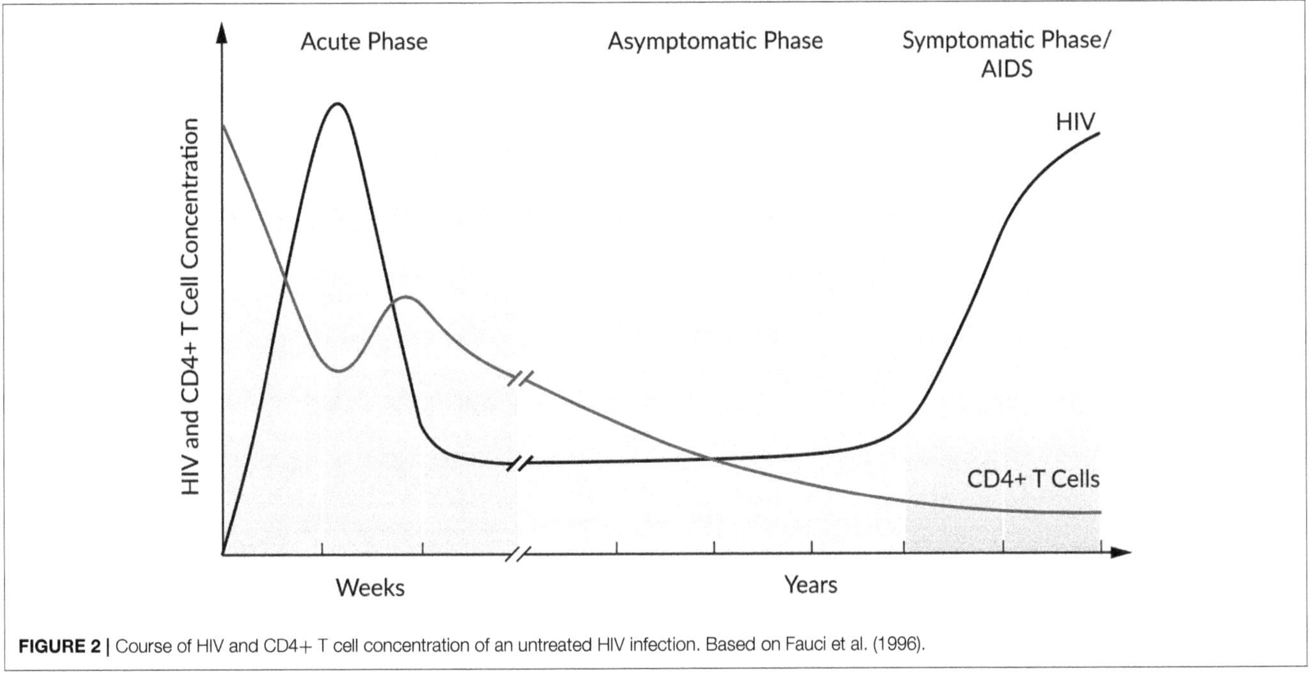

FIGURE 2 | Course of HIV and CD4+ T cell concentration of an untreated HIV infection. Based on Fauci et al. (1996).

the target cells of HIV. Soon after the infection, the immune response kicks in and initiates a decrease in viral load until a constant level, the so-called set point, is reached (Ho, 1996). Within this second asymptomatic phase, the virus persists for years while CD4+ T cells continuously and slowly decline. The third and final phase is characterized by a gradual depletion in CD4+ T cells that is correlated with a strong increase in the viral plasma concentration leading to AIDS (Alizon and Magnus, 2012; Maartens et al., 2014).

During the asymptomatic phase, the viral set point is maintained by a balance in viral clearance and the total virion production rate ($p_{total} = cV$). Therefore, a strong increase in viral load that is associated with a lower viral clearance rate indicates a stronger total viral production rate $p_{total} > cV$, while a decrease in viral load refers to a higher clearance rate, $p_{total} < cV$. Perturbations of this system equilibrium, e.g., by blocking viral production, lead to information on the rate constants and insights into the course of the viral infection and the potential of antiviral interventions (Perelson, 2002). At steady state and in the absence of ART, it has been estimated that HIV is a rapidly replicating virus that produces 10^{10} virions per day. Furthermore, a rapid virus replication also requires strong viral clearance to maintain the equilibrium (Perelson et al., 1996; Ramratnam et al., 1999).

HIV replicates in CD4+ T cells, which are represented by the target and infected cells in the target cell-limited model. With a modified target cell-limited model, Ribeiro et al. (2010) investigated the very early plasma viremia post exposure to HIV in 47 HIV-positive patients. After a time delay of 24 h where the virus became detectable (>50 RNA copies per mL), simulations have shown an initial viral doubling time of 0.65 days. Viral load peaked at 10^6 HIV RNA copies per mL after 14 days. The subsequent viral decline was characterized by a virion half-life of 1.2 days ($c = 0.6$ day^{-1}). Moreover, for this early infection stage, the authors calculated the basic reproductive ratio of $R_0 \sim 8$, indicating rapid viral spread and the necessity of an early intervention in order to reduce viral spread and to prevent development of chronicity (Ribeiro et al., 2010). By measuring the viral load in 10 HIV-positive patients for on average the first 100 days during primary infection, Stafford et al. (2000) have shown that the target cell-limited model is able to reproduce the interpatient variability within the highly dynamic initial phase post infection. The model simulations provided strong evidence that the initial viral load decline is due to a limitation in target cells with an estimated lifetime of 2.5 days ($\delta = 0.39$ day^{-1}) for infected virus-producing cells. However, the target cell-limited model was not able to mimic the data in all the patients equally well. Therefore, the authors suggested that processes not included in the model, such as an involvement of the immune response by CD8+ T cells or destruction of infected cells by cytotoxic T lymphocytes (CTL), might be associated with the stronger than predicted decrease of viral load observed in some patients (Stafford et al., 2000).

Antiretroviral Therapy

For more than 20 years, HIV-positive patients are treated with a combination of antiretroviral drugs. To analyze the effects of an antiviral treatment regimen, the target cell-limited model can be modified to include the effects of reverse transcriptase inhibitors (ε_k) that block viral infectivity (k) and protease inhibitors (ε_p) which reduce viral production (p) (Neumann, 1998). The effect of a protease inhibitor has been investigated within the first 7 days after the oral administration of Ritonavir (Perelson et al., 1996). Following a pharmacokinetic delay, the patients responded well to the Ritonavir treatment with a continuous decline in plasma viral load. In order to study the viral decline under ART,

Perelson et al. (1996) modified the target cell-limited model by the assumption that by the time of drug administration newly produced virions are non-infectious. After a pharmacokinetic delay of about 1.25 days, the model reproduced the strong decline in plasma viremia according to the Ritonavir-treated patients (**Figure 3A**). The model predicted lifetimes of 2.2 days for virus-producing infected cells and 0.3 days for virions (Perelson et al., 1996). Note that at the onset of ART, the system is assumed to be in steady state. By studying the long-term combination therapy of the protease inhibitor Nelfinavir and the reverse transcriptase inhibitors Zidovudine and Lamivudine, all the patients responded in a similar viral decline pattern (**Figure 3B**). After initiation of ART, a biphasic viral decline has been observed: a rapid initial reduction in viral load and productively infected cells (phase 1) followed by a slower decrease (phase 2). Perelson et al. (1997) integrated long-lived CD4+ T cells and latently infected lymphocytes that become productively virus-producing cells upon activation as second sources of virus into the target cell-limited model. The authors identified long-lived infected CD4+ T cells with a half-life of 14.1 days (compared to a half-life of 1.1 days of short-lived infected cells) and the continuous release of trapped virus as the main contributors for the second phase (Perelson et al., 1997). Subsequent studies have found more accurate estimates for the virion half-life with 28–110 min in HIV-positive patients under plasma apheresis (Ramratnam et al., 1999) and productively-infected CD4+ T cell half-life of 0.7 days under combination therapy (Markowitz et al., 2003). The continuous viral replication upon activation that is associated with viral persistence represents the challenge in finding a cure for HIV. Even highly active antiretroviral therapy (HAART) does not stop viral production completely, but can achieve a suppression of the viral load in plasma below levels of detection (<50 RNA copies per mL). It is assumed that the main reason for failure to achieve a cure is viral latency. At the same time, the transmission of drug-resistant virus strains is increasing, resulting in increasing treatment failure rates (Little et al., 2002).

In patients with multi-drug resistant virus, Raltegravir represents a promising new antiviral drug that inhibits integrase and hence prevents the strand transfer of proviral DNA into the host-cell genome (Steigbigel et al., 2008). Andrade et al. (2015) analyzed the effect of Raltegravir in monotherapy and in combination with the reverse transcript inhibitors Emtricitabine and Tenofovir Disoproxil Fumarate by an extended target cell-limited model that discriminates between infected cells with and without integrated viral DNA. The authors found a biphasic decline within the first phase during the first 10 days after onset of ART (**Figure 3C**). A loss in infected cells with integrated viral DNA and a half-life of ~0.8 days (in agreement with 0.7 days in Markowitz et al., 2003) has been identified as the main contributor to the first sub-phase (phase 1a). Cell loss and in addition the integration of provirus into pre-integrated infected cells have been identified as key contributors to the slower decay in the second sub-phase (phase 1b). Interestingly, the half-life of unintegrated infected cells depended strongly on the provirus integration rate and has been estimated to lie between 4 and 7 days (Andrade et al., 2015). Cardozo et al. (2017) generalized the model of Andrade et al. (2015) by taking long-lived infected cells and the effect of protease inhibitor into account in order to investigate the viral decay in presence or absence of Raltegravir therapy (Cardozo et al., 2017). Herein, the therapy containing

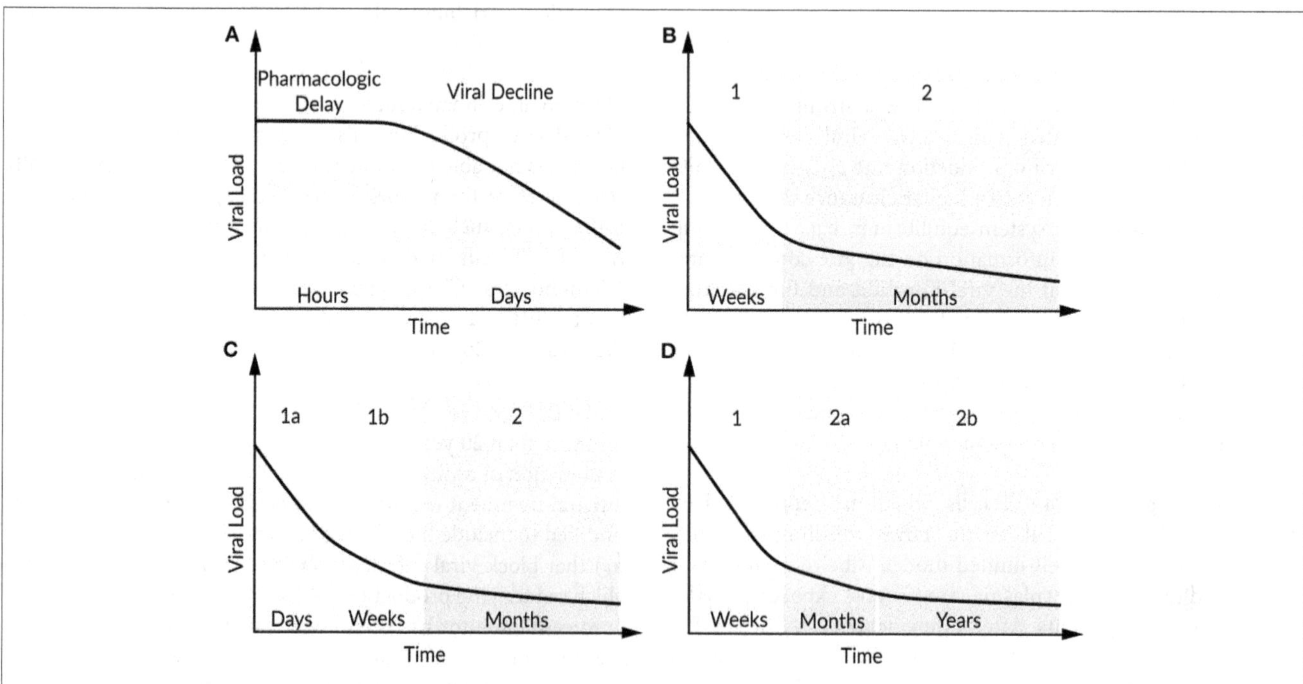

FIGURE 3 | Schematic illustration of viral load decline after onset of ART. **(A)** Viral decline following a pharmacokinetic delay, **(B)** characteristic biphasic decline (phase 1 and 2), **(C)** two sub-phases (1a and 1b) within the first phase, **(D)** two sub-phases (2a and 2b) within the second phase.

the integrase strand transfer inhibitor Raltegravir replaced as well the first phase by two sub-phases. The traditional therapy regimen without Raltegravir has shown the typical biphasic decline in viral load. Under Raltegravir therapy, the first phase was associated with the loss of short-lived cells while the second phase corresponded to the loss of long-lived cells with a half-life of ~33 days. The decline of the short-lived cell population within the first phase can be further separated by a loss of productively virus-producing cells with a half-life of ~0.8 days in sub-phase 1a and by pre-integration cells that showed a half-life of ~1.8 days. Furthermore, long-lived cells showed a shorter viral integration rate (0.05 day^{-1}) compared to short-lived cells with a viral integration rate of 2.6 day^{-1} (Cardozo et al., 2017).

Moreover, in patients under long-term ART, Palmer et al. (2008) studied a second biphasic decline within the second phase referring to two sources of viremia with persisting virus for more than 7 years (**Figure 3D**) (Palmer et al., 2008). Kim and Perelson (2006) introduced a model extended by the proliferation of latently infected CD4+ T cells without being activated (bystander proliferation) and explained the persistence of a latent reservoir (Kim and Perelson, 2006). Chomont et al. (2009) observed these results experimentally and identified two different memory T cells contributing to the long-lasting reservoir and thus the persistence of HIV for decades (Chomont et al., 2009). Therefore, an early antiretroviral intervention is necessary to limit the size of the latent reservoir.

However, to understand the effect of ART within the host cell, a comprehensive investigation of the viral life cycle is necessary. Reddy and Yin (1999) described a detailed model of the intracellular viral growth starting with reverse transcription to particle production and maturation. Their simulation results and sensitivity analysis predicted a higher monotherapeutic effect of reverse transcription inhibitors (ε_k) than protease inhibitors (ε_p). A 10-fold decrease in viral reverse transcriptase reduced the overall viral replication to <1%. Moreover, they found that the 10-fold inhibition of Rev—a regulator protein of virion production—increased the viral production, whereas a 100-fold inhibition decreased the production of virions (Reddy and Yin, 1999). These results indicate that incomplete inhibition might be compensated that might lead to adverse and unwanted effects.

As with other RNA viruses, the HIV genome is highly variable, posing its own challenges to treatment. For example, the trans-activating regulatory protein Tat controls gene expression and activates viral transcription by binding at the trans-activating response element TAR (Karn and Stoltzfus, 2012). It has been shown that point mutations in Tat may lead to more virulent HIV strains with higher stability and transcription efficiency which aggravate the development of novel antiretroviral drugs (Ronsard et al., 2014, 2017a; Ronsard, 2017b). On the other hand, Tat might be a promising vaccine candidate and has shown potential in the reduction of HIV plasma viremia associated with a reduced immune activation (Gray et al., 2016). Taking genomic variability and genetic drift of HIV under treatment into account is an important issue, and several authors have modeled the within-host evolution of HIV under selective pressure, see for example (Ribeiro and Bonhoeffer, 2000; Wodarz and Lloyd, 2004; Ball et al., 2007; Rong et al., 2007a,b; Xiao et al., 2013).

Role of CD8+ T Cells and the Latent Reservoir

Interestingly, within HIV cohort studies [VISCONTI (Goujard et al., 2012; Sáez-Ciríón et al., 2013) and SPARTAC (Salgado et al., 2011)] patients have been identified who were able to control HIV infection (<50 RNA copies per mL) after ART cessation, so-called post-treatment controllers. Moreover, there are HIV infected patients (elite controllers) which are able to control and suppress plasma viral load (<50 RNA copies per mL) naturally without ART. In HIV long-term non-progressors, significantly stronger and more complex CD8+ T cell responses associated with higher HIV directed CD8+ proliferation and more effective killing of infected CD4+ T cells have been observed (O'Connell et al., 2009). Recently, Conway and Perelson (2015) extended the target cell-limited model by CTL and latently infected CD4+ cells. Herein, for a very strong immune response, the same dynamics as in elite controllers has been observed. With respect to the size of the latent reservoir, an insufficient CTL response resulted either in viral rebound or post-treatment control. Therefore, post-treatment control after ART cessation depends strongly on a small latent reservoir. The authors suggested therapeutic vaccination to increase the strength of the CTL killing rate and latent reversing agents to decrease the size of the latent reservoir (Conway and Perelson, 2015).

Promising advances in the treatment of latent HIV have been made by an induction and clearing strategy of the latent reservoir, so-called "kick and kill." Kick refers to the activation of the HIV provirus replication of the latent reservoir, while kill refers to the clearance of reactivated cells by the immune system and/or ART (Barton et al., 2013). For example, vaccinating HIV-positive patients under HAART has shown a transient increase of CD4+ T cell killing and thus a temporary decrease of the latent reservoir (Persaud et al., 2011). Another possibility to activate HIV in latent CD4+ T cells may be achieved by Vorinostat, a histone deacetylase inhibitor. Vorinostat has been shown to be very effective in the induction of HIV transcription in resting memory CD4+ T cells in patients under ART (Archin et al., 2012). To understand the effect of Vorinostat on resting CD4+ cells and the whole latent reservoir, Ke et al. (2015) have developed mathematical models of latency under Vorinostat therapy. They could show that Vorinostat transiently activates HIV transcription but does not reduce the reservoir itself, indicating the necessity of a combination therapy (Ke et al., 2015). In 2015, HIV/AIDS disappeared from the list of the top 10 causes of deaths, indicating that substantial progress has been made by extensively investigating HIV, both experimentally and theoretically. Moreover, from 2000 to 2015 the number of people receiving ART increased from 770,000 to 18.2 million, with a projection of 30 million people on ART in 2020 (Boerma et al., 2015).

HEPATITIS C VIRUS

The blood-borne HCV is a plus-strand RNA virus that causes the acute hepatitis C infection, as well as life-threatening chronic hepatitis C-related diseases like liver cirrhosis or hepatocellular carcinoma. Worldwide, ~80 million people live with chronic hepatitis C with annually 400,000 deaths. For decades, the therapy of choice was based on standard or pegylated interferon (IFN/peg-IFN) and achieved a sustained virologic responses (SVR) between 30 and 60% for IFN and 40–65% for peg-IFN, depending on the HCV genotype and disease progression. Recently, DAAs were introduced to HCV treatment, and increased cure rates to over 90% (World Health Organization, 2016b).

Viral Dynamics

During an acute HCV infection, the viral load increases in a biphasic manner, reaching a peak of 10^5-10^7 IU per mL and is then cleared by the host immune response. However, 55–85% of HCV patients develop chronic hepatitis C with persisting virus (Hoofnagle, 2002). Thimme et al. (2001) found that the outcome of an acute infection and its correlation with HCV control is associated with a sustained CD4+ and CD8+ T cell response (Thimme et al., 2001). The biphasic increase in the plasma viral load has been characterized by a rapid viral rise followed by a slower increase, with viral doubling times in the two phases of 0.5 and 7.5 days, respectively (Major et al., 2004). In between these two phases, Dahari et al. (2005) observed a transient reduction in viremia and introduced a generalized model that allows the inhibition of virus production. Model simulations suggest that during that transient decrease of plasma viral load, the endogenous type I IFN response blocks virion production, but without controlling the HCV replication completely (Dahari et al., 2005).

Antiviral Treatment

To estimate the absolute efficacy of IFN therapy, Neumann (1998) integrated the effect of IFN-α into the target cell-limited model by inhibiting the virus production rate (p) or the *de novo* infection rate (k). After initiation of IFN-α therapy, plasma viral load declined in a similar biphasic manner as has been observed in HIV patients, with a strong first followed by a slower second decrease, resulting in persistence of HCV. Following a pharmacokinetic delay of ~9 h, this biphasic viral decline could be reproduced in the model by partial blocking of the viral production rate with $\varepsilon_p < 1$. Furthermore, the clearance of free virions (c) and therapy efficacy (ε) led to the initial rapid decline while the loss of infected cells (δ) represented the second slower phase. Due to a dose-dependent virus reduction, the authors suggested to increase IFN dosage in treatment for a better antiviral effect early in the infection. They estimated the virion half-life to be ~2.7 h ($c = 6.2$ day^{-1}) and the infected cell half-life of 1.7–70 days ($\delta = 0.14$ day^{-1}). Before the initiation of therapy, the estimated virion production and clearance rates were 10^{12} virions per day (Neumann, 1998).

In some patients, a triphasic decline with a more rapid third phase has been observed under treatment with pegylated IFN-α in monotherapy or in combination with Ribavirin. Herrmann et al. (2003) suggested the possibility that the third phase decline could be the result of an infected cell loss enhanced by immune-mediated clearance of Ribavirin (Herrmann et al., 2003). In some patients with the triphasic decline, the second phase represented a 4–28 days lasting shoulder phase where HCV was slowly decreasing or remained constant. With a modified model concerning the proliferation of uninfected and infected cells, Dahari et al. (2007b) could reproduce this triphasic pattern only if the majority of hepatocytes were assumed infected. Furthermore, an uninfected hepatocyte proliferation rate higher than the rate of infected cell loss resulted in that almost balanced shoulder phase. According to model simulations, the shoulder phase or even a biphasic viral decline are not observed if Ribavirin effects infected cell loss (δ) or inhibits the viral production rate (ε_p). The authors suggested that the rapidly decreasing third phase in patients with combination therapy of peg-IFN and Ribavirin might be explained by a mutagenic effect (Dahari et al., 2007b).

Direct Acting Antivirals

Combination therapy of peg-IFN with Ribavirin achieves a SVR in only around 50% of patients with HCV genotype 1 (Manns et al., 2001; Fried et al., 2002). With DAAs a new era began by targeting HCV-encoded proteins that are directly involved in the viral life cycle (**Figure 4**; Scheel and Rice, 2013). A combination of peg-IFN plus Ribavirin with the DAA Telaprevir—an HCV NS3/4A serine protease inhibitor—increased the SVR to around 70% (Jacobson et al., 2011). By modeling the antiviral effect of Telaprevir, Guedj and Perelson (2011) found a 4-fold higher viral decline during the second phase of the biphasic decline with Telaprevir ($\delta = 0.58$ day^{-1}) compared to the IFN-based therapy [$\delta = 0.14$ day^{-1}; Neumann, 1998]. The authors suggested a higher infected cell death as well as intracellular degradation of viral RNA as modes of action for Telaprevir (Guedj and Perelson, 2011).

Age-Based Multi-Scale Modeling

In 2010, a promising HCV NS5A inhibitor BMS-790052 (Daclatasvir; Kim et al., 2016) has been associated with a 3-log(10) reduction in viremia within the first 24 h, thus offering a highly potent drug (Gao et al., 2010). To understand and compare the mechanisms of action of Daclatasvir and IFN, Guedj et al. (2013) introduced an age-based multi-scale model by integrating intracellular processes, i.e., the antiviral effect on viral RNA replication and particle assembly/secretion, into the target cell-limited model (Equation 4, **Figure 2C**). For Daclatasvir, the model predicted a 99.0% effective blocking of viral RNA replication (ε_a) and 99.8% effective inhibition of assembly/secretion (ε_s). The viral clearance rate has been estimated as $c = 22.3$ day^{-1}, corresponding to an HCV half-life of 45 min, while the intracellular viral RNA had a half-life of on average 11 h. Compared to Daclatasvir, IFN showed a dose-dependent efficacy of 77–96% in blocking intracellular viral replication and only 39% in blocking assembly/secretion, which confirmed the IFN-mediated viral replication inhibition as the main mode of action. Interestingly, the strong antiviral effect of Daclatasvir has been observed only when efficiently blocking both, intracellular viral replication and assembly/secretion. If Daclatasvir was assumed to inhibit only the intracellular viral replication, the kinetics was comparable with that of IFN monotherapy (Guedj et al., 2013). With a similar age-based multi-scale model including intracellular viral RNA replication, viral

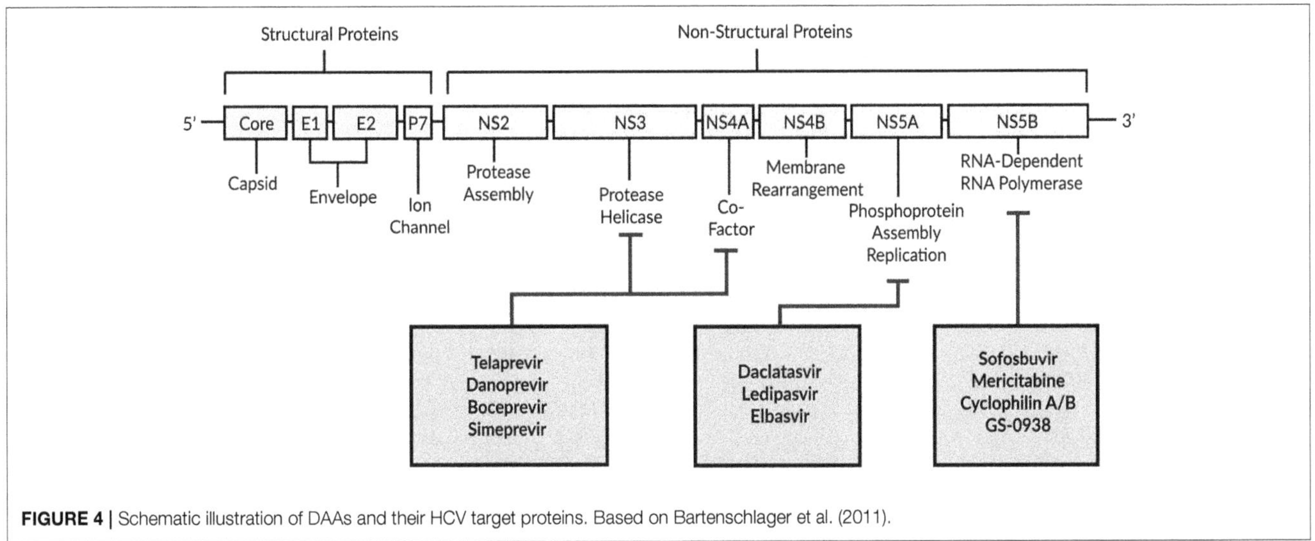

FIGURE 4 | Schematic illustration of DAAs and their HCV target proteins. Based on Bartenschlager et al. (2011).

RNA degradation, and assembly/secretion, Rong et al. (2013) investigated the antiviral effect of the HCV protease inhibitor Danoprevir. They found that Danoprevir was more efficient in inhibiting viral RNA replication (97%) and enhancing viral RNA degradation than inhibiting assembly/secretion (57%). However, for the Danoprevir monotherapy the viral clearance rate has been estimated with $c = 10.4$ day^{-1}, corresponding to a virion half-live of 1.6 h (Rong et al., 2013). The age-based multi-scale modeling strategy has shown huge potential in comparing treatment regimens and identifying modes of action of new DAAs.

IFN-Free Therapy

Regarding the severe side effects that have been reported with IFN-based therapy (Heim, 2013) and the improved therapeutic response to DAAs, an IFN-free therapy became more and more desirable. Patients treated with the DAA Mericitabine, a nucleoside NS5B HCV polymerase inhibitor, have shown a slower initial viral decline (phase 1) compared to, e.g., the IFN-based therapy, NS5A or non-nucleoside NS5B inhibitors. However, in 40% of the patients, a slow but monophasic viral decline has been observed within the 14 days of Mericitabine treatment. Model predictions have shown that Mericitabine blocks effective viral production whereas the efficacy increases with the accumulation of intracellular phosphates (Guedj et al., 2012). However, a faster initial decline compared to Mericitabine but slower than for other DAAs has been found by evaluating the efficacy of single and co-treatment with the nucleoside HCV NS5B polymerase inhibitors Sofosbuvir and GS-0938. By comparing mono and combination therapy of DAAs of the same family, it was shown that both drugs alone were highly effective and only minor more effective in combination, suggesting an antiviral combination therapy with DAAs of different families (Guedj et al., 2014).

Clinical trials investigating the combination of Sofosbuvir with Ledipasvir (an HCV NS5A inhibitor) with and without Ribavirin have proven highly effective and safe with a SVR >90% (Afdhal et al., 2014a,b; Kowdley et al., 2014). Using a mathematical model, Dahari et al. (2016) analyzed the curing time of Sofosbuvir in combination with either Daclatasvir, Simeprevir, or Ledipasvir within a 12-week treatment duration in 58 patients with chronic hepatitis C. Their simulations show that 98% of patients achieved a SVR with less than one remaining hepatitis C virion. Interestingly, after 6 weeks of treatment, 100% of patients have shown viral loads <15 IU per mL and no detectable virions in 91% of patients. Additionally, the model predicted that therapy could be shortened in more than 80% of the patients, resulting in a reduce in medication costs by 16–20% (Dahari et al., 2016).

Host Factor Targeting and Intracellular Models

A limitation of the DAA-based therapy is the possibility of developing viral resistance, i.e., emergence of drug-escaping variants dependent on patient groups, HCV genotype, and treatment regimen (Pawlotsky, 2016). In patients treated with Telaprevir over a period of 14-days, Kieffer et al. (2007) found not only an increase in plasma viral load, but also an increase in drug-resistant variants, which replaced the wild-type HCV almost completely at day 15 (Kieffer et al., 2007). Therefore, attention must be paid to finding an effective therapy regimen so that development of drug resistance is avoided. Another alternative treatment strategy is to not directly target the virus, but rather aim for cellular co-factors, since the virus depends strongly on the living host cell for efficient replication. As an example, Cyclophilin B has been identified as a cellular factor modulating the RNA binding activity to HCV NS5B polymerase and thus regulating the HCV replication (Watashi et al., 2005). Liu et al. (2009) reported an interaction of Cyclophilin A and the HCV NS5B polymerase, and predicted that Cyclophilin A as a major key host factor for an active replicase (Liu et al., 2009). Cyclophilin inhibitors such as Alisporivir (Gallay and Lin, 2013), SCY-635 (Hopkins et al., 2012), and NIM 88 (Lawitz et al., 2011) have confirmed the potential in disrupting the HCV replication. This and other findings on host factors have proven how important a detailed understanding of the HCV life cycle and the host interaction is.

To characterize the intracellular viral replication in more detail, Dahari et al. (2007c) developed a detailed mathematical model investigating the single steps of intracellular RNA replication. The model with cytoplasmic translation and RNA replication within a replication compartment has shown that HCV regulates the plus-strand to the minus-strand relation by a strand-specific affinity of HCV NS5B polymerase. Additionally, the authors have shown that the virus benefits from encapsulating its genome replication inside membranous replication sites (Dahari et al., 2007c). Using an extended model and based on detailed measurements of the initial replication kinetics, Binder et al. (2013) mimicked the highly dynamic initial phase within the first hours post infection until steady state of minus-strand RNA, plus-strand RNA, and protein activity. An important finding of this model is the role of the protective replication compartment in which HCV replicates its genome. On the one hand, this compartment appears to protect the virus from antiviral mechanisms and is required for the establishment of a successful replication, on the other hand, this compartment also seems to limit viral growth and thus exerts tight control over the viral dynamics. By the integration of host factors into the model, the authors showed that cellular co-factors that are involved in the formation of the membranous replication sites and the initiation of minus-strand synthesis are responsible for differences in replication efficacy in different cell lines (Binder et al., 2013).

Recently, Benzine et al. (2017) have estimated the half-lives of the replicase complex (a complex of viral and cellular proteins associated with viral genome synthesis) in slowly and rapidly replicating HCV strains. Their mathematical model distinguishes between different viral plus-strand RNA genomes—RNA associated with translation, RNA responsible for RNA synthesis in the membranous web and the replicase complex, as well as RNA that is assembled and packed into virions. The authors estimated replicase complex half-lives of 3.5 h for the fast replicating strain and 9.9 h for the slow replicating strain and speculated that differences in the amino-acids in non-structural (NS) proteins that are responsible for replicase complex formation as well as the interactions with each other or host proteins are underlying the observed differences in half-lives. Furthermore, the antiviral efficacy has been integrated by the effect of the NS5A inhibitor Elbasvir, the NS5B inhibitor Sofosbuvir, and Compound 23. Sofosbuvir inhibits the plus- and minus-strand synthesis, Elbasvir blocks the formation of new replicase complexes and the viral assembly while Compound 23 inhibits the formation of replicase complexes. For the slowly replicating strains, the model predicted that by blocking viral assembly, the RNA is increasingly used for translation while that redirection was very low in fast replicating viral strains (Benzine et al., 2017).

Clausznitzer et al. (2015) developed a multi-scale model combining the target cell-limited model with detailed intracellular replication to investigate the specific effect of Daclatasvir that targets HCV NS5A within the first 2 days post drug administration. For Daclatasvir, the exact mode of action is still unknown. The authors compared different putative mechanisms concerning the initial and long-term dynamics. Blocking viral replication affected the long-term dynamics, while blocking viral assembly/secretion had an effect on the initial and the long-term dynamics. Interestingly, a complete inhibition of viral assembly/secretion did not eradicate the virus. Additionally, it has been shown that the host factor affected the long-term dynamics and represented the main parameter in individual differences in the viral replication efficacy (Clausznitzer et al., 2015).

In a mouse model, Mailly et al. (2015) have shown that the inhibition of Claudin1-mediated viral entry by Claudin1-specific monoclonal antibodies has shown highly effective in preventing HCV infection without the emergence of resistance. By using the target cell-limited model that has been extended by the effect of monoclonal antibodies which inhibit the *de novo* infection rate (k), the model predicted the clearance of infected cells and the prevention of new infection (Mailly et al., 2015). Thus, the inhibition of cellular co-factors that mediate viral entry might be a promising strategy to prevent and eradicate HCV.

INFLUENZA VIRUS

The seasonal influenza is an acute infection of the respiratory tract caused by influenza virus of types A, B, and C. Annually, on average 3–5 million people worldwide are infected. The disease is often associated with severe symptoms and leads to 250,000–500,000 deaths per year. Two classes of antiviral drugs are available against influenza: neuraminidase inhibitors and M2 proton channel blockers. However, the most effective strategy against a seasonal influenza infection is the prevention by a vaccination, which has been proven to be safe and effective for more than 60 years (World Health Organization, 2017c).

Viral Dynamics and Immune Response

The course of infection with IAV is characterized by an exponential growth of viral load, reaching its maximum 2 days post infection (**Figure 5**). Within the following days, the viral load declines until the virus becomes undetectable within 6–8 days post infection (Wright et al., 2013). Baccam et al. (2006) modified the target cell-limited model, taking the rapid dynamics of IAV into account. Their model neglects the regeneration and death of target cells (Baccam et al., 2006). With the assumption that progeny virus is undetectable within the first 6–8 h (Sedmak and Grossberg, 1973), an eclipse phase was incorporated into the model that characterized the time delay from cell infection to virus production. In order to model the eclipse phase, the authors introduced two different infected cell populations: not yet virus producing infected cells that are in the eclipse phase (I_1) and actively virus producing infected cells (I_2, Equation 5). With data of patients experimentally infected with IAV, mathematical models with and without the eclipse phase have been analyzed. The authors could show that both models fit the patient data equally well, whereas the eclipse phase model estimated biologically more reasonable parameters with a half-life of free virion of 3.2 h. Furthermore, after a 6 h delay, the

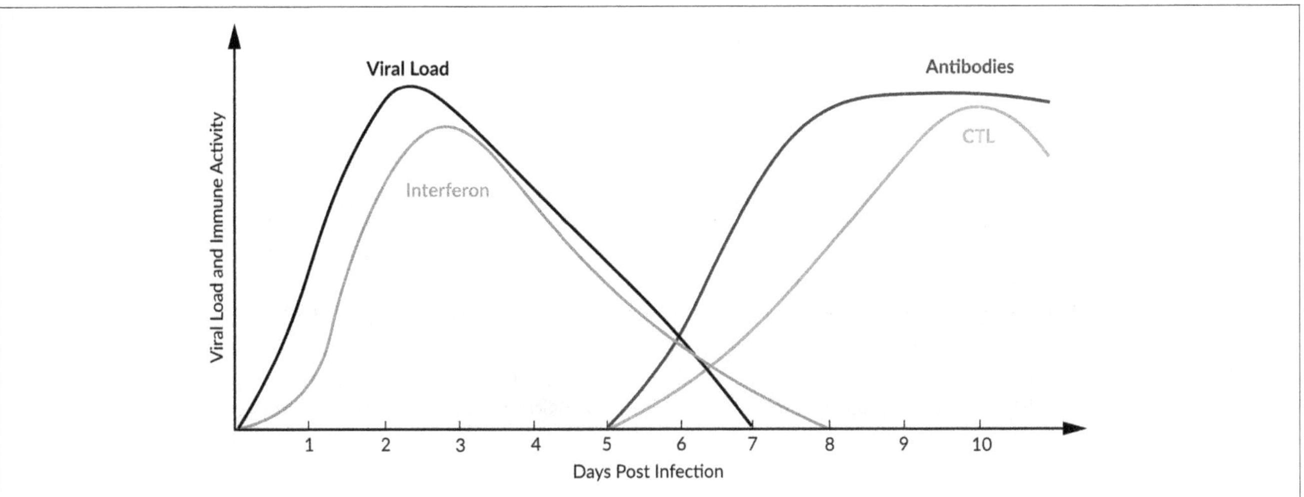

FIGURE 5 | Course of an IAV infection (viral load), the innate immune response (interferon), and the adaptive immune response (antibodies and CTL). Inspired by Beauchemin and Handel (2011) and Wright et al. (2013).

infected cells are producing virus for about 5 h, leading to an average lifetime of about 11 h for infected cells. Additionally, the authors calculated the basic reproductive ratio $R_0 \sim 22$ indicating a rapid viral spread ($R_0 \gg 1$) where 1 cell infects ~ 22 other epithelial cells in the upper respiratory tract, suggesting that an early initiation of treatment is crucial. Interestingly, in 50% of the patients a second peak in viral load has been observed. By extending the target cell-limited model by the effect of IFN (Equation 5), the second peak might be explained by a decreasing antiviral effect of IFN (Baccam et al., 2006).

During IAV infection, IFN is detectable 24 h post infection reaching a maximum after 72–96 h (Roberts et al., 1979). IFN plays a major role in the inhibition of viral infection and establishing an antiviral state (Samuel, 2001). In turn, the IAV protein NS1 has been identified as an IFN antagonist that circumvent the IFN-mediated antiviral response and correlates with pathogenicity (Garcia-Sastre et al., 1998). Saenz et al. (2010) extended the target cell-limited model by the regulation of the IIR. Herein, IFN is released by infected cells which induce an antiviral state by turning target cells into refractory cells. Model predictions demonstrated the major role of IFN in controlling early infection by protecting target cells (Saenz et al., 2010).

To capture the interaction of IAV with the IIR and AIR, Pawelek et al. (2012) included an antiviral state by refractory cells, as well as an IFN-induced infected cell killing into the target cell-limited model. The authors have shown that the early viral infection might be controlled by target cell depletion. The rapid viral post-peak decline could be explained by the enhanced infected cell killing mediated by cytokines, natural killer cells, or other cells activated by IFN. Moreover, the authors were able to mimic the bimodal pattern with a rebound of plasma viral load observed in 50% of the patients (Baccam et al., 2006). They assume that this second peak is due to a loss of the antiviral effect of IFN leading to a recovery of target cells (Pawelek et al., 2012). By comparing the dynamics of four different IAV strains in a mouse model, Manchanda et al. (2014) have shown a strain-specific rebound in viremia leading to a second peak. Furthermore, model predictions explained the rebound by persistent inflammation that correlated with disease severity (Manchanda et al., 2014).

The AIR is mainly mediated by CTLs and antibodies which appear at day 5 after primary infection and at day 3 after reinfection, resulting in a faster memory cell-mediated secondary response (Tamura and Kurata, 2004). Handel et al. (2010) extended the target cell-limited model by simple defense mechanisms of immune mediators, e.g., inflammatory cytokines, as well as antibodies or CTLs (Equation 6). It has been shown that the models with either antibody (killing of free virions) or the CTL-mediated immune response (killing of infected cells) fit the data equally well. A distinction of the underlying mechanisms of the AIR was not possible with the available data (Handel et al., 2010). Miao et al. (2010) combined CTL and antibodies, IgG and IgM, within a mathematical model and confirmed the necessity of CTL and IgM in infection clearance, leading to average half-lives for infected cells of $\sim$0.5 days and for free virions of $\sim$1.8 min. In the absence of an AIR (days 0–5), the half-lives for infected cells have been estimated with $\sim$1.2 days and for free virions $\sim$4 h. Furthermore, the model predicted the contribution of CTLs in killing infected cells while mainly IgM cleared the viral load. Due to a low contribution of IgG in primary infection clearance, the authors suggested a role of IgG together with CD4+ T cells in generating a memory and therefore a second immune response (Miao et al., 2010).

Risk Factor Age

The recommended prevention of an influenza infection is a vaccination that reduces severity, complications, and deaths especially in elderly. However, due to a lower antibody response in elderly (age >65 years) the vaccine efficacy is only 17–53% compared with 70–90% in young adults (Goodwin et al., 2006). Hernandez-Vargas et al. (2014) studied the impact of age on the immune response to the course of IAV infection and have shown a limited stimulation of the adaptive immune cells that led to a reduced viral growth with a 1.5 lower R_0 in immune naïve aged mice. Additionally, a delayed (1–2 days) infection clearance correlated with a delayed increase of CD8+ T cells in aged mice, indicating a key role of CD8+ T cells in infection clearance. Therefore, the 10-fold lower viral burden might trigger the immune response insufficiently, explaining the striking difference between infection control and viral titers in elderly and young mice (Hernandez-Vargas et al., 2014). However, these experimental results and modeling predictions are valid for immune naïve aged mice. To study the efficacy of vaccination in elderly, the validation of these results in humans would be appropriate, but is obviously more complicated.

Modeling the effect of CD8+ T cell populations to recurrent IAV infections, Zarnitsyna et al. (2016) have shown that an increase in CD8+ T cell levels led to a decreased viral load and a shorter recovery time. The model of Cao et al. (2016) confirmed the relationship of a faster recovery with an increased level of effector CD8+ T cells. Thus, the induction of CD8+ T cells might be a promising vaccination strategy instead of boosting the antibody response that might lead to antigenic mutations and constantly evolving new influenza strains (Cao et al., 2016; Zarnitsyna et al., 2016).

Antiviral Drugs

The effect of Amantadine, an antiviral agent acting as an M2 ion channel blocker, has been included into the eclipse model (Baccam et al., 2006) by affecting the infection rate (k) of target cells by virions. The authors show that the maximum drug efficacy for Amantadine is only 74%, this can be explained by a possible rapid development of drug resistance. For the characterization of the viral dynamics under Adamantane treatment (e.g., Amantadine), it is therefore important to take the emergence of drug-resistance into account (Beauchemin et al., 2008).

Canini et al. (2014) investigated the effect of Oseltamivir (a neuraminidase inhibitor) using a model combining antiviral treatment regimen, IIR, and AIR, as well as a scoring system for symptoms, and the emergence of drug resistance as a random event. The authors show that the prophylactic use (pre-symptomatic phase) of Oseltamivir in low doses may cause a 27% higher emergence of drug resistance during the incubation period, due to an insufficient AIR, e.g., by natural killer cells. The initiation and duration of treatment, drug doses, as well as treatment frequency have been identified as crucial factors for the emergence of drug resistance (Canini et al., 2014). Kamal et al. (2015) studied the time course of influenza infection with and without Oseltamivir that had an effect on the virion production rate by inhibiting the release of newly produced virions (viral shedding). They have shown that a sooner initiation of Oseltamivir treatment correlates with a decreased viral secretion duration. By investigating the effect of a combined treatment, they found that the effect of Oseltamivir together with an antiviral drug affecting viral clearance had significant better effects reducing viral load, regardless of the onset of therapy (Kamal et al., 2015).

Heldt et al. (2013) developed an age-based multi-scale model combining the viral life cycle with cell-to-cell transmission with the aim to investigate the effect of DAAs. The authors found the most promising antiviral strategy by interfering with viral transcription, replication, protein synthesis, nuclear export, and assembly/secretion, while inhibiting early steps in replication—virus entry—caused only a delayed virus production. They additionally showed that some drugs could in fact increase the virus production, indicating how important a detailed understanding of the dynamic events in the virus life cycle is (Heldt et al., 2013). Schelker et al. (2016) investigated early events in the viral life cycle within a 3D diffusion modeling approach that identified the time point of endocytosis and the distance of diffusion to the nucleus as a bottleneck, supporting cytosolic degradation as limiting factors for efficient virus replication (Schelker et al., 2016).

OTHER VIRUSES

Ebola Virus

From 2013 on, EBOV of the type Zaire has caused the largest outbreak to date in West Africa with reported 29,000 disease cases and 11,000 deaths. An untreated acute Ebola infection causes severe illness with a fatality rate of on average 50% (World Health Organization, 2017a). EBOV is a negative-stranded RNA virus that replicates in immune cells, with the ability to persist in immune-privileged sites such as the central nervous system and may thus lead to viral relapse (Jacobs et al., 2016). No specific treatment is currently available, but recently a clinical trial with a newly developed vaccine (rVSV-ZEBOV) has shown to be highly protective against the Ebola disease (Henao-Restrepo et al., 2017).

To capture the Ebola infection dynamics, Nguyen et al. (2015) used the target cell-limited model and compared EBOV to pandemic IAV. EBOV infection time is significantly slower than IAV infection time (9.5 h vs. 30–80 min) (Holder et al., 2011; Pinilla et al., 2012; Nguyen et al., 2015). Furthermore, the viral replication rate has been estimated as $\sim$63 ffu/mL day^{-1} cell^{-1}, EBOV is hence highly efficient with a virion half-live of $\sim$23 h ($c = 1.05$ day^{-1}) (Nguyen et al., 2015). Unfortunately, these results are uncertain due to parameter identifiability problems. Nonetheless, the target cell-limited model confirmed the viral growth seen in experimental data, starting at day 3 post infection with a complete target cell depletion at day 6. Madelain et al. (2015) extended the target cell-limited model by an eclipse phase (non-/virus-producing infected cells) and found a half-life for virus-producing infected cells of 6.4 h and a basic reproductive ratio of $R_0 \sim 9$. The authors furthermore studied the antiviral effect in mice treated with Favipiravir, an antiviral drug that blocks the RNA-dependent RNA polymerase in a broad spectrum of RNA viruses (Furuta et al., 2013). By inhibiting the virus production rate p, they found a sharp decrease in viral load that was associated with an increasing drug efficacy of 95, 98.5, and 99.6% at days 2, 3, and 6 after the onset of treatment. Since Favipiravir achieves its maximal efficacy after 3 days, an early treatment initiation is suggested (Madelain et al., 2015). With patient data of survivors and fatalities from the Uganda Ebola disease outbreak in 2000/2001, Martyushev et al. (2016)

studied the relationship between virus replication and disease severity. For this purpose, they extended the target cell-limited model by two target cell populations: potential target cells (T_2), that are recruited via proinflammatory cytokines (e.g., recruited macrophages, hepatocytes, splenocytes, and endotheliocytes), which become susceptible target cells (T_1), that are the primary target for viral replication (e.g., macrophages and dendritic cells). Ebola disease severity is described by a 2 log(10) higher plasma viral load, that is correlated with an extensive recruitment of potential target cells and a 2.2-fold higher basic reproductive ratio; $R_0 \sim 6$ for fatal cases and $R_0 \sim 2.8$ for nonfatal cases. Hence, the higher viral load in fatal cases and a massive infection/hypersecretion of cytokines by active virus-producing replication cells is associated with the potential severity of the Ebola disease (Wauquier et al., 2010; Martyushev et al., 2016). Additionally, antiviral intervention of (i) an antibody-based therapy that affects the *de novo* infection (k), (ii) a siRNA-based treatment that blocks viral production (p), and (iii) a nucleoside analog-based therapy (e.g., Favipiravir) have been evaluated in mono- and combination therapy. The combination of nucleoside analog-based therapy and siRNA-based turned out to be most efficient if initiated 4 days post symptom onset, while the antibody-based therapy seemed insufficient (Martyushev et al., 2016). The authors then demonstrated that a critical inhibition rate of 80.5% in fatal cases and 58.5% in nonfatal cases is needed to prevent fatal outcomes of the Ebola virus disease.

Dengue Virus

The DENV is a positive-stranded RNA virus, infecting annually 390 million people worldwide. DENV is spread mainly by the mosquitos *Aedes aegypty* and *Aedes albopictus*, which also transmit Chikungunya Virus, Yellow Fever Virus, and ZIKV. There are four serotypes of DENV, causing flu-like illness occasionally associated with severe complications like hemorrhagic fever. A cleared dengue infection provides a serotype-specific lifelong immunization, while secondary infections with another serotype can result in severe dengue disease. Currently, there is no antiviral treatment available, but a recently developed dengue vaccine (CYD-TDV; Villar et al., 2015) is suggested for endemic regions (World Health Organization, 2016a).

To explain inter-individual differences in DENV infection dynamics, Clapham et al. (2014) extended the target cell-limited model by a simple AIR. Moreover, differences between primary and secondary infection could be explained by the variations in the immune response. For a secondary infection, the immune response-related parameters have shown higher values, e.g., the immune cell proliferation rate and the virus clearance rate. Interestingly, the infectivity rate constant (k) has also reached higher values in a secondary infection compared to a primary infection, supporting the hypothesis of antibody-dependent enhancement where antibodies mediate virus entry and thus increase the viral infectivity in a secondary infection (Clapham et al., 2014). In a subsequent study, Clapham et al. (2016) investigated the antibody dynamics within a target cell-limited model predicting the role of IgM and IgG in the course of a dengue infection. They showed that a primary infection was mainly cleared by IgM while a secondary infection was cleared by IgG and IgM. These results refer to the key role of IgM in DENV infection clearance. Furthermore, best fitting results have been found by assuming that antibodies directly neutralize free virus compared to a clearance of infected cells, e.g., via antibody-dependent cell cytotoxicity. However, model predictions have shown a short life-span of infected cells with 0.3 days referring to additional immune-mediated clearance mechanisms (Clapham et al., 2016).

Ben-Shachar and Koelle (2014) developed a series of within-host dengue models integrating key players of the IIR and AIR in order to investigate the viral dynamics and development of severe dengue disease. They extended the target cell-limited model only by the IIR and were able to reproduce the viral dynamics in primary infection. Furthermore, they showed that higher rate constants for infectivity (k; evidence for antibody-dependent enhancement) and infected cell death (δ; evidence for T cell response with increasing severity) were necessary to mimic the viral dynamics of a secondary infection (Ben-Shachar and Koelle, 2014). Recently, Ben-Shachar et al. (2016) refined these results by investigating serotype-specific differences. The higher infectivity rate constants (k) estimated for DENV-2 and DENV-3 compared to DENV-1 in their model were consistent with varying replication efficacy of different dengue serotypes (Ben-Shachar et al., 2016).

With a population-based delay model coupled to the IIR, Schmid et al. (2015) studied the attenuated viral spread of a DENV mutant that is proposed as a vaccine candidate. In their work, they show that the DENV mutant has a faster IFN activation and production which establishes an antiviral state in infected cells and leads to an 8-fold decreased viral production and spread compared to the wildtype DENV. Furthermore, their model shows a stronger impact of the autocrine IFN in comparison to the paracrine effect on reducing viral spread (Schmid et al., 2015).

Zika Virus

ZIKV is a plus-stranded RNA virus that is mainly carried and transmitted by *Aedes* mosquitos, but sexual transmission has as well been reported (Foy et al., 2011; Musso et al., 2015; D'Ortenzio et al., 2016). Human infections with ZIKV usually cause only mild disease with similar symptoms as seen in DENV infections. However, during the recent outbreak in Brazil with estimated 440,000–1,300,000 Zika cases (Heukelbach et al., 2016), ZIKV has been associated with neurologic complications such as Guillain-Barré syndrome and fetal microcephaly (World Health Organization, 2017d).

Recently, Best et al. (2017) developed a series of models with and without incorporation of the immune response and fitted those to plasma viral load data of ZIKV-infected nonhuman primates. Within that model series, the target cell-limited model only extended by an eclipse phase that distinguishes between non-actively and actively virus-producing infected cells was the best-suited model to reproduce the data. Furthermore, the incorporation of key players of the IIR or AIR, e.g., by IFN or natural killer cells, respectively, did not improve the model fitting and thus has been neglected. The simple eclipse phase model estimated an eclipse phase of ~4 h (already observed via modeling in Osuna et al., 2016) and a basic reproductive ratio of $R_0 \sim 10.7$. The degradation rate of productively infected cells was estimated with $\delta = 4.5$ day^{-1}, corresponding to a lifetime of ~5 h. The authors furthermore included the effect of antiviral therapy by inhibition of the viral production rate. With the broad spectrum RNA polymerase inhibitor Favipiravir, the time to undetectable plasma viremia could be reduced by 2 days if the initiation of therapy starts at the time point of infection ($t = 0$ days post infection). The therapy initiation at day 2 post infection led to the same result compared to no drug treatment, leading to undetectable plasma viral load after 5 days post infection (Best et al., 2017). By integrating the immune response via IFN and neutralizing antibodies into the eclipse phase model, Aid et al. (2017) found a positive effect of both in controlling the viral infection in the periphery. The overall best fit was achieved by initiating IFN response at day 1.5 while the activity of neutralizing antibodies started at day 6 (Aid et al., 2017).

CONCLUSION

For more than 20 years, the population-based target cell-limited model has been used to describe the dynamics of a variety of viruses. The interdisciplinary research combining experimental measurements and mathematical modeling improved our understanding of virus-host interactions and helped to quantify key parameters of the viral life cycle. Simple mathematical models allowed the investigation of the circumstances that lead to viral eradication or the development of chronic infections with an equilibrium of virus production and immune-mediated clearance. Studying antiviral drug treatments with the target cell-limited model enabled the identification of drug efficacy and modes of action. Moreover, simple extensions of the model led to insights into the different patterns of viral decline during drug treatment and the evaluation of different treatment regimens. By taking the immune system into account, mathematical modeling helped to identify the key players for viral clearance.

A comprehensive and quantitative, dynamic understanding of virus-host interactions is vital for advances in antiviral therapy, and can be achieved by modeling the entire viral life cycle from virus entry to particle production. This would support not only the prediction of more precise modes of action of DAAs, it would also help to identify and evaluate new treatment opportunities or the potential of broad-spectrum antiviral drugs. Drugs that interact directly with viral proteins have shown enormous potential, but may lead to the emergence of virus strain mutations, multi-drug resistance, and treatment failure. Therefore, future research might focus more on resistance free antiviral drugs, e.g., by targeting host factors or by the prevention of viral diseases with vaccination. To support knowledge-based design of such drugs and vaccines, a more comprehensive view of the immune response to viral infections is necessary. Regarding the complex interplay of the first line of defense by the IIR and the establishment of an immune response memory by the AIR, questions arise how the virus hides and circumvents the immune response or why some patients are able to clear an infection that would develop to chronic infection in the majority of patients.

Furthermore, modeling techniques may consider not only the time-dependent dynamics but focus as well more on the spatial scale. By combining time and space scales, agent-based models may help to characterize viral spread in tissue, within organs or in the whole human body. Additionally, the complex interplay between the virus and the immune system may be studied by agent-based models with relatively simple rules (Bauer et al., 2009; Graw and Perelson, 2015; Kumberger et al., 2016). Mathematical modeling addressed important questions concerning the virus-host interactions and may contribute to answering open questions.

AUTHOR CONTRIBUTIONS

All authors listed have made a substantial, direct and intellectual contribution to the work, and approved it for publication.

FUNDING

LK received funding from the BMBF through the ERASysAPP project SysVirDrug (031A602A).

REFERENCES

Afdhal, N., Reddy, K. R., Nelson, D. R., Lawitz, E., Gordon, S. C., Schiff, E., et al. (2014a). Ledipasvir and sofosbuvir for previously treated HCV genotype 1 infection. *N. Engl. J. Med.* 370, 1483–1493. doi: 10.1056/NEJMoa1316366

Afdhal, N., Zeuzem, S., Kwo, P., Chojkier, M., Gitlin, N., Puoti, M., et al. (2014b). Ledipasvir and sofosbuvir for untreated HCV genotype 1 infection. *N. Engl. J. Med.* 370, 1889–1898. doi: 10.1056/NEJMoa1402454

Aid, M., Abbink, P., Larocca, R. A., Boyd, M., Nityanandam, R., Nanayakkara, O., et al. (2017). Zika virus persistence in the central nervous system and lymph nodes of rhesus monkeys. *Cell* 169, 610–620.e14. doi: 10.1016/j.cell.2017.04.008

Alizon, S., and Magnus, C. (2012). Modelling the course of an HIV infection: insights from ecology and evolution. *Viruses* 4, 1984–2013. doi: 10.3390/v4101984

Andrade, A., Guedj, J., Rosenkranz, S. L., Lu, D., Mellors, J., Kuritzkes, D. R., et al. (2015). Early HIV RNA decay during raltegravir-containing regimens exhibits two distinct subphases (1a and 1b). *AIDS* 29, 2419–2426. doi: 10.1097/QAD.0000000000000843

Archin, N. M., Liberty, A. L., Kashuba, A. D., Choudhary, S. K., Kuruc, J. D., Crooks, A. M., et al. (2012). Administration of vorinostat disrupts HIV-1 latency in patients on antiretroviral therapy. *Nature* 487, 482–485. doi: 10.1038/nature11286

Asselah, T., Boyer, N., Saadoun, D., Martinot-Peignoux, M., and Marcellin, P. (2016). Direct-acting antivirals for the treatment of hepatitis C virus infection: optimizing current IFN-free treatment and future perspectives. *Liver Int.* 36, 47–57. doi: 10.1111/liv.13027

Baccam, P., Beauchemin, C., Macken, C. A., Hayden, F. G., and Perelson, A. S. (2006). Kinetics of influenza A virus infection in humans. *J. Virol.* 80, 7590–7599. doi: 10.1128/JVI.01623-05

Ball, C. L., Gilchrist, M. A., and Coombs, D. (2007). Modeling within-host evolution of HIV: mutation, competition and strain replacement. *Bull. Math. Biol.* 69, 2361–2385. doi: 10.1007/s11538-007-9223-z

Bartenschlager, R., Penin, F., Lohmann, V., and André, P. (2011). Assembly of infectious hepatitis C virus particles. *Trends Microbiol.* 19, 95–103. doi: 10.1016/j.tim.2010.11.005

Barton, K. M., Burch, B. D., Soriano-Sarabia, N., and Margolis, D. M. (2013). Prospects for treatment of latent HIV. *Clin. Pharmacol. Ther.* 93, 46–56. doi: 10.1038/clpt.2012.202

Bauer, A. L., Beauchemin, C. A., and Perelson, A. S. (2009). Agent-based modeling of host-pathogen systems: the successes and challenges. *Inf. Sci.* 179, 1379–1389. doi: 10.1016/j.ins.2008.11.012

Beauchemin, C. A., and Handel, A. (2011). A review of mathematical models of influenza A infections within a host or cell culture: lessons learned and challenges ahead. *BMC Public Health* 11:S7. doi: 10.1186/1471-2458-11-S1-S7

Beauchemin, C. A. A., McSharry, J. J., Drusano, G. L., Nguyen, J. T., Went, G. T., Ribeiro, R. M., et al. (2008). Modeling amantadine treatment of influenza A virus *in vitro*. *J. Theor. Biol.* 254, 439–451. doi: 10.1016/j.jtbi.2008.05.031

Ben-Shachar, R., and Koelle, K. (2014). Minimal within-host dengue models highlight the specific roles of the immune response in primary and secondary dengue infections. *J. R. Soc. Interface* 12:20140886. doi: 10.1098/rsif.2014.0886

Ben-Shachar, R., Schmidler, S., and Koelle, K. (2016). Drivers of inter-individual variation in dengue viral load dynamics. *PLoS Comput. Biol.* 12:e1005194. doi: 10.1371/journal.pcbi.1005194

Benzine, T., Brandt, R., Lovell, W. C., Yamane, D., Neddermann, P., De Francesco, R., et al. (2017). NS5A inhibitors unmask differences in functional replicase complex half-life between different hepatitis C virus strains. *PLoS Pathog.* 13:e1006343. doi: 10.1371/journal.ppat.1006343

Best, K., Guedj, J., Madelain, V., de Lamballerie, X., Lim, S. Y., Osuna, C. E., et al. (2017). Zika plasma viral dynamics in nonhuman primates provides insights into early infection and antiviral strategies. *Proc. Natl. Acad. Sci. U.S.A.* 114, 8847–8852. doi: 10.1073/pnas.1704011114

Binder, M., Sulaimanov, N., Clausznitzer, D., Schulze, M., Hüber, C. M., Lenz, S. M., et al. (2013). Replication vesicles are load- and choke-points in the hepatitis C virus lifecycle. *PLoS Pathog.* 9:e1003561. doi: 10.1371/journal.ppat.1003561

Boerma, T., Mathers, C., AbouZahr, C., Somnath, C., Hogan, D., and Stevens, G. (2015). *WHO Health in 2015: From MDGs to SDGs*. World Health Organization Available online at: http://www.who.int/gho/publications/mdgs-sdgs/en/

Boianelli, A., Nguyen, V. K., Ebensen, T., Schulze, K., Wilk, E., Sharma, N., et al. (2015). Modeling influenza virus infection: a roadmap for influenza research. *Viruses* 7, 5274–5304. doi: 10.3390/v7102875

Bonhoeffer, S., May, R. M., Shaw, G. M., and Nowak, M. A. (1997). Virus dynamics and drug therapy. *Proc. Natl. Acad. Sci. U.S.A.* 94, 6971–6976. doi: 10.1073/pnas.94.13.6971

Braciale, T. J., Hahn, Y. S., and Burton, D. R. (2013). "Adaptive immune response to viral infections," in *Fields Virology*, eds B. N. Fields, D. M. Knipe, and P. M. Howley (Philadelphia, PA: Wolters Kluwer Health; Lippincott Williams & Wilkins), 214–285.

Buchholtz, F., and Schneider, F. W. (1987). Computer simulation of T3 / T7 phage infection using lag times. *Biophys. Chem.* 26, 171–179. doi: 10.1016/0301-4622(87)80020-0

Canini, L., Conway, J. M., Perelson, A. S., and Carrat, F. (2014). Impact of different oseltamivir regimens on treating influenza A virus infection and resistance emergence: insights from a modelling study. *PLoS Comput. Biol.* 10:1003568. doi: 10.1371/journal.pcbi.1003568

Canini, L., and Perelson, A. S. (2014). Viral kinetic modeling: state of the art. *J. Pharmacokinet. Pharmacodyn.* 41, 431–443. doi: 10.1007/s10928-014-9363-3

Cao, P., Wang, Z., Yan, A. W., McVernon, J., Xu, J., Heffernan, J. M., et al. (2016). On the role of CD8+ T cells in determining recovery time from influenza virus infection. *Front. Immunol.* 7:611. doi: 10.3389/fimmu.2016.00611

Cardozo, E. F., Andrade, A., Mellors, J. W., Kuritzkes, D. R., Perelson, A. S., and Ribeiro, R. M. (2017). Treatment with integrase inhibitor suggests a new interpretation of HIV RNA decay curves that reveals a subset of cells with slow integration. *PLoS Pathog.* 13:e1006478. doi: 10.1371/journal.ppat.1006478

Chomont, N., El-Far, M., Ancuta, P., Trautmann, L., Procopio, F. A., Yassine-Diab, B., et al. (2009). HIV reservoir size and persistence are driven by T cell survival and homeostatic proliferation. *Nat. Med.* 15, 893–900. doi: 10.1038/nm.1972

Ciupe, S. M., and Heffernan, J. M. (2017). In-host modeling. *Infect. Dis. Model.* 2, 188–202. doi: 10.1016/j.idm.2017.04.002

Clapham, H. E., Quyen, T. H., Kien, D. T., Dorigatti, I., Simmons, C. P., Ferguson, N. M., et al. (2016). Modelling virus and antibody dynamics during dengue virus infection suggests a role for antibody in virus clearance. *PLoS Comput. Biol.* 12:e1004951. doi: 10.1371/journal.pcbi.1004951

Clapham, H. E., Tricou, V., Van Vinh Chau, N., Simmons, C. P., and Ferguson, N. M. (2014). Within-host viral dynamics of dengue serotype 1 infection. *J. R. Soc. Interface* 11, 504–507. doi: 10.1098/rsif.2014.0094

Clausznitzer, D., Harnisch, J., and Kaderali, L. (2015). Multi-scale model for hepatitis C viral load kinetics under treatment with direct acting antivirals. *Virus Res.* 218, 96–101. doi: 10.1016/j.virusres.2015.09.011

Conway, J. M., and Perelson, A. S. (2015). Post-treatment control of HIV infection. *Proc. Natl. Acad. Sci. U.S.A.* 6, 4–9. doi: 10.1073/pnas.1419162112

D'Ortenzio, E., Matheron, S., Yazdanpanah, Y., de Lamballerie, X., Hubert, B., Piorkowski, G., et al. (2016). Evidence of sexual transmission of zika virus. *N. Engl. J. Med.* 374, 2195–2198. doi: 10.1056/NEJMc1604449

Dahari, H., Canini, L., Graw, F., Uprichard, S. L., Araujo, E. S. A., Penaranda, G., et al. (2016). HCV kinetic and modeling analyses indicate similar time to cure among sofosbuvir combination regimens with daclatasvir, simeprevir or ledipasvir. *J. Hepatol.* 64, 1232–1239. doi: 10.1016/j.jhep.2016.02.022

Dahari, H., Lo, A., Ribeiro, R. M., and Perelson, A. S. (2007a). Modeling hepatitis C virus dynamics: Liver regeneration and critical drug efficacy. *J. Theor. Biol.* 247, 371–381. doi: 10.1016/j.jtbi.2007.03.006

Dahari, H., Major, M., Zhang, X., Mihalik, K., Rice, C. M., Perelson, A. S., et al. (2005). Mathematical modeling of primary hepatitis C infection: noncytolytic clearance and early blockage of virion production. *Gastroenterology* 128, 1056–1066. doi: 10.1053/j.gastro.2005.01.049

Dahari, H., Ribeiro, R. M., and Perelson, A. S. (2007b). Triphasic decline of hepatitis C virus RNA during antiviral therapy. *Hepatology* 46, 16–21. doi: 10.1002/hep.21657

Dahari, H., Ribeiro, R. M., Rice, C. M., and Perelson, A. S. (2007c). Mathematical modeling of subgenomic hepatitis C virus replication in Huh-7 cells. *J. Virol.* 81, 750–760. doi: 10.1128/JVI.01304-06

Dee, K. U., and Shuler, M. L. (1997). A mathematical model of the trafficking of acid-dependent enveloped viruses: application to the binding, uptake, and nuclear accumulation of baculovirus. *Biotechnol. Bioeng.* 54, 468–490. doi: 10.1002/(SICI)1097-0290(19970605)54:5<468::AID-BIT7>3.0.CO;2-C

Dee, K. U., Hammer, D. A., and Shuler, M. L. (1995). A model of the binding, entry, uncoating, and RNA synthesis of Semliki Forest virus in baby hamster kidney (BHK-21) cells. *Biotechnol. Bioeng.* 46, 485–496. doi: 10.1002/bit.260460513

Eigen, M., Biebricher, C. K., Gebinoga, M., and Gardiner, W. C. (1991). The hypercycle. Coupling of RNA and protein biosynthesis in the infection cycle of an RNA bacteriophage. *Biochemistry* 30, 11005–11018. doi: 10.1021/bi00110a001

Endy, D., Kong, D., and Yin, J. (1997). Intracellular kinetics of a growing virus: a genetically structured simulation for bacteriophage T7. *Biotechnol. Bioeng.* 55, 375–389. doi: 10.1002/(SICI)1097-0290(19970720)55:2<375::AID-BIT15>3.0.CO;2-G

Fauci, A. S., Pantaleo, G., Stanley, S., and Weissman, D. (1996). Immunopathogenic mechanisms of HIV infection. *Ann. Intern. Med.* 124, 654–663. doi: 10.7326/0003-4819-124-7-199604010-00006

Foy, B. D., Kobylinski, K. C., Chilson Foy, J. L., Blitvich, B. J., Travassos da Rosa, A., Haddow, A. D., et al. (2011). Probable non-vector-borne transmission of Zika virus, Colorado, USA. *Emerg. Infect. Dis.* 17, 880–882. doi: 10.3201/eid1705.101939

Fried, M. W., Shiffman, M. L., Reddy, K. R., Smith, C., Marinos, G., Gonçales, F. L., et al. (2002). Peginterferon Alfa-2a plus ribavirin for chronic hepatitis C virus infection. *N. Engl. J. Med.* 347, 975–982. doi: 10.1056/NEJMoa020047

Furuta, Y., Gowen, B. B., Takahashi, K., Shiraki, K., Smee, D. F., and Barnard, D. L. (2013). Favipiravir (T-705), a novel viral RNA polymerase inhibitor. *Antiviral Res.* 100, 446–454. doi: 10.1016/j.antiviral.2013.09.015

Gallay, P. A., and Lin, K. (2013). Profile of alisporivir and its potential in the treatment of hepatitis C. *Drug Des. Devel. Ther.* 7, 105–115. doi: 10.2147/DDDT.S30946

Gao, M., Nettles, R. E., Belema, M., Snyder, L. B., Nguyen, V. N., Fridell, R. A., et al. (2010). Chemical genetics strategy identifies an HCV NS5A inhibitor with a potent clinical effect. *Nature* 465, 96–100. doi: 10.1038/nature08960

Garcia-Sastre, A., Egorov, A., Matassov, D., Brandt, S., Levy, D. E., Durbin, J. E., et al. (1998). Influenza A virus lacking the NS1 gene replicates in interferon-deficient systems. *Virology* 252, 324–330. doi: 10.1006/viro.1998.9508

Goodwin, K., Viboud, C., and Simonsen, L. (2006). Antibody response to influenza vaccination in the elderly: a quantitative review. *Vaccine* 24, 1159–1169. doi: 10.1016/j.vaccine.2005.08.105

Goujard, C., Girault, I., Rouzioux, C., Lécuroux, C., Deveau, C., Chaix, M. L., et al. (2012). HIV-1 control after transient antiretroviral treatment initiated in primary infection: role of patient characteristics and effect of therapy. *Antivir. Ther.* 17, 1001–1009. doi: 10.3851/IMP2273

Graw, F., and Perelson, A. S. (2015). Modeling viral spread. *Annu. Rev. Virol.* 3, 1–18. doi: 10.1146/annurev-virology-110615-042249

Gray, G. E., Laher, F., Lazarus, E., Ensoli, B., and Corey, L. (2016). Approaches to preventative and therapeutic HIV vaccines. *Curr. Opin. Virol.* 17, 104–109. doi: 10.1016/j.coviro.2016.02.010

Guedj, J., Dahari, H., Rong, L., Sansone, N. D., Nettles, R. E., Cotler, S. J., et al. (2013). Modeling shows that the NS5A inhibitor daclatasvir has two modes of action and yields a shorter estimate of the hepatitis C virus half-life. *Proc. Natl. Acad. Sci. U.S.A.* 110, 3991–3996. doi: 10.1073/pnas.1203110110

Guedj, J., Dahari, H., Shudo, E., Smith, P., and Perelson, A. S. (2012). Hepatitis C viral kinetics with the nucleoside polymerase inhibitor mericitabine (RG7128). *Hepatology* 55, 1030–1037. doi: 10.1002/hep.24788

Guedj, J., Pang, P. S., Denning, J., Rodriguez-Torres, M., Lawitz, E., Symonds, W., et al. (2014). Analysis of the hepatitis C viral kinetics during administration of two nucleotide analogues: sofosbuvir (GS-7977) and GS-0938. *Antivir. Ther.* 19, 211–220. doi: 10.3851/IMP2733

Guedj, J., and Perelson, A. S. (2011). Second-phase hepatitis C virus RNA decline during telaprevir-based therapy increases with drug effectiveness: implications for treatment duration. *Hepatology* 53, 1801–1808. doi: 10.1002/hep.24272

Guedj, J., Rong, L., Dahari, H., and Perelson, A. S. (2010). A perspective on modelling hepatitis C virus infection. *J. Viral Hepat.* 17, 825–833. doi: 10.1111/j.1365-2893.2010.01348.x

Handel, A., Longini, I. M., and Antia, R. (2010). Towards a quantitative understanding of the within-host dynamics of influenza A infections. *J. R. Soc. Interface* 7, 35–47. doi: 10.1098/rsif.2009.0067

Heim, M. H. (2013). 25 years of interferon-based treatment of chronic hepatitis C: an epoch coming to an end. *Nat. Rev. Immunol.* 13, 535–542. doi: 10.1038/nri3463

Heldt, F. S., Frensing, T., Pflugmacher, A., Gröpler, R., Peschel, B., and Reichl, U. (2013). Multiscale modeling of influenza A virus infection supports the development of direct-acting antivirals. *PLoS Comput. Biol.* 9:e1003372. doi: 10.1371/journal.pcbi.1003372

Henao-Restrepo, A. M., Camacho, A., Longini, I. M., Watson, C. H., Edmunds, W. J., Egger, M., et al. (2017). Efficacy and effectiveness of an rVSV-vectored vaccine in preventing Ebola virus disease: final results from the Guinea ring vaccination, open-label, cluster-randomised trial (Ebola Ça Suffit!). *Lancet* 389, 505–518. doi: 10.1016/S0140-6736(16)32621-6

Herrmann, E., Lee, J. H., Marinos, G., Modi, M., and Zeuzem, S. (2003). Effect of ribavirin on hepatitis C viral kinetics in patients treated with pegylated interferon. *Hepatology* 37, 1351–1358. doi: 10.1053/jhep.2003.50218

Hernandez-Vargas, E. A., Wilk, E., Canini, L., Toapanta, F. R., Binder, S. C., Uvarovskii, A., et al. (2014). Effects of aging on influenza virus infection dynamics. *J. Virol.* 88, 4123–4131. doi: 10.1128/JVI.03644-13

Heukelbach, J., Alencar, C. H., Kelvin, A. A., de Oliveira, W. K., and Pamplona de Góes Cavalcanti, L. (2016). Zika virus outbreak in Brazil. *J. Infect. Dev. Ctries.* 10, 116–120. doi: 10.3855/jidc.8217

Ho, D. D. (1996). Viral counts count in HIV infection. *Science* 272, 1124–1125. doi: 10.1126/science.272.5265.1124

Ho, D. D., Neumann, A. U., Perelson, A. S., Chen, W., Leonard, J. M., and Markowitz, M. (1995). Rapid turnover of plasma virions and CD4 lymphocytes in HIV-1 infection. *Nature* 373, 123–126. doi: 10.1038/373123a0

Holder, B. P., Simon, P., Liao, L. E., Abed, Y., Bouhy, X., Beauchemin, C. A., et al. (2011). Assessing the *in vitro* fitness of an oseltamivir-resistant seasonal A/H1N1 influenza strain using a mathematical model. *PLoS ONE* 6:e14767. doi: 10.1371/journal.pone.0014767

Holford, N. H., and Sheiner, L. B. (1982). Kinetics of pharmacologic response. *Pharmacol. Ther.* 16, 143–166. doi: 10.1016/0163-7258(82)90051-1

Hoofnagle, J. H. (2002). Course and outcome of hepatitis C. *Hepatology* 36(5 Suppl. 1), S21–S29. doi: 10.1053/jhep.2002.36227

Hopkins, S., DiMassimo, B., Rusnak, P., Heuman, D., Lalezari, J., Sluder, A., et al. (2012). The cyclophilin inhibitor SCY-635 suppresses viral replication and induces endogenous interferons in patients with chronic HCV genotype 1 infection. *J. Hepatol.* 57, 47–54. doi: 10.1016/j.jhep.2012.02.024

Iwasaki, A., and Medzhitov, R. (2013). "Innate Responses to Viral Infections," in *Fields Virology*, eds B. N. Fields, D. M. Knipe, and P. M. Howley (Philadelphia, PA: Wolters Kluwer Health; Lippincott Williams & Wilkins), 189–213.

Jacobs, M., Rodger, A., Bell, D. J., Bhagani, S., Cropley, I., Filipe, A., et al. (2016). Late Ebola virus relapse causing meningoencephalitis: a case report. *Lancet* 388, 498–503. doi: 10.1016/S0140-6736(16)30386-5

Jacobson, I. M., McHutchison, J. G., Dusheiko, G., Di Bisceglie, A. M., Reddy, K. R., Bzowej, N. H., et al. (2011). Telaprevir for previously untreated chronic hepatitis C virus infection. *N. Engl. J. Med.* 364, 2405–2416. doi: 10.1056/NEJMoa1012912

Kamal, M. A., Gieschke, R., Lemenuel-Diot, A., Beauchemin, C. A., Smith, P. F., and Rayner, C. R. (2015). A Drug-disease model describing the effect of oseltamivir neuraminidase inhibition on influenza virus progression. *Antimicrob. Agents Chemother.* 59, 5388–5395. doi: 10.1128/AAC.00069-15

Karn, J., and Stoltzfus, C. M. (2012). Transcriptional and posttranscriptional regulation of HIV-1 gene expression. *Cold Spring Harb. Perspect. Med.* 2:a006916. doi: 10.1101/cshperspect.a006916

Ke, R., Lewin, S. R., Elliott, J. H., and Perelson, A. S. (2015). Modeling the effects of vorinostat *in vivo* reveals both transient and delayed HIV transcriptional activation and minimal killing of latently infected cells. *PLoS Pathog.* 11:e1005237. doi: 10.1371/journal.ppat.1005237

Kieffer, T. L., Sarrazin, C., Miller, J. S., Welker, M. W., Forestier, N., Reesink, H. W., et al. (2007). Telaprevir and pegylated interferon-alpha-2a inhibit wild-type and resistant genotype 1 hepatitis C virus replication in patients. *Hepatology* 46, 631–639. doi: 10.1002/hep.21781

Kim, H., and Perelson, A. S. (2006). Viral and latent reservoir persistence in HIV-1-infected patients on therapy. *PLoS Comput. Biol.* 2:e20135. doi: 10.1371/journal.pcbi.0020135

Kim, S., Thiessen, P. A., Bolton, E. E., Chen, J., Fu, G., Gindulyte, A., et al. (2016). PubChem substance and compound databases. *Nucleic Acids Res.* 44, D1202–D1213. doi: 10.1093/nar/gkv951

Kowdley, K. V., Gordon, S. C., Reddy, K. R., Rossaro, L., Bernstein, D. E., Lawitz, E., et al. (2014). Ledipasvir and sofosbuvir for 8 or 12 weeks for chronic HCV without cirrhosis. *N. Engl. J. Med.* 370, 1879–1888. doi: 10.1056/NEJMoa1402355

Kumberger, P., Frey, F., Schwarz, U. S., and Graw, F. (2016). Multiscale modeling of virus replication and spread. *FEBS Lett.* 590, 1972–1986. doi: 10.1002/1873-3468.12095

Lawitz, E., Godofsky, E., Rouzier, R., Marbury, T., Nguyen, T., Ke, J., et al. (2011). Safety, pharmacokinetics, and antiviral activity of the cyclophilin inhibitor NIM811 alone or in combination with pegylated interferon in HCV-infected patients receiving 14 days of therapy. *Antiviral Res.* 89, 238–245. doi: 10.1016/j.antiviral.2011.01.003

Little, S. J., Holte, S., Routy, J. P., Daar, E. S., Markowitz, M., Collier, A. C., et al. (2002). Antiretroviral-drug resistance among patients recently infected with HIV. *N. Engl. J. Med.* 347, 385–394. doi: 10.1056/NEJMoa013552

Liu, Z., Yang, F., Robotham, J. M., and Tang, H. (2009). Critical role of cyclophilin A and its prolyl-peptidyl isomerase activity in the structure and function of the hepatitis C virus replication complex. *J. Virol.* 83, 6554–6565. doi: 10.1128/JVI.02550-08

Maartens, G., Celum, C., and Lewin, S. R. (2014). HIV infection: epidemiology, pathogenesis, treatment, and prevention. *Lancet* 384, 258–271. doi: 10.1016/S0140-6736(14)60164-1

Mackey, T. K., Liang, B. A., Cuomo, R., Hafen, R., Brouwer, K. C., and Lee, D. E. (2014). Emerging and reemerging neglected tropical diseases: a review of key characteristics, risk factors, and the policy and innovation environment. *Clin. Microbiol. Rev.* 27, 949–979. doi: 10.1128/CMR.00045-14

Madelain, V., Oestereich, L., Graw, F., Nguyen, T. H., de Lamballerie, X., Mentré, F., et al. (2015). Ebola virus dynamics in mice treated with favipiravir. *Antiviral Res.* 123, 70–77. doi: 10.1016/j.antiviral.2015.08.015

Mailly, L., Xiao, F., Lupberger, J., Wilson, G. K., Aubert, P., Duong, F. H. T., et al. (2015). Clearance of persistent hepatitis C virus infection in humanized mice using a claudin-1-targeting monoclonal antibody. *Nat. Biotechnol.* 33, 549–554. doi: 10.1038/nbt.3179

Major, M. E., Dahari, H., Mihalik, K., Puig, M., Rice, C. M., Neumann, A. U., et al. (2004). Hepatitis C virus kinetics and host responses associated with disease and outcome of infection in chimpanzees. *Hepatology* 39, 1709–1720. doi: 10.1002/hep.20239

Manchanda, H., Seidel, N., Krumbholz, A., Sauerbrei, A., Schmidtke, M., and Guthke, R. (2014). Within-host influenza dynamics: a small-scale mathematical modeling approach. *Biosystems* 118, 51–59. doi: 10.1016/j.biosystems.2014.02.004

Manns, M. P., McHutchison, J. G., Gordon, S. C., Rustgi, V. K., Shiffman, M., Reindollar, R., et al. (2001). Peginterferon alfa-2b plus ribavirin compared with interferonalfa-2b plus ribavirin for initial treatment of chronic hepatitis C: a randomised trial. *Lancet* 358, 958–965. doi: 10.1016/S0140-6736(01)06102-5

Markowitz, M., Louie, M., Hurley, A., Sun, E., Di Mascio, M., Perelson, A. S., et al. (2003). A novel antiviral intervention results in more accurate assessment of human immunodeficiency virus type 1 replication dynamics and T-cell decay *in vivo*. *J. Virol.* 77, 5037–5038. doi: 10.1128/JVI.77.8.5037-5038.2003

Martyushev, A., Nakaoka, S., Sato, K., Noda, T., and Iwami, S. (2016). Modelling Ebola virus dynamics: implications for therapy. *Antiviral Res.* 135, 62–73. doi: 10.1016/j.antiviral.2016.10.004

Miao, H., Hollenbaugh, J. A., Zand, M. S., Holden-Wiltse, J., Mosmann, T. R., Perelson, A. S., et al. (2010). Quantifying the early immune response and adaptive immune response kinetics in mice infected with influenza A virus. *J. Virol.* 84, 6687–6698. doi: 10.1128/JVI.00266-10

Munier, M. L., and Kelleher, A. D. (2007). Acutely dysregulated, chronically disabled by the enemy within: T-cell responses to HIV-1 infection. *Immunol. Cell Biol.* 85, 6–15. doi: 10.1038/sj.icb.7100015

Musso, D., Roche, C., Robin, E., Nhan, T., Teissier, A., and Cao-Lormeau, V. M. (2015). Potential sexual transmission of Zika virus. *Emerg. Infect. Dis.* 21, 359–361. doi: 10.3201/eid2102.141363

Nelson, P. W., Gilchrist, M. A., Coombs, D., Hyman, J. M., and Perelson, A. S. (2004). Age-structured model of HIV infection that allows for variations in the production rate of viral particles and the death rate of productively infected Cells. *Math. Biosci. Eng.* 1, 267–288. doi: 10.3934/mbe.2004.1.267

Neumann, A. U. (1998). Hepatitis C viral dynamics *in vivo* and the antiviral efficacy of interferon- therapy. *Science* 282, 103–107. doi: 10.1126/science.282.5386.103

Nguyen, V. K., Binder, S. C., Boianelli, A., Meyer-Hermann, M., and Hernandez-Vargas, E. A. (2015). Ebola virus infection modeling and identifiability problems. *Front. Microbiol.* 6:257. doi: 10.3389/fmicb.2015.00257

Nowak, M. A., and Bangham, C. R. (1996). Population dynamics of immune responses to persistent viruses. *Science* 272, 74–79.

Nowak, M. A., Bonhoeffer, S., Hill, A. M., Boehme, R., Thomas, H. C., and McDade, H. (1996). Viral dynamics in hepatitis B virus infection. *Proc. Natl. Acad. Sci. U.S.A.* 93, 4398–4402. doi: 10.1073/pnas.93.9.4398

Nowak, M. A., and May, R. (2001). *Virus Dynamics: Mathematical Principles of Immunology and Virology*. Oxford University Press.

O'Connell, K. A., Bailey, J. R., and Blankson, J. N. (2009). Elucidating the elite: mechanisms of control in HIV-1 infection. *Trends Pharmacol. Sci.* 30, 631–637. doi: 10.1016/j.tips.2009.09.005

Osuna, C. E., Lim, S. Y., Deleage, C., Griffin, B. D., Stein, D., Schroeder, L. T., et al. (2016). Zika viral dynamics and shedding in rhesus and cynomolgus macaques. *Nat. Med.* 22, 1448–1455. doi: 10.1038/nm.4206

Palmer, S., Maldarelli, F., Wiegand, A., Bernstein, B., Hanna, G. J., Brun, S. C., et al. (2008). Low-level viremia persists for at least 7 years in patients on suppressive antiretroviral therapy. *Proc. Natl. Acad. Sci. U.S.A.* 105, 3879–3884. doi: 10.1073/pnas.0800050105

Pawelek, K. A., Huynh, G. T., Quinlivan, M., Cullinane, A., Rong, L., and Perelson, A. S. (2012). Modeling within-host dynamics of influenza virus infection including immune responses. *PLoS Comput. Biol.* 8:e1002588. doi: 10.1371/journal.pcbi.1002588

Pawlotsky, J. M. (2016). Hepatitis C Virus resistance to direct-acting antiviral drugs in interferon-free regimens. *Gastroenterology* 151, 70–86. doi: 10.1053/j.gastro.2016.04.003

Perelson, A. S. (2002). Modelling viral and immune system dynamics. *Nat. Rev. Immunol.* 2, 28–36. doi: 10.1038/nri700

Perelson, A. S., Essunger, P., Cao, Y., Vesanen, M., Hurley, A., Saksela, K., et al. (1997). Decay characteristics of HIV-1-infected compartments during combination therapy. *Nature* 387, 188–191. doi: 10.1038/387188a0

Perelson, A. S., and Guedj, J. (2015). Modelling hepatitis C therapy-predicting effects of treatment. *Nat. Rev. Gastroenterol. Hepatol.* 12, 437–445. doi: 10.1038/nrgastro.2015.97

Perelson, A. S., Kirschner, D. E., and De Boer, R. (1993). Dynamics of HIV infection of CD4+ T cells. *Math. Biosci.* 114, 81–125. doi: 10.1016/0025-5564(93)90043-A

Perelson, A. S., Neumann, A. U., Markowitz, M., Leonard, J. M., and Ho, D. D. (1996). HIV-1 dynamics *in vivo*: virion clearance rate, infected cell life-span, and viral generation time. *Science* 271, 1582–1586. doi: 10.1126/science.271.5255.1582

Perelson, A. S., and Ribeiro, R. M. (2013). Modeling the within-host dynamics of HIV infection. *BMC Biol.* 11:96. doi: 10.1186/1741-7007-11-96

Persaud, D., Luzuriaga, K., Ziemniak, C., Muresan, P., Greenough, T., Fenton, T., et al. (2011). Effect of therapeutic HIV recombinant poxvirus vaccines on the size of the resting CD4+ T-cell latent HIV reservoir. *AIDS* 25, 2227–2234. doi: 10.1097/QAD.0b013e32834cdaba

Pinilla, L. T., Holder, B. P., Abed, Y., Boivin, G., and Beauchemin, C. A. (2012). The H275Y neuraminidase mutation of the pandemic A/H1N1 influenza virus lengthens the eclipse phase and reduces viral output of infected cells, potentially compromising fitness in ferrets. *J. Virol.* 86, 10651–10660. doi: 10.1128/JVI.07244-11

Poveda, E., Wyles, D. L., Mena, A., Pedreira, J. D., Castro-Iglesias, A., and Cachay, E. (2014). Update on hepatitis C virus resistance to direct-acting antiviral agents. *Antiviral Res.* 108, 181–191. doi: 10.1016/j.antiviral.2014.05.015

Quintela, B. M., Conway, J. M., Hyman, J. M., Reis, R. F., dos Santos, R. W., Lobosco, M., et al. (2017). "An Age-based multiscale mathematical model of the hepatitis c virus life-cycle during infection and therapy: including translation and replication," in *VII Latin American Congress on Biomedical Engineering CLAIB 2016*, eds I. Torres, J. Bustamante, and D. Sierra (Singapore: Springer), 508–511.

Ramratnam, B., Bonhoeffer, S., Binley, J., Hurley, A., Zhang, L., Mittler, J. E., et al. (1999). Rapid production and clearance of HIV-1 and hepatitis C virus assessed by large volume plasma apheresis. *Lancet* 354, 1782–1785. doi: 10.1016/S0140-6736(99)02035-8

Reddy, B., and Yin, J. (1999). Quantitative intracellular kinetics of HIV type 1. *AIDS Res. Hum. Retroviruses* 15, 273–283. doi: 10.1089/088922299311457

Ribeiro, R. M., and Bonhoeffer, S. (2000). Production of resistant HIV mutants during antiretroviral therapy. *Proc. Natl. Acad. Sci. U.S.A.* 97, 7681–7686. doi: 10.1073/pnas.97.14.7681

Ribeiro, R. M., Qin, L., Chavez, L. L., Li, D., Self, S. G., and Perelson, A. S. (2010). Estimation of the initial viral growth rate and basic reproductive number during acute HIV-1 infection. *J. Virol.* 84, 6096–6102. doi: 10.1128/JVI.00127-10

Roberts, N. J., Douglas, R. G., Simons, R. M., and Diamond, M. E. (1979). Virus-induced interferon production by human macrophages. *J. Immunol.* 123, 365–369.

Rong, L., Feng, Z., and Perelson, A. S. (2007a). Emergence of HIV-1 drug resistance during antiretroviral treatment. *Bull. Math. Biol.* 69, 2027–2060. doi: 10.1007/s11538-007-9203-3

Rong, L., Gilchrist, M. A., Feng, Z., and Perelson, A. S. (2007b). Modeling within-host HIV-1 dynamics and the evolution of drug resistance: trade-offs between viral enzyme function and drug susceptibility. *J. Theor. Biol.* 247, 804–818. doi: 10.1016/j.jtbi.2007.04.014

Rong, L., Guedj, J., Dahari, H., Coffield, D. J., Levi, M., Smith, P., et al. (2013). Analysis of hepatitis C virus decline during treatment with the protease inhibitor danoprevir using a multiscale model. *PLoS Comput. Biol.* 9:e1002959. doi: 10.1371/journal.pcbi.1002959

Rong, L., and Perelson, A. S. (2009). Modeling HIV persistence, the latent reservoir, and viral blips. *J. Theor. Biol.* 260, 308–331. doi: 10.1016/j.jtbi.2009.06.011

Ronsard, L., Ganguli, N., Singh, V. K., Mohankumar, K., Rai, T., Sridharan, S., et al. (2017a). Impact of genetic variations in HIV-1 tat on LTR-mediated transcription via TAR RNA interaction. *Front. Microbiol.* 8:706. doi: 10.3389/fmicb.2017.00706

Ronsard, L., Lata, S., Singh, J., Ramachandran, V. G., Das, S., and Banerjea, A. C. (2014). Molecular and genetic characterization of natural HIV-1 tat exon-1 variants from North India and their functional implications. *PLoS ONE* 9:e85452. doi: 10.1371/journal.pone.0085452

Ronsard, L., Rai, T., Rai, D., Ramachandran, V. G., and Banerjea, A. C. (2017b). *In silico* analyses of subtype specific HIV-1 Tat-TAR RNA interaction reveals the structural determinants for viral activity. *Front. Microbiol.* 8:1467. doi: 10.3389/fmicb.2017.01467.

Saenz, R. A., Quinlivan, M., Elton, D., Macrae, S., Blunden, A. S., Mumford, J. A., et al. (2010). Dynamics of influenza virus infection and pathology. *J. Virol.* 84, 3974–3983. doi: 10.1128/JVI.02078-09

Sáez-Cirión, A., Bacchus, C., Hocqueloux, L., Avettand-Fenoel, V., Girault, I., Lecuroux, C., et al. (2013). Post-treatment HIV-1 controllers with a long-term virological remission after the interruption of early initiated antiretroviral therapy ANRS VISCONTI Study. *PLoS Pathog.* 9:e1003211. doi: 10.1371/journal.ppat.1003211

Salgado, M., Rabi, S. A., O'Connell, K. A., Buckheit, R. W., Bailey, J. R., Chaudhry, A. A., et al. (2011). Prolonged control of replication-competent dual- tropic human immunodeficiency virus-1 following cessation of highly active antiretroviral therapy. *Retrovirology* 8:97. doi: 10.1186/1742-4690-8-97

Samuel, C. E. (2001). Antiviral actions of interferons. *Clin. Microbiol. Rev.* 14, 778–809. doi: 10.1128/CMR.14.4.778-809.2001

Scheel, T. K., and Rice, C. M. (2013). Understanding the hepatitis C virus life cycle paves the way for highly effective therapies. *Nat. Med.* 19, 837–849. doi: 10.1038/nm.3248

Schelker, M., Mair, C. M., Jolmes, F., Welke, R. W., Klipp, E., Herrmann, A., et al. (2016). Viral RNA degradation and diffusion act as a bottleneck for the influenza A virus infection efficiency. *PLoS Comput. Biol.* 12:e1005075. doi: 10.1371/journal.pcbi.1005075

Schmid, B., Rinas, M., Ruggieri, A., Acosta, E. G., Bartenschlager, M., Reuter, A., et al. (2015). Live cell analysis and mathematical modeling identify determinants of attenuation of dengue virus 2′-O-methylation mutant. *PLoS Pathog.* 11:e1005345. doi: 10.1371/journal.ppat.1005345

Sedmak, J. J., and Grossberg, S. E. (1973). Interferon bioassay: reduction in yield of myxovirus neuraminidases. *J. Gen. Virol.* 21, 1–7. doi: 10.1099/0022-1317-21-1-1

Shepard, D. S., Undurraga, E. A., Halasa, Y. A., and Stanaway, J. D. (2016). The global economic burden of dengue: a systematic analysis. *Lancet Infect. Dis.* 16, 935–941. doi: 10.1016/S1473-3099(16)00146-8

Simon, V., and Ho, D. D. (2003). HIV-1 dynamics *in vivo*: implications for therapy. *Nat. Rev. Microbiol.* 1, 181–190. doi: 10.1038/nrmicro772

Stafford, M. A., Corey, L., Cao, Y., Daar, E. S., Ho, D. D., and Perelson, A. S. (2000). Modeling plasma virus concentration during primary HIV infection. *J. Theor. Biol.* 203, 285–301. doi: 10.1006/jtbi.2000.1076

Steigbigel, R. T., Cooper, D. A., Kumar, P. N., Eron, J. E., Schechter, M., Markowitz, M., et al. (2008). Raltegravir with Optimized background therapy for resistant HIV-1 infection. *N. Engl. J. Med.* 359, 339–354. doi: 10.1056/NEJMoa0708975

Tamura, S., and Kurata, T. (2004). Defense mechanisms against influenza virus infection in the respiratory tract mucosa. *Jpn. J. Infect. Dis.* 57, 236–247.

Thimme, R., Oldach, D., Chang, K. M., Steiger, C., Ray, S. C., and Chisari, F., V (2001). Determinants of viral clearance and persistence during acute hepatitis C virus infection. *J. Exp. Med.* 194, 1395–1406. doi: 10.1084/jem.194.10.1395

United Nations (2017). *A Socio-economic Impact Assessment of the Zika Virus in Latin America and the Caribbean.* Available online at: http://www.undp.org/content/undp/en/home/librarypage/hiv-aids/a-socio-economic-impact-assessment-of-the-zika-virus-in-latin-am.html

Villar, L., Dayan, G. H., Arredondo-García, J. L., Rivera, D. M., Cunha, R., Deseda, C., et al. (2015). Efficacy of a tetravalent dengue vaccine in children in Latin America. *N. Engl. J. Med.* 372, 113–123. doi: 10.1056/NEJMoa1411037

Watashi, K., Ishii, N., Hijikata, M., Inoue, D., Murata, T., Miyanari, Y., et al. (2005). Cyclophilin B is a functional regulator of hepatitis C virus RNA polymerase. *Mol. Cell* 19, 111–122. doi: 10.1016/j.molcel.2005.05.014

Wauquier, N., Becquart, P., Padilla, C., Baize, S., and Leroy, E. M. (2010). Human fatal zaire ebola virus infection is associated with an aberrant innate immunity and with massive lymphocyte apoptosis. *PLoS Negl. Trop. Dis.* 4:e837. doi: 10.1371/journal.pntd.0000837

Wei, X., Ghosh, S. K., Taylor, M. E., Johnson, V. A., Emini, E. A., Deutsch, P., et al. (1995). Viral dynamics in human immunodeficiency virus type 1 infection. *Nature* 373, 117–122. doi: 10.1038/373117a0

Wodarz, D., and Lloyd, A. L. (2004). Immune responses and the emergence of drug-resistant virus strains *in vivo*. *Proc. Biol. Sci.* 271, 1101–1109. doi: 10.1098/rspb.2003.2664

Wodarz, D., and Nowak, M. A. (2002). Mathematical models of HIV pathogenesis and treatment. *BioEssays* 24, 1178–1187. doi: 10.1002/bies.10196

World Health Organization (2016a). *Dengue and Severe Dengue.* World Health Organization.

World Health Organization (2016b). *Guidelines for the Screening, Care and Treatment of Persons with Chronic Hepatitis C Infection.* WHO.

World Health Organization (2017a). *Ebola Virus Disease.* World Health Organization. Available online at: http://www.who.int/mediacentre/factsheets/fs103/en/

World Health Organization (2017b). *HIV/AIDS.* WHO. Available online at: http://www.who.int/mediacentre/factsheets/fs360/en/

World Health Organization (2017c). *Influenza (Seasonal).* World Health Organisation Available online at: http://www.who.int/mediacentre/factsheets/fs211/en/

World Health Organization (2017d). *Zika Virus.* World Health Organization. Available online at: http://www.who.int/mediacentre/factsheets/zika/en/

Wright, P. F., Neumann, G., and Kawaoka, Y. (2013). "Orthomyxoviruses," in *Fields Virology*, eds B. N. Fields, D. M. Knipe, and P. M. Howley (Philadelphia, PA: Wolters Kluwer Health/Lippincott Williams & Wilkins), 1186–1123.

Xiao, Y., Miao, H., Tang, S., and Wu, H. (2013). Modeling antiretroviral drug responses for HIV-1 infected patients using differential equation models. *Adv. Drug Deliv. Rev.* 65, 940–953. doi: 10.1016/j.addr.2013.04.005

Zarnitsyna, V. I., Handel, A., McMaster, S. R., Hayward, S. L., Kohlmeier, J. E., and Antia, R. (2016). Mathematical model reveals the role of memory CD8 T cell populations in recall responses to influenza. *Front. Immunol.* 7:165. doi: 10.3389/fimmu.2016.00165

Zeisel, M. B., Lupberger, J., Fofana, I., and Baumert, T. F. (2013). Host-targeting agents for prevention and treatment of chronic hepatitis C-Perspectives and challenges. *J. Hepatol.* 58, 375–384. doi: 10.1016/j.jhep.2012.09.022

8

Predictive Virtual Infection Modeling of Fungal Immune Evasion in Human Whole Blood

*Maria T. E. Prauße[1,2], Teresa Lehnert[1,3], Sandra Timme[1,2], Kerstin Hünniger[4,5], Ines Leonhardt[3,4], Oliver Kurzai[3,4,5] and Marc Thilo Figge[1,2,3]**

[1] Applied Systems Biology, Leibniz Institute for Natural Product Research and Infection Biology, Hans Knöll Institute (HKI), Jena, Germany, [2] Faculty of Biological Sciences, Friedrich Schiller University Jena, Jena, Germany, [3] Center for Sepsis Control and Care (CSCC), Jena University Hospital, Jena, Germany, [4] Fungal Septomics, Leibniz Institute for Natural Product Research and Infection Biology, Hans Knöll Institute (HKI), Jena, Germany, [5] Institute of Hygiene and Microbiology, University of Würzburg, Würzburg, Germany

***Correspondence:**
Marc Thilo Figge
thilo.figge@leibniz-hki.de

Bloodstream infections by the human-pathogenic fungi *Candida albicans* and *Candida glabrata* increasingly occur in hospitalized patients and are associated with high mortality rates. The early immune response against these fungi in human blood comprises a concerted action of humoral and cellular components of the innate immune system. Upon entering the blood, the majority of fungal cells will be eliminated by innate immune cells, i.e., neutrophils and monocytes. However, recent studies identified a population of fungal cells that can evade the immune response and thereby may disseminate and cause organ dissemination, which is frequently observed during candidemia. In this study, we investigate the so far unresolved mechanism of fungal immune evasion in human whole blood by testing hypotheses with the help of mathematical modeling. We use a previously established state-based virtual infection model for whole-blood infection with *C. albicans* to quantify the immune response and identified the fungal immune-evasion mechanism. While this process was assumed to be spontaneous in the previous model, we now hypothesize that the immune-evasion process is mediated by host factors and incorporate such a mechanism in the model. In particular, we propose, based on previous studies that the fungal immune-evasion mechanism could possibly arise through modification of the fungal surface by as of yet unknown proteins that are assumed to be secreted by activated neutrophils. To validate or reject any of the immune-evasion mechanisms, we compared the simulation of both immune-evasion models for different infection scenarios, i.e., infection of whole blood with either *C. albicans* or *C. glabrata* under non-neutropenic and neutropenic conditions. We found that under non-neutropenic conditions, both immune-evasion models fit the experimental data from whole-blood infection with *C. albicans* and *C. glabrata*. However, differences between the immune-evasion models could be observed for the infection outcome under neutropenic conditions with respect to the distribution of fungal cells across the immune cells. Based on these predictions, we suggested specific experimental studies that might allow for the validation or rejection of the proposed immune-evasion mechanism.

Keywords: *Candida albicans*, *Candida glabrata*, immune evasion, state-based model, innate immune response, polymorphonuclear neutrophils, whole-blood infection assay

INTRODUCTION

Even though pathogenic microbes constantly colonize the human skin or are inhaled, the human immune system is usually able to protect the body against infections. Thus, immunocompromised individuals have an increased risk for infections by opportunistic pathogens (1). In case of injuries or disturbed cellular integrity, the pathogens can easily overcome physical skin barriers and/or mucosal surfaces, and enter the host tissue or the blood stream (2, 3). Innate immune responses defend the host against microbial invaders (4–6), however, the exact interplay between pathogens and the immune defense is in many cases not fully resolved (7, 8). In order to investigate such unknown mechanisms, mathematical modeling is an appropriate approach to investigate complex biological systems at a quantitative level. Furthermore, mathematical models allow for hypothesis testing by varying single parameters or comparing various possible scenarios. This approach allows going beyond experimental limitations, for example, by quantifying biological processes that are not amenable to a direct measurement in experiment. Moreover, ethical concerns and financial efforts of experimental studies can be considerably reduced by computer simulations, because systematic variations of model parameters allow narrowing down the number and kind of further experimental investigations necessary to identify causal relationships responsible for experimentally observed effects (9). The iterative cycle of such a systems biology approach combines wet-lab and dry-lab experiments to their best advantage (10, 11).

In previous studies, we have applied a systems biology approach to investigate the complex interaction of the human-pathogenic fungus, *Candida albicans* with innate immune cells in human whole blood (12, 13). Interestingly, we observed that a relatively high proportion of *C. albicans* can survive in human blood and evades the immune response by a so far unknown mechanism. The experimental part of this study comprised human whole-blood infection assays, where blood samples from healthy donors were infected with fungal cells to acquire time-resolved data on the interaction of *C. albicans* with immune cells as well as fungal survival over the course of infection. Based on these experimental results, a bio-mathematical model was developed using a state-based modeling approach (12, 13). The model is composed of states that represent different *C. albicans* cell populations of the biological system. These include alive and killed *C. albicans* cells, which are either in extracellular space or phagocytosed by the immune cells, i.e., PMN or monocytes. Moreover, the model represents a population of fungal cells that can evade the immune defense, since these cells appear to be neither phagocytosed by immune cells nor killed extracellularly. Transitions between various states of cell populations can occur and these state changes represent biological processes like phagocytosis and killing. In the original state-based model (SBM), transition rates were defined to characterize the different transitions between the states, which represent the biological processes. The *a priori* unknown values for these transition rates were evaluated by applying the global parameter estimation algorithm *Simulated Annealing* that is based on the *Metropolis Monte Carlo* scheme (12, 13). This algorithm explores the space of transition rates and searches for the global minimum of the fitting error, i.e., the deviation between the simulated and experimentally measured kinetics, and by that yields values for the transition rates that together achieve optimal agreement between these kinetics. The resulting rates indicated that the larger number of *C. albicans* cells inside PMN, in comparison to the much smaller number of fungal cells inside monocytes, is not merely a consequence of the higher number of PMN than monocytes, but is also due to a larger phagocytosis rate of PMN compared to monocytes. This quantification, which is not directly accessible from the experimental data alone, allowed us to generally conclude that elimination of *C. albicans* cells in human blood is governed by PMN.

In the SBM, fungal cells that evaded the immune response were assumed to undergo a spontaneous process with a constant transition rate and we will refer to it as *spon-IE model* from now on (see **Figure 1A**). While the exact mechanism causing immune evasion of *C. albicans* in human blood has not been identified yet, our previous studies already allowed for the rejection of various hypotheses. In the work by Hünniger et al. (12) it has been shown that the non-filamentous *efg1*Δ, *cph1*Δ mutant of *C. albicans*, and even thimerosal-killed *C. albicans* yeast cells are both able to evade the immune response. These observations imply that the fungal cells do not play an active role in the acquisition of immune-evasive properties. Therefore, we addressed aspects of the host. However, we found that the addition of fresh blood of the same donor to an infected blood sample after 2 h did not result in higher elimination of fungal cells, implying that the hypothesis of early PMN exhaustion in the infection assay could be rejected. Additionally, we observed that during the 4 h of whole-blood infection the number of immune cells remained fairly constant. Thus, acquisition of immune evasion by fungal cells inside the phagocytes, which might then be followed by the destruction of phagocytic immune cells, appears to be unlikely. This lytic escape mechanism, which has been observed for macrophages (14), has not been reported for human PMN in *C. albicans* infection.

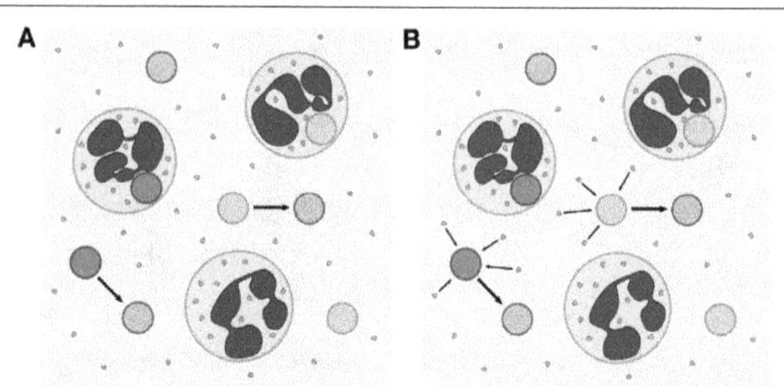

FIGURE 1 | Schematic depiction of two immune-evasion mechanisms. PMN (purple) with granula and fungal cells are either alive (green), killed (red), or immune evasive (gray). **(A)** Illustration of spontaneously evading fungal cells. **(B)** Illustration of the PMN-mediated immune-evasion mechanism, which is associated with degranulation on first-time phagocytosis of fungal cells by PMN. Degranulation is assumed to mediate the release of proteins into extracellular space that enables fungal cells to evade subsequent killing and phagocytosis by modification of their surface.

In this study, we investigate the unresolved mechanism of immune evasion by pathogens in human whole blood. This is realized by making predictions based on mathematical modeling of the infection kinetics and by comparing various infection scenarios that may be tested in experiment. Based on our previously developed state-based virtual infection model (12, 13), we hypothesize that the immune-evasion process is mediated by host factors and incorporate such a mechanism in the model. Our hypothesis is motivated by the experimental observation that even thimerosal-killed *C. albicans* cells can acquire immune-evasive properties. Thus, pathogen immune evasion may be actively driven by the host. Although PMN are the main actors in the defense against *C. albicans,* immune cells also have been shown to cause remodeling of the *C. albicans* cell wall (15). However, while it is known that PMN degranulation is associated with the release of antimicrobial effector proteins that can kill *C. albicans* cells in extracellular space (16, 17), the consequences of the cell wall remodeling is yet not clear, e.g., whether or not it enables the immune evasion by the pathogen. We here consider the possibility that PMN degranulation is associated with the secretion of effector molecules that may cause immune evasion. We investigate the possibility that these PMN-derived molecules may change the pathogen surface and thereby render the pathogen undetectable for immune cells (see **Figure 1B**). We will refer to the model that assumes a PMN-mediated evasion mechanism as *PMNmed-IE model* in the following.

The PMNmed-IE model will be compared with the spon-IE model by simulating the immune response to pathogens in healthy individuals as well as in virtual patients with neutropenia. Furthermore, we also extend this analysis to the fungus *C. glabrata*, which attributes to the rise of microbial infection in the clinics, especially in elderly individuals and immunocompromised patients (18). The two fungal pathogens are part of the normal microbial flora of the majority of people and remain in a commensal state under healthy conditions (19). *C. albicans* and *C. glabrata*, respectively, rank first and second in isolation frequency in humans (20) and in immunocompromised patients can switch into a pathogenic state, overcome physical barriers, enter the bloodstream, and disseminate throughout the body (4, 7). In blood, the microorganisms are attacked and cleared by the innate immune response. However, we find that both pathogens—albeit to a different quantitative extent—have the ability to evade the immune response. This emphasizes once more the importance of investigating immune-evasion mechanisms by mathematical modeling in order to generate testable hypothesis that may be checked in experiment and ultimately enable medical intervention that cuts the pathogen escape route in and subsequent dissemination from human whole blood.

MATERIALS AND METHODS

Ethics Statement

This study was conducted according to the principles expressed in the Declaration of Helsinki. All protocols were approved by the Ethics Committee of the University Hospital Jena (permit number: 273-12/09). Written informed consent was obtained from all blood donors.

Fungal Strains and Culture

The GFP expressing *C. albicans* strain was constructed as described in Hünniger et al. (12) and grown in liquid yeast extract-peptone-dextrose (YPD) medium at 30°C. The GFP expressing *C. glabrata* strain (21) was incubated at 37°C in YPD medium. After overnight culture both strains were reseeded in fresh YPD medium followed by growing at 30 and 37°C, respectively, until they reached the mid-log-phase. Finally, the fungal cells were washed and harvested in HBSS until use.

Human Whole Blood Infection Assay

Human peripheral blood samples from healthy individuals were infected with either *C. albicans* or *C. glabrata*. The assay was performed as described previously (12). In short, $1{\cdot}10^6$ *Candida* cells were added per ml of anti-coagulated blood and incubated at 37°C with gentle rotation for indicated time points. Subsequent to the confrontation, samples were maintained at 4°C and further analyzed by flow cytometry. Flow cytometry gating strategy was performed as previously described using FlowJo 7.6.4 software to investigate the distribution of fungal cells in human blood (12). Survival of fungal cells was determined in a plating assay by analysis of recovered colony forming units after plating appropriate dilutions of all time points on YPD agar plates.

SBM of Whole-Blood Infection

Recently, we established a virtual infection model to simulate the immune response against the fungal pathogen *C. albicans* in human whole blood (12, 13). This enabled us to quantify innate effector mechanisms as well as *C. albicans* immune evasion based on experimental data as obtained by FACS analysis and survival assays during a time course of 4 h. The time-resolved data comprised *C. albicans* viability as well as its association to innate immune cells, i.e., monocytes and PMN. In the SBM, immune cells and fungal cells can populate specific states. We identified five combined units of these states that could be directly compared with the experimentally measured cell populations. The combined unit P_E involves all extracellular pathogens and is given by

$$P_E \equiv P_{AE} + P_{KE} + P_{AIE} + P_{KIE} \quad (1)$$

Here, the states P_{AE} and P_{KE} represent extracellular cells that are alive and killed, respectively. The states P_{AIE} and P_{KIE} describe pathogens that are either alive and evade the immune response or kill and evade the immune response. Note that alive extracellular cells do not comprise alive immune-evasive cells and that these combined units are excluding each other.

Pathogens P_{AE} and P_{KE} can be phagocytozed by immune cells and in the SBM we account for phagocytosis by monocytes (M) and PMN (N), where the latter may also be referred to as neutrophils and are, therefore, labeled with N. An intracellular pathogen is either phagocytosed by a PMN

$$P_N \equiv \sum_{i\geq 0} \sum_{j\geq 0} (i+j) N_{i,j}, \quad (2)$$

or by a monocyte

$$P_M \equiv \sum_{i\geq 0} \sum_{j\geq 0} (i+j) M_{i,j}. \quad (3)$$

Here, the indices i and j refer to the immune cell state that is defined by the number of internalized alive and killed pathogens, respectively. The combined unit of killed pathogens is given by

$$P_K \equiv P_{KE} + P_{KIE} + \sum_{i\geq 0} \sum_{j\geq 0} (M_{i,j} + N_{i,j}) j, \quad (4)$$

whereas the combined unit of alive pathogens is defined by

$$P_A \equiv P_{AE} + P_{AIE} + \sum_{i\geq 0} \sum_{j\geq 0} (M_{i,j} + N_{i,j}) i. \quad (5)$$

Note that the total number of pathogens is given by $P \equiv P_E + P_N + P_M + P_{KIE}$ or $P \equiv P_K + P_A$.

The states are connected by transitions that indicate possible state changes and thereby enable to simulate the dynamics of the model (see Figure S1 in Supplementary Material). Transition rates characterize these state changes and are defined as the probability of a transition per simulation time step Δt. The SBM by Hünniger et al. (12) and Lehnert et al. (13) distinguished a rate for first and subsequent phagocytosis events by PMN, since it was assumed that a phagocytosis event activates the PMN and leads to a higher phagocytosis rate. Since this fact is not experimentally validated for whole-blood infection with *C. glabrata*, we here implement a single phagocytosis rate of PMN that accounts for both, first and subsequent phagocytosis events. Therefore, the SBM of whole-blood infection comprises seven different transition rates that are given by the phagocytosis rate ϕ_M of monocytes, the phagocytosis rate ϕ_N of PMN, the intracellular killing rates κ_M and κ_N of both monocytes and PMN, the transition rates γ and $\bar{\kappa}_{EK}$, which define the extracellular killing, and the spontaneous immune-evasion rate ρ (see Table S1 in Supplementary Material). As already noted in our previous study (12), occasional filamentation of fungal cells but no budding could be observed in samples of blood smears. Therefore, proliferation of fungal cells is not included in the SBM. An overview of the SBM simulation algorithm is briefly described in Section S1 in Supplementary Material and schematically illustrated in Figure S1 in Supplementary Material. For a detailed description of the SBM, including the definition of rates for state transitions and their estimation by the *Simulated Annealing* algorithm that is based on the *Metropolis Monte Carlo* scheme (22, 23), we refer to our previous studies by Hünniger et al. (12) and Lehnert et al. (13). Here, we briefly mention that the values of the transition rates in the virtual infection model were estimated such that deviations from the kinetics of the combined units as obtained from the experiments are minimized. A brief overview of the parameter estimation algorithm is given in Section S2 and Figure S2 in Supplementary Material.

Our object-oriented framework combining the SBM simulation algorithm and the parameter estimation is implemented in the programming language C++ and available for download from https://asbdata.hki-jena.de/publidata/PrausseEtAl2018_FrontImmunol/.

Modeling of Immune Evasion by Pathogens

As was observed in our previous analysis for *C. albicans*, pathogens can evade the immune response in the states alive (P_{AIE}) or killed (P_{KIE}), i.e., these cells can neither be phagocytosed nor killed by PMN and monocytes, and their total number is denoted by $P_{IE} \equiv P_{KIE} + P_{AIE}$ (12). Note that immune evasion of *C. albicans* in human whole blood was first predicted by our state-based virtual infection model and then also verified experimentally. Since the mechanisms of the immune evasion could not be identified yet, this process was assumed to occur spontaneously with time-independent transition rate

$$\rho = \text{constant} \quad (6)$$

and we refer to this model as spon-IE model. In this study, spontaneous immune evasion of pathogens (see **Figure 1A**) was compared to an immune-evasion mechanism, which was assumed to be mediated by PMN. Since PMN secrete antimicrobial peptides upon initial phagocytosis of pathogens, we speculated that these pathogens may also secrete proteins that can mediate the immune evasion (see **Figure 1B**), e.g., inducing alterations of pathogens by modulating its molecular surface. We accounted for this mechanism in the SBM by replacing the constant transition rate of the spon-IE model with the time-dependent rate

$$\rho(t = n\Delta t) = \bar{\rho} \sum_{m=0}^{n} \frac{N_{NP}(t' = m\Delta t)}{G_{(0,0)}(0)} \cdot \exp(-\gamma_R \cdot \Delta t(n-m)) \quad (7)$$

in the PMNmed-IE model. In close analogy to the rate of extracellular killing of pathogens by antimicrobial peptide-release from PMN (1), Eq. 7 represents the rate of pathogen immune evasion at time t as mediated by the sum of PMN-released proteins upon first phagocytosis events (N_{NP}) up to time point t. Note that the simulation algorithm performs n simulation steps with step size Δt to calculate the system dynamics at time point $t = n\Delta t$. The impact of secreted molecules is determined by the parameters $\bar{\rho}$ and γ_R, where the latter describes the half-life associated with the molecular degradation, such that the molecules' immune-evasive effect is exponentially decreasing after their release at time $t' = m\Delta t$. Therefore, the PMNmed-IE model comprises eight parameters, i.e., one more rate than the spon-IE model for spontaneous immune-evasion processes.

Simulation of Virtual Patients With Neutropenia

In order to study the difference between the two models, spon-IE and PMNmed-IE, we simulated infection scenarios in human whole blood under neutropenic conditions. More specifically, virtual patients were considered with gradually decreasing amounts of PMN within the range of medically established severity levels of neutropenia (24) (see **Table 1**) and the impact of these conditions was compared with regards to the two mechanisms of immune evasion. The simulation algorithm described in Lehnert et al. (13) was applied to human whole-blood samples of 1 ml containing $5 \cdot 10^5$ monocytes and $1 \cdot 10^6$ pathogens. For each infection

TABLE 1 | Number of PMN per ml blood for different severity levels of neutropenia.

State of disease	PMN (1/ml)
Healthy	$1.8 \cdot 10^6$–$8 \cdot 10^6$
Mild neutropenia	$<1.5 \cdot 10^6$
Moderate neutropenia	$<1 \cdot 10^6$
Severe neutropenia	$<5 \cdot 10^5$

scenario, we performed 50 simulations with transition rate values that were randomly sampled within their respective SD.

RESULTS

Whole-Blood Infection Show Pathogen-Specific Immune Response Kinetics

Whole-blood infection assays were performed for the two fungal pathogens, *C. albicans* and *C. glabrata*. At specific time points, whole-blood samples were analyzed using flow cytometry and survival assays to acquire time-resolved data for the association between pathogens and immune cells as well as viability of the pathogens. **Figures 2A,B,D,E** depict these experimental data (dashed lines) for *C. albicans* and *C. glabrata*, respectively.

Comparing the two pathogens, the fraction of extracellular fungal cells at 4 h post infection was highest for *C. albicans* with 15 ± 5.8%and lowest for *C. glabrata* with 8.9 ± 7.5%, where the sub-populations of alive and killed cells are comparable in size (see **Figures 2A,B,D,E**). In the case of an infection with *C. albicans*, a fraction of 6.5 ± 4.2% cells still remained alive at 4 h post infection, whereas survival assays revealed that 1.3 ± 1.5% of *C. glabrata* cells were not killed at that time point. Interestingly, the association of fungal cells to monocytes was markedly higher for *C. glabrata* with a fraction of 10.1 ± 2.7% compared to *C. albicans* with a fraction of 2.7 ± 1.9%. Furthermore, *C. albicans* showed only a slightly higher association of 82.3 ± 7.0% to PMN than *C. glabrata* (81.0 ± 8.1%), as was previously observed by Duggan et al. (25). Nevertheless, for both pathogens, the fraction of association to PMN was dominant over association to monocytes, i.e., by a factor eight for *C. glabrata* and by a factor 30 for *C. albicans*. Furthermore, Hopke et al. showed that degranulation of PMN has an impact on cell wall modulation in fungi, but whether this could enable pathogenic immune evasion is still unclear (15). These findings motivated our decision to focus on a PMN-mediated immune-evasion mechanism in comparison to spontaneous immune evasion.

Spontaneous and PMN-Mediated Immune Evasion in Agreement With Experimental Data

We investigated the possibility that PMN secrete upon initial phagocytosis of pathogen proteins that can mediate immune evasion, e.g., inducing alterations of the surface of pathogens (15) (see **Figure 1B**). This mechanism was studied by applying mathematical modeling for hypothesis testing, i.e., we compared the impact of spontaneous versus PMN-mediated immune evasion on the infection outcome. To this end, we modified a previously implemented state-based virtual infection model (12, 13) to realize the PMN-mediated evasion mechanism. We refer to this model as *PMNmed-IE model* to distinguish it from the previously modeled spontaneous immune evasion, which we refer to as *spon-IE model*.

The transition rate values of the SBM were determined by the global parameter estimation algorithm *Simulated Annealing* based on *Metropolis Monte Carlo* scheme. This algorithm aims at searching for the optimal agreement between the simulated kinetics and the experimental data obtained from the whole-blood infection assays. The resulting transition rate values of both models are given in the Tables S2 and S3 in Supplementary Material and the corresponding simulated kinetics are depicted in **Figure 2**. Here, the experimental kinetics correspond to the combined units introduced in the Section "Materials and Methods" plotted in **Figure 2**. The excellent agreement between experiment and simulation can be seen for the whole-blood infection assays with either *C. albicans* (see **Figures 2A,B**) or *C. glabrata* (see **Figures 2D,E**) with their transition rate values in **Figures 2C,F**.

For *C. albicans* infection, the comparison between the spon-IE model and the PMNmed-IE model revealed comparable values for most transition rates, such as ϕ_N, ϕ_M, κ_N, and $\bar{\kappa}_{EK}$ (see **Figure 2C**; Table S2 in Supplementary Material). The largest differences were observed for intracellular killing in monocytes $\left(\kappa_M^{\text{PMNmed-IE}}/\kappa_M^{\text{spon-IE}} = 1.66\right)$ and the decrease of the antimicrobial effect $\left(\gamma^{\text{PMNmed-IE}}/\gamma^{\text{spon-IE}} = 1.26\right)$. However, the whole-blood infection assay does not allow to directly measure differences in these values in order to distinguish between the two immune-evasion models. Similarly, quantitative differences could also be observed for the kinetics of extracellular killing due to antimicrobial peptides (see **Figure 3A**) as well as for the kinetics of immune evasion (see **Figure 3B**). However, these readouts of the simulations either yield only small quantitative differences (time-dependent killing by antimicrobial peptides) or are, despite the qualitatively different time course, again not directly accessible in experiment (time-dependent immune-evasion rate). Thus, while it is possible to reconcile both models with the experimental data, differences in directly measurable quantities could not be identified (see Figures S3 and S4 in Supplementary Material for *C. albicans*).

While the experimental kinetics for *C. glabrata* infection were also found to be in excellent agreement with both the spon-IE and the PMNmed-IE models (see **Figures 2D,E**), differences between the estimated transition rate values were relatively large with up to 23% (see **Figure 2F**; Table S3 in Supplementary Material). The time-dependent extracellular killing due to antimicrobial factors was found to be strongly different between the two models, i.e., the peak values were six times higher for spon-IE model than PMNmed-IE model (see **Figure 3A**) and also the kinetics of immune-evasion were indicative for a larger effect in the spon-IE model than the PMNmed-IE model (see **Figure 3B**). The amount of fungal cells that became immune-evasive increased until 45 min post infection and then leveled off at the predicted

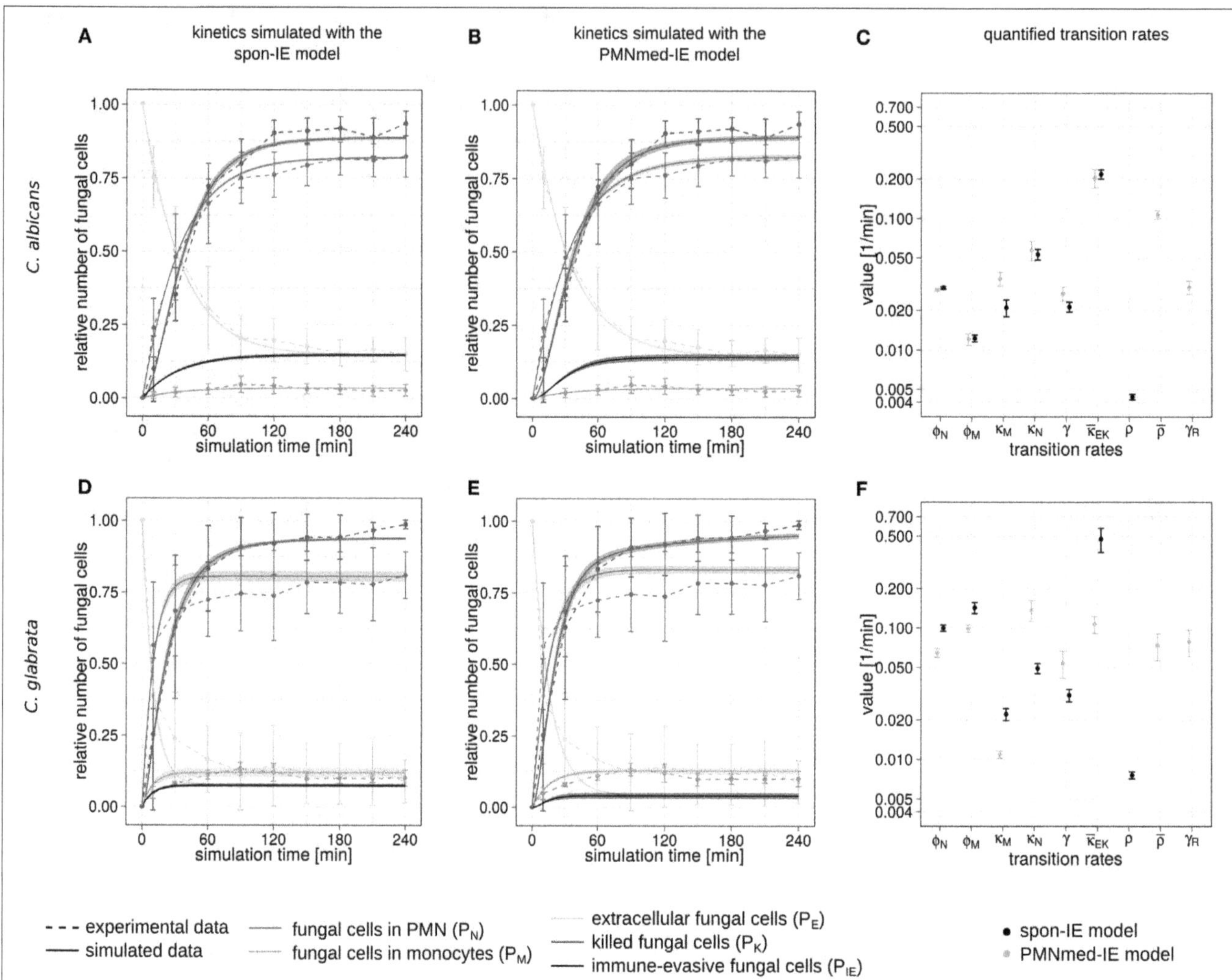

FIGURE 2 | Kinetics of combined units and corresponding transition rate values of the spon-IE model and the PMNmed-IE model. Experimental data from whole-blood infection assays (dashed lines) with corresponding SDs are compared to the simulated data (solid lines) by the spon-IE model (left column) and the PMNmed-IE model (middle column). The thickness of solid lines indicates the mean ± SD of 50 simulations with transition rate values that were randomly sampled within their corresponding SD. Mean values (data points) and SDs (error bars) of transition rates (right column) were quantified by the global parameter estimation algorithm *Simulated Annealing* based on *Metropolis Monte Carlo* scheme for the spon-IE model (black data points) and PMNmed-IE model (gray data points). The transition rates are given by the phagocytosis rate ϕ_N of PMN and the phagocytosis rate ϕ_M of monocytes, the intracellular killing rates κ_M and κ_N of both monocytes and PMN, the transition rates γ and $\bar{\kappa}_{EK}$ which define the extracellular killing, and the spontaneous immune-evasion rate ρ and the PMN-mediated immune-evasion rates $\bar{\rho}$ and γ_R, respectively. The time-course of the relative number of killed pathogens (P_K), which are indicated by red dashed lines, were experimentally measured by survival assays. The relative number of fungal cells that were associated with monocytes (P_M), PMN (P_N), or in extracellular space (P_E) were measured by association assays and indicated by orange, blue, or green dashed lines, respectively. The experimental results were compared with the corresponding combined units calculated for the simulated data. Black solid lines refer to the simulated time-course of immune-evasive fungal cells (P_{IE}). Kinetics of a *Candida albicans* infection simulated by **(A)** the spon-IE model and **(B)** the PMNmed-IE model. **(C)** Transition rates quantified by both models for a *C. albicans* infection. Kinetics of a *Candida glabrata* infection simulated by **(D)** the spon-IE model and **(E)** the PMNmed-IE model. **(F)** Transition rates quantified by both models for a *C. glabrata* infection.

value 7.47 ± 0.58% in the spon-IE model and 4.09 ± 1.0% in the PMNmed-IE model.

The comparison of whole-blood infections with the two pathogens revealed the estimated phagocytosis rate values ϕ_N and ϕ_M to be in both immune-evasion models lower for *C. albicans* than the phagocytosis rates of *C. glabrata*. Furthermore, for *C. albicans*, we found that $\phi_N > \phi_M$, whereas this relation is reversed for *C. glabrata*, reflecting the observed higher association of this pathogen to monocytes. Interestingly, the spon-IE model for infection with *C. glabrata* in comparison to infection with *C. albicans* predicted a higher peak value of the antimicrobial effect by a factor three (see **Figure 3A**). In contrast, the PMNmed-IE model predicted a peak value of the antimicrobial effect that is lower by a factor 0.5 for infection with *C. glabrata* compared to *C. albicans*. Apart from these observations, the two immune-evasion models could equally well explain the experimental

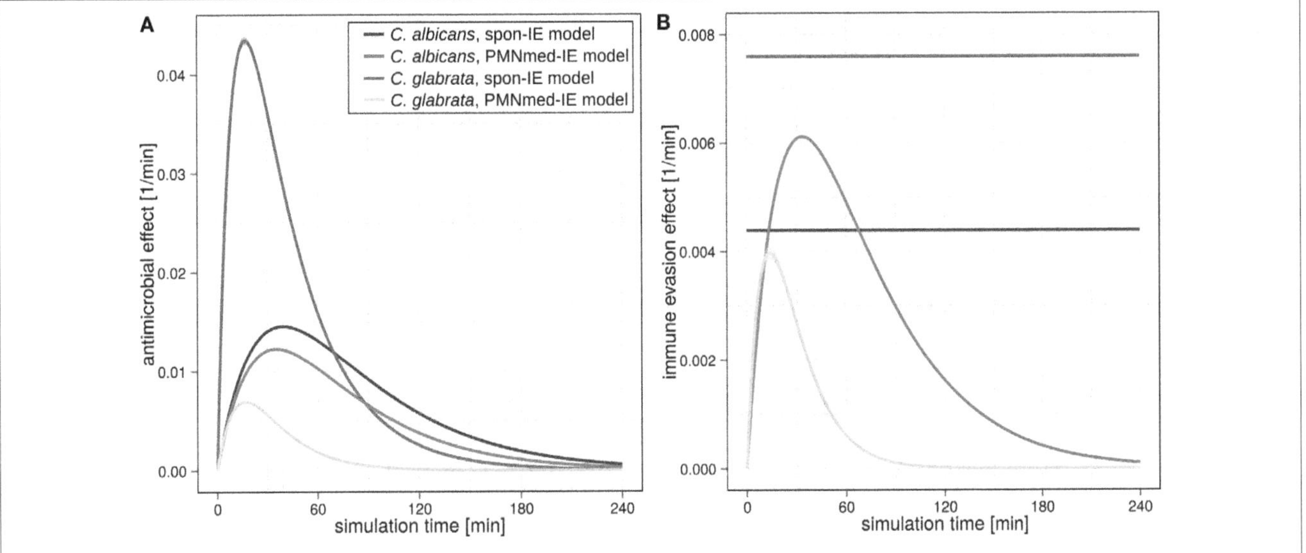

FIGURE 3 | Kinetics of the extracellular killing rate **(A)** and immune-evasion rate **(B)** predicted by spon-IE model and PMNmed-IE model. In both subfigures, purple lines represent results of infection with *Candida albicans* and blue lines depict results of infection with *Candida glabrata*. Predictions by the spon-IE model and PMNmed-IE model are indicated by dark colored lines and pale colored lines, respectively.

kinetics of infection in whole-blood samples as obtained from the healthy blood donors. To work out differences between the two immune-evasion models, we addressed the question how the models differ in their predictions on the infection kinetics for virtual patients with varying severity levels of neutropenia.

Simulations for Virtual Patients With Neutropenia Reveal Differences Between Immune-Evasion Models

The main difference between the spon-IE model and the PMNmed-IE model is that immune evasion in the latter is mediated by PMN and, therefore, is directly associated with the number of PMN in whole blood. Although most patients with candidemia are non-neutropenic, it is well known that neutropenia results in an impaired prognosis and facilitates disseminated infection and organ manifestation (16). Taking the previously estimated transition rate values for healthy blood donors as a reference, we gradually decreased the PMN number in the simulations within the range of medically established severity levels of neutropenia (see **Table 1**) and kept the number of monocytes and fungal cells fixed at $5 \cdot 10^5$ cells and $1 \cdot 10^6$ cells per milliliter, respectively. The predictions of simulations at 4 h post infection for the two immune-evasion models and for each of the two fungal pathogens are shown in **Figure 4**. As could be expected, an increase in the severity level of neutropenia was accompanied by a decreased interaction of fungal cells with PMN.

Virtual infections with *C. albicans* cells under neutropenic conditions revealed clear differences between the spon-IE model (see **Figure 4A**) and the PMNmed-IE model (see **Figure 4B**) at 240 min post infection. Differences in the models could be observed at the transition from moderate to severe neutropenia, where the fraction of immune-evasive fungal cells increased to 25.2 ± 1.0% in the spon-IE model and decreased to 10.4 ± 1.1% in PMNmed-IE model. These values for immune-evasive cells changed to 42.7 ± 1.6% for the spon-IE model and 0.24 ± 0.03% for the PMNmed-IE model in the simulations with the lowest PMN number ($5 \cdot 10^3$ cells/ml). Even though the latter immune-evasion model predicted the number of immune-evasive *C. albicans* cells after 240 min post infection to be vanishingly small, the fraction of extracellular alive fungal cells was larger with 24.5 ± 5.6% for the PMNmed-IE model than for the spon-IE model with 9.7 ± 1.1%. In the simulations with the lowest PMN number, the spon-IE model predicted an association of 46.4 ± 1.9% fungal cells to monocytes, which is clearly lower compared to 73.3 ± 5.8% in the PMNmed-IE model. Furthermore, the number of killed *C. albicans* cells differs between the two models with being predicted as 41.2 ± 2.3% in the spon-IE model and 67.1 ± 5.5% in the PMNmed-IE model. In general, we observed that the differences in various fractions of *C. albicans* cells between the two immune-evasion models clearly increase with progressing simulation time under neutropenic conditions. This can be seen in Video S1 in the Supplementary Material showing the development of the various fungal cell fractions at specific time points between time point 0 and 240 min post infection. Furthermore, differences between the models were observed for the distribution of fungal cells in immune cells for the condition of severe neutropenia with $5 \cdot 10^3$ PMN per milliliter. As shown in (**Figures 5A,B**), the distribution of alive and killed fungal cells across immune cells revealed differences between the immune-evasion models. Here it can be seen that the maximum of the distribution refers to PMN that contain two *C. albicans* cells for the spon-IE model (see **Figure 5A**) and three *C. albicans* cells for the PMNmed-IE model (see **Figure 5B**). Regarding the distribution of fungal cells in monocytes, the spon-IE model and the PMNmed-IE

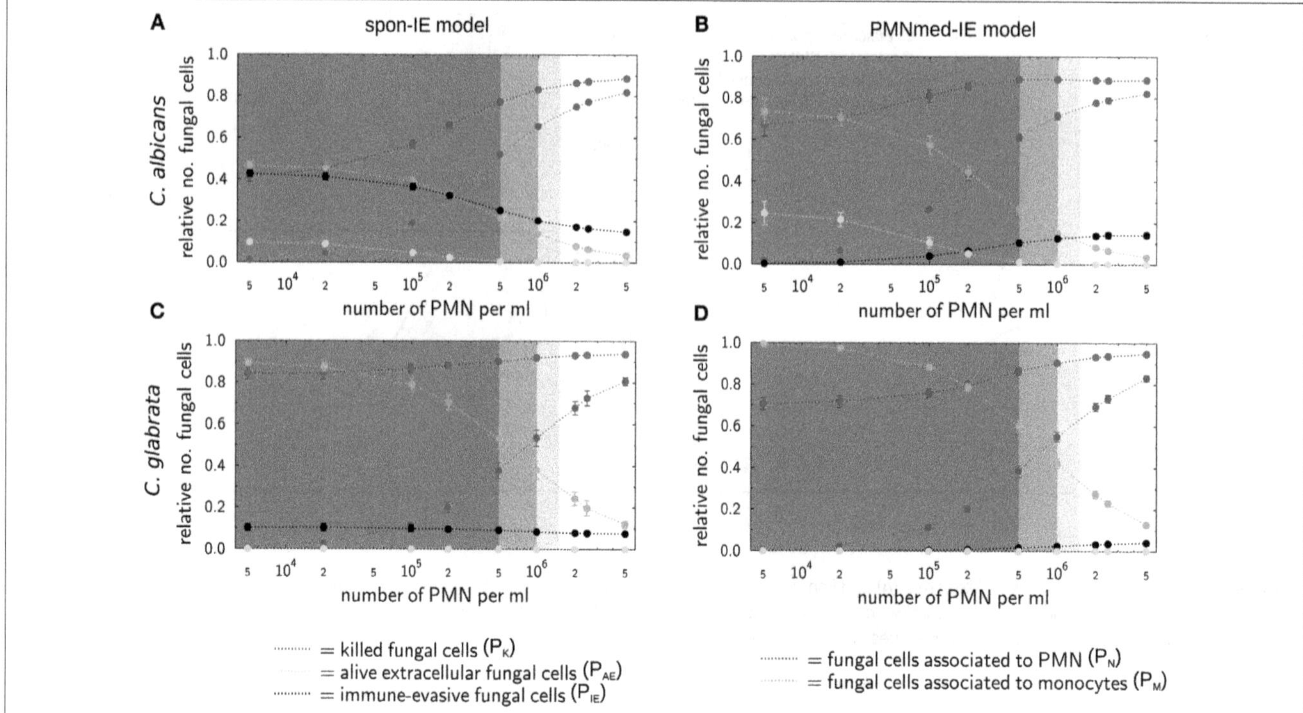

FIGURE 4 | Simulation results of the spon-IE model and of the PMNmed-IE model for different severity levels of neutropenia at the time point 240 min. The white region represents the physiological concentration of a whole-blood sample with 5·10^5 monocytes per milliliter and 5 ·10^6 PMN per milliliter. The PMN concentration declines with increasing severity levels of neutropenia: light gray area represents mild neutropenia (<1.5·10^6 PMN/ml), medium gray area represents moderate neutropenia (<1·10^6 PMN/ml), and dark gray area represents severe neutropenia (<5·10^5 PMN/ml). The error bars indicate SDs of 50 simulations with transition rate values that were randomly sampled within their corresponding SD. **(A,B)** Depict simulation results of a virtual *Candida albicans* infection, respectively, for the spon-IE model and of the PMNmed-IE model and **(C,D)** accordingly for *Candida glabrata* infection. The relative numbers of killed fungal cells (red), alive extracellular fungal cells (green), phagocytosed fungal cells by monocytes (yellow), and by PMN (blue), as well as fungal cells which evaded the immune defense (black) are depicted. Note that alive extracellular cells do not comprise alive immune-evasive cells and that these combined units are excluding each other.

model predicted that the maximum number of monocytes which contained no fungal cells (see **Figure 5C**) and one fungal cell (see **Figure 5D**), respectively. These differences are accompanied by an overall shift of the distributions to higher numbers of phagocytes with more fungal cells in the PMNmed-IE model relative to the spon-IE model (see **Figures 5A–D**). In addition, the spon-IE model predicted a fraction of 7.0 ± 0.5% PMN that contain alive *C. albicans* cells (see **Figure 5A**), whereas this fraction of PMN was predicted to be more than two times larger in the PMNmed-IE model (19.9 ± 1.5%) (see **Figure 5B**).

Simulations for *C. glabrata* infection revealed as well differences between the spon-IE model and the PMNmed-IE model (see **Figures 4C,D**). The fraction of immune-evasive cells attained the value 10.2 ± 1.6% for the spon-IE model and 0.02 ± 0.00% for the PMNmed-IE model in the limit of lowest PMN number (5 ·10^3 cells/ml). While these fractions reached different values, the fractions of extracellular alive cells were found to be vanishingly small in both models. At the PMN number of 5 ·10^3 cells/ml, the spon-IE model predicted 84.1 ± 1.6% of *C. glabrata* cells to be killed and the majority of cells were phagocytosed by monocytes (89.2 ± 1.7%). Analysis of simulations of the PMNmed-IE model revealed that 70.6 ± 2.8% of *C. glabrata* cells were killed and the majority of cells were phagocytosed by monocytes (99.3 ± 0.06%).

The time courses of each of these *C. glabrata* fractions at specific time points between 0 and 240 min post infection are shown in Video S2 in the Supplementary Material. Here it can be seen that at early time points post infection, the differences between the immune-evasion models is clearly visible. But with increasing simulation time these differences become smaller. While the distribution of killed and alive *C. glabrata* cells in PMN was similar for both immune-evasion models (see **Figures 5E,F**), differences in the distributions of fungal cells in monocytes, and their state of viability were observed (see **Figures 5G,H**). As can be seen in **Figure 5G**, the spon-IE model predicted that monocytes contained one to six fungal cells, where only a small fraction of fungal cells was alive, i.e., up to 7.1 ± 0.9% of monocytes contained alive fungal cells. This is in contrast to the PMNmed-IE model (see **Figure 5H**), which predicted a four times larger fraction of monocytes containing alive fungal cells (31.7 ± 1.0%). Thus, under severe neutropenic conditions, the most remarkable differences between the immune-evasion models were obtained with regard to the distribution of alive *C. glabrata* cells in monocytes.

Taken together, comparing the simulations of virtual patients under neutropenic conditions for the two immune-evasion models revealed, except for the number of immune-evaded cells,

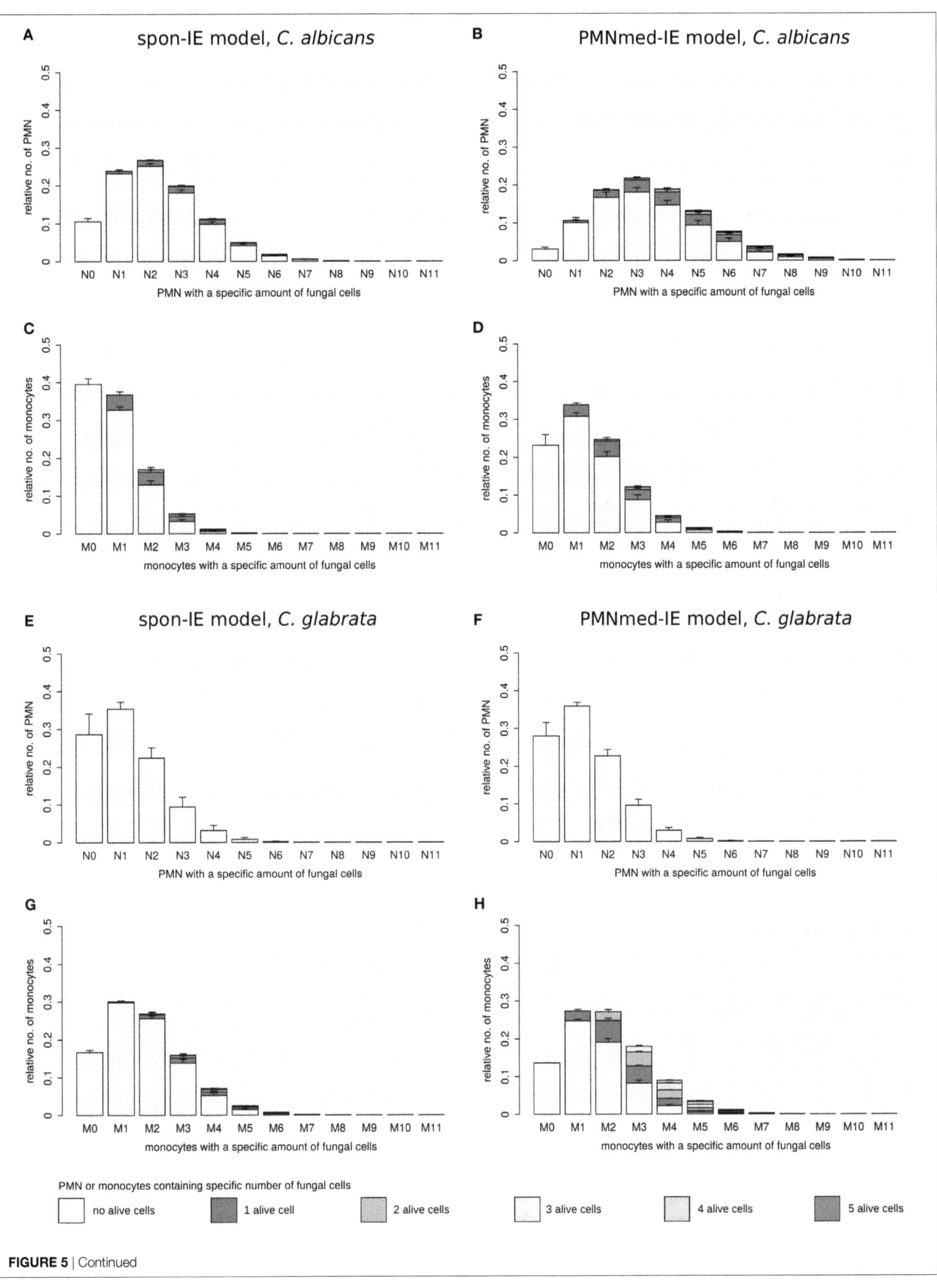

FIGURE 5 | Continued

FIGURE 5 | Distribution of total and alive fungal cells in PMN and monocytes for the most severe neutropenic condition 500 PMN/ml for the spon-IE model (left column) and PMNmed-IE model (right column). Relative numbers of PMN and monocytes are depicted corresponding to their association with fungal cells while each bar represents the immune cell type with the total number (0–11) of phagocytosed fungal cells. The error bars refer to SDs of 50 simulations with transition rate values that were randomly sampled within their corresponding SD. Gray-colored bars refer to "no alive" fungal cells, i.e., phagocytes contain killed cells only, bars in pink color refer to phagocytes with one alive fungal cell, orange bars refer to two alive fungal cells, green bars refer to phagocytes with three alive fungal cells, blue bars refer to phagocytes with four alive fungal cells, and purple bars refer to phagocytes with five alive fungal cells. **(A–D)** *Candida albicans* cell distribution for a virtual infection under the condition of severe neutropenia. **(E–H)** *Candida glabrata* cell distribution for a virtual infection under the condition of severe neutropenia.

a qualitative agreement for both pathogens (see **Figure 4**). Comparing the infection outcome between the two pathogens for each immune-evasion models revealed qualitative agreement, except for the alive extracellular fungal cells that increase (decrease) in the case of *C. albicans* (*C. glabrata*) with higher severity levels of neutropenia. As previously observed for whole blood from healthy donors, the fraction of immune-evasive cells for neutropenic patients was predicted to be higher for *C. albicans* than for *C. glabrata* in the spon-IE model. In contrast, the PMNmed-IE model predicted for both pathogens a quantitatively comparable fraction of immune-evasive cells that vanishes with the severity level of neutropenia. The phagocytosis by monocytes was found to be much lower for *C. albicans* than for *C. glabrata*, for both immune-evasion models, as previously observed for whole blood from healthy donors. This observation was also reflected by the distribution of fungal cells in immune cells (see **Figure 5**). *C. glabrata* was also represented by relatively large numbers of alive cells in monocytes at 4 h post infection. These findings indicate that infection in neutropenic whole blood could shed light on the mechanism of immune evasion by pathogens.

DISCUSSION

In this study, we applied mathematical modeling to investigate the yet unresolved mechanism of immune evasion by pathogens in human blood. The mechanism of immune evasion was first described in a systems biology study that quantified the immune response to *C. albicans* in human whole blood using a state-based virtual infection model (12, 13). Since the mechanism of immune evasion has not been identified so far, the immune evasion was assumed to occur spontaneously with a time-independent rate in the SBM (spon-IE model). In this study, we modified the spon-IE model by implementing a time-dependent immune-evasion mechanism mediated by PMN and refer to this virtual infection model as PMNmed-IE model. This is based on experimental findings, which show that neutrophils can modulate the composition of the fungal cell surface (15). The state-based modeling approach enables realization of such a process by a transition rate that is time-dependent and reflects PMN dynamics of phagocytosis and release of neutrophilic peptides. In order to verify the PMNmed-IE model and the spon-IE model, we estimated the *a priori* unknown transition rates of these models by fitting the simulated kinetics to the experimental data from human whole-blood infection assays with either *C. albicans* or *C. glabrata*. To further work out differences between the immune-evasion models, we simulated infection scenarios with reduced numbers of PMN that correspond to the range of medically established severity levels of neutropenia.

The comparison of the simulated kinetics for infections of blood with physiological and reduced numbers of PMN, the estimated transition rate values, as well as the pathogen distribution across immune cells revealed pathogen-specific differences between the two immune-evasion models. Based on these results, we suggest future experiments that could be performed to distinguish between the two immune-evasion mechanisms. While the kinetics of the experimental whole-blood infection assays for both pathogens could be reconciled with the virtual infection kinetics for both immune-evasion models, simulations for reduced PMN numbers revealed differences between the two immune-evasion models. These differences were largest for *C. albicans* infection and relatively small for infections with *C. glabrata*. In particular, the fractions of fungal cells that were killed, associated with monocytes or that became immune-evasive in simulations with reduced numbers of PMN, showed deviations between the two immune-evasion models most clearly for *C. albicans* (see **Figures 4A,B**). With decreasing PMN number, the PMNmed-IE model for this pathogen predicted that the fraction of immune-evasive pathogens remarkably decreased. Instead of becoming immune-evasive, *C. albicans* cells were mainly phagocytosed by monocytes and killed in this model. Furthermore, a significant fraction of fungal cells ($24.5 \pm 5.6\%$) was still alive and in extracellular space at 240 min post infection. In contrast to the PMNmed-IE model, the spon-IE model predicted the fractions of *C. albicans* cells that are (i) phagocytosed by monocytes, (ii) killed, or (iii) remained viable in extracellular space to be notably smaller, whereas the fraction of immune-evasive *C. albicans* cells is larger, because the constant rate of immune evasion does not depend on the decreasing number of PMN. Interestingly, both immune-evasion models predict even at 240 min post infection a remarkable fraction of *C. albicans* cells that are capable of dissemination. However, in the PMNmed-IE model these cells are mainly alive and extracellular due to absent phagocytosis whereas in the spon-IE model they are mostly immune-evasive fungal cells. Thus, both models would explain the observation that dissemination of *C. albicans* is more frequent in a neutropenic setting, albeit with different mechanisms (26–28). In order to verify the predicted differences for the two immune-evasion models, we suggest studying whole-blood infection assays either with depleted PMN numbers or with blood samples from neutropenic patients.

Regarding the pathogen distribution across immune cells, virtual infection scenarios for *C. albicans* with the low PMN number of $5 \cdot 10^3$ cells/ml revealed differences between the two immune-evasion models in the pathogen distributions within

PMN and monocytes as well as in the fraction of alive *C. albicans* cells in PMN (see **Figures 5A–D**). The experimental validation of the pathogen distribution in PMN and monocytes could be performed by Giemsa-stained blood smears obtained from *C. albicans*-infected blood samples of neutropenic patients. The overall distribution of *C. albicans* cells in PMN and monocytes could lead to further conclusions by comparing the experimental observations to simulated results, although information about viability cannot be obtained by Giemsa-stained blood smears. For the experimental validation of pathogen distribution across immune cells during infection of neutropenic blood samples it is necessary to differentiate between alive and killed fungal cells to unravel the immune-evasion mechanism of *C. glabrata*. The virtual infection of neutropenic blood by this pathogen showed clear differences between the immune-evasion models with regards to the distribution of alive pathogen cells in monocytes (see **Figures 5G,H**). The PMNmed-IE model predicted a relatively large fraction of alive fungal cells in monocytes at 240 min post infection. With increasing infection time in neutropenic patients, the high amount of alive fungal cells in monocytes may result in higher amounts of fungal cells in macrophages, which are professional phagocytes of the monocytic lineage. Since it is reported that *C. glabrata* cells are able to proliferate within macrophages and subsequently can leave these phagocytes (21, 29), this process could contribute to the increased risk for disseminated candidiasis in neutropenic patients (30).

Another suggestion for the experimental investigation of the immune-evasion mechanisms is to measure the activity of antimicrobial effector proteins inducing extracellular killing, because these kinetics are predicted to be different for the two immune-evasion models. This difference was observed to be relatively high for virtual *C. glabrata* infection at physiological numbers of PMN: in the spon-IE model the maximum value for the extracellular killing rate was much larger for *C. glabrata* infection compared to *C. albicans*, whereas in the PMNmed-IE model this peak value was predicted to be much smaller for *C. glabrata* infection (see **Figure 3A**). We, therefore, suggest measuring and comparing the activity of antimicrobial effector proteins inducing extracellular killing, such as lactoferrin, elastase 2 and myeloperoxidase, for both pathogens. In a previous study by Duggan et al. (25), where the differential recognition of *C. albicans* and *C. glabrata* by PMN was investigated, the concentration of these proteins were measured in supernatants of confrontation assays of PMN with the fungi 4 h after infection. For each of these antimicrobial proteins, the concentration in confrontation assays with *C. albicans* was observed to be higher than in confrontation assays with *C. glabrata*. We now suggest measuring not only the concentration of these antimicrobial peptides but also their fungicidal effect on the different pathogens in a comparative fashion. Moreover, our analysis predicts the time-window, where the largest difference for the kinetics of extracellular killing between both pathogens occurs, i.e., at 10 to 50 min post infection.

In future studies, the predictive power of virtual infection modeling can be further exploited by simulating infection scenarios with modified models that enable generating predictions for other hypotheses. For example, while the present study focused on the role of PMN-mediated immune evasion, a similar mechanism could be studied for monocytes, as well as a combination of contributions from both types of immune cells. Future computational studies could also benefit from spatial agent-based modeling. By applying a bottom-up approach, as previously performed by Lehnert et al. (13), the transition rate values of the SBM could be used as input for an agent-based model, where also spatial system properties are captured, such as the cells' morphology and/or migration pattern. This agent-based virtual infection model could, for example, be applied to investigate the impact of the various immune-evasion models on a hyper- and hypo-inflammatory immune response in human blood. In addition, the impact of the spatial distribution of PMN-secreted proteins causing immune evasion could be investigated by advancing the cellular agent-based virtual infection model to a hybrid agent-based model that simulates diffusion at the molecular level by partial differential equations. For example, in previous studies related to fungal infections, a hybrid agent-based model enabled to investigate the immune response against *Aspergillus fumigatus* in the alveoli of the human lung (31, 32). It could be shown that the migration pattern of immune cells is of high importance for the timely infection clearance and this lead to the prediction that chemotactic signaling molecules are essential for recruitment of phagocytes to the spatial position of fungal cells in the lung. Moreover, image-based systems biology approach combining mathematical modeling with microscopy experiments could be pursued (9, 33, 34).

While imaging in whole blood is not performed today, host–pathogen interactions can be investi-gated by microscopy experiments under controlled conditions in a Petri dish. Recently, we have developed algorithms for the fully automated analysis of host–pathogen confrontation from microscopic endpoint experiments (33, 35–38), as well as from live cell maging (39, 40). Similar to our recent comparative studies on *C. albicans* and *C. glabrata* phagocytosis (16, 41), host–pathogen confrontation assays could be performed and analyzed by automated image analysis to visualize surface alterations of immune-evading fungal cells.

AUTHOR CONTRIBUTIONS

Conceived and designed this study: TL and MF. Provision of computational resources: MF. Provision of materials: OK. Data processing, implementation, and application of the computational algorithm: MP, TL, and MF. Performed experiments: KH and IL. Evaluation and analysis of the results: MP, TL, ST, KH, IL, OK, and MF. Draft and revision of the manuscript: MP, TL, ST, KH, IL, OK, and MF.

ACKNOWLEDGMENTS

The authors thank all anonymous blood donors.

FUNDING

This work was financially supported by the Center for Sepsis Control and Care (CSCC) (FKZ 01EO1502, project Quantim to MTF and OK) that is funded by the Federal Ministry for Education and Research, and by the CRC/TR124 FungiNet (project B4 to MTF and project C3 to OK) that is funded by the Deutsche Forschungsgemeinschaft (DFG).

SUPPLEMENTARY MATERIAL

VIDEO S1 | Time-course of simulation results of both immune-evasion models for *C. albicans* infection for different severity levels of neutropenia. The error bars indicate standard deviations of 50 simulations with transition rate values that were randomly sampled within their corresponding standard deviation. The white region represents the physiological concentration of a whole-blood sample with 5 10^5 monocytes per milliliter and 5 10^6 PMN per milliliter. The PMN concentration declines with increasing severity levels of neutropenia: light gray area represents mild neutropenia (<1.5·10^6 PMN/ml), medium gray area represents moderate neutropenia (<1·10^6 PMN/ml) and dark gray area represents severe neutropenia (<5·10^5 PMN/ml). **(A,B)** depict simulation results of a virtual *C. albicans* infection, respectively, for the spon-IE model and of the PMNmed-IE model. The relative numbers of killed fungal cells (red), alive extracellular fungal cells (green), phagocytosed fungal cells by monocytes (yellow) and by PMN (blue), as well as fungal cells which evaded the immune defense (black) are depicted. Note that alive extracellular cells do not comprise alive immune-evasive cells and that these combined units exclude each other.

VIDEO S2 | Time-course of simulation results of both immune-evasion models for *C. glabrata* infection for different severity levels of neutropenia. The error bars indicate standard deviations of 50 simulations with transition rate values that were randomly sampled within their corresponding SD. The white region represents the physiological concentration of a whole-blood sample with 5·10^5 monocytes per milliliter and 5·10^6 PMN per milliliter. The PMN concentration declines with increasing severity levels of neutropenia: light gray area represents mild neutropenia (<1.5·10^6 PMN/ml), medium gray area represents moderate neutropenia (<1·10^6 PMN/ml) and dark gray area represents severe neutropenia (<5·10^5 PMN/ml). **(A,B)** depict simulation results of a virtual *C. glabrata* infection, respectively, for the spon-IE model and of the PMNmed-IE model. The relative numbers of killed fungal cells (red), alive extracellular fungal cells (green), phagocytosed fungal cells by monocytes (yellow) and by PMN (blue), as well as fungal cells which evaded the immune defense (black) are depicted. Note that alive extracellular cells do not comprise alive immune-evasive cells and that these combined units exclude each other.

REFERENCES

Kabir MA, Hussain MA, Ahmad Z. *Candida albicans*: a model organism for studying fungal pathogens. *ISRN Microbiol* (2012) 2012:1–15. doi:10.5402/2012/538694

Kühbacher A, Burger-Kentischer A, Rupp S. Interaction of *Candida* species with the skin. *Microorganisms* (2017) 5(2):32. doi:10.3390/microorganisms5020032

Lee SH, Jeong SK, Ahn SK. An update of the defensive barrier function of skin. *Yonsei Med J* (2006) 47(3):293–306. doi:10.3349/ymj.2006.47. 3.293

Turvey SE, Broide DH. Innate immunity. *J Allergy Clin Immunol* (2010) 125 (2 Suppl 2):S24–32. doi:10.1016/j.jaci.2009.07.016

Cheng S-C, Sprong T, Joosten LAB, van der Meer JWM, Kullberg B-J, Hube B, et al. Complement plays a central role in *Candida albicans*-induced cytokine production by human PBMCs. *Eur J Immunol* (2012) 42(4):993–1004. doi:10.1002/eji.201142057

Beutler BA. TLRs and innate immunity. *Blood* (2009) 113(7):1399–407. doi:10.1182/blood-2008-07-019307

Mogensen TH. Pathogen recognition and inflammatory signaling in innate immune defenses. *Clin Microbiol Rev* (2009) 22(2):240–73. doi:10.1128/CMR. 00046-08

Cheng SC, Joosten LAB, Kullberg BJ, Netea MG. Interplay between *Candida albicans* and the mammalian innate host defense. *Infect Immun* (2012) 80(4):1304–13. doi:10.1128/IAI.06146-11

Medyukhina A, Timme S, Mokhtari Z, Figge MT. Image-based systems biology of infection. *Cytometry A* (2015) 87(6):462–70. doi:10.1002/cyto. a.22638

Chavali AK, Gianchandani EP, Tung KS, Lawrence MB, Peirce SM, Papin JA. Characterizing emergent properties of immunological systems with multi-cellular rule-based computational modeling. *Trends Immunol* (2008) 29:589–99. doi:10.1016/j.it.2008.08.006

Materi W, Wishart DS. Computational systems biology in drug discovery and development: methods and applications. *Drug Discov Today* (2007) 12:295–303. doi:10.1016/j.drudis.2007.02.013

Hünniger K, Lehnert T, Bieber K, Martin R, Figge MT, Kurzai O. A virtual infection model quantifies innate effector mechanisms and *Candida albicans* immune escape in human blood. *PLoS Comput Biol* (2014) 10(2):e1003479. doi:10.1371/journal.pcbi.1003479

Lehnert T, Timme S, Pollmächer J, Hünniger K, Kurzai O, Figge MT. Bottom-up modeling approach for the quantitative estimation of parameters in pathogen-host interactions. *Front Microbiol* (2015) 6:608. doi:10.3389/fmicb.2015.00608

Erwig LP, Gow NAR. Interactions of fungal pathogens with phagocytes. *Nat Rev Microbiol* (2016) 14:163–76. doi:10.1038/nrmicro.2015.21

Hopke A, Nicke N, Hidu EE, Degani G, Popolo L, Wheeler RT. Neutrophil attack triggers extracellular trap-dependent *Candida* cell wall remodeling and altered immune recognition. *PLoS Pathog* (2016) 12(5):e1005644. doi:10.1371/journal.ppat.1005644

Duggan S, Leonhardt I, Hünniger K, Kurzai O. Host response to *Candida albicans* bloodstream infection and sepsis. *Virulence* (2015) 6(4):316–26. do i:10.4161/21505594.2014.988096

Gazendam RP, van de Geer A, Roos D, van den Berg TK, Kuijpers TW. How neutrophils kill fungi. *Immunol Rev* (2016) 273(1):299–311. doi:10.1111/imr.12454

Low C-Y, Rotstein C. Emerging fungal infections in immunocompromised patients. *F1000 Med Rep* (2011) 3(14). doi:10.3410/M3-14

Falagas ME, Roussos N, Vardakas KZ. Relative frequency of albicans and the various non-albicans *Candida* spp among candidemia isolates from inpatients in various parts of the world: a systematic review. *Int J Infect Dis* (2010) 14(11):e954–66. doi:10.1016/j.ijid.2010.04.006

Brunke S, Hube B. Two unlike cousins: *Candida albicans* and *C. glabrata* infection strategies. *Cell Microbiol* (2013) 15(5):701–8. doi:10.1111/cmi.12091

Seider K, Brunke S, Schild L, Jablonowski N, Wilson D, Majer O, et al. The facultative intracellular pathogen *Candida glabrata* subverts macrophage cytokine production and phagolysosome maturation. *J Immunol* (2011) 187(6):3072–86. doi:10.4049/jimmunol.1003730

de Vries G, Hillen T, Lewis M, Müller J, Schonfisch B. *A Course in Mathematical Biology: Quantitative Modeling with Computational Methods (Monographs on Mathematical Modeling and Computation)*. Philadelphia Society for Industrial and Applied Mathematics (2006).

Press W, Teukolsky S, Vetterling WT, Flannery BP. *Numerical Recipies: The Art of Scientific Computing*. 3rd ed. New York: Cambridge University Press (2007). 1256 p.

Boxer LA. How to approach neutropenia. *Hematology Am Soc Hematol Educ Program* (2012) 2012:174–82. doi:10.1182/asheducation-2012.1.174

Duggan S, Essig F, Hünniger K, Mokhtari Z, Bauer L, Lehnert T, et al. Neutrophil activation by *Candida glabrata* but not *Candida albicans* pro- motes fungal uptake by monocytes. *Cell Microbiol* (2015) 17(9):1259–76. doi:10.1111/cmi.12443

Guiot HFL, Fibbe WE, van't Wout JW. Risk factors for fungal infection in patients with malignant hematologic disorders: implications for empirical therapy and prophylaxis. *Clin Infect Dis* (1994) 18(4):525–32. doi:10.1093/clinids/18.4.525

Bow EJ, Loewen R, Cheang MS, Schacter B. Invasive fungal disease in adults undergoing remission-induction therapy for acute myeloid leukemia:

the pathogenetic role of the antileukemic regimen. *Clin Infect Dis* (1995) 21(2):361–9. doi:10.1093/clinids/21.2.361

Verduyn Lunel FM, Meis JF, Voss A. Nosocomial fungal infections: candidemia. *Diagn Microbiol Infect Dis* (1999) 34(3):213–20. doi:10.1016/S0732-8893(99)00035-8

Kasper L, Seider K, Hube B. Intracellular survival of *Candida glabrata* in macrophages: immune evasion and persistence. *FEMS Yeast Res* (2015) 15(5):1–12. doi:10.1093/femsyr/fov042

Perlroth J, Choi B, Spellberg B. Nosocomial fungal infections: epidemiology, diagnosis, and treatment. *Med Mycol* (2007) 45(4):321–46. doi:10.1080/13693780701218689

Pollmächer J, Figge MT. Agent-based model of human alveoli predicts chemotactic signaling by epithelial cells during early *Aspergillus fumigatus* infection. *PLoS One* (2014) 9(10):e111630. doi:10.1371/journal.pone.0111630

Pollmächer J, Figge MT. Deciphering chemokine properties by a hybrid agent-based model of *Aspergillus fumigatus* infection in human alveoli. *Front Microbiol* (2015) 6:503. doi:10.3389/fmicb.2015.00503

Mech F, Wilson D, Lehnert T, Hube B, Figge MT. Epithelial invasion outcompetes hypha development during *Candida albicans* infection as revealed by an image-based systems biology approach. *Cytometry A* (2014) 85(2):126–39. doi:10.1002/cyto.a.22418

Figge MT, Murphy RF. Image-based systems biology. *Cytometry A* (2015) 87:459–61. doi:10.1002/cyto.a.22663

Mech F, Thywißen A, Guthke R, Brakhage AA, Figge MT. Automated image analysis of the host-pathogen interaction between phagocytes and *Aspergillus fumigatus*. *PLoS One* (2011) 6(5):e19591. doi:10.1371/journal.pone.0019591

Kraibooj K, Schoeler H, Svensson C, Brakhage AA, Figge MT. Automated quantification of the phagocytosis of *Aspergillus fumigatus* conidia by a novel image analysis algorithm. *Front Microbiol* (2015) 6:549. doi:10.3389/fmicb.2015.00549

Cseresnyes Z, Kraibooj K, Figge MT. Hessian-based quantitative image analysis of host-pathogen confrontation assays authors. *Cytometry A* (2018). doi:10.1002/cyto.a.23201

Kraibooj K, Park H-R, Dahse H-M, Skerka C, Voigt K, Figge MT. Virulent strain of *Lichtheimia corymbifera* shows increased phagocytosis by macrophages as revealed by automated microscopy image analysis. *Mycoses* (2014) 57:56–66. doi:10.1111/myc.12237

Brandes S, Mokhtari Z, Essig F, Hünniger K, Kurzai O, Figge MT. Automated segmentation and tracking of non-rigid objects in time-lapse microscopy videos of polymorphonuclear neutrophils. *Med Image Anal* (2015) 20(1):34–51. doi:10.1016/j.media.2014.10.002

Brandes S, Dietrich S, Hünniger K, Kurzai O, Figge MT. Migration and inter- action tracking for quantitative analysis of phagocyte-pathogen confrontation assays. *Med Image Anal* (2017) 36:172–83. doi:10.1016/j.media.2016.11.007

Essig F, Hünniger K, Dietrich S, Figge MT, Kurzai O. Human neutrophils dump *Candida glabrata* after intracellular killing. *Fungal Genet Biol* (2015) 84:37–40. doi:10.1016/j.fgb.2015.09.008

9

Development of a Computational Model of Abscess Formation

Alexandre B. Pigozzo[1]*, Dominique Missiakas*[2]*, Sergio Alonso*[3]*, Rodrigo W. dos Santos*[4] *and Marcelo Lobosco*[4*]

[1] Department of Computer Science, Federal University of São João Del-Rei, São João Del-Rei, Brazil, [2] Department of Microbiology, University of Chicago, Chicago, IL, United States, [3] Department of Physics, Universitat Politècnica de Catalunya, Barcelona, Spain, [4] Graduate Program in Computational Modeling, Federal University of Juiz de Fora, Juiz de Fora, Brazil

***Correspondence:**
Marcelo Lobosco
marcelo.lobosco@ice.ufjf.br

In some bacterial infections, the immune system cannot eliminate the invading pathogen. In these cases, the invading pathogen is successful in establishing a favorable environment to survive and persist in the host organism. For example, *S. aureus* bacteria survive in organ tissues employing a set of mechanisms that work in a coordinated and highly regulated way allowing: (1) efficient impairment of the immune response; and (2) protection from the immune cells and molecules. *S. aureus* secretes several proteins including coagulases and toxins that drive abscess formation and persistence. Unless staphylococcal abscesses are surgically drained and treated with antibiotics, disseminated infection and septicemia produce a lethal outcome. Within this context, this paper develops a simple mathematical model of abscess formation incorporating characteristics that we judge important for an abscess to be formed. Our aim is to build a mathematical model that reproduces some characteristics and behaviors that are observed in the process of abscess formation.

Keywords: *S. aureus* infection, abscess formation, fibrin network, partial differential equation, computational modeling

1. INTRODUCTION

In some *Staphylococcus aureus* infections, neutrophils cannot completely eliminate the invading pathogen. In such cases, a lesion known as abscess may form, especially in skin or in soft tissue organs. An abscess is characterized by an area comprising invading pathogens, fibrin, immune cells (mainly neutrophils) and many types of dead cells, and it may be formed in response to viral or bacterial infections in various organs. Abscess formation is often a defense mechanism elicited by the host to prevent dissemination of pathogens. However, in some instances, such as mycobacterial and staphylococcal infections, the pathogen appears to have subverted this defense and paradoxically uses this environment to thrive and persist (Cheng et al., 2009, 2010; Graves et al., 2010; Kim et al., 2011, 2012; McAdow et al., 2012).

Following intravenous infection of mice, *S. aureus* starts to leave the vasculature to colonize the renal tissue a few hours later. In the vasculature, *S. aureus* begins to produce toxins[1]. Some, like α-toxin, can target various cell types and lead to massive damage in infected sites. Other, like the leukotoxins, are more specific and target mainly leukocytes (Kwiecinski, 2013). The function

[1] "Lysing toxins" or membrane-active toxins that interact with membranes of host cells and - under some conditions - can cause lysis of those cells.

of these toxins is thought to primarily kill immune cells, but also to alter host responses. For example, interaction of α-toxin with its receptor ADAMS10 causes tissue barrier disruption that may facilitate dissemination from the vasculature to organs (Berube and Bubeck Wardenburg, 2013). *S. aureus* also induces the clotting of blood and plasma in the vasculature (Cheng et al., 2009, 2010). Presumably this mechanism prevents immune cells, in the bloodstream, to phagocytose the bacteria. Further, this mechanism is responsible for the formation of bacterial agglutinates or micro-emboli that may help to mechanically disrupt the endothelial barrier and thereby allow the bacteria to gain access into tissues. Despite these strategies, few bacteria manage to survive in the vasculature and establish lesions in the kidney successfully. Within 3 h of infection, the bacteria load in both blood and kidneys are high (Cheng et al., 2009, 2010). Then bacteria loads decrease until 12 h post inoculation (Cheng et al., 2009, 2010). This is due to the fact that immune cells, mainly neutrophils, are successfully eliminating the majority of bacteria. Other host defense mechanisms, such as complement system, also contribute to bacterial killing (Foster, 2005). Then after 12 h, we can clearly view a pattern of logistic growth of the bacteria load. This pattern appears as a result of the abscess formation dynamics (Cheng et al., 2009).

After 12 h, *S. aureus* starts to replicate forming a *Staphylococcus* abscess community (SAC) inside the abscess lesion. During this process, the bacteria employ a variety of mechanisms to kill and evade immune cells. But equally important is a mechanism used by *S. aureus* to isolate themselves from immune cells conferring an even greater protection. This mechanism is the result of the deposition of fibrin clots around the SAC, and around the entire lesion (Cheng et al., 2009, 2010; McAdow et al., 2012). *S. aureus* secretes coagulases, Coa and vWbp, that bind to and activate prothrombin, thereby converting fibrinogen to fibrin. The coagulases diffuse throughout the tissue from the SAC, inducing the conversion of fibrinogen to fibrin in the regions around the bacteria colonies. As a result, a fibrin network is formed around the SAC (Foster, 2005; Cheng et al., 2010; McAdow et al., 2012). *S. aureus* encodes a surface protein called Clumping Factor A (ClfA) (Foster and Höök, 1998), which is responsible for the recognition and binding to fibrin. ClfA-mediated binding of fibrin delineates the first margin of the SAC. The resultant fibrin polymer forms the structure of fibrin around the staphylococci (Foster, 2005; Cheng et al., 2010; McAdow et al., 2012), and *S. aureus* persists in the center of abscess lesions protected from the immune system. Unless staphylococcal abscesses are surgically drained and treated with antibiotics, disseminated infection and septicemia produce a lethal outcome (Kim et al., 2011). Therefore it is important to gain a deep understanding of how an abscess is formed in order to develop vaccines and treatments to *S. aureus* infections. *In vivo* experiments have been performed to identify the factors necessary for abscess formation, but the search for its determinants is a complex task, since it requires studying the interaction between hundreds or even thousands of components that participate in the process and analyzing how observed behavior emerges from these interactions. Mathematical and computational modeling (Bender, 2000; Meerschaert, 2013; Shiflet and Shiflet, 2014) can help in this search, contributing to a better comprehension of some aspects of abscess formation as, for example, the importance of different mechanisms employed by pathogens to survive in the host.

A set of related works developed mathematical models of the immune response with the objective of studying the following subjects: (1) the innate immune response to a bacterial infection, (2) the formation of bacteria colonies, and (3) the dynamics of interaction between the host and the pathogen. The related works bear some similarities to this paper, such as for instance, the modeling of bacteria and neutrophil cells and the modeling of processes such as bacteria replication, neutrophil migration, phagocytosis and diffusion. However, none of them are capable of reproducing the formation of a stable abscess pattern.

In Keener and Sneyd (1998) a unidimensional model developed by Alt and Lauffenburger (1987) is presented to study under what conditions Polymorphonuclear leukocytes (PMNs), more commonly called neutrophils, are successful in controlling a bacterial infection. The model is comprised of three variables: bacteria (b), cytokine (c) and neutrophil (n). The authors performed a linear stability analysis of the model [more details can be obtained in section 16.3 of the book Mathematical Physiology Keener and Sneyd, 1998] and the results obtained can be summarized in three cases: (1) bacteria are completely eliminated and the neutrophil concentration stabilizes to a normal value; (2) neutrophils cannot control the growth of bacteria and bacteria grow without limitation; (3) neutrophils control the growth of bacteria, but they cannot completely eliminate them. In this case, there is a state of persistent infection where both are present and maintain a balance. These three behaviors are also obtained in the bacteria-neutrophil model developed here. The paper concludes that a bacterial infection can be controlled when the rate of phagocytosis is sufficiently large and the immune response is most effective when neutrophils are able to recruit more cells and move chemotactically. As will be shown, the same behavior is observed in this paper for models that consider the dynamics of neutrophils. The model of Alt and Lauffenburger (1987) does not consider the dynamics of fibrin as this paper does. Here, we study and analyze the effects of fibrin in a mathematical model of the abscess formation process.

Kawasaki et al. (1997) have developed a reaction-diffusion system for bacterial and nutrient concentrations that reproduces various observed growth patterns in colonies of bacteria. One of the important elements of the model is a non-linear diffusion term that depends on both concentrations of bacteria and nutrients. The model simulates the fact that, in regions devoid of nutrients, the bacteria cannot move, becoming more inactive. They were able to produce highly branched patterns only with the presence of a minimal anisotropy coming from the square *lattice* used in simulations. In spite of reproducing several patterns, the model was not able to reproduce the pattern of concentric rings because, according to the authors, this pattern requires additional mechanisms. The model of Kawasaki et al. (1997) does not study the immune response to a bacterial infection, the dynamics of fibrin and toxins as this paper does. Besides, the model does not consider diffusion to be dependent on the amount of available space as the models presented in this paper do.

An additional mechanism was proposed by Lacasta et al. (1999). They presented a model of reaction-diffusion for the growth of colonies of bacteria of the species *Bacillus subtilis.* The model is comprised of two equations for the concentrations of bacteria and nutrients. Like the previous model of Kawasaki et al. (1997), the model of Lacasta and co-authors was able to reproduce different growth patterns of species *B. subtilis*, which resulted in a rich variety of structures. Certain structures, such as concentric rings, were only obtained because they considered in the model a cooperative behavior among bacteria. This behavior was modeled considering a global phenomenological variable that represents the number of bacteria most active in the colony, that is, the bacteria that move more in search of nutrients. In addition, they considered a nonlinear diffusion coefficient that depends on this variable.Lacasta et al. (1999) did not consider the immune response, the dynamics of fibrin and toxins in their model as this paper does.

Smith et al. (2011) developed a number of models to gain a greater understanding of how different layers of host defense in the lower respiratory tract, including resident cells and recruited cells, combine to form a response against a pneumococcal lung infection. In this study, the immune response is divided into three stages: (1) the response given by resident alveolar macrophages; (2) the response given by neutrophils; and (3) the response given by macrophages derived from monocytes from the bloodstream. Mathematical models that describe the dynamics of each of these three stages were developed (Smith et al., 2011). Smith and co-authors studied the relationship between the inoculated concentration of bacteria and two outcomes: (1) the establishment or (2) the eradication of an infection. First, they used a single alveolar macrophage response equation to study how a threshold dose determines whether the result will be the establishment or eradication of the infection. This model was then extended to incorporate pro-inflammatory cytokine production accompanied by neutrophil recruitment. Finally, they examined the possibility of elimination of the bacteria given by an influx of monocyte-derived macrophages. The authors argue that through these models it was possible to better understand the contribution of each of the variables considered for the initiation and resolution of pneumococcal pulmonary infection and were able to capture the qualitative behavior of the experimental data.The work of Smith et al. (2011) does not consider the dynamics of fibrin formation and toxin production by the bacteria and the interactions between fibrin, toxin and neutrophils.

Other studies examine the dynamics of parasites in the immune system. The first work (Antia et al., 1994) considers the dynamics of parasites during an acute infection. The model considers a generic population of parasites and it assumes that the virulence of parasites is proportional to the rate of parasite growth in the host. The results indicated that the transmission would be more efficient if the parasite had an intermediate growth rate (not as high as, for example, *E. coli*, and not as low as *M. tuberculosis*). The authors argued that this would result in an evolution and maintenance of an intermediate level of parasitic virulence. A second work by Antia et al. (1996) considered a different set of hypotheses for the dynamics of persistent parasitic infections. This model predicts that initial persistence in the host can be achieved by parasites that grow very slowly or by parasites that have a niche that is inaccessible to the immune response. In addition, the authors suggested that the evasion of immune response by the pathogen at a time well after the onset of infection may be a consequence of two processes: (1) deletion of T cells in the thymus caused by the antigens; and (2) presence of a maximum limit on the number of divisions of a T cell. In this paper, we show that a refuge mechanism used by some bacteria to persist in the host is the formation of a fibrin network that confers protection against the immune response.

In our previous paper (Pigozzo et al., 2012), we were capable of reproducing the initial formation of an abscess, but the abscess pattern did not remain stable. One possible explanation is the fact that *S. aureus* abscesses are encapsulated within a fibrin capsule triggered upon secretion of two coagulases, Coa and vWbp (Cheng et al., 2010; McAdow et al., 2012), which were not modeled in our previous paper.

The objective of this paper is to construct a mathematical model, based on partial differential equations (PDEs), that essentially reproduces a pattern that is observed in histology images of renal abscesses in mice (Cheng et al., 2009, 2010; Graves et al., 2010; Kim et al., 2011; McAdow et al., 2012; Kim et al., 2012). The pattern is comprised by the following regions:)1) some region occupied by the bacteria colony (SAC); (2) some region containing fibrin that forms a network around a bacteria colony; and (3) surrounding the fibrin network, a region comprised mainly of necrotic neutrophils and some live neutrophils. **Figure 1** shows these regions and how they appear in the results of the computational simulations of this paper. In addition, we study and analyze the characteristics of distinct models involving the interactions between bacteria, the two coagulases or coagulation factors, Coa and vWbp, fibrin and neutrophils. This paper shows that it is possible to reproduce some aspects of abscess formation through computational models that are able to capture the spatiotemporal dynamics of the fibrin network formation around the bacteria colony as well as the neutrophil response to the bacterial infection. The computational models were implemented using an explicit Euler method for time discretization and, for the spatial discretization, the Finite Volume Method (Versteeg and Malalasekera, 2011), as will be described in the following section.

The rest of the text is organized as follow. First, we describe the characteristics of the mathematical models developed in this paper and the numerical methods employed in the implementation. Then, we present the results of computational simulations with the models and, finally, we discuss limitations and future work and draw our conclusions.

2. MATERIALS AND METHODS

This paper introduces a mathematical model composed of a system of Partial Differential Equations (PDEs) to describe the abscess formation. PDE-based models usually include terms such

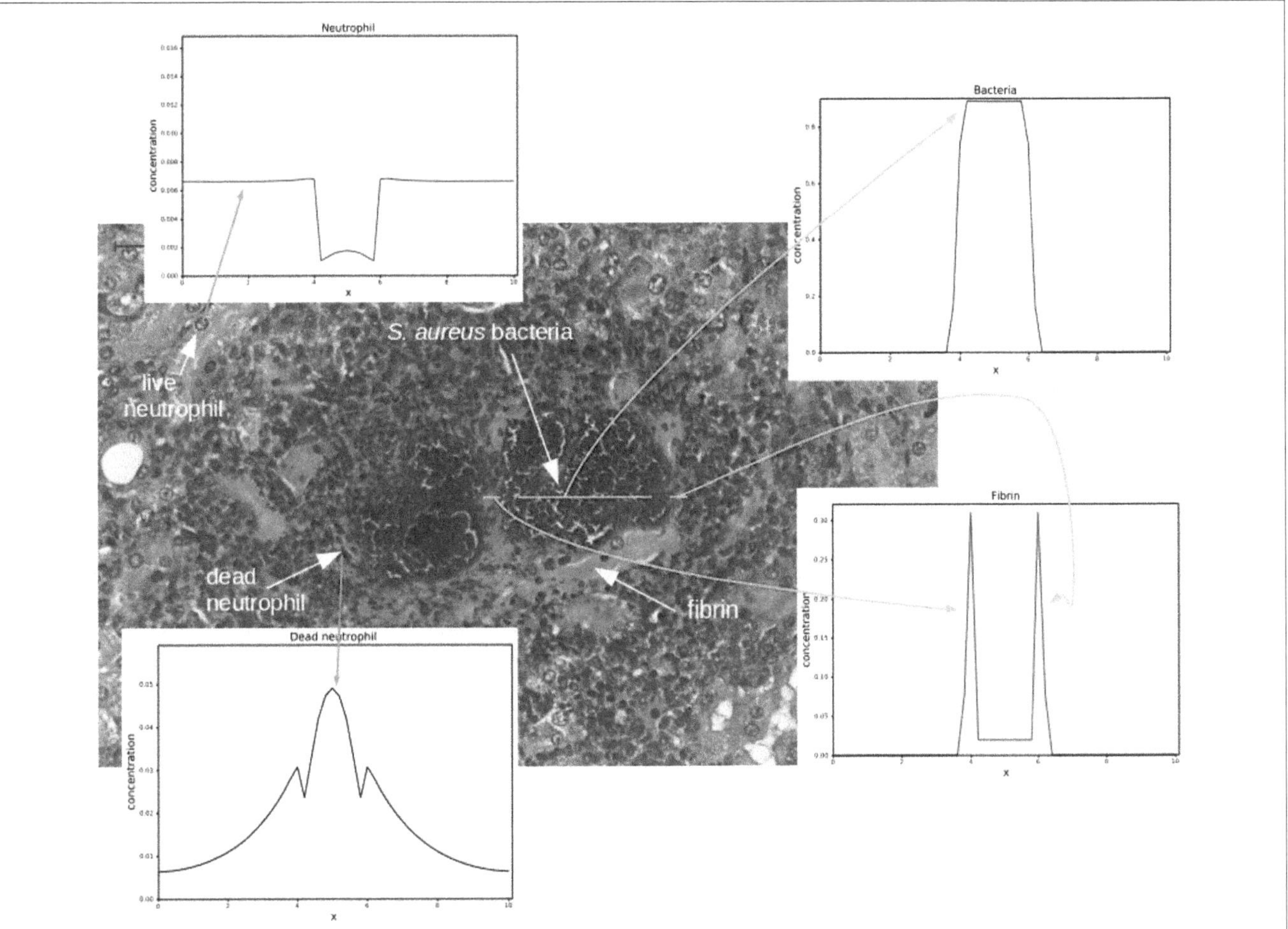

FIGURE 1 | Histology image provided by the Laboratory of Microbiology of the University of Chicago. Adapted with permission of Dominique Missiakas and Olaf Schneewind. The histology image shows a mouse renal tissue infected with *S. aureus* and the corresponding spatial distributions for each cell type. The spatial distributions were obtained by the computational simulation that will be presented in this paper. The darker purple region is the colony of staphylococci and the pink region around the staphylococci colony is the fibrin network. Some dark points around the fibrin are necrotic neutrophils and some points in the "periphery" of the abscess are live neutrophils. These regions form the abscess. For each region highlighted in this figure, an example of a result obtained by the implementation of the mathematical models presented in this paper is shown with a yellow arrow.

as growth, death and interaction terms and they have terms that are responsible for modeling the movement of cells, molecules and bacteria through the diffusion process. The majority of PDEs presented in this paper have the following structure in common:

$$\frac{\partial u}{\partial t} = f\,g + D\nabla \cdot (g\,\nabla u),$$
$$u(x,0) = u_0, \frac{\partial u(.,t)}{\partial \vec{n}}|_{\partial\Omega} = 0, \tag{1}$$

where u is a variable that refers to a given population, the term f is a function that models the growth of u and the term $D\nabla \cdot (g\,\nabla u)$ models the nonlinear diffusion of u. Function g is equivalent to the g function proposed in (Painter and Sherratt, 2003). This function was originally developed to model the movement of interacting cell populations (Painter and Sherratt, 2003). We extended it to model interactions that also occur in other cellular processes. For example, we use the g function to model interactions that occur during bacterial growth or neutrophil migration. The g function is used to account for different interaction strengths between the populations and the effects of these in processes of growth, phagocytosis, migration, death and diffusion.

The g function is defined as the heaviside function of $\overline{g}$:

$$g(w) = \begin{cases} \overline{g}(w), & 0 \leq \overline{g}(w) \leq 1 \\ 0, & otherwise. \end{cases} \tag{2}$$

Function $\overline{g}(w)$ is defined as:

$$\overline{g}(w) = 1 - \frac{w}{total}, \tag{3}$$

where w is a term that models the interactions between distinct populations and *total* is a parameter that denotes the maximum population supported in a discretized region of the domain. In this work, we consider that the value of *total* is constant and is equal to 1 for all discretized regions.

The interactions between the populations can be stimulatory or inhibitory. In this paper, we consider only inhibitory interactions in the w term. To illustrate the meaning of w, consider, for example, a system with two types of populations: u and v. The interactions that each population has with the other one are modeled by the w term. Therefore, the w term is defined for each distinct population in the system. For example, the w for the u population is defined as:

$$w_u = w_{uu}\, u + w_{vu}\, v, \tag{4}$$

where $w_{uu}\, u$ is the inhibition that u exerts on itself and $w_{vu}\, v$ is the inhibition that v exerts on u. These inhibitory relations will affect all processes in u dynamics. w_{uu} and w_{vu} are constant parameters. We call these parameters "weights" to refer to the fact that they control the strength of the inhibition that one population exerts on the other.

The $\bar{g}$ function for the u population is:

$$\bar{g}(w_u) = 1 - w_u. \tag{5}$$

For the v population, we have:

$$w_v = w_{vv}\, v + w_{uv}\, u, \tag{6}$$

where $w_{vv}\, v$ is the inhibition that v exerts on itself and $w_{uv}\, u$ is the inhibition that u exerts on v. These inhibitory relations will affect all processes in v dynamics. w_{vv} and w_{uv} are constant parameters. The $\bar{g}$ function for the v population is:

$$\bar{g}(w_v) = 1 - w_v. \tag{7}$$

We can extend the definition of w for a system with n distinct populations. Considering the u population again, w_u is defined as:

$$w_u = w_{uu}\, u + \sum_{\substack{j \in C,\\ j \neq u}} w_{ju}\, j, \tag{8}$$

where C is the set of all distinct populations in the system and j is one of these populations that is different from u. The summation accounts for the inhibition that u suffers from all other populations, with w_{ju} being the strength of the inhibition that j population exerts on u.

We can also interpret the g function as a way to model the effect that the lack of space has in the dynamics of a population because its value can be seen as the amount of available space in a discretized region of the domain. Considering that all regions in the domain support a maximum number of cells, molecules and/or bacteria (denoted by *total*), diffusion cannot occur for fully occupied regions where there is no available space. In these regions, we have $w \geq$ *total* which implies that $\frac{w}{total} \geq 1$ and $\bar{g}(w) \leq 0$ and, as a result, $g(w)$ of Equation 2 is zero.

The diffusion of bacteria has another term, $h(b)$, that models their cooperative behavior. The bacteria diffusion term is defined as:

$$D_b \nabla \cdot (g_b(w_b)\, h(b)\, \nabla b), \tag{9}$$

where $g_b(w_b)$ is the bacteria g function and w_b is the bacteria interaction term. The function $h(b)$ models a behavior where the bacteria colony grows when conditions are favorable and the colony density is high. The bacteria will only colonize nearby regions when they were successful in establishing a colony in their current location. As a consequence of this, in our model, the diffusion of bacteria only occurs when bacteria concentration is above a threshold. The function $h(b)$ is defined as:

$$h(b) = \frac{(\alpha + 1)\, b^{\gamma}}{\alpha + b^{\gamma}}. \tag{10}$$

This equation is a hyperbolic saturation function (Haefner, 2005) and it is known as Hill equation in this form (Goutelle et al., 2008). The Hill equation is used, for example, to model the relationship between drug concentration and its effects (Wagner, 1968). In this equation, the term $\alpha + 1$ scales the maximum value to which the function is asymptotic, parameter α is a half saturation constant and γ is a shape parameter (Haefner, 2005). It is important to mention that the term $h(b)$ is only present in the diffusion of bacteria. If we consider that the cooperative behavior is absent by doing $h(h) = 1$, we have a situation where, even for a region with very few bacteria, the bacteria can diffuse to neighboring regions with available space and, as a result, it is hard for the bacteria to form a colony surrounded by fibrin because some bacteria will always "escape." Therefore, in our model, such cooperative behavior as well as the nonlinear diffusion are important to the formation of the abscess pattern.

In all models, the exchange between the vascular system (arterioles and vessels) and the tissue was assumed to occur in all points of the one-dimensional space. This is a reasonable first approach because the kidney is highly vascularized.

The numerical methods used were the following: (1) explicit Euler method for time discretization; and (2) for spatial discretization, we used the Finite Volume Method (FVM) (Versteeg and Malalasekera, 2011). The nonlinear diffusion was implemented with a method based on FVM, where the calculus of the divergent operator is based on the quantities calculated at the two interfaces (left and right) of the finite volume. The derivatives and the gradient operator are approximated with numerical fluxes calculated at the interfaces. The quantities at each interface are an average of the quantities on the neighboring nodes. In summary, FVM is based on the evaluation of influx and outflux in a control volume around each node in the mesh. The code was implemented in C and the graphs were generated with a script in Python.

3. RESULTS

In this paper, we incrementally build a mathematical model of abscess formation. The interactions between the model's components are depicted in **Figure 2**. It is important to highlight that the intensity of a particular inhibitory relation (in **Figure 2**, inhibitory relations are represented by red arrows with the word inhibition) depends on concentrations of the cellular types that are exerting the inhibition. In the next sections, we will discuss

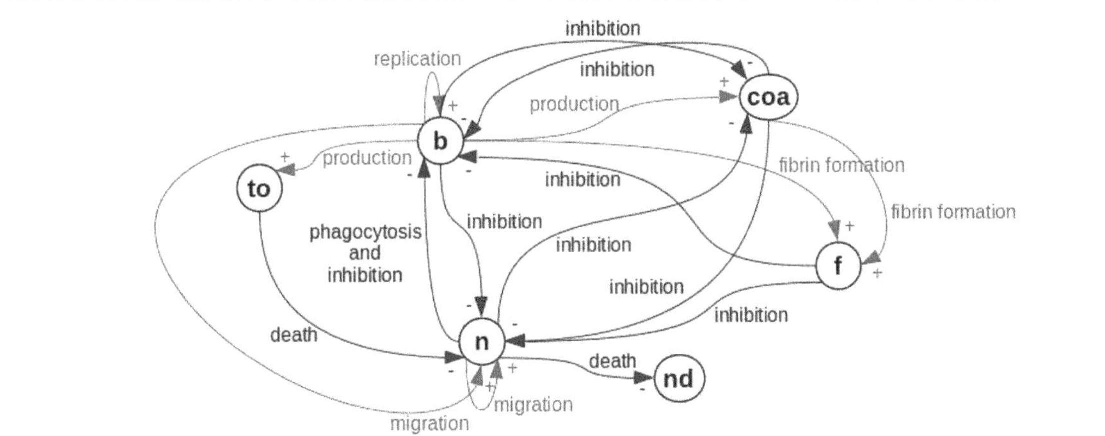

FIGURE 2 | Interactions in the abscess formation model. In this figure, we use the notation of Causal Loop Diagrams (CLD) of System Dynamics. Bacteria are represented by *b*, Coa/vWbp are represented by *coa*, fibrin is represented by *f*, neutrophils are represented by *n*, dead neutrophils are represented by *nd* and toxins are represented by *to*. Bacteria have a replication process forming new bacteria. Bacteria produce Coa/vWbp and participate together with Coa/vWbp in fibrin network formation. Bacteria are phagocytosed by neutrophils. In addition, bacteria produce toxins that cause neutrophil death and inhibit all processes in neutrophil dynamics. The processes present in the bacteria dynamics are all inhibited by Coa/vWbp, fibrin and neutrophil. Coa production is inhibited by the neutrophil and by the bacteria. Neutrophil migration depends on neutrophils and on bacteria. All processes in neutrophil dynamics are inhibited by bacteria, fibrin and Coa/vWbp. In this diagram, we are not representing self-inhibitions that are also present in the mathematical models of this paper.

each of these relations and we will present the characteristics of each submodel that is part of the abscess formation model.

3.1. Bacteria-Coa/vWbp-Fibrin Model

The first model accounts for the interaction between bacteria, Coa/vWbp and fibrin. The objective of this model is to reproduce the formation of a fibrin network around the bacteria colony. In this model, we have the bacteria replicating and producing two coagulation factors: *coagulase* (Coa) and von Willebrand factor Binding Protein (*vWbp*). These coagulation factors are responsible for converting fibrinogen into fibrin.

The model is comprised by the following system of equations:

$$\begin{aligned} \frac{\partial coa}{\partial t} &= k\, b\, g_{coa}(b,f,coa) + D_{coa}\, \text{coa\_diffusion}(), \\ coa(x,0) &= coa_0, \frac{\partial coa(.,t)}{\partial \vec{n}}|_{\partial\Omega} = 0, \\ \frac{\partial b}{\partial t} &= r\, b\, g_b(b,f,coa) + D_b\, \text{b\_diffusion}(), \\ b(x,0) &= b_0, \frac{\partial b(.,t)}{\partial \vec{n}}|_{\partial\Omega} = 0, \\ f &= b\, coa, \end{aligned} \tag{11}$$

where the term *coa* denotes the coagulation factors Coa and vWbp, b denotes the bacteria and f denotes fibrin. The functions $g_{coa}(b,f,coa)$ and $g_b(b,f,coa)$ are the g functions of Coa and bacteria, respectively. The functions coa_diffusion() and b_diffusion() models Coa/vWbp and bacteria diffusion, respectively. The diffusion is modeled in two ways: (1) with the classic diffusion operator (diffusion terms in the System of Equation 14); and (2) with the nonlinear diffusion given by 15 and 16. In the next section, we show the simulation results with both diffusion operators. Diffusion is the net movement of molecules or atoms from a region of high concentration (or high chemical potential) to a region of low concentration (or low chemical potential) as a result of random motion of the molecules or atoms.

The equation $f = b\, coa$ models fibrin formation. We assume that fibrin formation depends on the interaction between the bacteria and the coagulation factors.

The term $k.b.g_{coa}(b,f,coa)$ denotes the Coa/vWbp production, where k is the production rate. The function $g_{coa}(b,f,coa)$ is given by:

$$g_{coa}(b,f,coa) = 1 - (w_{bcoa}\, b + w_{fcoa} f + w_{coacoa}\, coa). \tag{12}$$

The parameters w_{bcoa}, w_{coacoa} and w_{fcoa} represent the influence of bacteria, Coa/vWbp and fibrin in Coa/vWbp dynamics.

The Coa/vWbp production is limited by the available space and is inhibited by bacteria and Coa/vWbp molecules that are in the same discretized region. This inhibition is considered to simulate the coagulation factors spreading from the border of the bacteria colony and also to simulate the fibrin network formation on this border.

The term $r.b.g_b(b,f,coa)$ denotes the bacteria replication, where r is the replication rate. The function $g_b(b,f,coa)$ is given by:

$$g_b(b,f,coa) = 1 - (w_{bb}\, b + w_{fb} f + w_{coab}\, coa). \tag{13}$$

The parameters w_{bb}, w_{coab} and w_{fb} represent the influence of bacteria, Coa/vWbp and fibrin in bacteria dynamics.

The bacteria replication is limited by the available space and is inhibited by Coa/vWbp molecules and the fibrin network. The Coa/vWbp inhibition is justified by the fact that, when the colony is being formed, the bacteria inside the colony will alter their behavior and, consequently, will decrease replication and focus on protecting themselves with the fibrin network. The fibrin network inhibition is considered to simulate that bacteria colony cannot replicate and expand over fibrin to other regions after the formation of the fibrin network.

3.1.1. One-Dimensional Simulations

With the objective of understanding the spatiotemporal behavior of the bacteria-Coa/vWbp-fibrin model, the diffusion process was added to the model (Equation 14) and numerical simulations were carried out on a one-dimensional domain:

$$\begin{aligned} \frac{\partial coa}{\partial t} &= k\, b\, g_{coa}(b,f,coa) + D_{coa}\frac{\partial^2 coa}{\partial x^2} \\ coa(x,0) &= coa_0,\ \frac{\partial coa(.,t)}{\partial \vec{n}}|_{\partial\Omega} = 0 \\ \frac{\partial b}{\partial t} &= r\, b\, g_b(b,f,coa) + D_b\frac{\partial^2 b}{\partial x^2} \\ b(x,0) &= b_0,\ \frac{\partial b(.,t)}{\partial \vec{n}}|_{\partial\Omega} = 0 \\ f &= b\, coa \end{aligned} \tag{14}$$

$D_{coa}\frac{\partial^2 coa}{\partial x^2}$ and $D_b\frac{\partial^2 b}{\partial x^2}$ are the diffusion terms of Coa/vWbp and bacteria, respectively, where D_{coa} and D_b are the diffusion coefficients.

In spite of *S. aureus* not being a motile organism, we considered a diffusion process for *S. aureus* to simulate the bacterial expansion as the bacteria replicate and increase in number, having as a consequence an increase in the region occupied by the bacteria colony. We chose a small diffusion coefficient for the bacteria ($D_b = 0.05$) to simulate the aforementioned aspect of *S. aureus* infections.

The model's initial conditions and parameters are presented in **Tables 1**, **2**, respectively. In our simulations, we assumed a one-dimensional domain of 10 *mm* length and a simulation time of 20 days. In fact, this one-dimensional model is a simplification of a 3D block model in that we have assumed that the lengths associated with *y* and *z* are much smaller than the length associated with *x*. In all PDEs, the domain is homogeneous and the boundary conditions are of Neumann type.

Bacteria are initially placed in the middle of the domain, neutrophils and the coagulation factors are placed initially with a small concentration all over the domain. The bacteria initial location can be seen as the set of points (arterioles) where bacteria extravasate from the vasculature to the kidney tissue.

In all computational simulations we used the parameters values presented in **Table 2**, except when we vary some parameters to simulate different scenarios and, in these cases, we highlight what are the new values employed.

Due to the lack of experimental data and the difficult in making a direct correlation between some measured biological quantities and the parameters of the models, the parameters values were chosen to illustrate the different behaviors that the models are capable of reproducing.

We observe in **Figure 3A** that, with time, the bacteria replicate and the bacteria colony increases in size. As a result, the production of the coagulation factors Coa/vWbp increases. With time, Coa/vWbp is converted to fibrin. The fibrin has some influence in bacteria's growth but fibrin was not able to prevent the spread of bacteria around the initial site of infection. We believe this happened because fibrin is not influencing bacteria diffusion as it influences bacterial growth. Therefore the bacteria colony can spread to other areas of the tissue. The spatial pattern seen in this result does not resemble the abscess pattern because we cannot observe the formation of one or more colonies of bacteria surrounded by fibrin.

In the simulated scenario described previously, we implemented the classical diffusion operator that does not consider any external influence in the diffusion of a population. In some situations, this hypothesis that the diffusion of a cell is not influenced by any other cell or molecule present in the system is not true. In the human body, a cell can interact with

TABLE 1 | Initial conditions.

Variable	Value	Unit
b_0	$\begin{cases} 0.6: & 4 \le x \le 6 \\ 0: & otherwise \end{cases}$	amount/mm^3
n_0	$0.01: \ 0 \le x \le 10$	amount/mm^3
coa_0	$0.01: \ 0 \le x \le 10$	amount/mm^3
f_0	$0: \ 0 \le x \le 10$	amount/mm^3
nd_0	$0: \ 0 \le x \le 10$	amount/mm^3
to_0	$0: \ 0 \le x \le 10$	amount/mm^3

The amount refers to the amount of one particular population (e.g., in b_0 it refers to bacteria, in n_0 it refers to neutrophils, and so on).

TABLE 2 | Set of parameters used in simulations.

Parameter	Value	Unit
r	1.3	1/day
α	0.1	dimensionless
γ	5	dimensionless
k	2	1/day
D_{coa}	0.05	mm/day
s	10	1/((amount/mm^3).day)
l	40	1/((amount/mm^3).day)
D_n	3	mm/day
w_{bb}	1	1/(amount/mm^3)
w_{coab}	4	1/(amount/mm^3)
w_{nb}	1.1	1/(amount/mm^3)
w_{fb}	1	1/(amount/mm^3)
w_{bcoa}	1.5	1/(amount/mm^3)
w_{coacoa}	1	1/(amount/mm^3)
w_{ncoa}	1.2	1/(amount/mm^3)
w_{fcoa}	0	1/(amount/mm^3)
w_{bn}	1.2	1/(amount/mm^3)
w_{coan}	0.5	1/(amount/mm^3)
w_{nn}	1	1/(amount/mm^3)
w_{fn}	2	1/(amount/mm^3)
β_{to}	0.5	1/((amount/mm^3).day)
μ_{to}	0.5	1/day
D_{to}	2	mm/day
α_{to}	0.7	1/((amount/mm^3).day)

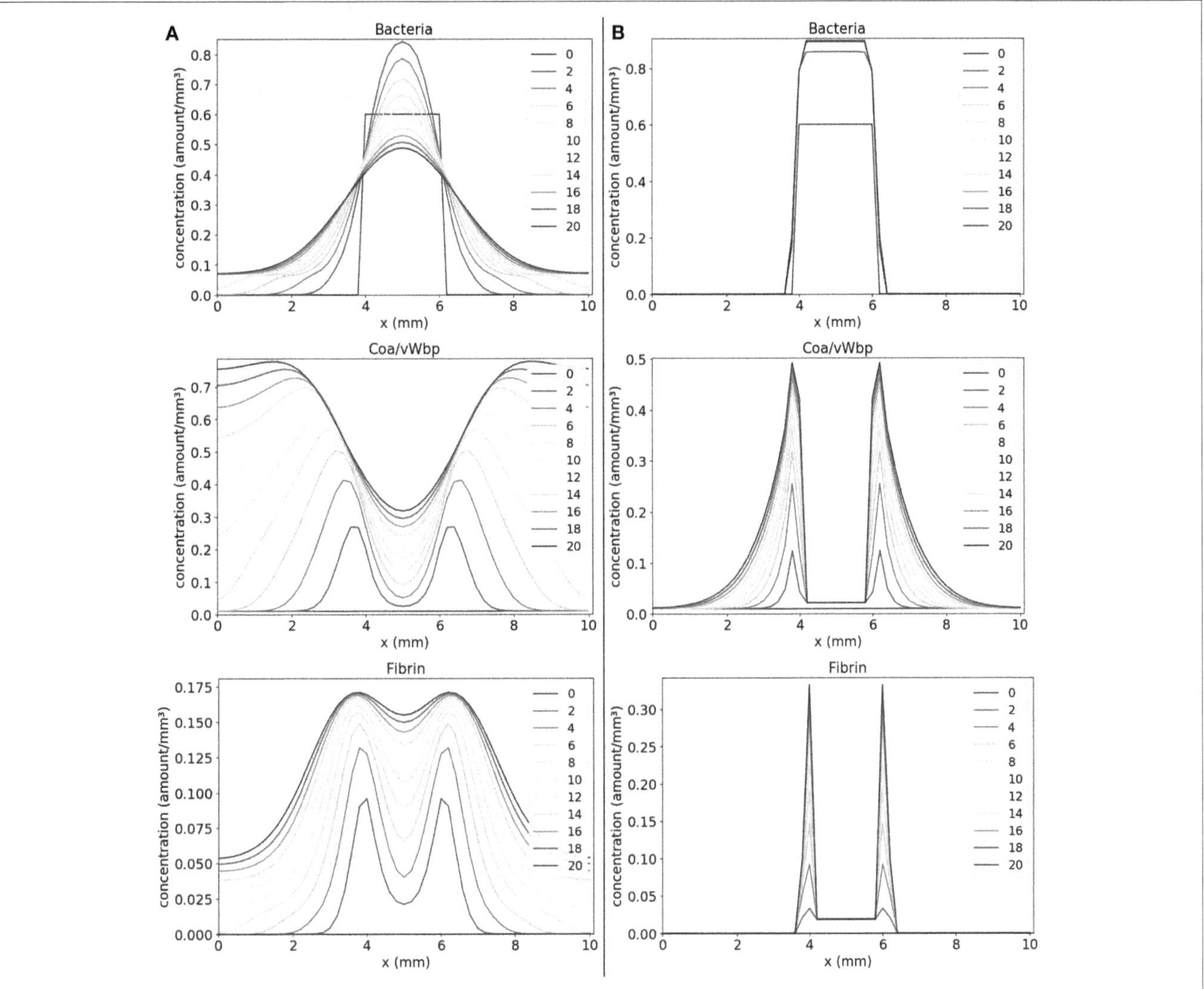

FIGURE 3 | Spatial distribution of bacteria, Coa/vWbp and fibrin concentrations in the comparison between the classic (**A** on the left) and the nonlinear (**B** on the right) diffusion scenarios. The y-axis (concentration) represents the fraction occupied by a particular population in a discretized region of the domain. The x-axis (x) represents the space in *mm*. The simulated time correspond to 20 days. Each line represents a particular day. The simulation starts at day 0 and finishes at day 20. In classic diffusion scenario **(A)**, it is observed that the bacteria spread throughout the domain and cannot establish a colony surrounded by fibrin as in the nonlinear diffusion scenario **(B)**.

dozens of cells in a short period of time. Due to this fact, a cell can have many of its processes influenced by these interactions. Besides, space in the body is limited therefore the volume of some part of a tissue supports a maximum concentration of cells, molecules, liquids and other substances. The nonlinear diffusion models the influence of a cell population in the diffusion of other cell population. To represent the influence of both fibrin and Coa/vWbp in bacteria diffusion, the diffusion term of bacteria is defined as:

$$D_b \nabla \cdot (g_b(b, f, coa)\, h(b)\, \nabla b), \tag{15}$$

where $g_b(b, f, coa)$ models the influence resulting from the interactions between bacteria, Coa/vWbp and fibrin. The term $h(b)$ models the cooperative behavior of bacteria and was defined in Equation 10. The diffusion of Coa/vWbp is defined as:

$$D_{coa} \nabla \cdot (g_{coa}(b, f, coa)\, \nabla coa). \tag{16}$$

The nonlinear diffusion simulates the fact that bacteria colonies will be unable to expand to some points where fibrin concentration is sufficiently high reproducing, in this way, the formation of a fibrin network around the colonies. The fibrin network acts like a barrier preventing any cell to cross it. We will show that these hypotheses are important in the development of a mathematical model of abscess formation.

Incorporating the nonlinear diffusion terms in the PDEs, we obtain the following system:

$$\begin{aligned}\frac{\partial coa}{\partial t} &= k\, b\, g_{coa}(b,f,coa) + D_{coa}\nabla \cdot (g_{coa}(b,f,coa)\,\nabla coa),\\ \frac{\partial b}{\partial t} &= r\, b\, g_b(b,f,coa) + D_b\nabla \cdot (g_b(b,f,coa)\, h(b)\,\nabla b),\\ f &= b\, coa. \end{aligned} \tag{17}$$

The results obtained with numerical simulations of these equations are shown in **Figure 3B**. We observe that, initially, the bacteria colony grows and starts to expand. At the same time, the bacteria produce the coagulation factors Coa/vWbp. The concentration of these factors increases and they convert fibrinogen, present in the body and that is not explicitly considered here, to fibrin. In addition, the fibrin concentration increases and we can see that fibrin is located around the bacteria colony. Both coagulation factors and fibrin interacts with bacteria preventing them to colonize other parts of the tissue. This process reflects the quorum sensing behavior seen in *S. aureus* infections.

Quorum sensing (Painter and Hillen, 2002; Yarwood and Schlievert, 2003; Le and Otto, 2015) is the process by which microorganisms regulate population density through chemical signaling. Chemical molecules secreted by microorganisms are a form of intra- and interspecies communication that helps bacteria coordinate their behavior. Quorum sensing allows to modulate diverse characteristics of the microorganisms, such as the motility, production of virulence factors and the formation of biofilms. In staphylococci, the ability to sense the bacterial density, or quorum, and to respond with genetic adaptations is an important mechanism to bacteria survival in the host (Le and Otto, 2015).

The nonlinear diffusion improved the model result, making it possible to obtain a pattern more similar to an abscess. However, abscesses are also composed by dead and live neutrophils. To reproduce the complete pattern, it is necessary to include these types of cell in the model. We will start including live neutrophils, and then dead neutrophils and toxins will be included. We will use the PDEs system given by Equations 17 as a base for further developments of our mathematical model of abscess formation.

3.2. Bacteria-Neutrophil Model

The model of interaction between bacteria and neutrophil, called bacteria-neutrophil model, is similar to the bacteria-Coa/vWbp-fibrin model presented previously in section 3.1. The neutrophil migration depends on bacteria concentration as the production of Coa/vWbp. The neutrophil has also a *g* function that is present in both growth and diffusion terms.

The bacteria-neutrophil model is comprised by the following set of PDEs:

$$\begin{aligned}\frac{\partial b}{\partial t} &= (r - l\,n)\, b\, g_b(b,n) + D_b\nabla \cdot (g_b(b,n)\, h(b)\,\nabla b)),\\ \frac{\partial n}{\partial t} &= s\, b\, n\, g_n(b,n) + D_n\nabla \cdot (g_n(b,n)\,\nabla n)).\end{aligned} \tag{18}$$

The variable *n* denotes neutrophil concentration and the variable *b* denotes bacteria concentration. The term $s.b.n.g_n(b,n)$ models neutrophil migration. Product $b.n$ in term $s.b.n.g_n(b,n)$ can be interpreted as the pro-inflammatory cytokine production. The pro-inflammatory cytokines would have the effect of attracting more neutrophils to the infection site. For the sake of simplicity, these cytokines are not considered explicitly in this model. The term $r.b.g_b(b,n)$ represents bacteria replication. Bacteria phagocytosis is denoted by the term $l.n.b.g_b(b,n)$. The model has two *g* functions: (1) $g_b(b,n)$ for bacteria; and (2) $g_n(b,n)$ for neutrophils.

The *g* functions equations are given by:

$$\begin{aligned} g_b(b,n) &= 1 - (w_{bb}.b + w_{nb}.n),\\ g_n(b,n) &= 1 - (w_{bn}.b + w_{nn}.n).\end{aligned} \tag{19}$$

The model's parameters are: (1) r is the bacteria replication rate; (2) l is the phagocytosis rate; (3) w_{bb} is the influence of bacteria on its own dynamics; (4) w_{nb} is the influence of neutrophils on bacteria dynamics; (5) s is the neutrophil migration rate; (6) w_{bn} is the influence of bacteria on neutrophils dynamics; and (7) w_{nn} is the influence of neutrophils on its own dynamics.

3.2.1. One-Dimensional Simulations

With the objective of analyzing the spatiotemporal behavior of bacteria-neutrophil model, one-dimensional simulations of the Equation 18 were performed. In the simulations performed, we observed three main behaviors: (1) the formation of a bacteria colony when considering a small phagocytosis rate; (2) a disseminated infection when small rates for phagocytosis and for neutrophil migration are considered; and (3) infection control with complete elimination of bacteria when considering a "normal" immune response.

Values of parameters s (rate of neutrophil migration) and l (rate of phagocytosis) were varied in three different scenarios: (1) small phagocytosis rate: $s = 10$ and $l = 20$ (**Figure 4A**); (2) small rates for phagocytosis and neutrophil migration: $s = 5$ and $l = 20$ (**Figure 4B**); and (3) "normal" values for phagocytosis and neutrophil migration: $s = 10$ and $l = 40$ (**Figure 4C**).

The first scenario is presented in **Figure 4A**. This scenario simulates the mechanisms employed by bacteria to escape phagocytosis by immune cells. We observe that neutrophils begin to migrate to the tissue in an attempt to control the infection, but they are not able to phagocytose bacteria efficiently. As a consequence, the bacteria colony grows and expands around the initial site of infection.

The second scenario (**Figure 4B**) simulates a deficient immune response where it is considered an impairment in neutrophil migration caused by bacteria, besides the impairment in phagocytosis. It is observed that the bacteria colony can rapidly expand to other areas of the tissue without the presence of neutrophils. Neutrophil migration is impaired and there are almost no neutrophils to fight the infection. Eventually, with time, the bacteria will spread to larger areas of the tissue.

In the last simulated scenario (**Figure 4C**), we considered a normal immune response. We observe that the bacteria were completely eliminated by neutrophils. Neutrophils were successful in controlling the infection due to rapid migration and efficient killing of bacteria. After bacteria elimination, the spatial

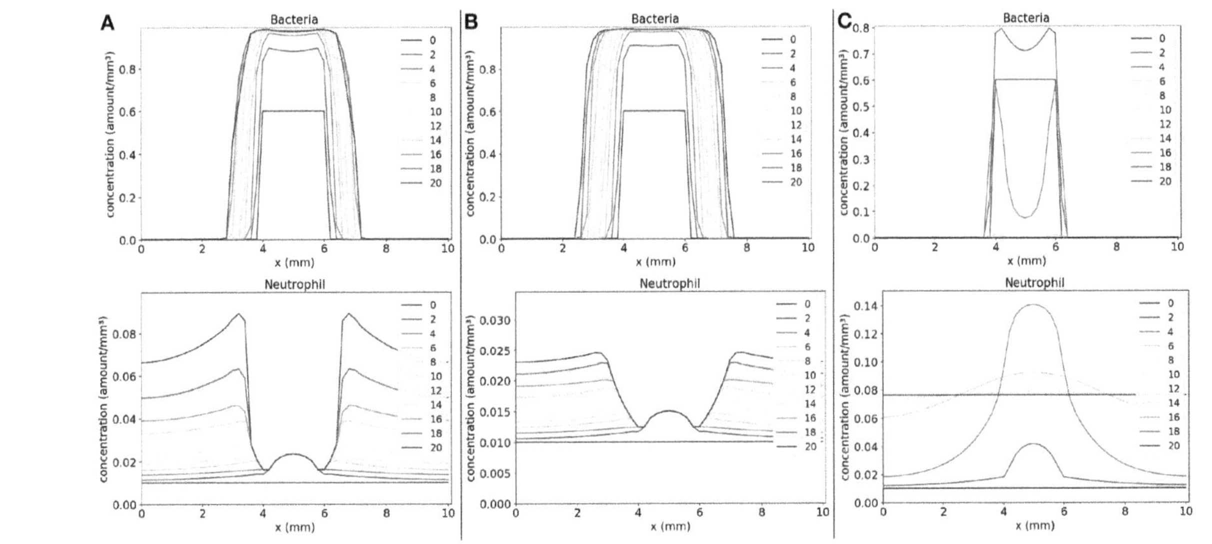

FIGURE 4 | Spatial distribution of bacteria and neutrophil concentrations in three distinct scenarios: (a) the scenario with small phagocytosis rate (**A** on the left), (b) the scenario with small rates for phagocytosis and neutrophil migration (**B** on the middle), and (c) the scenario with "normal" values for phagocytosis and neutrophil migration (**C** on the right). The y-axis (concentration) represents the fraction occupied by a particular population in a discretized region of the domain. The x-axis (x) represents the space in *mm*. The simulated time correspond to 20 days. Each line represents a particular day. The simulation starts at day 0 and finishes at day 20. In **(A)**, we observe that the bacteria colony grows and infects other regions because the neutrophil response is very ineffective. The same occurs in **(B)** where, besides an impairment in phagocytosis, there are very few neutrophils to fight the infection. A different situation occurs in **(C)** where neutrophils are capable of eliminating bacteria completely, controlling the infection.

distribution of neutrophils tend to stabilize throughout the tissue due to the fact that we have not modeled the neutrophil apoptosis.

3.3. Bacteria-Coa/vWbp-Fibrin-Neutrophil Model

The bacteria-Coa/vWbp-fibrin-neutrophil model is an extension combining the two models presented previously: the bacteria-Coa/vWbp-fibrin model and the bacteria-neutrophil model. The objective of this model is to reproduce, in addition to the formation of one or more colonies of bacteria surrounded by fibrin, the spatial distribution of neutrophils inside the abscess lesion. The model is comprised by the following PDEs system:

$$\begin{aligned}\frac{\partial coa}{\partial t} &= k\, b\, g_{coa}(b,f,coa,n) + D_{coa}\nabla\cdot(g_{coa}(b,f,coa,n)\,\nabla coa),\\ \frac{\partial b}{\partial t} &= (r - l\, n)\, b\, g_b(b,f,coa,n) + D_b\nabla\cdot(g_b(b,f,coa,n)\, h(b)\,\nabla b),\\ f &= b\, coa,\\ \frac{\partial n}{\partial t} &= s\, b\, n\, g_n(b,f,coa,n) + D_n\nabla\cdot(g_n(b,f,coa,n)\,\nabla n).\end{aligned} \quad (20)$$

The equation $f = b\, coa$ models fibrin formation. The g functions now depend on four types of populations: bacteria, Coa/vWbp, fibrin and neutrophil. The new g functions are given by:

$$\begin{aligned} g_{coa}(b,f,coa,n) &= (1 - w_{bcoa}\, b - w_{fcoa} f - w_{coacoa}\, coa - w_{ncoa}\, n),\\ g_b(b,f,coa,n) &= (1 - w_{bb}\, b - w_{fb} f - w_{coab}\, coa - w_{nb}\, n),\\ g_n(b,f,coa,n) &= (1 - w_{bn}\, b - w_{fn} f - w_{coan}\, coa - w_{nn}\, n).\end{aligned} \quad (21)$$

It is important to highlight that when choosing $n = 0$ in Equation 20, we obtain the bacteria-Coa/vWbp-fibrin model presented in Equation 17. In addition, when we consider $coa = 0$ and $f = 0$ in Equation 20, we obtain the bacteria-neutrophil model presented in Equation 18.

The parameters of the model are: (1) k is the Coa/vWbp production rate; (2) r is the rate of bacteria replication; (3) l is the rate of phagocytosis; (4) s is the neutrophil migration rate; (5) w_{bcoa}, w_{fcoa}, w_{coacoa} and w_{ncoa} are the influence of bacteria, fibrin, Coa/vWbp and neutrophil, respectively, in Coa/vWbp dynamics; (6) w_{bb}, w_{fb}, w_{coab} and w_{nb} are the influence of bacteria, fibrin, Coa/vWbp and neutrophil, respectively, in bacteria dynamics; (7) w_{bn}, w_{fn}, w_{coan} and w_{nn} are the influence of bacteria, fibrin, Coa/vWbp and neutrophil, respectively, in neutrophil dynamics; and (8) D_{coa}, D_b and D_n are the diffusion coefficients of Coa/vWbp, bacteria and neutrophil, respectively.

In this model, we consider, besides fibrin influence in the dynamics of bacteria, also their influence in the dynamics of neutrophil. The influence is reflected in the fact that when fibrin concentration is sufficiently high, fibrin prevents neutrophils from getting closer to the bacteria colonies. It is important to highlight that phagocytosis is also influenced by fibrin. Depending on fibrin's location in the domain, for example, if fibrin is located around a bacteria colony it will protect bacteria from being phagocytized by neutrophils outside the colony. Neutrophils inside the colony are not capable of handling the infection alone.

3.3.1. One-Dimensional Simulations

We first present and compare the results of two scenarios: (1) a scenario with the coagulation factors production rate k equals to

2; and (2) a scenario with the coagulation factors production rate k equals to 0.4.

The first scenario is presented in **Figure 5A**. We can observe that neutrophils have been able to enter the site of the colony of bacteria, but were not able to eliminate them after saturation of several points of the domain. The saturation ocurred also due to the production of the coagulation factors and fibrin formation. This scenario illustrates a limitation of the model: after saturation of a domain position, neutrophils cannot phagocytose bacteria there anymore. We observed that saturation occurred because parameter w_{bn} has a great impact in the model results together with the initial condition. If the product $w_{bn}.b$ is sufficiently high, in some points of the domain, few neutrophils can migrate to the tissue before it saturates. As a consequence, these neutrophils are not in sufficient number to eliminate all bacteria there. Another limitation is the fact that we are not considering any mechanism used by the bacteria to kill neutrophils. As a result, we have the stabilization of cells populations with a considerable amount of neutrophils inside the bacteria colony. These limitations were the primary motivation for the development of an extension of the current model by adding a variable that represents the toxins produced by the bacteria. Toxins are also important for the persistence of bacteria in the host. Basically, we can assume that toxins interact with neutrophils causing their death.

The second scenario (**Figure 5B**) shows that when we decrease the value of Coa/vWbp production (parameter k) to 0.4 and, consequently, decreasing the fibrin formation, the bacteria are completely eliminated. This scenario illustrates the importance of fibrin in protecting the bacteria.

The simulations with bacteria-Coa/vWbp-fibrin-neutrophil model allowed us to better understand the effect of each parameter in the dynamics of the model. We have observed that, for the immune response to be effective, the rate of neutrophil migration cannot be so high because the regions with bacteria

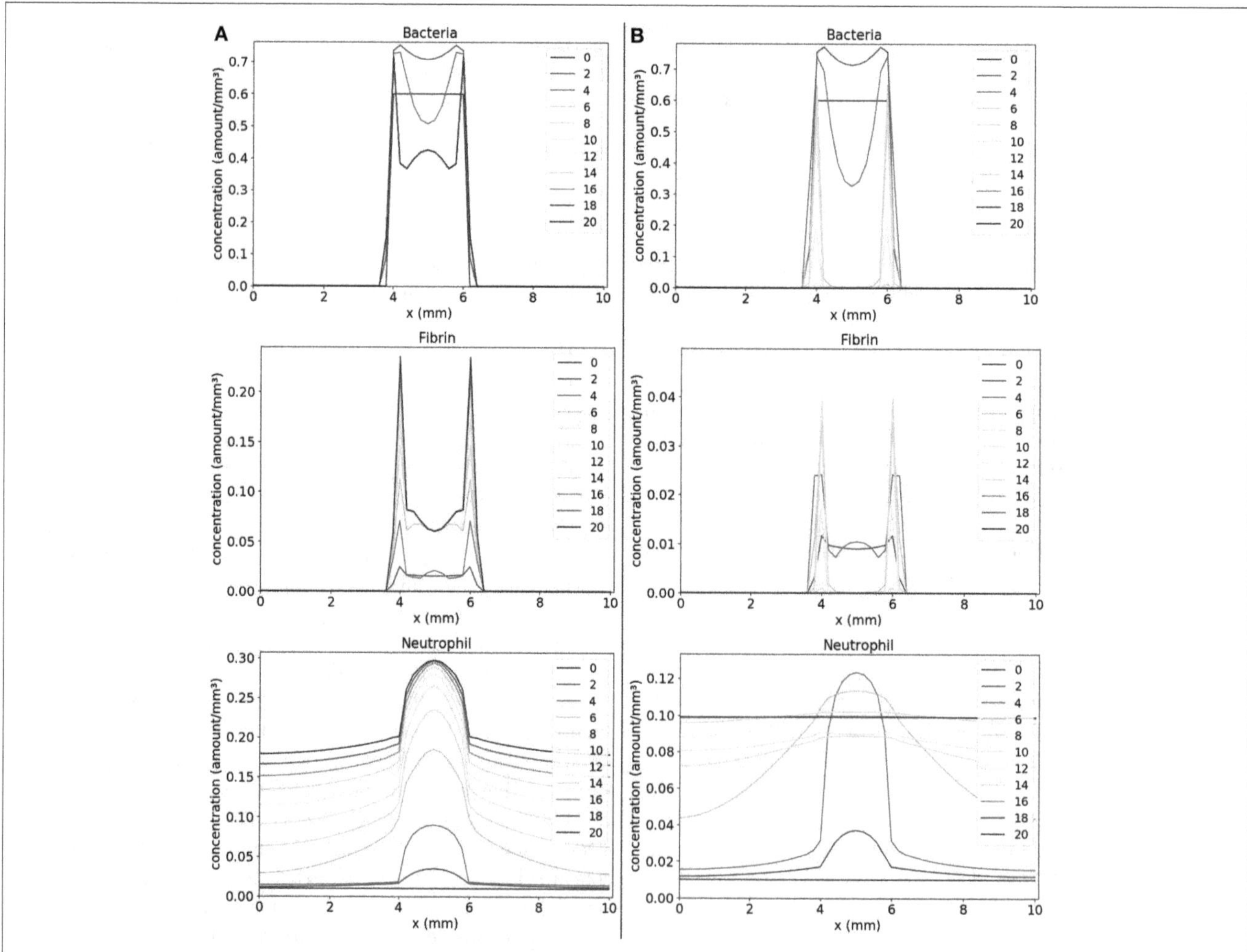

FIGURE 5 | Spatial distribution of bacteria, fibrin and neutrophil concentrations in the comparison between the scenario with $k = 2$ (**A** on the left) and the scenario with $k = 0.4$ (**B** on the right). The y-axis (concentration) represents the fraction occupied by a particular population in a discretized region of the domain. The x-axis (x) represents the space in *mm*. The simulated time correspond to 20 days. Each line represents a particular day. The simulation starts at day 0 and finishes at day 20. **(A)** shows that the neutrophils that migrate into the tissue phagocytose part of the colony of bacteria until saturation occurs in regions where there are neutrophils and bacteria. At this time, no more phagocytosis occurs. In **(B)**, the colony of bacteria cannot produce fibrin fast enough to protect itself and it is eliminated.

could saturate rapidly and, in this case, neutrophils could no longer eliminate the bacteria. We have also observed that the rate of phagocytosis has an important role in model dynamics. The elimination of bacteria was only obtained when we considered a high phagocytosis rate combined with a moderate migration rate and a small rate for Coa/vWbp production.

3.4. Bacteria-Coa/vWbp-Fibrin-Neutrophil-Toxin Model

The previous model (Equation 20) can be modified to better understand the effects of toxins produced by *Staphylococcus aureus*. The toxins also contribute to the persistence of *S. aureus* in the host (Cheng et al., 2009, 2010). The role of toxins is to mantain cells of the immune system, mainly neutrophils, away from the colony of *S. aureus*. Even after the formation of the fibrin network, *S. aureus* bacteria continue to produce several types of toxins, which, because of their small volume, are able to pass through the fibrin network and reach the regions where most living neutrophils are migrating to the infected tissue.

It is important to highlight that the immune system of wild type mice as well as the immune system of humans is efficient in eliminating dead cells from tissue, cleaning the infection site. This cleansing would allow neutrophils and other immune system cells to approach the fibrin network around the bacterial colony, threatening to dissolve (to break down) this network to gain access to the colony of bacteria, but the toxins may prevent this process (Guggenberger et al., 2012; McAdow et al., 2012).

It was considered a simplified model of toxin's dynamics based on the following hypothesis:

- The production of toxins depends on bacteria concentration, having a saturation. This production is not influenced by other cells;
- The toxins cause the death of neutrophils at a rate that is proportional to the concentration of both;
- It is considered that the diffusion of toxins is not influenced by the presence of other cells;
- Both toxins and dead neutrophils do not influence the growth and diffusion of other cell types.

It is assumed that the volume of toxins and of dead neutrophils are negligible in relation to the volumes of other cells, therefore they are not considered in the g functions.

The model is composed by the following PDEs system:

$$\begin{aligned}
\frac{\partial coa}{\partial t} &= k.b.g_{coa}(b,f,coa,n) + D_{coa}\nabla\cdot(g_{coa}(b,f,coa,n).\nabla coa),\\
\frac{\partial b}{\partial t} &= (r-l.n).b.g_b(b,f,coa,n) + D_b\nabla\cdot(g_b(b,f,coa,n).h(b).\nabla b),\\
f &= b\,coa,\\
\frac{\partial n}{\partial t} &= s.b.n.g_n(b,f,coa,n) - \alpha_{to}.to.n + D_n\nabla\cdot(g_n(b,f,coa,n).\nabla n),\\
\frac{\partial to}{\partial t} &= \beta_{to}.b.(1-to) - \mu_{to}.to + D_{to}.\Delta to,\\
\frac{\partial nd}{\partial t} &= \alpha_{to}.to.n,
\end{aligned} \tag{22}$$

where toxins represented by *to* and dead neutrophils represented by *nd* are the new populations added to the model. Term $\beta_{to}.b.(1-to)$ denotes toxin production, where β_{to} is the production rate. Term $\mu_{to}.to$ denotes toxin decay and term $D_{to}.\Delta to$ denotes toxin diffusion with μ_{to} being the decay rate and D_{to} being the diffusion coefficient. Neutrophils in contact with toxins die at a rate α_{to} that is proportional to the concentration of both (term $\alpha_{to}.to.n$). The g functions are the same as in the previous model.

3.4.1. One-Dimensional Simulations

Simulations in one dimension were carried out to understand the new behaviors that can be obtained after the introduction of the toxin. In simulations with the toxin model, we have used the parameter values of the "normal" immune response ($s = 10$ and $l = 40$) scenario (**Table 2**) with the exception of Coa/vWbp production rate k which we varied in the two scenarios presented here. The values of the new parameters that were incorporated into the model are: $\beta_{to} = 0.5, \mu_{to} = 0.5, D_{to} = 2$, and $\alpha_{to} = 0.7$.

In the first scenario presented in **Figure 6A**, we considered $k = 2$. We observe, in Panel A, that as the toxin diffuses through the tissue, it causes a lot of death in the region occupied by the bacteria colony. As a consequence, a concentration of dead neutrophils is observed at the infection site. The toxins helped bacteria to establish a favorable environment to persist.

One interesting result is observed when we consider a smaller Coa/vWbp production rate ($k = 0.5$) in second scenario (**Figure 6B**). In this case, we see the formation of two abscesses next to each other. Neutrophils migrate in the middle of the domain where the concentration of bacteria is high and phagocyte bacteria there. Neutrophils start to die due to the action of toxins. The toxins together with saturation after fibrin formation prevent neutrophils to eliminate bacteria completely and, as a result, there are the formation of two abscesses. In histology images of mice kidneys infected with *S. aureus*, it is also observed, in many situations, the formation of one or more abscesses (Cheng et al., 2009, 2010; Kim et al., 2011, 2012)

4. DISCUSSION

In the mathematical models developed in this paper, we have considered the influence of a population on the dynamics of other population. This influence represents not only the lack of available space due to the volume occupied by distinct populations in a discretized region but also represents other types of interactions such as inhibitory or stimulatory interactions. These interactions are modeled through the use of the g function presented first in section 2. The interactions between different populations were modeled through the product of their concentration by constant parameters. We can also model these interactions by considering some function of various parameters. However, in order to avoid introducing complexity into the model and trying to better understand its behavior, we have chosen more simplified interactions.

Numerical simulations were important for us to understand the effects of the g function not only on the growth terms but also on the processes of movement. As shown in **Figure 3A**,

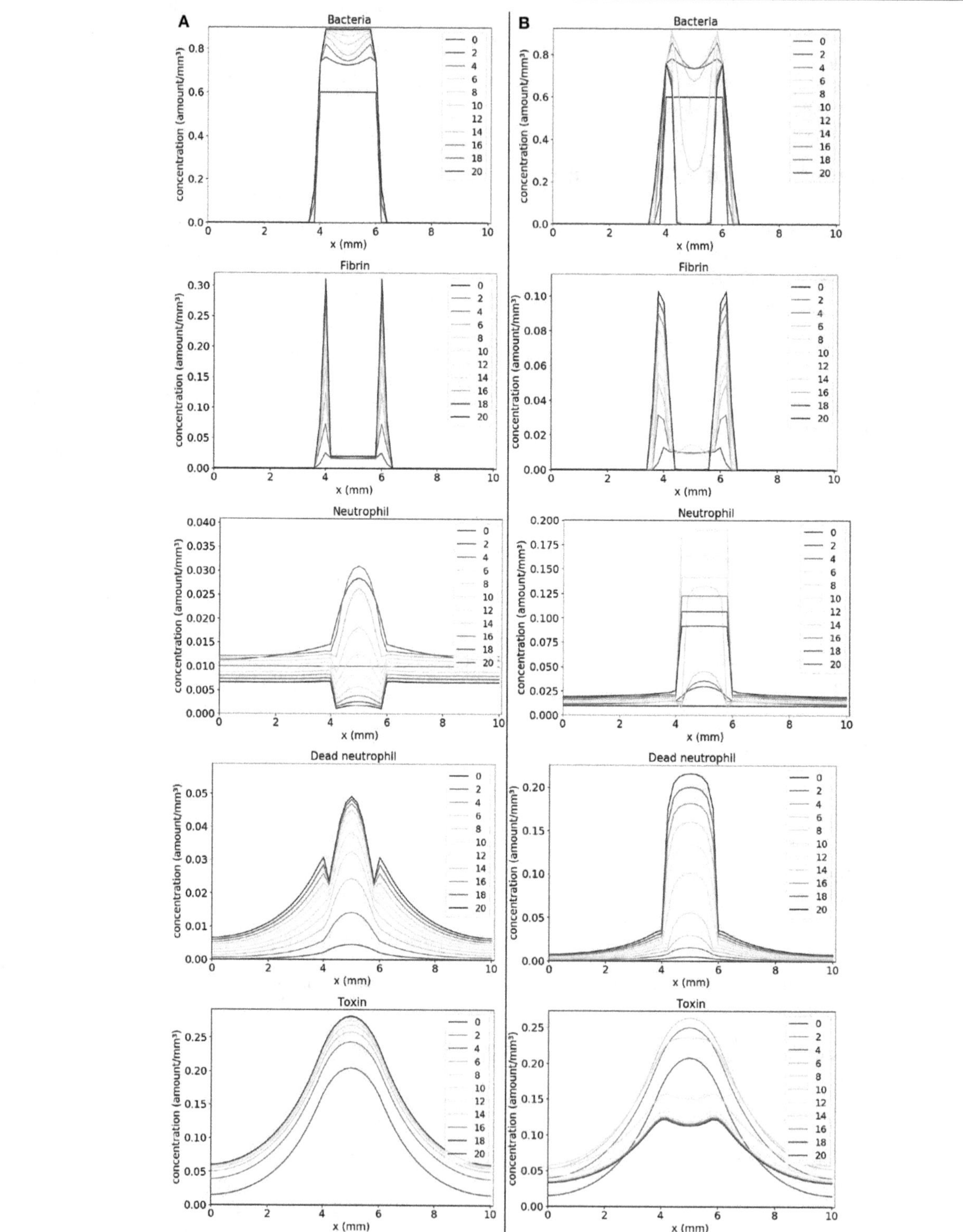

FIGURE 6 | Spatial distribution of bacteria, fibrin, live neutrophil, dead neutrophil and toxin concentrations in the comparison between two scenarios: a scenario where the bacteria persist forming one colony **(A)** and a scenario where the bacteria persist forming two colonies **(B)**. The y-axis (concentration) represents the fraction occupied by a particular population in a discretized region of the domain. The x-axis (x) represents the space in *mm*. The simulated time correspond to 20 days. Each line represents a particular day. The simulation starts at day 0 and finishes at day 20. **(A)** shows that bacteria rapidly produce toxins killing neutrophils, and ensuring that they form a colony protected by fibrin. **(B)** shows a similar behavior, but, this time, neutrophils manage to phagocytose a great number of bacteria located near the middle of the domain. This results in a separation of the initial colony in two. These newly formed colonies have time to produce sufficient fibrin to protect themselves, surviving in the host.

without considering the g function in the diffusion terms, it was not possible to obtain a pattern similar to an abscess. This happened because bacteria and fibrin could move freely through the domain. There was nothing to stop them from moving to a location already containing a large concentration of cells, molecules and other substances. The incorporation of the g function into the diffusion, in this case, allowed us to model a behavior that is believed to be more real in this situation: an adaptive behavior in which populations adapt to the environment around them. This adaptation occurs due to the lack of space, but it could be due to the lack of nutrients, for example. With the g function, it is possible to react to changes in the environment avoiding a situation where more populations are created in a place where this creation would not be possible anymore.

We think that the effect of the g function on the movement of populations contributes to stabilize their spatial distributions. Studies on parasitoid–host interaction and on predator-prey models (Briggs and Hoopes, 2004, and references therein) found some spatial mechanisms resulting on stability or increased persistence. One of these mechanisms is the limited dispersion of populations. One of the effects of the g function, in this paper, is to limit the diffusion at the cellular level. In the case of models that consider patch dynamics, other important mechanisms that contribute to persistence are: spatial heterogeneity and asynchronous dynamics between patches (Briggs and Hoopes, 2004, and references therein).

It was possible to observe, with the simulations, that the parameter w_{bn} is important for the persistence of bacteria in the host, because this parameter represents the influence that the bacteria exert in neutrophil migration. The higher the value of w_{bn}, the lower the migration of neutrophils and the lower the efficiency of neutrophil response. Another important parameter is the rate of neutrophil migration s. We have observed that this rate cannot be very high because a great concentration of neutrophils would saturate rapidly the regions with bacteria before eliminating them. But this rate cannot be small because bacteria would spread throughout the domain. The model results are also affected considerably by the rate of Coa/vWbp production k. If this rate is below a threshold then we have a scenario where bacteria are completely eliminated. Otherwise, we have a scenario where bacteria persist in the host.

4.1. Limitations and Future Work

As limitations of this paper, we can note the fact that the use of models based on differential equations requires detailed knowledge about the parameters that are included in the equations. Some of these parameters can be measured experimentally, while others need to be estimated. In this paper, we used parameter values for illustration purposes, they were not estimated due to lack of sufficient experimental data.

As future work, we plan to better study the effects of toxins and the different behaviors that could be obtained by considering it. We also plan to study the effect of considering the migration of cells ocurring only at some points of the domain, simulating the presence of blood vessels at those points. Some numerical simulations already performed using this specific scenario have shown that the chemotaxis process of neutrophils has a major impact in the result because the chemotaxis allows neutrophils to reach the bacterial colony faster than when diffusion only applies. This observation is in good agreement with our previous observations (Pigozzo et al., 2013). Besides, we plan to add pro-inflammatory cytokines to the model and to consider their chemoattractant effect on immune system cells.

As a future work, we plan to build a more complete model and validate it with distinct experimental data such as histology images, values of bacteria load in the tissue, size of abscess diameter, among others, obtained from various *in vivo* experiments including the leukocyte depletion experiment (Robertson et al., 2008; Navarini et al., 2009; Attia et al., 2013) and the Coa/vWbp inhibition experiment (Vanassche et al., 2011, 2012; Flick et al., 2013). We plan to consider, in our model, the use by the bacteria *S. aureus* of its sensory/regulatory systems to adapt the production of virulence factors, specifically to a triggering signal, e.g., neutrophils (Guerra et al., 2017). The idea is to study how the interaction between *S. aureus* and neutrophils provokes certain sensing and adaptive responses used by *S. aureus* (Guerra et al., 2017).

In addition, we plan to extend the model to two and three-dimensional domains, but we think that the behaviors that could be obtained with two or three dimensions are the same that we can obtain with the one-dimensional models because the spatial mechanisms considered are not altered with the increase in the number of dimensions.

5. CONCLUSIONS

In this paper, we have developed computational models based on partial differential equations that were able to reproduce some characteristics observed in the abscess formation process.

The study comprised the analysis of the spatiotemporal behavior of bacteria, the coagulation factors Coa/vWbp, fibrin, toxins and neutrophils. These analyses were important and helped to understand how the modeled processes interact, the effects of the incorporation of certain processes, among other factors.

It was shown, in this paper, that the use of the g function in the growth and diffusion terms of the populations was one of the characteristics that allowed the mathematical models to reproduce some key aspects of the abscess formation process. Other important characteristic was the fibrin network formation. The fibrin network protected bacteria from the immune response given by the neutrophils. The formation of the fibrin network was modeled considering the production of coagulation factors and the interaction of these factors with the colony of bacteria.

More tests and refinement of the model may be needed, but this initial model was capable of reproducing some characteristics found in the abscess pattern such as: the formation of a fibrin network around the colonies of bacteria and an accumulation of necrotic neutrophils and live neutrophils in the abscess region.

Based on simulations results and on analyses done so far, we believe that the fibrin network is essential for bacteria persistence inside the abscess lesion together with the mechanisms used by the bacteria to kill neutrophils such as the production of toxins and mechanisms used to evade phagocytosis.

The abscess pattern can also be obtained by models other than those based on PDEs. For example, Cellular Automata (Zorzenon dos Santos and Coutinho, 2001; Moreira and Deutsch, 2002; Xiao et al., 2006), Colored Petri Nets (Carvalho et al., 2015; Pennisi et al., 2016) and models based on Agents (Gopalakrishnan et al., 2013; Chiacchio et al., 2014; Abar et al., 2017) can also be used to capture this pattern of formation.

AUTHOR CONTRIBUTIONS

DM have helped the understanding of histopathology of abscesses. AP, RS, ML, and SM have defined the methods and experiments. AP has written the software code to implement the model and has performed all simulations. AP, RS and ML have analyzed and interpreted the results. All authors have written, read and approved the final version of the paper.

FUNDING

The funding will come from Universidade Federal de Juiz de Fora where is located the Graduate Program in Computational Modeling.

ACKNOWLEDGMENTS

The authors would like to thank CAPES, FAPEMIG, UFJF, and UFSJ for supporting this work. Work described in this study was supported in part by grant AI110937 from the National Institute of Allergy and Infectious Diseases to DM.

REFERENCES

Abar, S., Theodoropoulos, G. K., Lemarinier, P., and OâHare, G. M. (2017). Agent based modelling and simulation tools: a review of the state-of-art software. *Comp. Sci. Rev.* 24, 13–33. doi: 10.1016/j.cosrev.2017.03.001

Alt, W., and Lauffenburger, D. (1987). Transient behavior of a chemotaxis system modelling certain types of tissue inflammation. *J. Math. Biol.* 24, 691–722. doi: 10.1007/BF00275511

Antia, R., Koella, J. C., and Perrot, V. (1996). Models of the within-host dynamics of persistent mycobacterial infections. *Proc. R. Soc. Lond B Biol. Sci.* 263, 257–263. doi: 10.1098/rspb.1996.0040

Antia, R., Levin, B. R., and May, R. M. (1994). Within-host population dynamics and the evolution and maintenance of microparasite virulence. *Am. Nat.* 144, 457–472. doi: 10.1086/285686

Attia, A. S., Cassat, J. E., Aranmolate, S. O., Zimmerman, L. J., Boyd, K. L., and Skaar, E. P. (2013). Analysis of the staphylococcus aureus abscess proteome identifies antimicrobial host proteins and bacterial stress responses at the host-pathogen interface. *Pathog. Dis.* 69, 36–48. doi: 10.1111/2049-632X.12063

Bender, E. A. (2000). *An Introduction to Mathematical Modeling.* Mineola, NY: Dover Publications (Educa Books).

Berube, B. J., and Bubeck Wardenburg, J. (2013). Staphylococcus aureus alpha-toxin: Nearly a century of intrigue. *Toxins* 5, 1140–1166. doi: 10.3390/toxins5061140

Briggs, C. J., and Hoopes, M. F. (2004). Stabilizing effects in spatial parasitoid–host and predator-prey models: a review. *Theor. Popul. Biol.* 65, 299–315. doi: 10.1016/j.tpb.2003.11.001

Carvalho, R. V., van den Heuvel, J., Kleijn, J., and Verbeek, F. J. (2015). Coupling of petri net models of the mycobacterial infection process and innate immune response. *Computation* 3, 150–176. doi: 10.3390/computation3020150

Cheng, A. G., Kim, H. K., Burts, M. L., Krausz, T., Schneewind, O., and Missiakas, D. M. (2009). Genetic requirements for staphylococcus aureus abscess formation and persistence in host tissues. *FASEB J.* 23, 3393–3404. doi: 10.1096/fj.09-135467

Cheng, A. G., McAdow, M., Kim, H. K., Bae, T., Missiakas, D. M., and Schneewind, O. (2010). Contribution of coagulases towards staphylococcus aureus disease and protective immunity. *PLoS Pathog* 6:e1001036. doi: 10.1371/journal.ppat.1001036

Chiacchio, F., Pennisi, M., Russo, G., Motta, S., and Pappalardo, F. (2014). Agent-based modeling of the immune system: netlogo, a promising framework. *BioMed Res. Int.* 2014:907171. doi: 10.1155/2014/907171

Flick, M. J., Du, X., Prasad, J. M., Raghu, H., Palumbo, J. S., Smeds, E., et al. (2013). Genetic elimination of the binding motif on fibrinogen for the *s. aureus* virulence factor clfa improves host survival in septicemia. *Blood* 121, 1783–1794. doi: 10.1182/blood-2012-09-453894

Foster, T. J. (2005). Immune evasion by staphylococci. *Nat. Rev. Micro.* 3, 948–958. doi: 10.1038/nrmicro1289

Foster, T. J., and Höök, M. (1998). Surface protein adhesins of staphylococcus aureus. *Trends Microbiol.* 6, 484–488. doi: 10.1016/S0966-842X(98)01400-0

Gopalakrishnan, V., Kim, M., and An, G. (2013). Using an agent-based model to examine the role of dynamic bacterial virulence potential in the pathogenesis of surgical site infection. *Adv. Wound Care* 2, 510–526. doi: 10.1089/wound.2012.0400

Goutelle, S., Maurin, M., Rougier, F., Barbaut, X., Bourguignon, L., Ducher, M., et al., (2008). The hill equation: a review of its capabilities in pharmacological modelling. *Fundam. Clin. Pharmacol.* 22, 633–648. doi: 10.1111/j.1472-8206.2008.00633.x

Graves, S., Kobayashi, S., and DeLeo, F. (2010). Community-associated methicillin-resistant staphylococcus aureus immune evasion and virulence. *J. Mol. Med.* 88, 109–114. doi: 10.1007/s00109-009-0573-x

Guerra, F. E., Borgogna, T. R., Patel, D. M., Sward, E. W., and Voyich, J. M. (2017). Epic immune battles of history: neutrophils vs. staphylococcus aureus. *Front. Cell. Inf. Microbiol.* 7:286. doi: 10.3389/fcimb.2017.00286

Guggenberger, C., Wolz, C., Morrissey, J. A., and Heesemann, J. (2012). Two distinct coagulase-dependent barriers protect staphylococcus aureus from neutrophils in a three dimensional <italic>in vitro</italic> infection model. *PLoS Pathog* 8:e1002434. doi: 10.1371/journal.ppat.1002434

Haefner, J. W. (2005). *Modeling Biological Systems: Principles and Applications.* New York, NY: Springer.

Kawasaki, K., Mochizuki, A., Matsushita, M., Umeda, T., and Shigesada, N. (1997). Modeling spatio-temporal patterns generated bybacillus subtilis. *J. Theor. Biol.* 188, 177–185. doi: 10.1006/jtbi.1997.0462

Keener, J., and Sneyd, J. (1998). *Mathematical Physiology.* New York, NY: Springer-Verlag New York, Inc.

Kim, H. K., Kim, H.-Y., Schneewind, O., and Missiakas, D. (2011). Identifying protective antigens of staphylococcus aureus, a pathogen that suppresses host immune responses. *FASEB J.* 25, 3605–3612. doi: 10.1096/fj.11-187963

Kim, H. K., Thammavongsa, V., Schneewind, O., and Missiakas, D. (2012). Recurrent infections and immune evasion strategies of staphylococcus aureus. *Curr. Opin. Microbiol.* 15, 92–99. doi: 10.1016/j.mib.2011.10.012

Kwiecinski, J. (2013). *Bacteria-Host Interplay in Staphylococcus aureus Infections.* Ph.D. thesis, University of Gothenburg; Göteborgs Universitet.

Lacasta, A. M., Cantalapiedra, I. R., Auguet, C. E., Peñaranda, A., and Ramírez-Piscina, L. (1999). Modeling of spatiotemporal patterns in bacterial colonies. *Phys. Rev. E* 59, 7036–7041. doi: 10.1103/PhysRevE.59.7036

Le, K. Y., and Otto, M. (2015). Quorum-sensing regulation in staphylococci-an overview. *Front. Microbiol.* 6, 1174. doi: 10.3389/fmicb.2015.01174

McAdow, M., Missiakas, D. M., and Schneewind, O. (2012). Staphylococcus aureus secretes coagulase and von willebrand factor binding protein to modify the coagulation cascade and establish host infections. *J. Innate Immun.* 4, 141–148. doi: 10.1159/000333447

Meerschaert, M. M. (2013). *Mathematical Modeling*. 4th Edn. Waltham, MA: Academic Press.

Moreira, J., and Deutsch, A. (2002). Cellular automaton models of the tumor development: a critical review. *Adv. Complex Syst.* 05, 247–267. doi: 10.1142/S0219525902000572

Navarini, A. A., Lang, K. S., Verschoor, A., Recher, M., Zinkernagel, A. S., Nizet, V., et al. (2009). Innate immune-induced depletion of bone marrow neutrophils aggravates systemic bacterial infections. *Proc. Natl. Acad. Sci. U.S.A.* 106, 7107–7112. doi: 10.1073/pnas.0901162106

Painter, K. J., and Hillen, T. (2002). Volume-filling and quorum-sensing in models for chemosensitive movement. *Can. Appl. Math. Q.* 10, 501–543.

Painter, K. J., and Sherratt, J. A. (2003). Modelling the movement of interacting cell populations. *J. Theor. Biol.* 225, 327–339. doi: 10.1016/S0022-5193(03)00258-3

Pennisi, M., Cavalieri, S., Motta, S., and Pappalardo, F. (2016). A methodological approach for using high-level petri nets to model the immune system response. *BMC Bioinformatics* 17(Suppl. 19):498. doi: 10.1186/s12859-016-1361-6

Pigozzo, A., Macedo, G., dos Santos, R., and Lobosco, M. (2013). On the computational modeling of the innate immune system. *BMC Bioinformatics*, 14(Suppl. 6):S7. doi: 10.1186/1471-2105-14-S6-S7

Pigozzo, A. B., Macedo, G. C., Weber dos Santos, R., and Lobosco, M. (2012). Computational modeling of microabscess formation. *Comput. Math. Methods Med.* 2012:736394. doi: 10.1155/2012/736394

Robertson, C. M., Perrone, E. E., McConnell, K. W., Dunne, W. M., Boody, B., Brahmbhatt, T., et al. (2008). Neutrophil depletion causes a fatal defect in murine pulmonary staphylococcus aureus clearance. *J. Surg. Res.* 150, 278–285. doi: 10.1016/j.jss.2008.02.009

Shiflet, A. B., and Shiflet, G. W. (2014). *Introduction to Computational Science: Modeling and Simulation for the Sciences*, 2nd Edn. Princeton, NJ: Princeton University Press.

Smith, A. M., McCullers, J. A., and Adler, F. R. (2011). Mathematical model of a three-stage innate immune response to a pneumococcal lung infection. *J. Theor. Biol.* 276, 106–116. doi: 10.1016/j.jtbi.2011.01.052

Vanassche, T., Kauskot, A., Verhaegen, J., Peetermans, W. E., van Ryn, J., Schneewind, O., et al. (2012). Fibrin formation by staphylothrombin facilitates staphylococcus aureus-induced platelet aggregation. *Thromb. Haemost.* 107, 1107–1121. doi: 10.1160/TH11-12-0891

Vanassche, T., Verhaegen, J. L., Peetermans, W. E., van Ryn, J., Cheng, A., Schneewind, O., et al. (2011). Inhibition of staphylothrombin by dabigatran reduces staphylococcus aureus virulence. *J. Thromb. Haemost.* 12, 2436–2446. doi: 10.1111/j.1538-7836.2011.04529.x

Versteeg, H., and Malalasekera, W. (2011). *An Introduction to Computational Fluid Dynamics: The Finite Volume Method*. Upper Saddle River, NJ: Pearson Education, Limited.

Wagner, J. G. (1968). Kinetics of pharmacologic response i. proposed relationships between response and drug concentration in the intact animal and man. *J. Theor. Biol.* 20, 173–201. doi: 10.1016/0022-5193(68)90188-4

Xiao, X., Shao, S.-H., and Chou, K.-C. (2006). A probability cellular automaton model for hepatitis b viral infections. *Biochem. Biophys. Res. Commun.* 342, 605–610. doi: 10.1016/j.bbrc.2006.01.166

Yarwood, J. M., and Schlievert, P. M. (2003). Quorum sensing in staphylococcus infections. *J. Clin. Investig.* 112, 1620–1625. doi: 10.1172/JCI2003 20442

Zorzenon dos Santos, R., and Coutinho, S. (2001). Dynamics of hiv infection: a cellular automata approach. *Phys. Rev. Lett.* 87, 168102. doi: 10.1103/PhysRevLett.87.168102

10

Influenza Virus Infection Model with Density Dependence Supports Biphasic Viral Decay

Amanda P. Smith [1], *David J. Moquin* [2], *Veronika Bernhauerova* [3] *and Amber M. Smith* [1*]

[1] *Department of Pediatrics, University of Tennessee Health Science Center, Memphis, TN, United States,* [2] *Department of Internal Medicine, University of Tennessee Health Science Center, Memphis, TN, United States,* [3] *Viral Populations and Pathogenesis Unit, Institut Pasteur, Paris, France*

***Correspondence:**
Amber M. Smith
amber.smith@uthsc.edu

Mathematical models that describe infection kinetics help elucidate the time scales, effectiveness, and mechanisms underlying viral growth and infection resolution. For influenza A virus (IAV) infections, the standard viral kinetic model has been used to investigate the effect of different IAV proteins, immune mechanisms, antiviral actions, and bacterial coinfection, among others. We sought to further define the kinetics of IAV infections by infecting mice with influenza A/PR8 and measuring viral loads with high frequency and precision over the course of infection. The data highlighted dynamics that were not previously noted, including viral titers that remain elevated for several days during mid-infection and a sharp 4–5 $\log_{10}$ decline in virus within 1 day as the infection resolves. The standard viral kinetic model, which has been widely used within the field, could not capture these dynamics. Thus, we developed a new model that could simultaneously quantify the different phases of viral growth and decay with high accuracy. The model suggests that the slow and fast phases of virus decay are due to the infected cell clearance rate changing as the density of infected cells changes. To characterize this model, we fit the model to the viral load data, examined the parameter behavior, and connected the results and parameters to linear regression estimates. The resulting parameters and model dynamics revealed that the rate of viral clearance during resolution occurs 25 times faster than the clearance during mid-infection and that small decreases to this rate can significantly prolong the infection. This likely reflects the high efficiency of the adaptive immune response. The new model provides a well-characterized representation of IAV infection dynamics, is useful for analyzing and interpreting viral load dynamics in the absence of immunological data, and gives further insight into the regulation of viral control.

Keywords: influenza virus infection, viral kinetics, mathematical model, density dependence, biphasic viral decay

1. INTRODUCTION

Influenza A virus (IAV) is a leading cause of lower respiratory tract infections and causes a significant amount of morbidity and mortality (Simonsen et al., 2000; Taubenberger and Morens, 2008; Medina and García-Sastre, 2011), with over 15 million individuals infected and more than 200,000 hospitalizations each year in the U.S. (Thompson et al., 2004). Vaccination against influenza viruses remains the most effective measure to prevent infection, but the large number of antigenically distinct strains, the emergence of new strains, and the low efficacy of antivirals make combatting the disease challenging. New therapeutic strategies are thus necessary and may require modulation of different viral control mechanisms, which are not entirely understood for IAV infection. Thus, it is critical to gain a deeper understanding of the infection kinetics, including determining the time scales, magnitudes, contribution, and interrelatedness of different control processes throughout IAV infection.

Kinetic modeling of *in vivo* infection processes provides important insight into viral growth and decay, host immune responses, antiviral actions, and multi-pathogen interactions. Remarkably, as few as 3–4 equations for target cells, infected cells, and virus can accurately describe viral load dynamics for a variety of virus infections [e.g., IAV, HIV, HCV, Zika virus, and West Nile Virus (Perelson et al., 1996; Neumann et al., 1998; Baccam et al., 2006; Banerjee et al., 2016; Best et al., 2017)]. For IAV infections, numerous studies have used these simple models with great success to elucidate mechanisms during IAV infection and during IAV coinfection with bacterial pathogens (reviewed in Smith and Ribeiro, 2010; Beauchemin and Handel, 2011; Smith and Perelson, 2011; Smith and McCullers, 2014; Boianelli et al., 2015). However, investigating mechanisms of immune control is often inhibited by insufficient data, which limits effective model calibration and selection. Further, it can be difficult to distinguish between mechanisms because a viral kinetic model that excludes equations and terms for specific immune responses can fit viral load dynamics with ease.

To aid interpretation of model results and gain insight into the mechanisms of infection, previous studies have used linear regression and approximate solutions to the viral kinetic model (derived by Smith et al., 2010) to identify how different processes (e.g., virus infection, production, and clearance) contribute to viral load dynamics throughout the course of infection (Miao et al., 2010; Smith et al., 2010, 2011a; Holder et al., 2011a,b; Halloran et al., 2012; Li and Handel, 2014; Kakizoe et al., 2015; Pinky and Dobrovolny, 2016; Best et al., 2017; Palmer et al., 2017; Smith, 2017). In the initial hours of infection, virus quickly infects cells or is cleared. Following an eclipse phase, virus production begins and virus increases exponentially for ~2 d. This initial growth can be approximated by a linear function of the $\log_{10}$ viral titers or by $V(t) = e^{\lambda t}$, where λ is a combination of all infection processes and is equivalent to the log-linear slope (Smith et al., 2010, 2011a). After this growth phase, virus peaks and begins to decline until the infection is resolved. Virus decay is typically exponential in nature and can be approximated in a similar fashion as the growth phase. That is, $V(t) = e^{-\delta t}$, where δ is the infected cell death rate and the sole process dictating the viral decay dynamics. Here, the log-linear slope is an estimate of the infected cell death rate (Smith et al., 2010, 2011a).

Although these dynamics and approximations have improved our knowledge of viral kinetics, some dynamical features, such as the plateauing of virus following the peak (reviewed in Smith and Perelson, 2011) cannot be explained by current kinetic models that exclude equations for immune factors. One model could reproduce the plateauing of virus through modeling interferon and an interferon-induced adaptive immune response (Pawelek et al., 2012). The study concluded that specific equations for the innate and adaptive responses were necessary. However, quantitative immunological data was not used to support model selection, parameterization, and conclusions. This type of data is scarce and has been a limiting factor of modeling studies. With viral loads as the most prevalent type of data, models that limit the number of parameters and equations remain desirable. However, even most viral load data is insufficiently quantitative to confidently detect features like a mid-infection plateau and build appropriate mathematical models.

Here, we first sought to increase the quality and quantity of viral load data in order to improve predictive power of mathematical models and gain a deeper insight into the kinetics of viral resolution. To do this, we measured viral loads daily from groups of BALB/cJ mice infected with influenza A/Puerto Rico/8/34 (H1N1) (PR8). In addition, we tightly controlled the experimental conditions and repeated the experiment numerous times to ensure reproducibility and identify data with meaningful biological heterogeneity (i.e., due to an underlying mechanism) vs. data with experimental heterogeneity (i.e., due to poor technique). The high resolution of these data defined important dynamical features, including a long plateau phase followed by a rapid decay phase. Because current viral kinetic models cannot reproduce these data, we developed a new model that incorporated a density-dependent decay of infected cells and could accurately describe the observed viral load dynamics. We used a rigorous fitting scheme to estimate the model parameters and infer important dynamics. Subsequent linear regression analysis and sensitivity analysis aided effective interpretation of the model results and direct comparison with published results. The data, model, and analyses provide a robust quantification of IAV infection kinetics and indicate that the rate of virus clearance changes with respect to the density of infected cells.

2. MATERIALS AND METHODS

2.1. Use of Experimental Animals

All experimental procedures were approved by the Animal Care and Use Committee at SJCRH under relevant institutional and American Veterinary Medical Association guidelines and were performed in a Biosafety level 2 facility that is accredited by AALAAS.

2.2. Mice

Adult (6 week old) female BALB/cJ mice were obtained from Jackson Laboratories (Bar Harbor, ME). Mice were housed in groups of 5 mice in high-temperature 31.2 × 23.5 × 15.2 cm polycarbonate cages with isolator lids. Rooms used for housing mice were maintained on a 12:1 2-h light:dark cycle at 22 ± 2°C with 50% humidity in the biosafety level 2 facility at St. Jude Children's Research Hospital (Memphis, TN). Prior to inclusion in the experiments, mice were allowed at least 7 days to acclimate to the animal facility such that they were 7 weeks old at the time of infection. Laboratory Autoclavable Rodent Diet (PMI Nutrition International, St. Louis, MO) and autoclaved water were available *ad libitum*. All experiments were performed under an approved protocol and in accordance with the guidelines set forth by the

Animal Care and Use Committee at St. Jude Children's Research Hospital.

2.3. Infectious Agents

All experiments were done using the mouse adapted influenza A/Puerto Rico/8/34 (H1N1) (PR8).

2.4. Infection Experiments

The viral infectious dose ($TCID_{50}$) was determined by interpolation using the method of Reed and Muench (Reed and Muench, 1938) using serial dilutions of virus on Madin-Darby canine kidney (MDCK) cells. Mice were intranasally inoculated with 75 $TCID_{50}$ PR8 in 100 µl. Mice were weighed at the onset of infection and each subsequent day for illness and mortality. Mice were euthanized if they became moribund or lost 30% of their starting body weight. Each experiment was repeated numerous times to ensure reproducibility. Two complete experiments (10 animals per time point) were used for these studies. The raw data is shown in **Figure 1A** and is available upon request.

2.5. Lung Titers

Mice were euthanized by CO_2 asphyxiation. Lungs were aseptically harvested, washed three times in PBS, and placed in 500 µl sterile PBS. Whole lungs were digested with collagenase (1 mg/ml, Sigma C0130), and physically homogenized by syringe plunger against a 40 µm cell strainer. Cell suspensions were centrifuged at 4°C, 500 × g for 7 min. The supernatants were used to determine the viral titers using serial dilutions on MDCK monolayers.

2.6. Mathematical Model

The standard viral kinetic model used to describe IAV infection kinetics tracks 4 populations: susceptible epithelial ("target") cells (T), two classes of infected cells (I_1 and I_2), and virus (V) (Baccam et al., 2006):

$$\frac{dT}{dt} = -\beta TV \tag{1}$$

$$\frac{dI_1}{dt} = \beta TV - kI_1 \tag{2}$$

$$\frac{dI_2}{dt} = kI_1 - \delta(I_2)I_2 \tag{3}$$

$$\frac{dV}{dt} = pI_2 - cV \tag{4}$$

In this model, target cells become infected with virus at rate βV per cell. Once infected, these cells enter an eclipse phase (I_1) before transitioning at rate k per cell to produce virus (I_2). Virus production occurs at rate p per cell. Virus is cleared at rate c and virus-producing infected cells (I_2) are cleared according to the function $\delta(I_2)$. The standard viral kinetic model assumes that infected cells are cleared at a constant rate ($\delta(I_2) = \delta_s$) (Baccam et al., 2006). The subscript s is used to denote "standard." This model could not recapitulate the data (see Table S1 and Figure S1) and a modification of the model was necessary. Given that the rate of infected cell clearance ($\delta(I_2)$) drives the virus decay dynamics (Smith et al., 2010), we let the clearance rate vary with the number of infected cells such that

$$\delta(I_2) = \frac{\delta_d}{K_\delta + I_2}, \tag{5}$$

where δ_d/K_δ is the maximum rate of infected cell clearance and K_δ is the half-saturation constant. The subscript d is used to denote "density-dependent." Modifications to other terms were examined, but none could replicate the data.

2.7. Parameter Estimation

Given a parameter set θ, the cost $C(\theta) = \sum_{v_i}(V(\theta, t_i) - v_i)^2$ was minimized across parameter ranges using an Adaptive Simulated Annealing (ASA) global optimization algorithm (details in the Supplementary Material) to compare experimental and predicted values of $\log_{10}$ $TCID_{50}$/lung. A sample search pattern is shown in Figure S2. Errors of the $\log_{10}$ data were assumed to be normally distributed. To explore and visualize the regions of parameters consistent with the models, we fit Equations 1–5 to 1,000 bootstrap replicates of the data. For each bootstrap data set, the model was fit 10 times beginning from the best-fit parameters estimate $\boldsymbol{\theta}^{\text{best}}$ that was found by fitting the model to the data then perturbing each parameter estimate uniformly within ±50% of its best-fit value. If the three best bootstrap fits were within $\chi^2 = 0.05$ of the best-fit, then the bootstrap was considered successful (Smith et al., 2011a, 2013). For each best fit estimate, we provide 95% confidence interval (CI) computed from the bootstrap replicates. All calculations were performed in MATLAB.

Estimated parameters included the rates of virus infection (β), virus production (p), virus clearance (c), eclipse phase transition (k), infected cell clearance (δ_d), and the half saturation constant (K_δ). Bounds were placed on the parameters to constrain them to physically realistic values. Because biological estimates are not available for all parameters, ranges were set reasonably large based on preliminary results and previous estimates (Smith et al., 2011a). The rate of infection (β) was allowed to vary between 10^{-6} $TCID_{50}^{-1}$ d^{-1} and 10^{-1} $TCID_{50}^{-1}$ d^{-1}, and the rate of viral production (p) between 10^{-1} $TCID_{50}$ $cell^{-1}$ d^{-1} and 10^3 $TCID_{50}$ $cell^{-1}$ d^{-1}. Bounds for the viral clearance rate (c) were 1 d^{-1} ($t_{1/2}$ = 16.7 h) and 10^3 d^{-1} ($t_{1/2}$ = 1 min). Previous estimates of the eclipse phase rate (k) for IAV infection in mice resulted in estimates that fell outside the biologically feasible range of 4–6 h (Smith et al., 2011a). To insure biological feasibility, the lower and upper bounds for the eclipse phase rate (k) were 4 d^{-1} and 6 d^{-1}. Limits for the half-saturation constant (K_δ) were $10^2 - 10^6$ cells, and limits for the infected cell clearance parameter (δ_d) were $1 \times 10^6 - 4 \times 10^6$ cells/d.

The initial number of target cells (T_0) was set to 10^7 cells (Smith et al., 2011a, 2013). Because the initial viral inoculum rapidly infects cells and/or is cleared within 4 h pi, as indicated by the undetectable viral titers at this time point (**Figure 1**), the initial number of infected cells $I_1(0)$ was set to 75 cells to reflect an initial dose of 75 $TCID_{50}$. This is an alteration from previous studies, including our own, that either estimate the initial amount

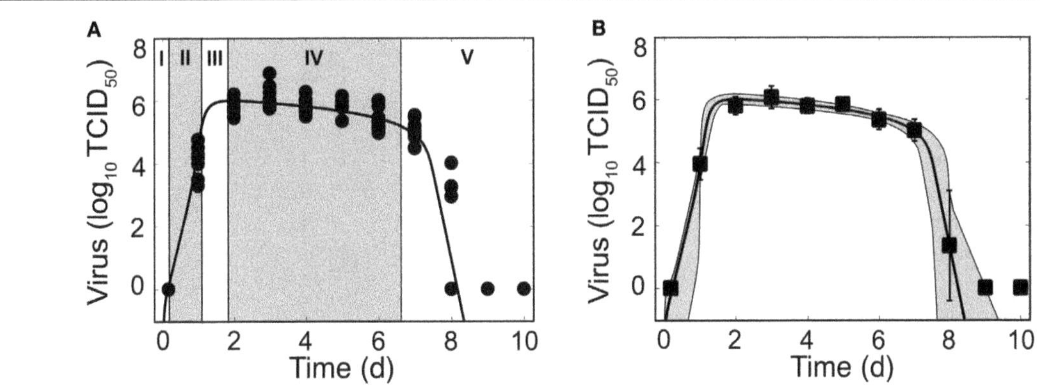

FIGURE 1 | Phases of viral kinetics and fit of the density-dependent viral kinetic model. **(A)** Fit of the density-dependent viral kinetic model (Equations 1–5) to viral titers from the lungs of individual mice (10 mice per time point) infected with 75 $TCID_{50}$ PR8. Each dot is an individual mouse and the solid black line is the optimal solution of the model. Phases I–V of the viral kinetics are illustrated, where virus (I) quickly infects cells, (II) increases exponentially, (III) peaks, (IV) decays slowly, then (V) decays rapidly and clears. **(B)** Optimal fit of the model (solid black line) shown with the model solutions using parameter sets within the 95% CIs (gray shading). Data are shown as the mean ± standard deviation. Parameters are given in **Table 1**.

of virus (V_0) or set its value to the true viral inoculum. Fixing $V(0) = 75$ $TCID_{50}$ or estimating its value did not improve the fit and could not be statistically justified (see, for example, Table S1). Further, fixing $V(0) = 75$ $TCID_{50}$ yielded an unreasonably high estimate for the rate of virus clearance (c) due to the attempt to fit the sharp decay between 0–4 h pi. Estimating $I_1(0)$ could also not be justified and did not improve the model fit (e.g., as in Table S1 and Figure S1). The initial number of productively infected cells ($I_2(0)$) and the initial free virus (V_0) were set to 0.

2.8. Linear Regression

We used the function *polyfit* in MATLAB to perform linear regression of the $\log_{10}$ values of viral titer during the growth phase (4 h, 1 d pi) and the two decay phases (2–6 d pi and 7–8 d pi).

3. RESULTS

3.1. Phases of Viral Load Kinetics

Mice infected with 75 $TCID_{50}$ PR8 have viral load kinetics that can be separated into five distinct phases (**Figure 1A**). This is in contrast to the three phases that we previously defined (Smith et al., 2010). In the first phase, virus quickly infects cells and is undetectable within 4 h pi. In the second and third phases, virus increases exponentially and peaks after ~2 d pi. Following the peak, the viral decline can be separated into two phases. In the first decay phase (2–6 d pi), virus decays slowly at a relatively constant rate. In the second decay phase (7–8 d pi), virus declines rapidly (4–5 $\log_{10}$ $TCID_{50}$). Sixty percent of mice had no detectable virus by 8 d pi. The remaining mice resolved the infection by 9 d pi.

These data reduced the heterogeneity observed in a previous data set from infection with the same virus (Smith et al., 2011a). We discovered that the majority of heterogeneity in the previous data set could be attributed to inconsistent infections and, thus, inocula that varied. We further reduced heterogeneity by normalizing the viral titer to the total lung volume, rather than using units of $TCID_{50}$/ml lung homogenate. As expected, some heterogeneity remains at 1 d pi and at 8 d pi. These time points correspond to when virus is rapidly increasing and decreasing, respectively.

3.2. Kinetic Model With Density Dependent Viral Clearance

We first fit the standard viral kinetic model, which is given by Equations (1)–(4) and assumes only one mechanism of constant clearance ($\delta(I_2) = \delta_s$) (Baccam et al., 2006), to the viral load data (see Supplementary Material). This model was unable to capture the entire time course of viral load dynamics, but was able to fit the data from infection initiation to 7 d pi (Figure S1). To more accurately model IAV kinetics and simultaneously recapitulate the two phases of viral decline, we modified the rate of infected cell clearance ($\delta(I_2)$) so that the rate changes with respect to the density of the infected cell population. That is, $\delta(I_2) = \delta_d/(K_\delta + I_2)$ (Equation 5), where δ_d/K_δ is the maximum rate of clearance and K_δ is the number of productively infected cells where the rate is half of its maximum.

Fitting this new model to the viral load data illustrated that the model can accurately reproduce the data and simultaneously capture both phases of viral decline while excluding specific immune responses. The resulting dynamics are shown in **Figure 1**, the parameter values and 95% confidence intervals (CIs) are given in **Table 1**, and the parameter ensembles are shown in **Figure 2** and Figure S3. For this model, the basic reproduction number (R_0) is given by

$$R_0 = \frac{\beta p T_0 K_\delta}{c \delta_d} \tag{6}$$

Given the parameters in **Table 1**, $R_0 = 8.8$.

To understand how the addition of $\delta(I_2) = \delta_d/(K_\delta + I_2)$ influences the other parameters during the fitting scheme, we

TABLE 1 | Parameter values and 95% confidence intervals obtained from fitting the density-dependent viral kinetic model (Equations 1–5) to viral titers from mice infected with 75 $TCID_{50}$ PR8.

Parameter	Description	Units	Value	95% CI
β	Virus infectivity	$TCID_{50}^{-1}$ d^{-1}	2.4×10^{-4}	$[5.0 \times 10^{-5}, 7.8 \times 10^{-2}]$
p	Virus production	$TCID_{50}$ $cell^{-1}$ d^{-1}	1.6	[0.82, 125.3]
c	Virus clearance	d^{-1}	13.0	[6.3, 943.1]
k	Eclipse phase	d^{-1}	4.0	[4.0, 6.0]
δ_d	Infected cell clearance	$cell^{-1}$ d^{-1}	1.6×10^{6}	$[1.4 \times 10^{6}, 1.7 \times 10^{6}]$
K_δ	Half saturation constant	cells	4.5×10^{5}	$[1.2 \times 10^{2}, 1.7 \times 10^{5}]$
$T(0)$	Initial uninfected cells	cells	1×10^{7}	-
$I_1(0)$	Initial infected cells	cells	75	-
$I_2(0)$	Initial infected cells	cells	0	-
$V(0)$	Initial virus	$TCID_{50}$	0	-

plotted the resulting histograms and 2D parameter projections (**Figure 2**). As expected, strong correlations exist between the rates of virus production (p) and virus clearance (c) and between the rate of infection (β) and the infected cell death rate (δ_d/K_δ). The other correlations visible in **Figure 2** were a consequence of these two relations. Of note, δ_d was not strongly correlated with any of the other model parameters (Figure S3). In addition, the confidence interval was small, particularly compared to the other parameters. Estimates for the other parameters (β, p, c, and K_δ) with the exception of the eclipse phase rate (k) were well bounded such that the 95% CIs fell within the upper and lower bounds imposed in the estimation scheme. Similar to previous studies (Baccam et al., 2006; Smith et al., 2011a), the eclipse phase rate (k) was restricted to biologically realistic values and was not well defined on the given interval. In support, the ASA algorithm search patterns show a longer search time for k compared to the other parameters (Figure S2).

To further determine how the addition of $\delta(I_2) = \delta_d/(K_\delta + I_2)$ influences the sensitivity of the model solution to changes in parameter values, we performed a one-at-a-time sensitivity analysis (**Figure 3**). The infected cell clearance parameter (δ_d) is the most sensitive parameter and largely dictates the viral decay. Decreasing δ_d significantly delays viral clearance while increasing δ_d leads to rapid viral resolution (**Figure 3**). In accordance with previous results (Smith et al., 2010), all other parameters are less sensitive and collectively affect the exponential growth phase and peak.

As illustrated in **Figure 4A**, the rate of infected cell clearance is rapid when these cells are in small numbers. Given the parameters in **Table 1**, the maximum clearance rate is $\delta(I_2) = 12.7$ d^{-1}, which corresponds to half-life $t_{1/2} = 1.3$ h. The rate begins to slow when $I_2 > 10^4$ cells and is minimal when I_2 is at its maximum (8×10^6 cells). When I_2 is maximal, $\delta(I_2) = 0.21$ d^{-1} and $t_{1/2} = 78$ h. In our previous work, we discovered that linear regression analysis could be used to accurately estimate the exponential growth rate, which was a combination of all model parameters, and that the slope of the viral decay could provide an estimate of $\delta(I_2)$ (Smith et al., 2010, 2011a). To evaluate how these relations correlate to parameters in the model with density dependence, we performed a linear regression on the data during the growth phase (4 h–1 d pi) and the two decay phases (2–6 d pi and 7–8 d pi) (**Figure 4B**). The slope of the growth phase is 4.7 $\log_{10}$ $TCID_{50}$/d (red line in **Figure 4B**). In accordance with the previous studies, this slope is a good approximation to the model until shortly before the peak. The model deviates slightly from this estimate and suggests that the virus growth rate briefly increases prior to the peak and that the decay phase begins prior to 2 d pi. This nonlinearity in the growth can be attributed to the decreasing infected cell clearance rate as the number of infected cells increases. These results are in contrast to the standard viral kinetic model, which suggests that the virus growth rate strictly decreases following exponential growth (Smith et al., 2010, 2011a). In the first phase of decay, the slope is -0.2 $\log_{10}$ $TCID_{50}$/d (green line in **Figure 4B**), which corresponds to $\delta(I_2) = 0.4$ d^{-1} (green diamond in **Figure 4A**). In the second phase of decay, the slope is -3.8 $\log_{10}$ $TCID_{50}$/d (blue line in **Figure 4B**), which corresponds to $\delta(I_2) = 8.7$ d^{-1} (blue dot in **Figure 4A**).

4. DISCUSSION

Mathematical models have been widely used to investigate IAV dynamics (reviewed in Smith and Ribeiro, 2010; Beauchemin and Handel, 2011; Smith and Perelson, 2011; Smith and McCullers, 2014; Boianelli et al., 2015). The viral kinetic model given by Equations (1)–(4) with $\delta(I_2) = \delta_s$ (Baccam et al., 2006) has been the standard in the field for over 10 years. We previously used this model together with data from murine infection to gain insight into IAV virulence factors (Smith et al., 2011a) and into coinfection with bacterial pathogens (Smith et al., 2013; Smith and Smith, 2016; Smith, 2017). Although some predictions made using this model have been experimentally tested and deemed accurate (Ghoneim et al., 2013; Smith and McCullers, 2014; Warnking et al., 2015; Smith and Smith, 2016), the data here suggested that some dynamical features could not be accounted for and thus a new model was necessary. The model we introduced here includes density-dependent infected cell clearance and better captures the entire course of IAV infection dynamics, including the two-phase viral decay following the peak (**Figure 1**). Importantly, the model added only a single parameter (the half-saturation constant, K_δ)

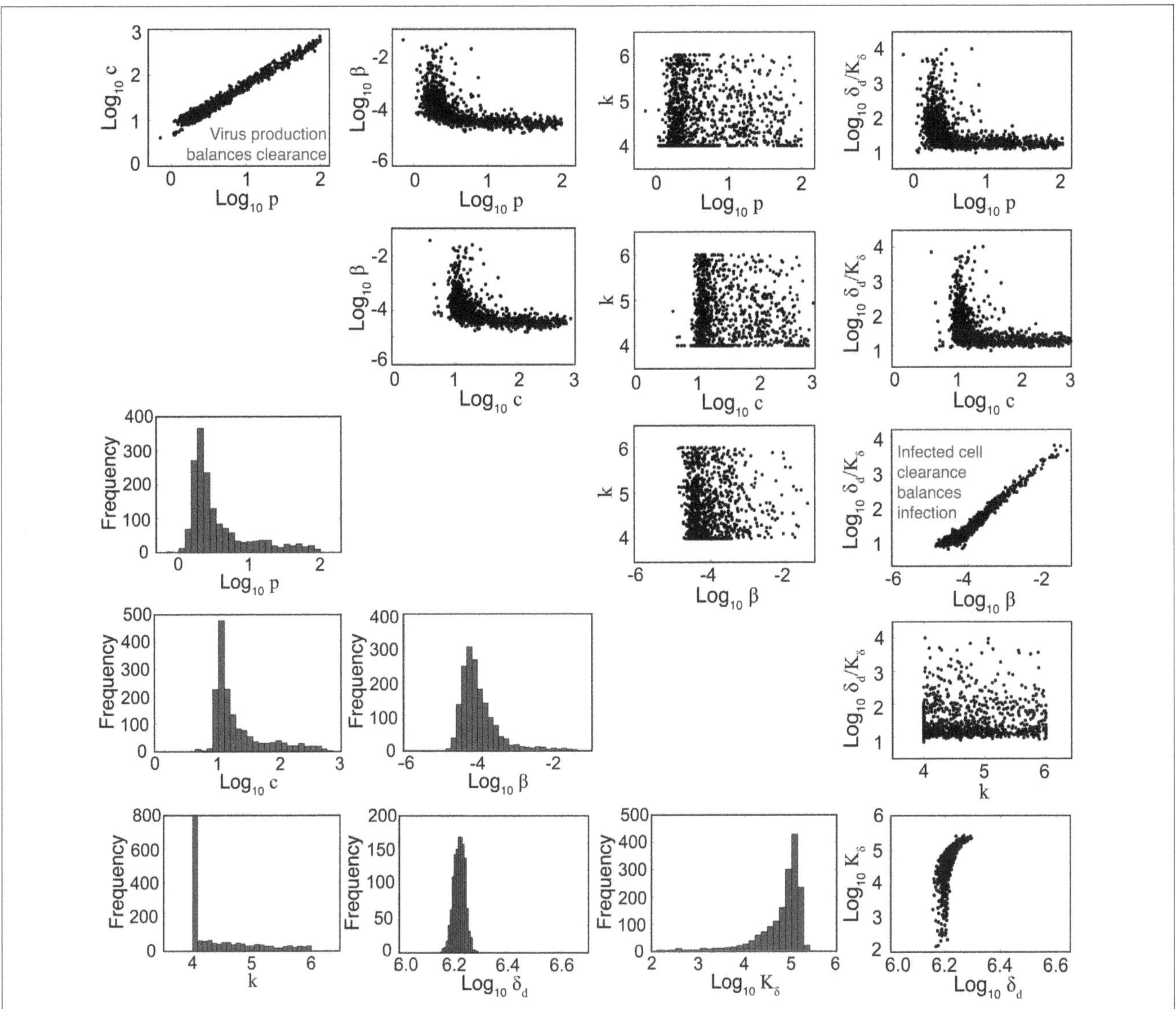

FIGURE 2 | Parameter ensembles and histograms. Parameter ensembles and histograms resulting from fitting the density-dependent viral kinetic model (Equations 1–5) to viral titers from mice infected with 75 $TCID_{50}$ PR8. Two main correlations are evident between the rates of virus production (*p*) and clearance (*c*) and between the rates of infection (β) and infected cell clearance (δ_d/K_δ). The axes limits reflect imposed bounds (except $k \in [4, 6]$). All parameters except the eclipse phase rate (*k*) are well bounded (i.e., the 95% CIs do not reach the imposed bounds). Additional ensemble plots (e.g., for R_0) are in Figure S3.

while significantly improving the model fit to viral loads from IAV infection without including additional equations detailing immune responses

By sampling with high frequency and controlling for experimental heterogeneity, we were able to obtain more accurate data (i.e., smaller standard deviations and better reproducibility) that highlighted several important dynamics, some of which were not previously observed. Our data showed that viral loads are maintained at a high level between 2 d and 7 d pi (**Figure 1**). Sustained viral loads have been observed in several studies (Jao et al., 1970; Douglas et al., 1975; Larson et al., 1976; Reuman et al., 1989; Bjornson et al., 1991; Toapanta and Ross, 2009; Smith et al., 2011a). In some data sets, the peak appears more pronounced and is often followed by the plateau phase or a second, lower peak (Jao et al., 1970; Douglas et al., 1975; Larson et al., 1976; Bjornson et al., 1991; Bender and Small, 1993; Hayden et al., 1998; Baccam et al., 2006). Our murine data do not indicate a second peak, although there is a subtle increase in viral loads at 5 d pi that may be biologically significant. Previous influenza modeling studies suggest that these dynamics required equations/terms for the innate and adaptive immune responses (Baccam et al., 2006; Pawelek et al., 2012; Cao et al., 2016). However, HIV modeling studies have used similar density-dependent terms to achieve a two-phase viral load decay (Holte et al., 2006; Burg et al., 2009). Importantly, the model here provides a means for capturing the changes in viral load decay

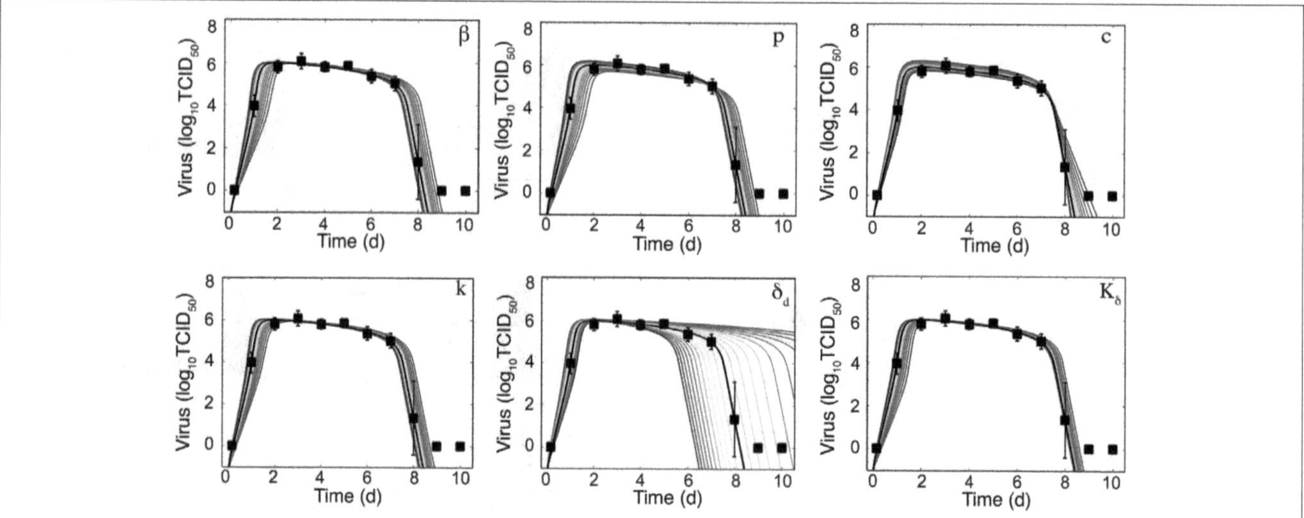

FIGURE 3 | Sensitivity of the density-dependent viral kinetic model. Solutions of the density-dependent viral kinetic model (Equations 1–5) for the best-fit parameters (black line, **Table 1**) and with the indicated parameter increased (red) or decreased (blue) 50% from the best-fit value.

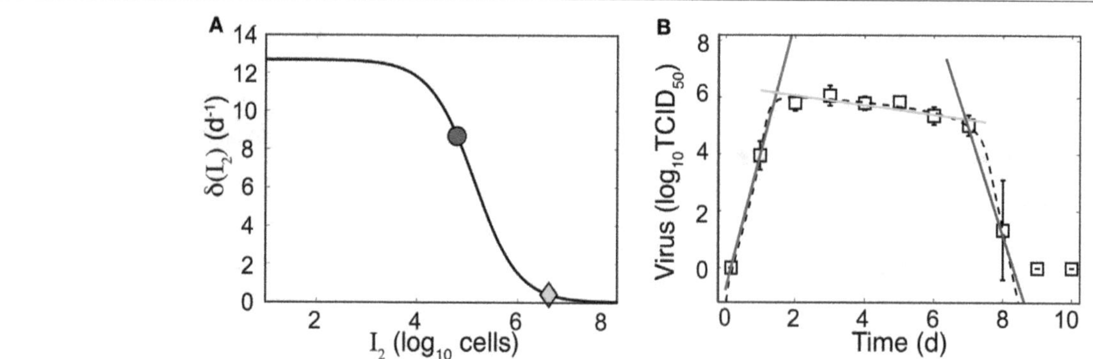

FIGURE 4 | Density-dependent infected cell clearance rate and correlation to linear regression. **(A)** The infected cell clearance rate ($\delta(I_2)$, Equation 5) is plotted for different values of infected cells (I_2). The green diamond and the blue dot indicate the corresponding infected cell clearance rates during the slow and fast phases of virus clearance, respectively. These correspond to linear regression estimates in **(B)**. **(B)** Linear regression fits to the viral load data (white squares) during the growth phase (4 h–1 d pi, red line), the first phase of virus decay (2–6 d pi, green line), or the second phase of virus decay (7–8 d pi, blue line). The dashed black line is the fit of the density-dependent viral kinetic model (Equations 1–5) to the viral load data.

without complicating the model or inferring information about specific immune mechanisms, which are not well understood. However, the change in clearance rate could reflect the change from innate to adaptive immunity. If this is the case, our estimates would suggest that the adaptive response is 25 times more effective than the innate response (-0.2 log_{10} $TCID_{50}/d$ between 2–6 d pi vs. -3.8 log_{10} $TCID_{50}/d$ between 7–8 d pi; **Figure 4B**).

It is well accepted that the rapid decline in virus during the second decay phase is due to the infiltration of $CD8^+$ T cells (reviewed in McMichael et al., 1983; Kim et al., 2011; Grant et al., 2016). These cells typically enter the infection site between 5–6 d pi and peak between 8–9 d pi (e.g., as in Toapanta and Ross, 2009). The rapid rate of viral decline between 7–8 d pi suggests that these cells are highly effective. However, the initial infiltration begins at least 1–2 d before a change in the rate of virus decay is visible. Thus, there may be a nonlinearity to this response or it may reflect a simultaneous increase in infections and killing of infected cells or a change in effectiveness proportional to the density of infected cells or to the density of $CD8^+$ T cells. A handling-time effect, which can represent the time required for immune cells to kill each infected cell and/or the time for immune cells to become activated (e.g., as in Pilyugin et al., 1997; Graw and Regoes, 2009; Smith et al., 2011b; Gadhamsetty et al., 2014; Li and Handel, 2014; Le et al., 2015), can slow the per capita rate of clearance. Spatial constraints (e.g., crowding effect), where the number of immune cells within an area is limited, may also play a role. In contrast, numerous clearance mechanisms (e.g., interferons, macrophages, neutrophils, natural killer (NK) cells) are thought to be important during early- and mid-infection, but their contribution to the viral load kinetics is unclear. Using a model to distinguish between these mechanisms is challenging given the close fit of simple kinetic models to viral load data (**Figure 1** and Figure S1). Further, neither the data nor the models can discriminate whether the maintenance of high viral loads is due to a lack of clearance of infected cells (i.e., long infected cell lifespan/ineffective clearance) or to the balance of new infections and clearance (i.e., short infected cell lifespan/rapid clearance coupled with rapid virus infection/production). Thus, new experimental designs and more diverse data are necessary.

Viral titers remain the most frequently used data to calibrate models and assess infection dynamics. This is because collecting immunological data is more laborious and expensive. Thus, we seek models that are simple yet accurate and that can be used in the absence of immunological data. The standard viral kinetic model includes the minimal number of parameters and equations needed to recapitulate viral load dynamics. However, viral load data is typically insufficient to uniquely define all 6 parameters (Miao et al., 2011; Smith et al., 2011a). Fortunately, this has not limited our ability to make robust predictions about the underlying biology or to estimate accurate parameter values even when correlations are present (Gutenkunst et al., 2007; Smith et al., 2013; Smith and Smith, 2016). Here, the resulting parameter ensembles were well-bounded (i.e., the 95% CIs did not include the imposed bounds) and correlations were observed in two sets of parameters (**Figure 2**). The correlation between the rates of virus production (p) and virus clearance (c) indicates the balance of these processes. This is expected because viral loads measure the amount of virus present and slow virus production/clearance would be indistinguishable from fast production/clearance. Similarly, the rates of infection (β) and infected cell clearance (δ_d/K_δ) were correlated, which indicates a balance of cells becoming infected and being cleared. This is visible in **Figure 4B**, where the log-linear fit to the data in the growth phase (red line) deviates from the model solution (black dashed line).

Analyzing infection kinetics with mathematical models provides a means to quantify different infection processes. By modeling viral load data, we can make meaningful predictions about the time scales, magnitudes, and rates of different processes even if we cannot directly define specific mechanisms. Further, having a well-characterized model allows us to design new experiments and to perform *in silico* experiments that evaluate situations where data is challenging to obtain. Here, our data, model, and analyses suggest that the clearance rate of infected cells is variable and depends on their density such that clearance slows when infected cells are numerous and is fast when they are in low numbers. Determining what processes give rise to this density dependence remains an open question. Understanding how and why the rate changes should facilitate a deeper understanding of other viral infections and of immunological data, as it becomes available. Further establishing how the virus and host components work together and how they can be manipulated will undoubtedly aid the development of therapies that prevent or treat IAV infections.

AUTHOR CONTRIBUTIONS

AMS conceived the idea, performed the experiments, developed the model, ran the simulations, performed the analysis, and wrote the manuscript. APS and DM performed the experiments. VB implemented the code and ran the simulations.

ACKNOWLEDGMENTS

This work was supported by NIH grants AI100946 and AI125324, and by ALSAC. A portion of this work was completed while all authors were at St. Jude Children's Research Hospital. We thank Alan Perelson and Laura Liao for their helpful comments.

REFERENCES

Baccam, P., Beauchemin, C., Macken, C., Hayden, F., and Perelson, A. (2006). Kinetics of influenza A virus infection in humans. *J. Virol.* 80, 7590–7599. doi: 10.1128/JVI.01623-05

Banerjee, S., Guedj, J., Ribeiro, R., Moses, M., and Perelson, A. (2016). Estimating biologically relevant parameters under uncertainty for experimental within-host murine West Nile virus infection. *J. R. Soc. Interface* 13:20160130. doi: 10.1098/rsif.2016.0130

Beauchemin, C., and Handel, A. (2011). A review of mathematical models of influenza A infections within a host or cell culture: lessons learned and challenges ahead. *BMC Public Health* 11(Suppl 1):S7. doi: 10.1186/1471-2458-11-S1-S7

Bender, B., and Small, P. Jr. (1993). Heterotypic immune mice lose protection against influenza virus infection with senescence. *J. Infect. Dis.* 168, 873–880. doi: 10.1093/infdis/168.4.873

Best, K., Guedj, J., Madelain, V., de Lamballerie, X., Lim, S., Osuna, C., et al. (2017). Zika plasma viral dynamics in nonhuman primates provides insights into early infection and antiviral strategies. *Proc. Natl. Acad. Sci. U.S.A.* 114, 8847–8852. doi: 10.1073/pnas.1704011114

Bjornson, A., Mellencamp, M., and Schiff, G. (1991). Complement is activated in the upper respiratory tract during influenza virus infection. *Am. Rev. Respir. Dis.* 143(5 Pt 1):1062–1066.

Boianelli, A., Nguyen, V., Ebensen, T., Schulze, K., Wilk, E., Sharma, N., et al. (2015). Modeling influenza virus infection: a roadmap for influenza research. *Viruses* 7, 5274–5304. doi: 10.3390/v7102875

Burg, D., Rong, L., Neumann, A., and Dahari, H. (2009). Mathematical modeling of viral kinetics under immune control during primary HIV-1 infection. *J. Theor. Biol.* 259, 751–759. doi: 10.1016/j.jtbi.2009.04.010

Cao, P., Wang, Z., Yan, A., McVernon, J., Xu, J., Heffernan, J., et al. (2016). On the role of CD8+ T cells in determining recovery time from influenza virus infection. *Front. Immunol.* 7:611. doi: 10.3389/fimmu.2016.00611

Douglas, R. Jr., Betts, R., Simons, R., Hogan, P., and Roth, F. (1975). Evaluation of a topical interferon inducer in experimental influenza infection in volunteers. *Antimicrob. Agents Ch.* 8, 684–687. doi: 10.1128/AAC.8.6.684

Gadhamsetty, S., Marée, A., Beltman, J., and de Boer, R. (2014). A general functional response of cytotoxic T lymphocyte-mediated killing of target cells. *Biophys. J.* 106, 1780–1791. doi: 10.1016/j.bpj.2014.01.048

Ghoneim, H., Thomas, P., and McCullers, J. (2013). Depletion of alveolar macrophages during influenza infection facilitates bacterial superinfections. *J. Immunol.* 191, 1250–1259. doi: 10.4049/jimmunol.1300014

Grant, E., Quiñones-Parra, S., Clemens, E., and Kedzierska, K. (2016). Human influenza viruses and CD8+ T cell responses. *Curr. Opin. Virol.* 16, 132–142. doi: 10.1016/j.coviro.2016.01.016

Graw, F., and Regoes, R. (2009). Investigating CTL mediated killing with a 3D cellular automaton. *PLoS Comput. Biol.* 5:e1000466. doi: 10.1371/journal.pcbi.1000466

Gutenkunst, R., Waterfall, J., Casey, F., Brown, K., Myers, C., and Sethna, J. (2007). Universally sloppy parameter sensitivities in systems biology models. *PLoS Comput. Biol.* 3:e189. doi: 10.1371/journal.pcbi.0030189

Halloran, S., Wexler, A., and Ristenpart, W. (2012). A comprehensive breath plume model for disease transmission via expiratory aerosols. *PLoS ONE* 7:e37088. doi: 10.1371/journal.pone.0037088

Hayden, F., Fritz, R., Lobo, M., Alvord, W., Strober, W., and Straus, S. (1998). Local and systemic cytokine responses during experimental human influenza A virus infection. Relation to symptom formation and host defense. *J. Clin. Investig.* 101:643.

Holder, B., Liao, L., Simon, P., Boivin, G., and Beauchemin, C. (2011a). Design considerations in building *in silico* equivalents of common experimental influenza virus assays. *Autoimmunity* 44, 282–293. doi: 10.3109/08916934.2011.523267

Holder, B., Simon, P., Liao, L., Abed, Y., Bouhy, X., Beauchemin, C., et al. (2011b). Assessing the *in vitro* fitness of an oseltamivir-resistant seasonal A/H1N1 influenza strain using a mathematical model. *PLoS ONE* 6:e14767. doi: 10.1371/journal.pone.0014767

Holte, S., Melvin, A., Mullins, I., Tobin, N., and Frenkel, L. (2006). Density-dependent decay in HIV-1 dynamics. *JAIDS* 41, 266–276. doi: 10.1097/01.qai.0000199233.69457.e4

Jao, R., Wheelock, E., and Jackson, G. (1970). Production of interferon in volunteers infected with Asian influenza. *J. Infect. Dis.* 121, 419–426. doi: 10.1093/infdis/121.4.419

Kakizoe, Y., Nakaoka, S., Beauchemin, C., Morita, S., Mori, H., Igarashi, T., et al. (2015). A method to determine the duration of the eclipse phase for *in vitro* infection with a highly pathogenic SHIV strain. *Sci. Rep.* 5:10371. doi: 10.1038/srep10371

Kim, T., Sun, J., and Braciale, T. (2011). T cell responses during influenza infection: getting and keeping control. *Trends Immunol.* 32, 225–231. doi: 10.1016/j.it.2011.02.006

Larson, E., Dominik, J., Rowberg, A., and Higbee, G. (1976). Influenza virus population dynamics in the respiratory tract of experimentally infected mice. *Infect. Immun.* 13, 438–447.

Le, D., Miller, J., and Ganusov, V. (2015). Mathematical modeling provides kinetic details of the human immune response to vaccination. *Front. Cell. Infect. Microbiol.* 4:177. doi: 10.3389/fcimb.2014.00177

Li, Y., and Handel, A. (2014). Modeling inoculum dose dependent patterns of acute virus infections. *J. Theor. Biol.* 347, 63–73. doi: 10.1016/j.jtbi.2014.01.008

McMichael, A., Gotch, F., Noble, G., and Beare, P. (1983). Cytotoxic T-cell immunity to influenza. *New Engl. J. Med.* 309, 13–17. doi: 10.1056/NEJM198307073090103

Medina, R., and García-Sastre, A. (2011). Influenza A viruses: new research developments. *Nat. Rev. Microbiol.* 9, 590–603. doi: 10.1038/nrmicro2613

Miao, H., Hollenbaugh, J., Zand, M., Holden-Wiltse, J., Mosmann, T., Perelson, A., et al. (2010). Quantifying the early immune response and adaptive immune response kinetics in mice infected by influenza A virus. *J. Virol.* 84, 6687–6698. doi: 10.1128/JVI.00266-10

Miao, H., Xia, X., Perelson, A., and Wu, H. (2011). On identifiability of nonlinear ODE models and applications in viral dynamics. *SIAM Rev.* 53, 3–39. doi: 10.1137/090757009

Neumann, A., Lam, N., Dahari, H., Gretch, D., Wiley, T., Layden, T., et al. (1998). Hepatitis C viral dynamics *in vivo* and the antiviral efficacy of interferon-α therapy. *Science* 282, 103–107. doi: 10.1126/science.282.5386.103

Palmer, J., Dobrovolny, H., and Beauchemin, C. (2017). The *in vivo* efficacy of neuraminidase inhibitors cannot be determined from the decay rates of influenza viral titers observed in treated patients. *Sci. Rep.* 7:40210. doi: 10.1038/srep40210

Pawelek, K., Huynh, G., Quinlivan, M., Cullinane, A., Rong, L., and Perelson, A. (2012). Modeling within-host dynamics of influenza virus infection including immune responses. *PLoS Comput. Biol.* 8:e1002588. doi: 10.1371/journal.pcbi.1002588

Perelson, A., Neumann, A., Markowitz, M., Leonard, J., and Ho, D. (1996). HIV-1 dynamics *in vivo*: virion clearance rate, infected cell life-span, and viral generation time. *Science* 271, 1582–1586. doi: 10.1126/science.271.5255.1582

Pilyugin, S., Mittler, J., and Antia, R. (1997). Modeling T-cell proliferation: an investigation of the consequences of the Hayflick limit. *J. Theor. Biol.* 186, 117–129. doi: 10.1006/jtbi.1996.0319

Pinky, L., and Dobrovolny, H. (2016). Coinfections of the respiratory tract: viral competition for resources. *PLoS ONE* 11:e0155589. doi: 10.1371/journal.pone.0155589

Reed, L., and Muench, H. (1938). A simple method of estimating fifty percent endpoints. *Am. J. Epidemiol.* 27, 493–497. doi: 10.1093/oxfordjournals.aje.a118408

Reuman, P., Bernstein, D., Keefer, M., Young, E., Sherwood, J., Schiff, G. M., et al. (1989). Efficacy and safety of low dosage amantadine hydrochloride as prophylaxis for influenza A. *Antivir. Res.* 11, 27–40. doi: 10.1016/0166-3542(89)90018-1

Simonsen, L., Fukuda, K., Schonberger, L., and Cox, N. (2000). The impact of influenza epidemics on hospitalizations. *J. Infect. Dis.* 181, 831–837. doi: 10.1086/315320

Smith, A. (2017). Quantifying the therapeutic requirements and potential for combination therapy to prevent bacterial coinfection during influenza. *J. Pharmacokinet. Pharm.* 48:81. doi: 10.1007/s10928-016-9494-9

Smith, A., Adler, F., McAuley, J., Gutenkunst, R., Ribeiro, R., McCullers, J., et al. (2011a). Effect of 1918 PB1-F2 expression on influenza A virus infection kinetics. *PLoS Comput. Biol.* 7:e1001081. doi: 10.1371/journal.pcbi.1001081

Smith, A., Adler, F., and Perelson, A. (2010). An accurate two-phase approximate solution to an acute viral infection model. *J. Math. Biol.* 60, 711–726. doi: 10.1007/s00285-009-0281-8

Smith, A., Adler, F., Ribeiro, R., Gutenkunst, R., McAuley, J., McCullers, J., et al. (2013). Kinetics of coinfection with influenza A virus and *Streptococcus pneumoniae*. *PLoS Pathog.* 9:e1003238. doi: 10.1371/journal.ppat.1003238

Smith, A., and McCullers, J. (2014). "Secondary bacterial infections in influenza virus infection pathogenesis," in *Influenza Pathogenesis and Control*, Vol. 1. *Current Topics in Microbiology and Immunology*, vol. 385. (Cham: Springer), 327–356.
Smith A.M., McCullers J.A. (2014) Secondary Bacterial Infections in Influenza Virus Infection Pathogenesis. In: Compans R., Oldstone M. (eds) Influenza Pathogenesis and Control - Volume I. Current Topics in Microbiology and Immunology, vol 385. Springer, Cham

Smith, A., McCullers, J., and Adler, F. (2011b). Mathematical model of a three-stage innate immune response to a pneumococcal lung infection. *J. Theor. Biol.* 276, 106–116. doi: 10.1016/j.jtbi.2011.01.052

Smith, A., and Perelson, A. (2011). Influenza A virus infection kinetics: quantitative data and models. *WIREs Sys. Biol. Med.* 3, 429–445. doi: 10.1002/wsbm.129

Smith, A., and Ribeiro, R. (2010). Modeling the viral dynamics of influenza A virus infection. *Crit. Rev. Immunol.* 30, 291–298. doi: 10.1615/CritRevImmunol.v30.i3.60

Smith, A., and Smith, A. (2016). A critical, nonlinear threshold dictates bacterial invasion and initial kinetics during influenza. *Sci. Rep.* 6:38703. doi: 10.1038/srep38703

Taubenberger, J., and Morens, D. (2008). The pathology of influenza virus infections. *Annu. Rev. Pathmechdis. Mech. Dis.* 3, 499–522. doi: 10.1146/annurev.pathmechdis.3.121806.154316

Thompson, W., Shay, D., Weintraub, E., Brammer, L., Bridges, Cox, C. B., et al. (2004). Influenza-associated hospitalizations in the United States. *J. Am. Med. Assoc.* 292, 1333–1340. doi: 10.1001/jama.292.11.1333

Toapanta, F., and Ross, T. (2009). Impaired immune responses in the lungs of aged mice following influenza infection. *Respir. Res.* 10:112. doi: 10.1186/1465-9921-10-112

Warnking, K., Klemm, C., Löffler, B., Niemann, S., Krüchten, A., Peters, G., et al. (2015). Super-infection with Staphylococcus aureus inhibits influenza virus-induced type I IFN signalling through impaired STAT1-STAT2 dimerization. *Cell. Microbiol.* 17, 303–317. doi: 10.1111/cmi.12375

11

A Quasi-Steady-State Approximation to the Basic Target-Cell-Limited Viral Dynamics Model with a Non-Cytopathic Effect

Richard A. Cangelosi[1], Elissa J. Schwartz[2,3] and David J. Wollkind[2]*

[1] Department of Mathematics, Gonzaga University, Spokane, WA, United States, [2] Department of Mathematics and Statistics, Washington State University, Pullman, WA, United States, [3] School of Biological Sciences, Washington State University, Pullman, WA, United States

Correspondence:
Richard A. Cangelosi
cangelosi@gonzaga.edu

Analysis of previously published target-cell limited viral dynamic models for pathogens such as HIV, hepatitis, and influenza generally rely on standard techniques from dynamical systems theory or numerical simulation. We use a quasi-steady-state approximation to derive an analytic solution for the model with a non-cytopathic effect, that is, when the death rates of uninfected and infected cells are equal. The analytic solution provides time evolution values of all three compartments of uninfected cells, infected cells, and virus. Results are compared with numerical simulation using clinical data for equine infectious anemia virus, a retrovirus closely related to HIV, and the utility of the analytic solution is discussed.

Keywords: quasi-steady-state approximation, viral dynamics, equine infectious anemia virus, HIV, dynamical systems, matched asymptotic expansion

1. INTRODUCTION

Mathematical models have proven valuable in understanding the dynamics of viral infections *in vivo* within host cells and were originally devised to examine HIV infection (reviewed by Perelson and Ribeiro, 2013). For interactions of that sort, a basic three-component dynamical systems model consisting of an uninfected target-cell population, an infected cell population, and the free virus population was proposed (see **Figure 1**). This model implied that the propagation of the virus was limited by the availability of susceptible target-cells and hence is now characterized as target-cell-limited (Phillips, 1996). Assuming a rapid enough time-scale for the free virus dynamics so that a quasi-steady-state approximation could be employed, Tuckwell and Wan (2004) formally reduced this basic target-cell-limited viral model system to a two-component one consisting of the uninfected and infected target-cells. They then showed that there were no periodic solutions for the two-component model and that the trajectories of both systems remained quite close. DeLeenheer and Smith (2003) and Prüss et al. (2008) studied the global stability of the biologically relevant equilibrium points for this basic target-cell-limited viral model system and found that its behavior depended upon the size of a particular non-dimensional parameter R_0, the basic reproductive number, to be defined in the next section. If $R_0 < 1$, they demonstrated that the virus-free equilibrium point was globally asymptotically stable, while if $R_0 > 1$, this property shifted to the disease-persistence equilibrium point.

The results cited above use either standard techniques of dynamical systems theory or numerical simulations. Defining α as the ratio of the death rates of the infected to the uninfected cells,

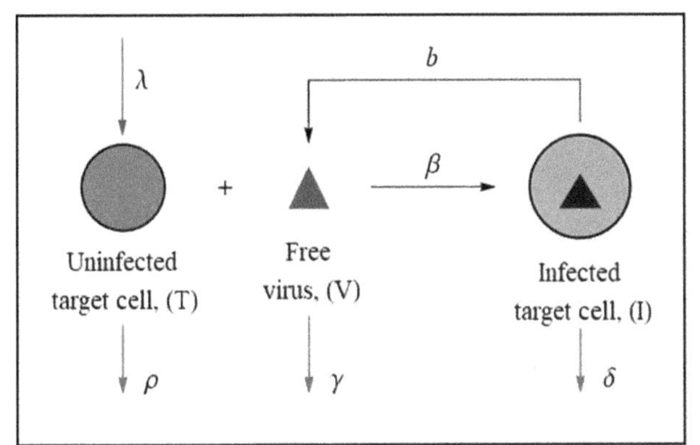

FIGURE 1 | Schematic diagram of the basic target-cell-limited viral dynamics model illustrating cell-virus interactions. Uninfected target-cells (T) can be infected by the virus (V) to create productively infected cells (I) (see e.g., Perelson and Ribeiro, 2013). In the case of a non-cytopathic virus $\rho \approx \delta$. The associated mathematical model (Equation 1) is described and analyzed in section 2.

Burg et al. (2009) classified such viral interactions to be either cytopathic or non-cytopathic depending upon whether $\alpha > 1$ or $\alpha = 1$, respectively. During cytopathic viral interactions the infected cells are killed by the virus during the course of infection. Some viruses are intrinsically non-cytopathic because they replicate in a relatively benign manner while others actively maintain such a state by shutting down all destructive processes, activating non-destructive mechanisms, or inducing alternate non-damaging replication programs (Plesa et al., 2006).

In what follows, we shall consider non-cytopathic retroviral interactions; that is, interactions that satisfy $\alpha = 1$, which is believed to be the case for the equine infectious anemia virus (EIAV) (Schwartz et al., 2018). EIAV shows many characteristics similar to other retroviruses, including a very rapid replication rate and high levels of antigenic variation. It, however, is unusual among retroviruses in that most infected animals, after a few episodes of fever and high viral load, progress to a stage with low viral load and an absence of clinical disease symptoms. The horses effectively control viral replication through adaptive immune mechanisms. Given that this differs from the retroviruses human immunodeficiency virus (HIV) and simian immunodeficiency virus (SIV), in which the infected develop immunodeficiency and disease, EIAV is especially interesting to study in clinical research as well as by using mathematical models. When adopting the mathematical model depicted in **Figure 1**, the viral clearance rate γ captures these adaptive immune system response mechanisms. In section 2, we shall employ a systematic two-time method (Matkowsky, 1970) to deduce a quasi-steady-state asymptotic closed-form analytic solution of that basic target-cell-limited viral dynamics model.

Although such non-linear problems can be solved numerically the computation must be performed sequentially for each different set of parameter values. The advantage of this asymptotic approach is that it yields an analytic representation, involving the parameters as well as time, required for least-squares parameter-identification curve-fitting procedures to experimental data. We conclude by applying this approach to an experimental data set on EIAV infection.

2. THE BASIC TARGET-CELL-LIMITED MODEL

The basic model for viral dynamics (see Anderson and May, 1992; Tuckwell and Wan, 2004; Burg et al., 2009; Stancevic et al., 2013) that describes the interactions of a virus with target-cells is given by

$$\frac{dT}{dt} = \lambda - \rho T - \beta TV \tag{1a}$$

$$\frac{dI}{dt} = \beta TV - \delta I \tag{1b}$$

$$\frac{dV}{dt} = bI - \gamma V \tag{1c}$$

where T represents the uninfected target-cell population, I is the population of infected cells, and V is quantity of free virus while t, as usual, represents time. It is assumed that the target-cells are produced at a constant rate λ and die at a rate ρT. Free virus infects target-cells at a rate βTV and infected cells die at a rate δI. New virus particles are produced at a rate bI and are cleared at a rate γV. For the model under consideration, we assume that the viral interaction is non-cytopathic and therefore take $\rho = \delta$ in the analysis which follows.

We begin by introducing the dimensionless quantities

$$x(\tau;\varepsilon) = \frac{\rho}{\lambda}T(t), \quad y(\tau;\varepsilon) = \frac{\rho}{\lambda}I(t), \quad v(\tau;\varepsilon) = \frac{\beta}{\rho}V(t), \quad \tau = \rho t,$$

$$\varepsilon = \rho/\gamma \quad \text{and} \quad R_0 = \frac{\lambda\beta b}{\rho\delta\gamma},$$

which upon substitution in Equations (1) yields the dimensionless system

$$\frac{dx}{d\tau} = 1 - x - xv \tag{2a}$$

$$\frac{dy}{d\tau} = xv - y \tag{2b}$$

$$\varepsilon\frac{dv}{d\tau} = R_0 y - v. \tag{2c}$$

2.1. The Method of Matched Asymptotic Expansions

The parameter, ε in Equations (2) is negligible when compared to terms of $O(1)$ if the intrinsic death rate of the target-cell population is small when compared to the clearance rate of the virus. We proceed under this assumption and seek a solution of the form

$$[x, y, v](\tau;\varepsilon) = [x_0, y_0, v_0](\tau) + O(\varepsilon). \tag{3}$$

Upon substituting Equation (3) into the dimensionless system (Equations 2) and retaining terms of order $O(1)$, we obtain the differential-algebraic system

$$\frac{dx_0}{d\tau} = 1 - x_0 - x_0 v_0 \tag{4a}$$

$$\frac{dy_0}{d\tau} = x_0 v_0 - y_0 \tag{4b}$$

$$v_0 = R_0 y_0. \tag{4c}$$

We now construct the inner (or boundary layer) solution, the outer (or quasi-steady-state) solution, and the uniformly valid additive composite.

2.1.1. The Inner or Boundary Layer Solution

The presence of ε in Equations (2) suggests that the system contains interactions that occur on two widely different time scales—one fast and one slow. In light of this, we introduce the "transient time" variables

$$\eta = \tau/\varepsilon = \gamma t, \quad \mathcal{X}(\eta;\varepsilon) = x(\tau;\varepsilon), \quad \mathcal{Y}(\eta;\varepsilon) = y(\tau;\varepsilon), \quad \mathcal{V}(\eta;\varepsilon) = v(\tau;\varepsilon). \tag{5}$$

Upon substituting these into Equations (2) and noting that $d/d\eta = \varepsilon\, d/d\tau$ we obtain the boundary layer equations

$$\frac{d\mathcal{X}}{d\eta} = \varepsilon(1 - \mathcal{X} - \mathcal{X}\mathcal{V}), \tag{6a}$$

$$\frac{d\mathcal{Y}}{d\eta} = \varepsilon(\mathcal{X}\mathcal{V} - \mathcal{Y}), \tag{6b}$$

$$\frac{d\mathcal{V}}{d\eta} = R_0\mathcal{Y} - \mathcal{V}. \tag{6c}$$

The ratio of the time scales $\varepsilon = \rho/\gamma << 1$, is both a consequence of the fact that the virus acts on a fast time scale $\eta = \gamma t$ and the target-cells, on a slower time scale $\tau = \rho t$, and a necessary condition for the employment of a quasi-steady-state approach.

Seeking a solution of Equations (6) of the form

$$[\mathcal{X}, \mathcal{Y}, \mathcal{V}](\eta;\varepsilon) = [\mathcal{X}_0, \mathcal{Y}_0, \mathcal{V}_0](\eta) + O(\varepsilon)$$

we find that

$$\frac{d\mathcal{X}_0}{d\eta} = \frac{d\mathcal{Y}_0}{d\eta} = 0, \quad \frac{d\mathcal{V}_0}{d\eta} = R_0\mathcal{Y}_0 - \mathcal{V}_0,$$

which upon integration yields

$$\mathcal{X}_0(\eta) \equiv x^{(0)}, \quad \mathcal{Y}_0(\eta) \equiv y^{(0)}, \quad \mathcal{V}_0(\eta) = R_0 y^{(0)} + [v^{(0)} - R_0 y^{(0)}]e^{-\eta}, \tag{7}$$

where $x^{(0)}, y^{(0)}$ and $v^{(0)}$ are the $O(1)$ values as $\varepsilon \to 0$ of the prescribed initial conditions

$$\mathcal{X}(0;\varepsilon) = x^{(0)}, \quad \mathcal{Y}(0;\varepsilon) = y^{(0)}, \quad \mathcal{V}(0;\varepsilon) = v^{(0)}.$$

2.1.2. The Outer Solution or the Quasi-Steady-State Approximation

We determine the proper initial conditions to impose for the one-term outer solution functions satisfying Equations (4) by employing the one-term matching rule

$$x_0(0) = \lim_{\eta\to\infty}\mathcal{X}_0(\eta), \; y_0(0) = \lim_{\eta\to\infty}\mathcal{Y}_0(\eta), \; v_0(0) = \lim_{\eta\to\infty}\mathcal{V}_0(\eta),$$

which in conjunction with the results of Equation (7) yields

$$x_0(0) = x^{(0)}, \quad y_0(0) = y^{(0)}, \quad v_0(0) = R_0 y^{(0)},$$

where the target-cell initial values can be normalized to satisfy

$$x^{(0)} + y^{(0)} = 1.$$

Since the target-cell populations for both their infected and uninfected states have been non-dimensionalized by employing the same scale factor, this may be accomplished if that common scaling is identified with the initial value of the sum of these populations.

Now returning to Equations (4) and taking the sum of its differential equations, we find that

$$\frac{d(x_0 + y_0)}{d\tau} + (x_0 + y_0) = 1 \tag{8}$$

with initial condition just determined of

$$x^{(0)} + y^{(0)} = 1. \tag{9}$$

Solving this differential equation problem (Equations 8 and 9), we obtain

$$x_0(\tau) + y_0(\tau) \equiv 1 \quad \text{or} \quad y_0 = 1 - x_0, \tag{10}$$

which from Equation(4c) implies

$$v_0 = R_0 y_0 = R_0(1 - x_0). \tag{11}$$

Finally, substituting Equation (11) into Equation (4a) yields the Ricatti equation for $x_0 = x_0(\tau; R_0)$:

$$\frac{dx_0}{d\tau} = 1 - (R_0 + 1)x_0 + R_0 x_0^2, \; \tau > 0; \; 0 \le x_0(0; R_0) = x^{(0)} \le 1, \tag{12}$$

where the initial condition follows from Equation (9). We note that $x_0 = 1$ is a particular solution of Equation (12), thus we introduce the variable

$$z \equiv x_0 - 1 \tag{13}$$

which upon substituting into the above Riccati equation yields the Bernoulli equation

$$\frac{dz}{d\tau} + (1 - R_0)z = R_0 z^2 \tag{14}$$

that can be solved by introducing the variable $w = z^{-1}$ to obtain

$$z^{-1} = \frac{R_0}{1 - R_0} + ce^{(1-R_0)\tau}. \tag{15}$$

Making use of Equation (13) and the initial condition $x_0(0) = x_i \equiv x^{(0)}$, we arrive at the quasi-steady-state approximation for the uninfected target-cell population

$$x_0(\tau) = \begin{cases} f(\tau) & \text{if} \quad R_0 = 1, \\ g(\tau) & \text{if} \quad R_0 \neq 1, \end{cases} \tag{16}$$

where

$$f(\tau) = \frac{x_i + (1 - x_i)\tau}{1 + (1 - x_i)\tau}$$

and

$$g(\tau) = 1 + \frac{(1 - R_0)(x_i - 1)}{R_0(x_i - 1) + (1 - R_0 x_i)e^{(1-R_0)\tau}}.$$

Note that expressions for $y_0(\tau)$ and $v_0(\tau)$ follow directly from Equations (10) and (11), respectively. For ease of exposition in what follows we set $y_i \equiv y^{(0)}$ and $v_i \equiv v^{(0)}$. Many similar three-component model systems assume that initially the target-cells are free of the viral infection. If an assumption of that sort were made for our model by taking $y_i = 0$ or equivalently $x_i = 1$ then Equation (16) would yield the unrealistic result that $x_0(\tau) \equiv 1$. Hence, we shall approximate that situation by adopting the initial condition $y_i = a$ or equivalently $x_i = 1 - a$ instead where the perturbation infected population density a satisfies the condition $0 < a << 1$. Specifically, for the relevant plots of **Figures 2, 3**, we shall take $a = 0.0001$ which implies that $x_i = 0.9999$.

2.1.3. The Uniformly Valid Additive Composite

Constructing the one-term uniformly valid additive composites defined by

$$x_u^{(0)}(\tau) = x_0(\tau) + \mathcal{X}_0(\tau/\varepsilon) - x_i,$$
$$y_u^{(0)}(\tau) = y_0(\tau) + \mathcal{Y}_0(\tau/\varepsilon) - y_i,$$
$$v_u^{(0)}(\tau) = v_0(\tau) + \mathcal{V}_0(\tau/\varepsilon) - R_0 y_i;$$

we obtain, from the results of sections 2.1.1 and 2.1.2, that

$$x_u^{(0)}(\tau) = x_0(\tau), \quad y_u^{(0)}(\tau) = y_0(\tau),$$
$$v_u^{(0)}(\tau) = v_0(\tau) + [v_i - R_0 y_i]e^{-\tau/\varepsilon}, \quad (18)$$

where

$$y_0(\tau) = 1 - x_0(\tau) \quad \text{and} \quad v_0(\tau) = R_0 y_0(\tau) = R_0[1 - x_0(\tau)]. \quad (19)$$

Observe, for the target-cell variables, the outer solution is actually uniformly valid to this order.

3. RESULTS

In this section we examine the qualitative behavior of the quasi-steady-state approximation given by Equations (18) and (19). We then compare the quasi-steady-state approximation with a numerical simulation of Equations (2) using equine infectious anemia virus (EIAV) data (Schwartz et al., 2018).

From the form of $x_0(\tau)$, it is readily seen that when $R_0 = 1$, $x_0(\tau) = f(\tau) \to 1$ as $\tau \to \infty$. If $R_0 < 1$ then $x_0(\tau) = g(\tau) \to 1$ while if $R_0 > 1$, $x_0(\tau) = g(\tau) \to 1/R_0$ as $\tau \to \infty$, where $x_0(\tau)$ is expressed as a percent of its initial population. This is consistent with the global stability results mentioned in section 1.

Figure 2 is a plot of the three uniformly valid composite functions $x_u^{(0)}(\tau)$, $y_u^{(0)}(\tau)$, and $v_u^{(0)}(\tau)$. Parameter values used are median values reported in Schwartz et al. (2018) for the equine infectious anemia virus. Specifically, we take

$$\lambda = 2019 \text{ cells/(ml} * \text{day)},$$
$$\beta = 3.25 \times 10^{-7} \text{ ml/(viral RNA copies} * \text{day)},$$
$$b = 505 \text{ viral RNA copies/(cell} * \text{day)},$$
$$\rho = \delta = 1/21 \text{ per day}, \quad \text{and} \quad \gamma = 6.73 \text{ per day}.$$

Given that a dimensionless time unit ($\tau = 1$) corresponds to 21 days, we see that the uninfected cell population remains relatively constant for approximately 7 days ($\tau = 0.33$). This is followed by a period of eight to ten days of rapid infection of the uninfected cell population at the end of which approximately 95% of the population has been infected by the EIAV.

Figure 3A provides a comparison of the one-term asymptotic representation of the cell population (solid black curve) given by Equation (16) with a numerical simulation (dashed curve) of Equation (2) using the parameter values given above. **Figure 3B** provides a comparison of the one-term asymptotic representation of the free virus population (solid black curve) with its numerical simulation (dashed curve). The initial virus population was taken to be $450 \times \beta/\rho \approx 0.00307$ viral RNA copies/ml. We note the excellent agreement between the analytic asymptotic representation and numerical simulations.

4. DISCUSSION

Researchers that employ the basic viral dynamics model now have an analytic representation involving the parameters that provides a vehicle for least-squares parameter-identification curve-fitting procedures to experimental data. In particular, given a time series population data set $\{(t_n, T_n)\}_{n=1}^{N}$ and our analytic solution for uninfected target-cells in dimensional variables denoted by $T(t; \lambda, \rho, \beta, b, \gamma)$, a parameter identification residual least squares fit to that data is determined by defining (Torres-Cerna et al., 2016)

$$E(\lambda, \rho, \beta, b, \gamma) = \sum_{n=1}^{N}[T(t_n; \lambda, \rho, \beta, b, \gamma) - T_n]^2$$

and minimizing this function by solving for $\lambda_c, \rho_c, \beta_c, b_c, \gamma_c$ such that

$$\frac{\partial E}{\partial \lambda}(\lambda_c, \rho_c, \beta_c, b_c, \gamma_c) = \frac{\partial E}{\partial \rho}(\lambda_c, \rho_c, \beta_c, b_c, \gamma_c)$$
$$= \frac{\partial E}{\partial \beta}(\lambda_c, \rho_c, \beta_c, b_c, \gamma_c)$$
$$= \frac{\partial E}{\partial b}(\lambda_c, \rho_c, \beta_c, b_c, \gamma_c)$$
$$= \frac{\partial E}{\partial \gamma}(\lambda_c, \rho_c, \beta_c, b_c, \gamma_c) = 0.$$

employing the appropriate algorithm. This procedure can be accomplished much more efficiently if one has a closed form representation for $T(t; \lambda, \rho, \beta, b, \gamma)$ as in our case.

We note that for the basic target-cell-limited viral dynamics model, the deduction of an analytic solution for

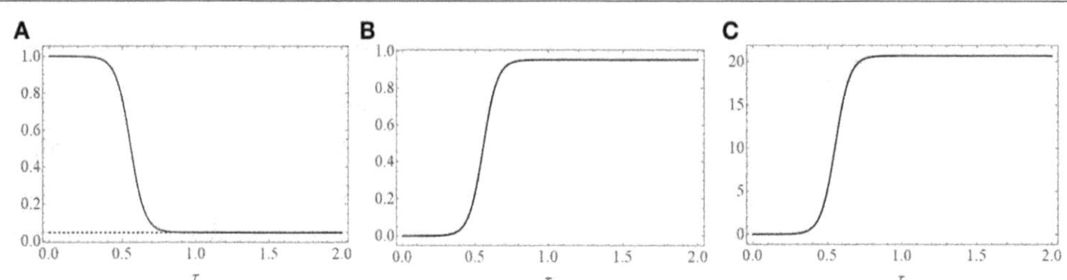

FIGURE 2 | Plots of the uniformly valid additive composite solutions. **(A)** Uninfected cell population, $x_U^{(0)}(\tau)$, **(B)** infected cell population, $y_U^{(0)}(\tau)$, and **(C)** free virus population, $v_U^{(0)}(\tau)$. Populations are expressed as a percent of their initial population values. One dimensionless time unit ($\tau = 1$) corresponds to 21 days. Parameters used to create the plots are given in the text and correspond to $R_0 = 21.7$ and $\varepsilon = 0.007$.

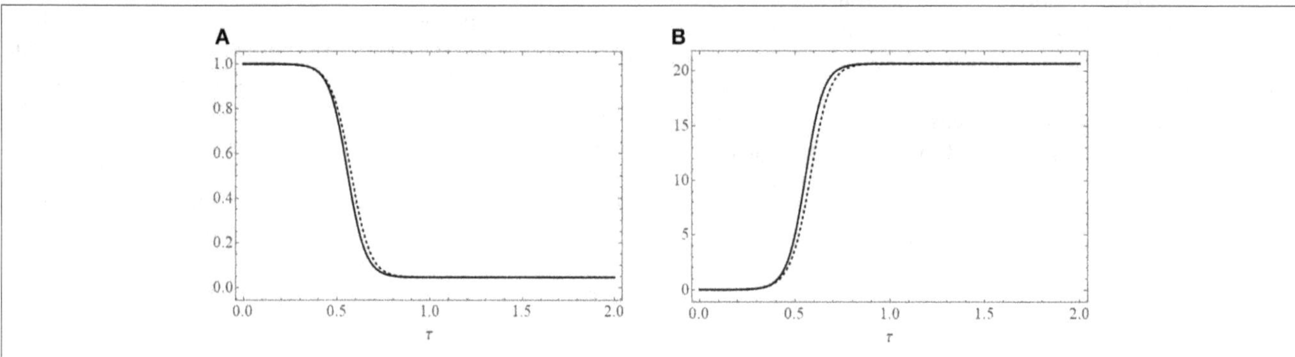

FIGURE 3 | Comparison of the asymptotic solution of the cell population (solid black line), **(A)**, and EIAV population (solid black line), **(B)**, with a numerical simulation (dashed line) of Equations (2). Parameters used to create the plots are given in the text and correspond to $R_0 = 21.7$ and $\varepsilon = 0.007$.

the quasi-steady-state approximation is crucially dependent on the non-cytopathic condition $\alpha = \delta/\rho = 1$ and we have selected parameter values relevant to this scenario for EIAV. If this were the only non-cytopathic virus, our development restricted to the spread of infection in horse populations might not be representative enough to enlist general interest from virologists. Besides EIAV, however, it has been shown that this non-cytopathic assumption is reasonable for a fairly wide class of important viral interactions in human and other animal populations as well, for example, Hepatitis B and C viruses (Wieland and Chisari, 2005). In addition, non-cytopathic enteroviruses such as the coxsackie virus B, one of the agents suspected to be responsible for chronic fatigue syndrome (Landay et al., 1991), cause persistent infections in their host's cells. Another non-cytopathic virus infecting human populations is the Newcastle disease virus (Carver et al., 1967). Finally, Table II in Marcus and Carver (1967) lists a collection of similar non-cytopathic viruses inducing intrinsic interference, among which is the hemadsorption simian virus.

We have been investigating the non-cytopathic interaction of EIAV infection. While similar to human immunodeficiency virus (HIV), EIAV differs from the latter in that it is not fatal, partially because the horses' immune systems help to effectively control the virus. Thus, studies of EIAV infection are of importance since they serve as useful prototypes of viral dynamics and immune control, which may have implications in the development of vaccines for HIV and other retroviral infections.

AUTHOR CONTRIBUTIONS

RAC led the project, performed model analysis, ran numerical simulations, and wrote the paper. EJS initiated the project, gathered data for application of the model, and assisted with the interpretation of results and writing the paper. DJW introduced the non-cytopathic assumption, performed model analysis, and assisted with writing the paper.

FUNDING

One of us (EJS) wishes to acknowledge the African Institute for Mathematical Sciences for partial support.

REFERENCES

Anderson, R. M., and May, R. M. (1992). *Infectious Diseases of Humans: Dynamics and Control.* Oxford: Oxford University Press.

Burg, D., Rong, L., Neumann, A. U., and Dahari, H. (2009). Mathematical modeling of viral kinetics under immune control during primary HIV-1 infection. *J. Theor. Biol.* 259, 751–759. doi: 10.1016/j.jtbi.2009.04.010

Carver, D. H., Marcus, P. I., and Seto, D. S. Y. (1967). Intrinsic interference: a unique interference system used in assaying non-cytopathic viruses. *Archiv für die Gesamte Virusforschung* 22, 55–60. doi: 10.1007/BF01240502

DeLeenheer, P., and Smith, H. L. (2003). Virus dynamics: a global analysis. *SIAM J. Appl. Math.* 63, 1313–1327. doi: 10.1137/S0036139902406905

Landay, A. L., Jessop, C., and Lennette, E. T. (1991). Chronic fatigue syndrome: clinical conditions associated with immune activation. *Lancet* 338, 707–712. doi: 10.1016/0140-6736(91)91440-6

Marcus, P. I., and Carver, D. H. (1967). "Hemadsorption-negative plaque test for viruses inducing intrinsic interference," in *Fundamental Techniques in Virology*, eds K. Habel, and N. P. Salzmann (New York and London: Academic Press), 161–183.

Matkowsky, B. J. (1970). Nonlinear dynamic stability: a formal theory. *SIAM J. Appl. Math.* 18, 872–883. doi: 10.1137/0118079

Perelson, A. S., and Ribeiro, R. M. (2013). Modeling the within-host dynamics of HIV infection. *BMC Biol.* 11:96. doi: 10.1186/1741-7007-11-96

Phillips, A. N. (1996). Reduction of HIV concentration during acute infection: independence from a particular immune response. *Science* 271, 497–499. doi: 10.1126/science.271.5248.497

Plesa, G., McKenna, P. M., Schnell, M. J., and Eisenlohr, L. C. (2006). Immunogenicity of cytopathic and noncytopathic viral vectors. *J. Virol.* 80, 6259–6266. doi: 10.1128/JVI.00084-06

Prüss, J., Zacher, R., and Schnaubelt, R. (2008). Global asymptotic stability of equilibria in models for virus dynamics. *Math. Model. Nat. Phenom.* 3, 126–142. doi: 10.1051/mmnp:2008045

Schwartz, E. J., Vaidya, N. K., Dorman, K., Carpender, S., and Mealey, R. H. (2018). Dynamics of lentiviral infection *in vivo* in the absence of adaptive host immune responses. *Virology* 513, 108–113. doi: 10.1016/j.virol.2017.09.023

Stancevic, O., Angstmann, C. N., Murray, J. M., and Henry, B. I. (2013). Turing patterns from dynamics of early HIV infection. *Bull. Math. Biol.* 75, 774–795. doi: 10.1007/s11538-013-9834-5

Torres-Cerna, C. E., Alanis, A. Y., Poblete-Castro, T., Bermejo-Jambrina, M., and Hernandez-Vargas, E. A. (2016). A comparative study of differential evolution algorithms for parameter fitting procedures. *IEEE CEC* 1:4662. doi: 10.1109/CEC.2016.7744385

Tuckwell, H. C., and Wan, F. Y. M. (2004). On the behaviour of solutions in viral dynamical models. *BioSystems* 73, 157–161. doi: 10.1016/j.biosystems.2003.11.004

Wieland, S. F., and Chisari, F. (2005). Stealth and cunning: hepatitis B and hepatitis C viruses. *J. Virol.* 79, 9369–9380. doi: 10.1128/JVI.79.15.9369-9380.2005

12

miPepBase: A Database of Experimentally Verified Peptides Involved in Molecular Mimicry

*Anjali Garg, Bandana Kumari, Ravindra Kumar and Manish Kumar**

Department of Biophysics, University of Delhi, New Delhi, India

***Correspondence:**
Manish Kumar
manish@south.du.ac.in

Autoimmune diseases emerge due to several reasons, of which molecular mimicry i.e., similarity between the host's and pathogen's interacting peptides is an important reason. In the present study we have reported a database of only experimentally verified peptide sequences, which exhibit molecular mimicry. The database is named as **miPepBase (Mi**micry **Pep**tide Data**base)** and contains comprehensive information about mimicry proteins and peptides of both host (and model organism) and pathogen. It also provides information about physicochemical properties of protein and mimicry peptides, which might be helpful in predicting the nature of protein and optimization of protein expression. The **miPepBase** can be searched using a keyword or, by autoimmune disease(s) or by a combination of host and pathogen taxonomic group or their name. To facilitate the search of proteins and/or epitope in miPepBase, which is similar to the user's interest, BLAST search tool is also incorporated. **miPepBase** is an open access database and available at http://proteininformatics.org/mkumar/mipepbase.

Keywords: autoimmune disease, molecular mimicry, database, peptide, cross-reactivity

INTRODUCTION

Mimicry is a very common phenomenon in which a living being pretends to be what it is not. By adopting mimicry, an animal get protection by not hiding, rather being mistaken for something a predator will avoid because either it look dangerous or tastes bad. Hence, it is not surprising that similar strategy has been exploited at the molecular level as well. The obvious benefit molecular mimicry confers to pathogens is to fool the host's defenses and survive. The presence of a molecule in a pathogen that is similar with a host antigen could inhibit the immune response of the host against the pathogen because of the immune tolerance toward self-antigens (Davies, 1997; Gowthaman and Eswarakumar, 2013). For example, *Helicobacter pylori* infection in human triggers two autoimmune diseases namely autoimmune gastritis and pernicious anemia. It occurs because activated $CD4^+$ Th1 cells infiltrates into gastric mucosa and they cross-recognize the self-epitopes of H^+K^+ ATPase and *H. pylori* antigens (D'Elios et al., 2004).

There are number of well documented molecular mimicry events, using which bacteria, viruses, or parasites evade the host's immune response (Oldstone, 2005). The pathogen's protein having similar epitope to that of the host results in cross-reactivity that generates immunological response against self (i.e., host), which ultimately leads to autoimmune diseases (Oldstone, 1998; Cusick et al., 2012). The peptides, which display this property, are called mimicry peptides and the phenomenon is called molecular mimicry (Davies, 1997). The role of molecular mimicry in autoimmune disease was getting strengthen when it was observed that the antibody against the phosphoprotein of measles virus and Herpes simplex type I can cross-react with human intermediate filament protein vimentin (Fujinami et al., 1983). Molecular mimicry can cause several immune-mediated disease such as Grave's disease (Kohn et al., 2000; Chen et al., 2001), Insulin-dependent diabetes (Rose and Mackay, 2000; Hiemstra et al., 2001), Multiple sclerosis (Banki et al., 1994; Wucherpfennig and Strominger, 1995; Appelmelk et al., 1996; Talbot et al., 1996; Rose and Mackay, 2000), Peptic ulcer (Appelmelk et al., 1996), Rheumatoid arthritis (Tiwana et al., 1999; Balandraud et al., 2004; Bridges, 2004), Systemic lupus erythematosus (Rönnblom and Alm, 2001; Kaufman et al., 2003; McClain et al., 2005), Myocarditis (Neu et al., 1987; Huber et al., 1994; Gauntt et al., 1995; Schulze and Schultheiss, 1995; Ang et al., 2004), and cancer as well, by modulating key signaling pathways, such as those involving Ras (Guven-Maiorov et al., 2016). A number of studies have deciphered various prospects and aspects of molecular mimicry, but these are scattered in numerous research papers. Compilation of the available information from literature can greatly facilitate the researchers who work in this domain. At present there is no data repository, which contains all the information related to autoimmune diseases caused due to molecular mimicry because piecing, together of this scattered data and discerning the accompanying details is complicated and tedious. To the best of our knowledge, only one database namely mimicDB (Ludin et al., 2011) is available which provides information about proteins or epitopes involved in host-pathogen interactions. But mimicDB is restricted to information pertaining to only a few human parasites. Also, the mimicry candidates of mimicDB were predicted through a computational pipeline.

In the present study we have reported a freely accessible database, which can serve as a comprehensive and high quality resource of peptides involved in molecular mimicry. We have also incorporated the information related to autoimmune diseases as well as in-depth information about mimicry peptide and proteins. The database is named, **miPepBase** (**Mi**micry **Pep**tide Data**base**), which is available at http://proteininformatics.org/mkumar/mipepbase. All molecular mimicry based autoimmunity events compiled in miPepBase were experimentally verified by the respective researchers and are supported by peer-reviewed publications. **MiPepBase** is an open access database that provides comprehensive information about the mimicry proteins and peptides of both host (and model) and pathogen. The information includes the names of host and pathogen proteins, sequences of mimicry peptide, autoimmune disease caused due to mimicry peptide, gene ontology information of the protein, PDB ID of the structure of protein (if present), type of immunological response generated by mimicry peptide and much more. We anticipate that miPepBase will help researchers to generate new hypothesis about different aspects of molecular mimicry and also act as a unified resource of information about molecular mimicry. The miPepBase can be searched using keyword(s) or by autoimmune disease(s) or by a combination of host and pathogen taxonomic groups or their names. The database also includes BLAST search tool to facilitate sequence similarity search against the mimicry proteins and/or peptide contained in it. Each miPepBase entry is also linked to many popular global repositories such as UniProt (Apweiler et al., 2004), PDB (Berman et al., 2000), EMBL-EBI QuickGO (Binns et al., 2009), and PubMed. MiPepBase also provides information about physicochemical properties of proteins containing mimicry peptides, which might be helpful in predicting the nature of protein and optimization of its expression. The basic architecture of miPepBase is shown in **Figure 1**. The data of miPepBase can also be downloaded in text file. Overall, mimicry peptides which are compiled in miPepBase might help in opening new gateways to explore the role of molecular mimicry in autoimmune diseases that are yet unaddressed. It is anticipated that miPepBase would be helpful in understanding the details of molecular mimicry and expedite the process of disease detection, diagnosis, prognosis, and even deciding the therapeutic regimen of autoimmune diseases.

MATERIALS AND METHODS

Data Collection and Compilation

The main aim of miPepBase was to collect, compile and curate all the information related to autoimmune disease caused by molecular mimicry. Therefore, experimentally verified data was collected after an extensive search of published research papers with the help of PubMed and Google Scholar using keywords "molecular mimicry," "host-pathogen cross-reactivity," and "autoimmune diseases." We also mined other additional relevant information such as gene and protein names, mimicry peptide sequence, name of autoimmune diseases, and immunological response by T-cells or antibodies. The information regarding proteins, taxonomic classification of pathogen, gene ontology information, PDB ID, annotation status of protein (review status) and protein sequences was obtained from the UniProt protein repository. The miPepBase also provides PubMed link with each entry from which the molecular mimicry and autoimmune disease information was extracted.

Web Interface and Database Architecture

The inner framework of miPepBase is built using MySQL (http://www.mysql.org), Perl (http://www.perl.org), and Apache (http://www.apache.org) on Cent OS Linux platform. The interface component consists of webpages designed in HTML/CSS in a Linux environment. To provide convenience in usage, the database was developed in a user-friendly manner. The "Browse" and "Search" options were provided to search and access the information content of miPepBase. The home page of miPepBase has a very short introduction about molecular mimicry based autoimmune diseases. It also provides a brief description of the database content and clickable icons with direct links to the database and its different utilities.

Database Accessibility

The miPepBase provides interactive access to the data and the users can connect and access the database using any one among different search options. The search options have been designed in a simple and intuitive manner so that the users can search the database either by keyword or predefined combinations of fields (advanced search).

Keyword search assists users to search the database by following fields: database ID or organism's name or protein's

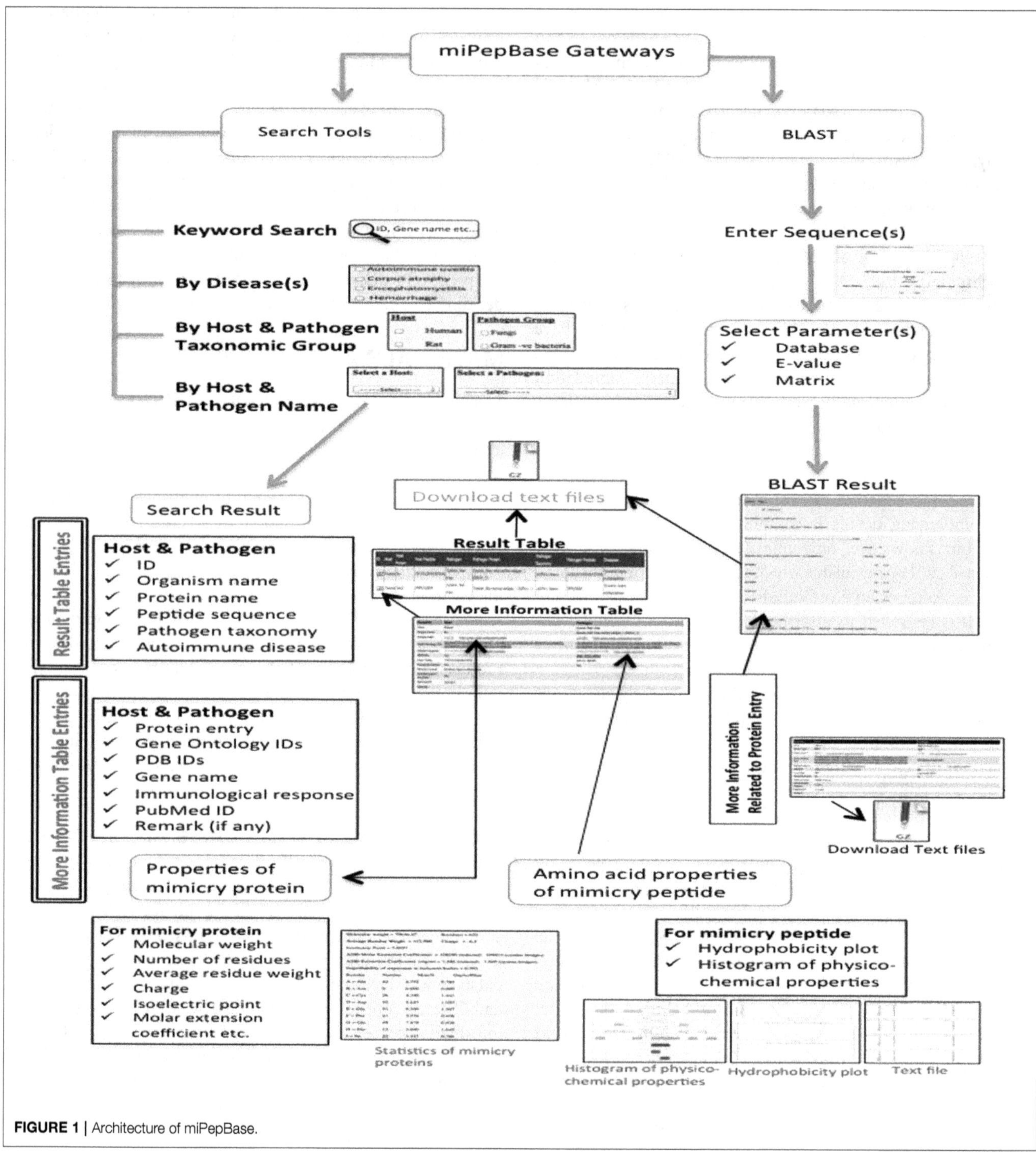

FIGURE 1 | Architecture of miPepBase.

name or entry or autoimmune disease or UniProt ID or taxonomic classification or gene ontology ID or PDB ID or peptide sequence or PubMed ID. It also permits free-floating Google like search over entire database.

Advanced search provides three different types of search options for users to access the data: First, search by one or multiple autoimmune disease(s) caused due to molecular mimicry. Second, search on the basis of host and pathogen taxonomic group, which allows users to explore one or multiple host(s) and pathogen taxonomic group(s) involved in molecular mimicry. The third and last option of advanced search is a drop down menu of host and pathogen name, which allows searching restricted to a specific set of host and pathogen. Irrespective of the mode of search chosen to query the miPepBase, the search result will be displayed in the tabular format. In the search result, the ID (shown in red color) is a clickable link and can display detailed information of corresponding entry. All the information can be downloaded in the text format, using the "download button" in result table. Additionally, different information related to protein sequence, structure, gene ontology and source of article, were linked to UniProt, RCSB PDB, EMBL-EBI QuickGO, and PubMed, respectively. A detailed step-by-step manual is also provided to assist users in smooth and efficient searching of miPepBase.

Tools Integrated in miPepBase

Different tools are also incorporated in the miPepBase to help users to search related proteins and/or peptides and analyze their different physicochemical properties. BLAST searches similar sequence(s) with in the database (Altschul et al., 1997, 2005) while pepstats and pepinfo utilities of EMBOSS package provides information about physicochemical properties of protein and peptides (Rice et al., 2000). The information derived from these tools might be helpful in predicting the nature of protein and optimization of protein expression.

Pepstats was used to calculate physicochemical properties of amino acids (such as molecular weight, number of residues) present in mimicry protein.

Pepinfo was used to calculate properties of mimicry peptide which include two types of plots: (i) Hydrophobicity plot (on the basis of Kyte and Doolittle parameters) and (ii) Histogram of presence of amino acid with the physico-chemical properties such as tiny, small, aliphatic, aromatic, non-polar, polar, charged, positive, and negative.

Basic Local Alignment Search Tool (BLAST): It is incorporated to find homologous sequence(s) and similar peptide(s) present within miPepBase database. User has to simply paste the sequence in the text box or upload sequence in the FASTA file to find similar sequence(s). Option to specify search parameters like database, *E*-value cutoff and alignment scoring matrix value is also present. The default cut-off *E*-value is 100 and alignment-scoring matrix is BLOSUM62. In the miPepBase BLAST tool, four different types of databases namely Host protein, Host peptide, Pathogen protein, and Pathogen peptide are present. Hence, similarity search can be carried out against any of the four databases.

RESULTS

Data Statistics and Content

In the miPepBase, only experimentally verified mimicry peptides from published papers are incorporated. The first release of miPepBase has 261 entries in total. It does not mean that miPepBase contains 261 host-pathogen peptide pairs. This is due to existence of multiple mimicry peptides in a single protein. Analysis of the miPepBase data shows that in both host and pathogen proteins more than one stretch of amino acids might be involved in molecular mimicry. The following information is associated with each entry:

ID: It is a unique identifier assigned to each entry of the miPepBase database. Each ID is linked to the detailed information of that entry, which includes details of host and pathogen proteins, their gene ontology information, PDB ID of structure (if known), gene name, annotation status of protein (reviewed/not reviewed), PubMed ID, and remark (if any).

Organism's name: With each event of molecular mimicry two different organisms are associated. Organism in which autoimmune response is generated was designated as host. Organism, which encodes the mimicry peptide, was designated as pathogen.

Protein names: Two different proteins are associated with each event of molecular mimicry. One that is encoded by the host and second which is encoded by the pathogen. Names of both the proteins are present with each entry.

Peptide sequence: This contains the stretch of amino acids (the peptide) present in both host's and pathogen's protein that actually leads to molecular mimicry.

Pathogen taxonomic group: Organisms from all taxonomic groups such as bacteria, viruses, fungi, and protozoa exhibit molecular mimicry. MiPepBase contains information of molecular mimicry based autoimmunity events caused by organisms from all taxonomic groups.

Broadly, pathogens are divided into four taxonomic groups namely bacteria, fungi, protozoa, and viruses. Bacteria is further subcategorized into gram-positive, gram-negative, and others i.e., diderms. Further, viruses are categorized according to the classification system purposed by David Baltimore (reviewed in Baltimore, 1971), namely retro transcribing virus, dsDNA virus, dsRNA virus, and ssRNA virus. The total numbers of entries belonging to pathogens of different categories is shown in **Figure 2A**.

Autoimmune disease: This field provides the information about disease caused due to molecular mimicry. Our analysis revealed that very diverse types of autoimmune diseases might occur due to molecular mimicry. Data content of miPepBase shows total 23 types of autoimmune diseases are associated with molecular mimicry. Multiple sclerosis was the most frequent disease followed by encephalomyelitis. The different types of autoimmune diseases and the number of times they were associated with molecular mimicry is shown in **Figure 2B**.

How to Search Query into miPepBase?

Using a Keyword

Any data in miPepBase can be search and access by five different ways. It is illustrated here using one protein (UniProt accession number **P10809**). Users can get the information associated to this protein by querying miPepBase submission of UniProt accession number as a keyword to the "Keyword search option" (**Figure 3A**) and click the search button (Step a1). The search result page showed a single hit and the information related to P10809 protein was presented in tabulated form. The search result contains following information: unique miPepBase ID (1217), host name (human), host protein name (HSP60), host mimicry peptide sequence (HRKPLVIIAEDVDGE), pathogen name (*Mycobacterium bovis*), pathogen protein name (HSP65), pathogen taxonomy (Gram positive bacteria), pathogen mimic

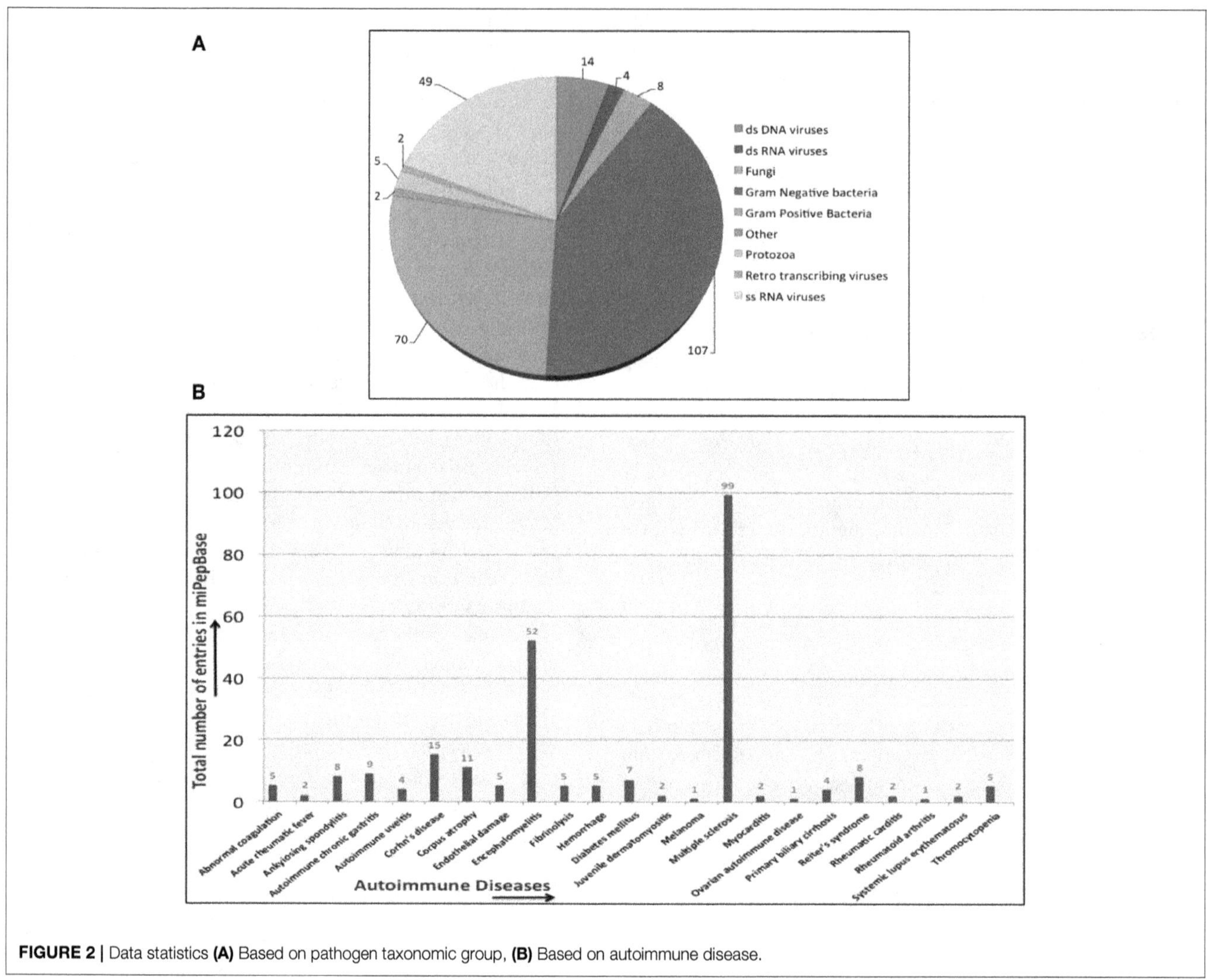

FIGURE 2 | Data statistics **(A)** Based on pathogen taxonomic group, **(B)** Based on autoimmune disease.

sequence (AGKPLLIIAEDVEGE), and autoimmune disease (Rheumatoid arthritis) caused due to host and pathogen cross reactivity. All these details can also be downloaded as text file (Step a2). More detailed information related to P10809 can be retrieved through miPepBase ID of P10809 (i.e., 1,217, displayed in red font in the search table) (Step a3). Further, it will give more information about the host's and pathogen's: protein entry (host-P10809 and pathogen-P0A521), gene ontology (available for both), PDB ID (host- 4PJ1 and pathogen-NA), gene name (host-HSPDI, HSP60 and pathogen-groL2, groEL2, groEL2, hsp65, Mb0448), protein reviewed (host-yes and pathogen-yes), immunological response (Helper T cell), PubMed ID (1577070), and remark (NA). In addition to these details the miPepBase also provide direct link to UniProt, EMBL-EBI, RCSB PDB, and PubMed. All information described above can also be downloaded as "Text File" (Step a6).

Apart from above described information users can also get the amino acids composition profiles for P10809 (host's protein) and P0A521 (pathogen's protein) entries and their hydrophobicity graph and other physico-chemical information for mimicry peptides through "View amino acids composition profile" (Step a4) and "View peptide properties" (Step a5), respectively. All graphs and text file related to physico-chemical properties of protein and peptide can be downloaded in text format.

By Disease

To retrieve the information related to mimicry proteins involved in a particular set of autoimmune diseases, users could use an advanced search option i.e., "Search by Diseases." This option lists a set of disease caused due to molecular mimicry and whose information is present in miPepBase. Here, it is demonstrated using **Rheumatoid arthritis** as an example (**Figure 3B**). On selection of rheumatoid arthritis as the disease whose information is desired (Step b1 and b2), search result page (Step b3) would be displayed. The search page would list the information related to proteins involved in the rheumatoid arthritis in a tabulated form. The information content and ways to navigate different sections remain same (Step a3–a6) as explained above for P10809 protein using Keyword search option.

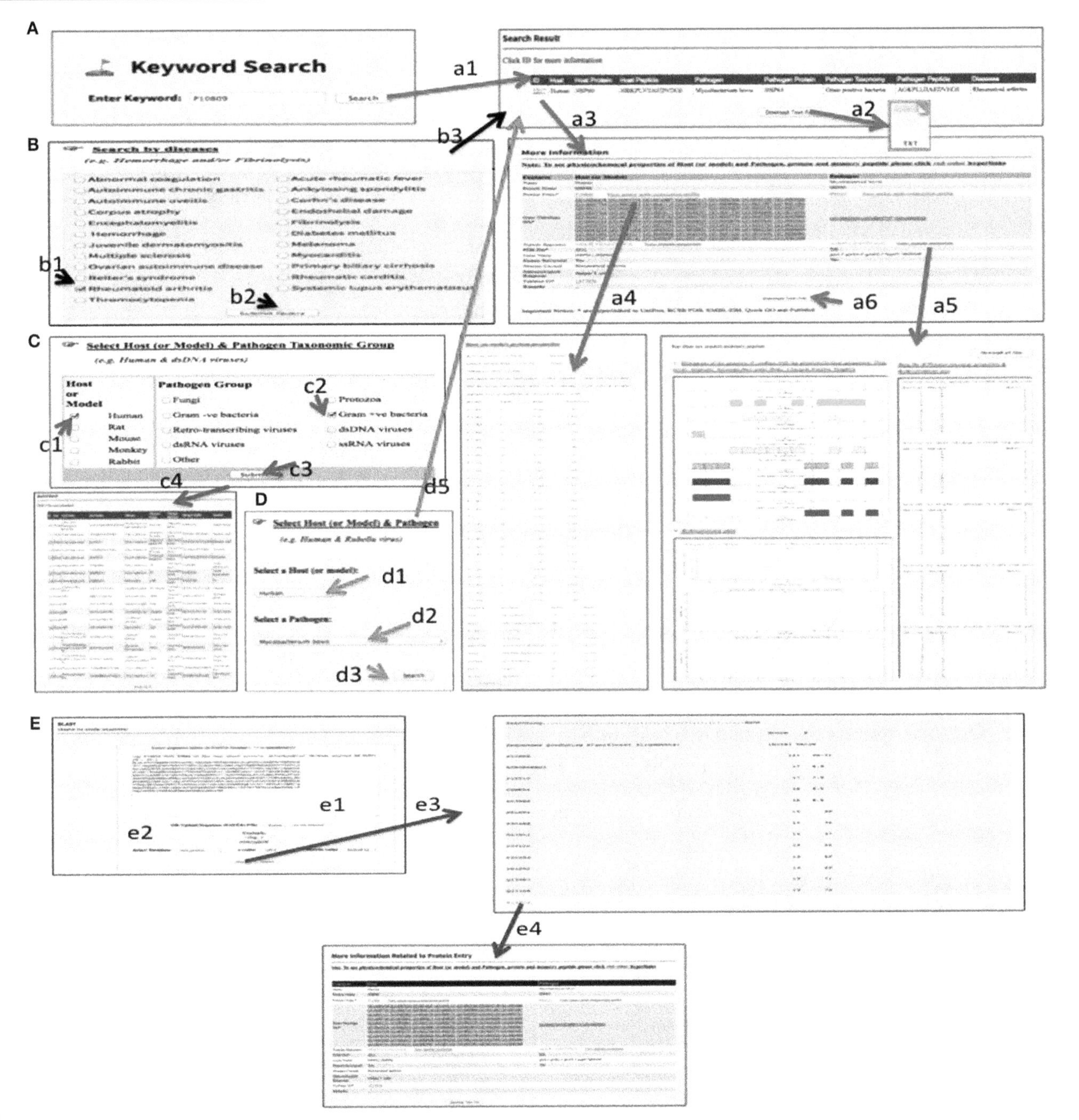

FIGURE 3 | Process of stepwise data retrieval and analysis in miPepBase. The user can search query with following options: **(A)** Keyword search, **(B)** Search by disease, **(C)** Search by host and pathogen taxonomic group, **(D)** Search by host and pathogen name. The search from **(A–D)** options display search result table and from that user can select the entry/displayed result for further detailed analysis. Sequence based search can also be searched by **(E)** BLAST search option and each hit is further linked to its details information page. The detail of result obtained from search options **(A–E)** is displayed by corresponding small case (the number indicates step number). From example a1–a6 denotes the results that can be obtained using keyword search option **(A)**.

By Host and Pathogen Taxonomic Group

This option provides a list of pathogens and host taxonomic group within which the search will be restricted. This search option gives an easy way to do comparative analysis among mimics encoded by different pathogens of same or different taxonomic group(s) (**Figure 3C**). Searching (Step c3) with "**Human" as host** (Step c1) **and "Gram-positive bacteria" as pathogen taxonomic group** (Step c2), total 19 entries related to gram-positive bacteria group (Step C4). Here also the presentation of search result data and further information (from

Step a3 to a6) were remaining same as discussed for above two searching methods.

By Host and Pathogen Name

The information related to event of cross reactivity between a specific host and pathogen that leads to autoimmune disease(s) can be achieved using another advanced options i.e., "Select host and pathogen." The names of host and pathogen can be selected from the dropdown menu present in this section. Here, it is exemplified (**Figure 3D**) using **Human as host** (Step d1) **and *Mycobacterium bovis* as pathogen** (Step d2). After submission of query (Step d3) a result page would be display that contains the search result information in tabulated form. The information content of search page will remain same as explained earlier for keyword search (Step a3–a6).

By Blast Search

This is not a direct way to search the data content of miPepBase. Rather it searches similar sequences and peptides in the miPepBase. The BLAST search option is available at menu bar (**Figure 3E**). The query sequence in FASTA format can either be pasted in the text box or uploaded as sequence file (Step e1). Three parameters have to be optimized for efficient BLAST search (i) the database in which related sequence will be searched; (ii) *E*-value, and (iii) Scoring Matrix. The default *e*-value and scoring matrix are 100 and BLOSUM 62, respectively (Step e2). As shown in section E, when **P10809** protein sequence was searched against host protein database, total 13 hits were obtained which are arranged on the basis of ascending *e*-value (Step e3). Also every BLAST hit protein entry is further linked (in blue color) to detailed information page, which provide tabulated detailed information of corresponding BLAST hit (Step e4). These information are the same as described above for keyword search option (Step a4–a6).

DISCUSSION

During the last few years, much active research and experimental verification has shed light on various aspects of molecular mimicry and it's role in autoimmune diseases. With the passage of time, number of autoimmune diseases caused due to molecular mimicry is increasing. Since, a unified repository of the available information related to molecular mimicry based autoimmune diseases is not available, hence we have built a database (miPepBase) which not only contains the information regarding proteins and peptides associated with the process, but several other important details also. In-depth analysis of this information might lead to the elucidation of mechanisms of autoimmune diseases controlled by mimicry peptides. Each entry in the miPepBase database is linked to many other molecular biology data repositories. Further, the database also includes inbuilt tools, which can help to fetch other relevant information related to the mimicry proteins and peptides. As more data will accumulate by the use of high throughput molecular, genomic and metagenomic methods, we anticipate that the release of miPepBase will facilitate comprehensive analyses of different factors involved in autoimmune diseases caused by the mimicry peptides. We also hope that miPepBase would be helpful for the scientific community in understanding the host-pathogen interactions, as well as how the pathogens evade host immune systems.

COMPARISON WITH OTHER AVAILABLE DATABASE OF ANTIGENIC PEPTIDES

Several web-based antigen/epitope databases are available the content of which is freely available to the users. A brief description of **MimicDB** along with comparison with miPepBase is as follows:

MimicDB

mimicDB (Ludin et al., 2011) is a database of linear amino acid epitopes derived from a comparative genomics approach. These epitopes were predicted to be a potential molecular mimicry peptide and derived from a computational prediction pipeline. Further mimicDB is focused on a few selected human endoparasites namely *Brugia malayi, Schistosoma mansoni, Plasmodium falciparum, Leshmania major, Cryptosporidium parvum, Trichomonas vaginalis,* and *Trypanosoma cruzi.* In miPepBase the information is not restricted to any particular class of pathogen and/or disease. It contains information related to all autoimmune diseases caused by pathogens, which may belong to viruses, or prokaryotes, or eukaryotes. miPepBase host's and pathogen's mimicry peptides were curated from literature. The respective researchers have already experimentally established the role of these mimicry epitopes in generating autoimmune disease.

LIMITATIONS AND FUTURE PROSPECTS

Although, we have made outmost effort to compile all available data at one place, it cannot be claimed that miPepBase contains information about each and every peptide/protein involved in molecular mimicry based autoimmune diseases. It is certainly possible that few peptides might have been missed and not included in the miPepBase. In future, we would make our best efforts to include the missing as well as newly added data in miPepBase. The motivation behind establishment of miPepBase was to establish a knowledgebase for proteins/peptides involved in molecular mimicry. We will continue to add new information, which may include but not limited to interaction partners of mimicry proteins and their role in disease. This will enable us to provide a platform for study of the mimicry peptides and pathways through which they trigger autoimmune diseases. We believe the miPepBase database would helpful to the scientific community in exploring the various prospect and aspects of molecular mimicry.

DATABASE UPDATE

An important aspect of any database is to keep it up to date by adding new data. We would constantly add information about newly discovered peptides, which exhibit molecular mimicry and cause autoimmune diseases.

AUTHOR CONTRIBUTIONS

AG and BK prepared the manuscript, collected and organized the data. AG and RK developed the web interface. AG, BK, RK, and MK analyzed the data. MK conceived the idea. All authors reviewed the manuscript.

FUNDING

AG is supported by ICMR-JRF [3/1/3 J.R.F.-2016/LS/HRD-(32262)], BK is a recipient of ICMR-SRF [BIC/11(33)/2014], and RK is supported by UGC-SRF [20-12/2009(ii) EU-IV].

ACKNOWLEDGMENTS

Authors are thankful to Dr. Neelja Singhal for proofreading the manuscript.

REFERENCES

Altschul, S. F., Madden, T. L., Schäffer, A. A., Zhang, J., Zhang, Z., Miller, W., et al. (1997). Gapped BLAST and PSI-BLAST: a new generation of protein database search programs. *Nucleic Acids Res.* 25, 3389–3402. doi: 10.1093/nar/25.17.3389

Altschul, S. F., Wootton, J. C., Gertz, E. M., Agarwala, R., Morgulis, A., Schäffer, A. A., et al. (2005). Protein database searches using compositionally adjusted substitution matrices. *FEBS J.* 272, 5101–5109. doi: 10.1111/j.1742-4658.2005.04945.x

Ang, C. W., Jacobs, B. C., and Laman, J. D. (2004). The Guillain-Barre syndrome: a true case of molecular mimicry. *Trends Immunol.* 25, 61–66. doi: 10.1016/j.it.2003.12.004

Appelmelk, B. J., Simoons-Smit, I., Negrini, R., Moran, A. P., Aspinall, G. O., Forte, J. G., et al. (1996). Potential role of molecular mimicry between *Helicobacter pylori* lipopolysaccharide and host Lewis blood group antigens in autoimmunity. *Infect. Immun.* 64, 2031–2040.

Apweiler, R., Bairoch, A., Wu, C. H., Barker, W. C., Boeckmann, B., Ferro, S., et al. (2004). UniProt: the Universal Protein knowledgebase. *Nucleic Acids Res.* 32, D115–D119. doi: 10.1093/nar/gkh131

Balandraud, N., Roudier, J., and Roudier, C. (2004). Epstein-Barr virus and rheumatoid arthritis. *Autoimmun. Rev.* 3, 362–367. doi: 10.1016/j.autrev.2004.02.002

Baltimore, D. (1971). Expression of animal virus genomes. *Bacteriol. Rev.* 35, 235–241.

Banki, K., Colombo, E., Sia, F., Halladay, D., Mattson, D. H., Tatum, A. H., et al. (1994). Oligodendrocyte-specific expression and autoantigenicity of transaldolase in multiple sclerosis. *J. Exp. Med.* 180, 1649–1663. doi: 10.1084/jem.180.5.1649

Berman, H. M., Westbrook, J., Feng, Z., Gilliland, G., Bhat, T. N., Weissig, H., et al. (2000). The protein data bank. *Nucleic Acids Res.* 28, 235–242. doi: 10.1093/nar/28.1.235

Binns, D., Dimmer, E., Huntley, R., Barrell, D., O'Donovan, C., and Apweiler, R. (2009). QuickGO: a web-based tool for Gene Ontology searching. *Bioinformatics* 25, 3045–3046. doi: 10.1093/bioinformatics/btp536

Bridges, S. L. (2004). Update on autoantibodies in rheumatoid arthritis. *Curr. Rheumatol. Rep.* 6, 343–350. doi: 10.1007/s11926-004-0008-1

Chen, C. R., Tanaka, K., Chazenbalk, G. D., McLachlan, S. M., and Rapoport, B. (2001). A full biological response to autoantibodies in Graves' disease requires a disulfide-bonded loop in the thyrotropin receptor N terminus homologous to a laminin epidermal growth factor-like domain. *J. Biol. Chem.* 276, 14767–14772. doi: 10.1074/jbc.M008001200

Cusick, M. F., Libbey, J. E., and Fujinami, R. S. (2012). Molecular mimicry as a mechanism of autoimmune disease. *Clin. Rev. Allergy Immunol.* 42, 102–111. doi: 10.1007/s12016-011-8294-7

Davies, J. M. (1997). Molecular mimicry: can epitope mimicry induce autoimmune disease? *Immunol. Cell Biol.* 75, 113–126. doi: 10.1038/icb.1997.16

D'Elios, M. M., Appelmelk, B. J., Amedei, A., Bergman, M. P., and Del Prete, G. (2004). Gastric autoimmunity: the role of *Helicobacter pylori* and molecular mimicry. *Trends Mol. Med.* 10, 316–323. doi: 10.1016/j.molmed.2004.06.001

Fujinami, R. S., Oldstone, M. B., Wroblewska, Z., Frankel, M. E., and Koprowski, H. (1983). Molecular mimicry in virus infection: crossreaction of measles virus phosphoprotein or of herpes simplex virus protein with human intermediate filaments. *Proc. Natl. Acad. Sci. U.S.A.* 80, 2346–2350. doi: 10.1073/pnas.80.8.2346

Gauntt, C. J., Tracy, S. M., Chapman, N., Wood, H. J., Kolbeck, P. C., Karaganis, A. G., et al. (1995). Coxsackievirus-induced chronic myocarditis in murine models. *Eur. Heart J.* 16(Suppl. O), 56–58. doi: 10.1093/eurheartj/16.suppl_O.56

Gowthaman, U., and Eswarakumar, V. P. (2013). Molecular mimicry: good artists copy, great artists steal. *Virulence* 4, 433–434. doi: 10.4161/viru.25780

Guven-Maiorov, E., Tsai, C. J., and Nussinov, R. (2016). Pathogen mimicry of host protein-protein interfaces modulates immunity. *Semin. Cell Dev. Biol.* 58, 136–145. doi: 10.1016/j.semcdb.2016.06.004

Hiemstra, H. S., Schloot, N. C., van Veelen, P. A., Willemen, S. J., Franken, K. L., van Rood, J. J., et al. (2001). Cytomegalovirus in autoimmunity: T cell crossreactivity to viral antigen and autoantigen glutamic acid decarboxylase. *Proc. Natl. Acad. Sci. U.S.A.* 98, 3988–3991. doi: 10.1073/pnas.071050898

Huber, S. A., Moraska, A., and Cunningham, M. (1994). Alterations in major histocompatibility complex association of myocarditis induced by coxsackievirus B3 mutants selected with monoclonal antibodies to group A streptococci. *Proc. Natl. Acad. Sci. U.S.A.* 91, 5543–5547. doi: 10.1073/pnas.91.12.5543

Kaufman, K. M., Kirby, M. Y., Harley, J. B., and James, J. A. (2003). Peptide mimics of a major lupus epitope of SmB/B'. *Ann. N.Y. Acad. Sci.* 987, 215–229. doi: 10.1111/j.1749-6632.2003.tb06051.x

Kohn, L. D., Napolitano, G., Singer, D. S., Molteni, M., Scorza, R., Shimojo, N., et al. (2000). Graves' disease: a host defense mechanism gone awry. *Int. Rev. Immunol.* 19, 633–664. doi: 10.3109/08830180009088516

Ludin, P., Nilsson, D., and Mäser, P. (2011). Genome-wide identification of molecular mimicry candidates in parasites. *PLoS ONE* 6:e17546. doi: 10.1371/journal.pone.0017546

McClain, M. T., Heinlen, L. D., Dennis, G. J., Roebuck, J., Harley, J. B., and James, J. A. (2005). Early events in lupus humoral autoimmunity suggest initiation through molecular mimicry. *Nat. Med.* 11, 85–89. doi: 10.1038/nm1167

Neu, N., Rose, N. R., Beisel, K. W., Herskowitz, A., Gurri-Glass, G., and Craig, S. W. (1987). Cardiac myosin induces myocarditis in genetically predisposed mice. *J. Immunol.* 139, 3630–3636.

Oldstone, M. B. (2005). Molecular mimicry, microbial infection, and autoimmune disease: evolution of the concept. *Curr. Top. Microbiol. Immunol.* 296, 1–17. doi: 10.1007/3-540-30791-5_1

Oldstone, M. B. (1998). Molecular mimicry and immune-mediated diseases. *FASEB J.* 12, 1255–1265.

Rice, P., Longden, I., and Bleasby, A. (2000). EMBOSS: the European Molecular Biology Open Software Suite. *Trends Genet.* 16, 276–277. doi: 10.1016/S0168-9525(00)02024-2

Rönnblom, L., and Alm, G. V. (2001). An etiopathogenic role for the type I IFN system in SLE. *Trends Immunol.* 22, 427–431. doi: 10.1016/S1471-4906(01)01955-X

Rose, N. R., and Mackay, I. R. (2000). Molecular mimicry: a critical look at exemplary instances in human diseases. *Cell. Mol. Life Sci.* 57, 542–551. doi: 10.1007/PL00000716

Schulze, K., and Schultheiss, H. P. (1995). The role of the ADP/ATP carrier in the pathogenesis of viral heart disease. *Eur. Heart J.* 16(Suppl. O), 64–67. doi: 10.1093/eurheartj/16.suppl_O.64

Talbot, P. J., Paquette, J. S., Ciurli, C., Antel, J. P., and Ouellet, F. (1996). Myelin basic protein and human coronavirus 229E cross-reactive T cells in multiple sclerosis. *Ann. Neurol.* 39, 233–240. doi: 10.1002/ana.410390213

Tiwana, H., Wilson, C., Alvarez, A., Abuknesha, R., Bansal, S., and Ebringer, A. (1999). Cross-reactivity between the rheumatoid arthritis-associated motif EQKRAA and structurally related sequences found in *Proteus mirabilis*. *Infect. Immun.* 67, 2769–2775.

Wucherpfennig, K. W., and Strominger, J. L. (1995). Molecular mimicry in T cell-mediated autoimmunity: viral peptides activate human T cell clones specific for myelin basic protein. *Cell* 80, 695–705. doi: 10.1016/0092-8674(95)90348-8

13

Integrating Non-Human Primate, Human and Mathematical Studies to Determine the Influence of BCG Timing on H56 Vaccine Outcomes

Louis R. Joslyn[1,2], Elsje Pienaar[1,2], Robert M. DiFazio[3], Sara Suliman[4], Benjamin M. Kagina[4], JoAnne L. Flynn[3], Thomas J. Scriba[4], Jennifer J. Linderman[1] and Denise E. Kirschner[2]**

[1] Department of Chemical Engineering, University of Michigan, Ann Arbor, MI, United States, [2] Department of Microbiology and Immunology, University of Michigan Medical School, Ann Arbor, MI, United States, [3] Department of Microbiology and Molecular Genetics, University of Pittsburgh School of Medicine, Pittsburgh, PA, United States, [4] South African Tuberculosis Vaccine Initiative and Institute of Infectious Disease and Molecular Medicine, Division of Immunology, Department of Pathology, University of Cape Town, Cape Town, South Africa

***Correspondence:**
Jennifer J. Linderman
linderma@umich.edu
Denise E. Kirschner
kirschne@umich.edu

Tuberculosis (TB) is the leading cause of death by an infectious agent, and developing an effective vaccine is an important component of the WHO's EndTB Strategy. Non-human primate (NHP) models of vaccination are crucial to TB vaccine development and have informed design of subsequent human trials. However, challenges emerge when translating results from animal models to human applications, and connecting post-vaccination immunological measurements to infection outcomes. The H56:IC31 vaccine is a candidate currently in phase I/IIa trials. H56 is a subunit vaccine that is comprised of 3 mycobacterial antigens: ESAT6, Ag85B, and Rv2660, formulated in IC31 adjuvant. H56, as a boost to Bacillus Calmette-Guérin (BCG, the TB vaccine that is currently used in most countries world-wide) demonstrates improved protection (compared to BCG alone) in mouse and NHP models of TB, and the first human study of H56 reported strong antigen-specific T cell responses to the vaccine. We integrated NHP and human data with mathematical modeling approaches to improve our understanding of NHP and human response to vaccine. We use a mathematical model to describe T-cell priming, proliferation, and differentiation in lymph nodes and blood, and calibrate the model to NHP and human blood data. Using the model, we demonstrate the impact of BCG timing on H56 vaccination response and reveal a general immunogenic response to H56 following BCG prime. Further, we use uncertainty and sensitivity analyses to isolate mechanisms driving differences in vaccination response observed between NHP and human datasets. This study highlights the power of a systems biology approach: integration of multiple modalities to better understand a complex biological system.

Keywords: tuberculosis, non-human primate, H56, mathematical modeling, bacillus calmette–guerin (BCG), vaccination

INTRODUCTION

Among infectious diseases, tuberculosis (TB) remains the leading cause of death due to a single agent. Its infectious agent, *Mycobacterium tuberculosis* (Mtb), kills approximately three individuals per minute (WHO, 2016). Additionally, in 2015, there were an estimated 480,000 incident cases of multi-drug resistant TB. The morbidity and mortality due to tuberculosis, including drug resistant strains, require renewed investment and research for an effective vaccine.

While Bacillus Calmette-Guérin (BCG) is widely used to prevent TB disease in infants, its efficacy amongst the adult population is highly variable (Colditz et al., 1995; Fine, 1995; Lanckriet et al., 1995; Mittal et al., 1996; Sterne et al., 1998; Zodpey et al., 1998). Originally developed in the early 1900s, the first clinical trials for BCG began in France in the 1920s and proved its efficacy in children (Andersen and Doherty, 2005). By 1973, BCG was compulsory for South Africa (Fourie, 1987) and emerged as the most widely used of all vaccines, due to ease of testing for vaccination via the tuberculin skin test. However, BCG efficacy fails to protect both infants and adults; with protection varying from 0-80% (Andersen and Doherty, 2005; Tameris et al., 2013). Thus, the search for a more effective vaccine continues.

Improved management of the TB epidemic could stem from vaccinations that prevent infection, active disease, or reactivation from latent infection, or ameliorate active infections. Currently, more than 13 TB vaccine candidates have entered clinical trials (Evans et al., 2016; Gonzalo-Asensio et al., 2017). These candidates include attenuated versions of Mtb, mycobacterial whole cell vaccines, viral vectored vaccines, and subunit vaccines (Ahsan, 2015).

Subunit vaccination strategies emerged when the Mtb genome was sequenced in 1998 (Cole et al., 1998). One such promising subunit vaccine candidate is H56 formulated with adjuvant IC31. H56 is a multistage vaccine composed of three antigens: ESAT6, Ag85B, and Rv2660c (Aagaard et al., 2011). ESAT6 and Ag85B are early secreted antigens that have been used before as individual vaccine antigens (Horwitz et al., 1995; Brandt et al., 2000; Olsen et al., 2001, 2004; Langermans et al., 2005). Ag85B is an antigen that is present in both BCG and H56 vaccine formulations. Both Ag85B and ESAT6 have been shown to be highly immunogenic antigens that are targeted by T cell populations (Mustafa et al., 2000a,b). Rv2660c was included in the vaccine because of its association with T cell responses from LTBI (Latent Tuberculosis Infection) individuals and its expression under starvation or hypoxic conditions, although its function has not yet been determined (Betts et al., 2002; Govender et al., 2010; Lin et al., 2012). Finally, all three antigens are thought to play a role in a variety of methods that mycobacteria likely employs to survive the intracellular environment (Ronning et al., 2000; Wilkinson et al., 2001; Ganguly et al., 2008; Lin et al., 2012; Rohde et al., 2012).

Common formulations of the H56 vaccine include the adjuvants IC31 and Cationic Adjuvant Formulation (CAF01). Human clinical trials used the IC31 adjuvant, a two-component adjuvant that includes the KLK peptide (an anti-microbial peptide) and oligodeoxynocleotide (a Toll-like receptor nine agonist) (Luabeya et al., 2015). IC31 was used in an NHP study that showed H56 limited reactivation of clinical latent TB (Lin et al., 2012), while CAF01 has been used in NHP studies herein. CAF01 is composed primarily of DDA (liposomes prepared in dimethyl dioctadecyl ammonium) and TDB (a component of the mycobacterial cell wall, trehalose dimycolate) (Agger, 2016). Both adjuvants support a Th1 CD4 T cell response (Luabeya et al., 2015; Agger, 2016).

While H56 represents a new vaccine candidate, it also provides an opportunity for a case study. Before evaluating the success of a vaccine via challenge, can we compare vaccine immunogenicity in humans and NHPs to further characterize the inherent differences between each species? Furthermore, can we utilize antigen specificity to explore the impact and role of prior BCG vaccination on H56 immunogenicity?

We use a systems biology approach employing mathematical modeling to relate pre-exposure vaccination dynamics in humans and non-human primates. We describe T-cell responses in lymph nodes and blood using a 2-compartment mathematical model, demonstrate the impact of BCG timing on subsequent H56 vaccination, and reveal basic mechanisms that dictate vaccine outcomes in NHPs and humans. We propose that timing of BCG vaccination and inherent differences between species could play an important role in the immune responses to the H56 vaccine candidate. Having this knowledge could improve the vaccine pipeline.

METHODS

Non-human Primate Data Collection and Analysis

Animals

The Institutional Animal Care and Use Committee of the University of Pittsburgh approved all experiments (protocol number 12080653). The animals were housed and maintained in accordance with standards established in the Animal Welfare Act and the Guide for the Care and Use of Laboratory Animals.

Vaccination

Cynomolgus macaques (*Macaca fascicularis*) imported from China and in the United States for at least a year (Valley Biosystems) were used for these studies (n=8). BCG and H56:CAF01 animals were primed with 0.1 mL BCG Danish intramuscularly followed by two doses of the vaccine H56 (Ag85B-ESAT6-Rv2660c; 50 μg) mixed with CAF01 (625 μg dimethyldioctadecyl-ammonium (DDA) and 125 μg trehalose-6,6-dibehenate (TDB)) at weeks 10 and 14 after BCG priming. Timing and doses of vaccination are based on previous studies by our collaborators and others in the field who perform protein-based boosting of BCG in macaques (Langermans et al., 2005; Lin et al., 2012).

Necropsy

For this study, macaques were euthanized approximately 44-48 weeks post-BCG prime (macaques received Mtb challenge 22 weeks following BCG prime, but Mtb-challenge data response was not included in this study and is therefore not outlined in this section). All animals were euthanized with an intravenous overdose of sodium pentobarbital (Beuthanasia) at 15mg/kg and maximally bled.

ELISPOT

ELISPOT for IFN-γ was performed using 96-well opaque multiscreen immunoprecipitation filtration plates (Merck Millipore) that were hydrated, washed, and coated with 7.5 μg/mL of anti-human/nonhuman primate IFN-γ (GZ-4: Mabtech) for 2 h at 37°C with 5% CO_2. Plates were then blocked with complete RPMI containing 10% human AB serum for 2 h at 37°C with 5% CO_2. Each stimulation condition was performed in duplicate. Medium only was used as a negative control, and phorbol dibutyrate/ionomycin (P&I) and anti-CD3 were used as positive controls. CFP and peptide pools of H56 vaccine antigens (ESAT-6, Ag85B, Rv2660c) were used at 10 μg/mL. PBMCs were then added, and the plate was incubated for 48 h at 37°C with 5% CO_2. The plate was then washed and detection antibody (7-B6: Mabtech) was added at 2.5 μg/mL and incubated for 2 h at 37°C with 5% CO_2. The plate was washed and streptavidin-conjugated horseradish peroxidase was added at a 1:100 dilution and incubated for 45 min at 37°C with 5% CO_2. The plate was washed and then developed using AEC substrate. The plate was dried overnight and read using an ImmunoSpot analyzer (Cellular Technologies Limited).

Figure 1 shows the timeline of experimental protocol, with blood draw events for NHP studies (bottom timeline). We represent the data from Difazio et al. in a manner consistent with the standardization of the phase I clinical trial data provided by Luabeya et al. Like Luabeya et al., we analyzed the antigen specific T cell response for CD4+ effector (CD27-CD45+), effector memory (CD27-CD45-), and central memory (CD27+CD45-) subtypes. ESAT6- or Ag85B-specific cellular concentrations were calculated. Finally, we converted the antigen-specific responses for each T-cell subtype to represent a percentage of total CD4+ T cells in blood.

Phase I Clinical Trial Data Collection and Analysis

For model calibration, we used data described previously (Luabeya et al., 2015). Briefly, the data is from the first in-human phase I clinical trial of candidate TB vaccine, H56 in IC31 adjuvant. The authors tested the safety and immunogenicity of H56:IC31 in adults with or without Mtb infection. Across 112 days, eight individuals without evidence of Mtb infection were injected with 3 doses of H56 (50 μg H56, 500 nmol IC31) at 56 day intervals. Blood was drawn from individuals on days 0, 14, 56, 70, 112, 126, and 210. Antigen-specific T-cell responses were isolated and collected at each sample collection time point. Every individual in the study received BCG vaccination as a child (approximately 30 years prior to this study). **Figure 1** shows the timeline of experimental protocol for the human trial (top timeline).

We standardized the results of Luabeya et al. in a manner that allows for eventual comparison to NHP data. The study revealed that the H56 vaccine does not induce a robust CD8+ T cell response. Therefore, we focused all data analysis, model calibration, and results on individual subtypes of the CD4+ T cell response to vaccination. That is, we examined effector ($CD45RA^+$ $CCR7^-$), effector memory ($CD45RA^-CCR7^-$), central memory ($CD45RA^-CCR7^+$), and total CD4+ T cell populations. Luabeya et al. also discovered that a dose of 50 μg of H56 was not optimal; however, we have selected the 50 μg dataset so that we can directly compare human responses to the NHP studies described above.

For each T cell subtype, we normalized the response by subtracting the number of unstimulated, cytokine-producing T cells from the quantity of T cells that produced cytokines in response to antigen. We converted this metric to represent a percentage of the total number of CD4+ T cells. This calculation was performed for responses to both the ESAT6 and Ag85B antigens.

Note that the adjuvants used in these two studies (NHP and human) are different and could contribute significantly to the results observed. In this work, we do not examine adjuvant differences but focus instead on the impact of BCG timing and differences in T cell responses between species. See below for further discussion of how we indirectly capture adjuvants.

Mathematical Model

In recent studies (Gong et al., 2014; Marino and Kirschner, 2016; Marino et al., 2016; Ziraldo et al., 2016), we captured lymph node and blood dynamics in response to Mtb infection using a mathematical model. We used a compartmentalized system of 16 non-linear, autonomous ordinary differential equations (ODEs) to track specific and non-specific CD4+ effector, effector memory, and central memory T cell responses. In these previous works we represent Mtb-specific T-cells as a generic class of antigen-specific cells; thus, it was simple to retool this class of cells and track them as ESAT6- or Ag85B-specific. We assume that all antigen-specific T cells are equally immune responsive. **Figure 2** displays the model schematic, **Supplementary Materials 1** details the system of ODEs, and **Supplementary Table 1** gives the list of all parameters, definitions, and values.

Our key assumption is that the *in silico*, exogenous introduction of antigen loaded, antigen-presenting cells (APCs) will act as a reasonable proxy for vaccination. This is valid for two reasons: First, it is well known that vaccine peptides are presented to T cells by APCs. Second, while we did not mechanistically model the impact of an adjuvant in this study, this assumption indirectly evaluates the impact of an adjuvant on T-cell responses. APCs require adjuvant to properly process and present vaccine peptides (Kamath et al., 2008). Therefore, to account for variability in individual response to an adjuvant and to represent variability across adjuvants (IC31 vs. CAF01), the quantity of APCs pulsed during vaccination events was assigned to a single quantity within a range of values. Thus, we simulated vaccination events by pulsing the APC equation in the system of ODEs at a time point equal to the day of H56 vaccination, according to each experimental protocol.

The non-linear ODE model system was implemented and solved in Matlab (R2016b v 9.1). Experimental and simulation

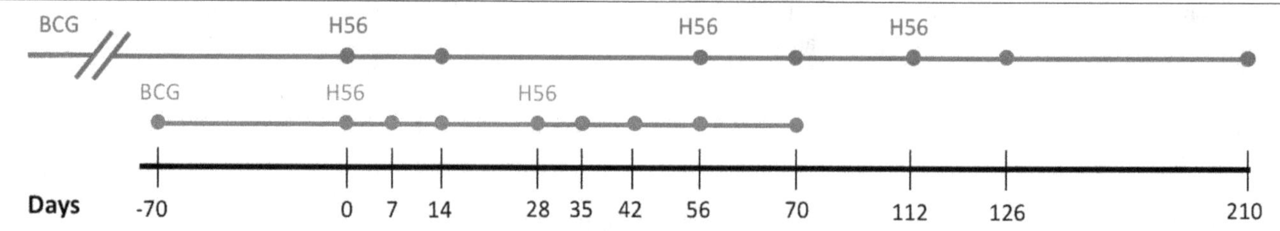

FIGURE 1 | Vaccination Experimental Protocol. Comparison of the Human (red) and Non-Human Primate (blue) study protocols. Dots along the respective timelines represent blood sample data collection time points. BCG, Bacillus Calmette–Guerin; H56, vaccination with H56 and adjuvant (IC31 in Human, CAF01 in Non-Human Primate).

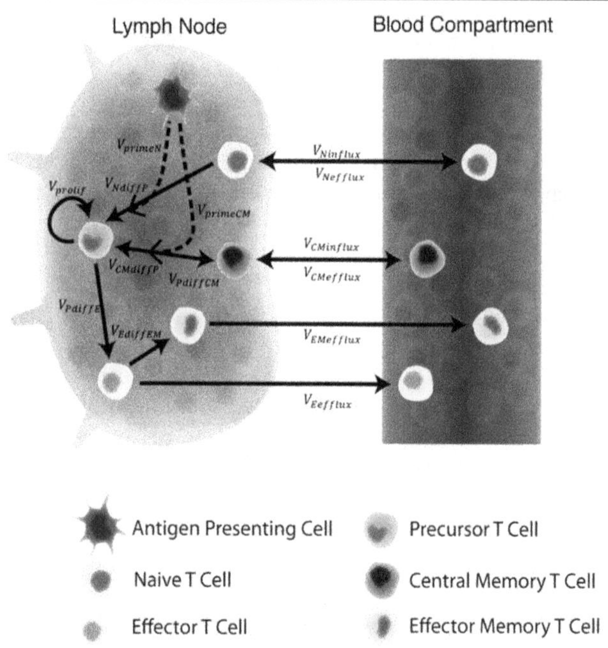

FIGURE 2 | Schematic of the two-compartment model. Each equation represents a concentration of a particular cell type, as outlined in the legend. These concentrations are dependent on other cell concentrations and interactions (as shown by arrows) between cells or compartments. Arrow labels are defined in greater detail in **Supplementary Materials 1**. Briefly, V_{primeN} and $V_{primeCM}$ represents the impact of APCs on naïve and central memory cell recruitment. V_{NdiffP} and $V_{CMdiffP}$ shows the transformation of naïve and central memory T cells to the precursor T cell population. V_{prolif}, V_{PdiffE}, $V_{PdiffCM}$, and $V_{EdiffEM}$ represents precursor proliferation and differentiation to effector, central memory and effector memory cell types, respectively. Finally, influx and efflux rates between LN and blood are shown as $V_{Ninflux}$, $V_{CMinflux}$, $V_{CMefflux}$, $V_{Eefflux}$, and $V_{EMefflux}$.

Box 1 | Important terms.

Immunogenicity Dataspace: The space defined by experimental results that contains the T-cell response to each antigen.

Parameter Range: The range of values for a parameter that are biologically feasible and are assigned to represent values of the mechanism for which that parameter represents. Values (and ranges) are assigned according to biological observations, experimental results, or mathematical estimation.

Parameter Space: The set of all combinations of parameter values for a particular model, as defined by the parameter ranges for each parameter.

Uncertainty and Sensitivity Analysis: A series of techniques used to evaluate the influence a parameter has on model outcomes. Influence of individual mechanism can be assessed (see Methods for more details).

Calibration: The process of varying parameters until the model behavior reaches a preferred end state or predetermined goal (usually the dataspace).

Initial Conditions: The predefined initial values of each variable in a mathematical model prior to simulating the model. In this work, initial conditions were also varied during model calibration as initial condition could represent pre-existing immune memory cells.

Radar Charts: A graphical visualization of multivariate data across multiple axis. We use radar charts to display the parameter space of our simulations.

data cleaning, visualization, and post-processing was performed in R (R version 3.4.0, RStudio version 1.0.143) using ggplot2 (Wickham, 2009), plyr (Wickham, 2011), and tidyr (Wickham and Henry, 2017) packages. See **Supplementary Materials 1** for equations and model parameters.

Model Calibration and Sensitivity Analysis

We first sought to define the parameter space that best represents each "immunogenicity dataspace" to calibrate to the human and NHP datasets (see **Box 1** for a description of several important terms for this section of our work). The parameter space was identified by a two-step process. First, for each immunogenicity space, we ran 1500 simulations with a 50% range around the baseline parameters outlined in our previous model construction (shown in Marino and Kirschner, 2016). A Latin hypercube sampling (LHS) algorithm was used to sample the multi-dimensional parameter space (Marino et al., 2008). This wide range of simulations yielded multiple candidates of baseline parameters that might best represent each immunogenicity dataspace. In the second step, we simulated 500 runs (sampling parameters in approximately 20% range) around these candidates' baseline values, again using LHS to sample the parameter space. We accepted the candidate parameter sets if all 500 runs fulfilled two criteria: (1) the simulations' minimum and maximum run must remain within the immunogenicity dataspace. That is, all simulations from the parameter ranges needed to remain within the logarithmic scale of the data. (2) the median simulation run across all 500 runs must cross the interquartile range of the majority of experimental time points (4 of 7 for human data, 4 of 8 for NHP data). This ensured that our model mimics at least the majority of both experimentally-determined dynamics. **Supplementary Table 1** displays the parameter range values after calibration to each immunogenicity dataspace.

We quantify the importance of each host mechanism involved in vaccination dynamics by finding correlations between model parameters and outputs. Correlations between specific model outputs and parameters were determined by using Partial Rank Correlation Coefficient (PRCC), where−1 denotes a perfect negative correlation between a model output and parameter (+1 denotes a perfect positive correlation between model output and parameter). Marino et al. completed a review of the statistical tests available to access significance of PRCC (Marino et al., 2008). PRCC results performed a dual role: not only do they reveal the relationship between model outcomes and parameters, they also inform calibration of the model to the immunogenicity dataspace. As the model is tuned, manipulations to the more sensitive parameters ameliorate model fitting according to the criteria above.

Since our model provides measurements in the form of cell counts in lymph node and cells/mm∧3 in the blood, we performed post-processing of the simulations to ensure that units matched those provided by the H56 vaccination data (See **Supplementary Materials 1** for details).

Parameter Space Visualization

We utilized radar charts to illustrate parameter range comparisons between species and the impact of BCG on cellular responses. Radar charts are a graphical visualization of multivariate data across multiple axis. In this work, we plotted radar charts using *R's* radarchart function in the fmsb package (Nakazawa, 2017). Each axis represents a parameter of interest in our ODE model. Points near the center of each axis represent a lower value for that parameter whereas points near the outer edges of each axis represent larger values. To compare parameter ranges across species, we calculate the minimum and maximum for each axis on the charts as the minimum and maximum value for each parameter across all species and antigen-specific fits (see **Supplementary Materials 2**). To compare the impact of BCG memory on the H56 immune response, we created the human radar charts with a minimum and maximum for each axis defined by the minimum and maximum parameter value across human model fits to ESAT6 or Ag85B. We created the NHP radar charts by displaying the parameter ranges within the minimum and maximum values across NHP model fits to either antigen.

RESULTS

Humans and Non-human Primates Exhibit Different T-Cell Responses to ESAT6 Following H56 Vaccination

In response to H56 vaccination, humans and NHPs showed large variability within and across species. While some of this variability can be attributed to the different experimental protocols used (**Figure 1**), the magnitudes of responses between species still differ. Several differences in the magnitude and timing of response across species are notable (**Figure 3**). The total response of CD4+ ESAT6+ T cells in NHPs is larger and more variable than the response in humans. For example, an *F* test to compare variances between the two species at day 14 reveals a significant difference ($p = 0.0003$; variance of NHPs was approximately 25 times greater than the humans). Day 14 is the final day that protocols follow the same timelines. Therefore we selected day 14 for this statistical test in order to exclude variability due to different experimental protocols.

Furthermore, the magnitude of effector and central memory population responses is larger in NHPs than humans. Between species, the effector memory subpopulation responses are most similar. The major contributors to the total NHP CD4+ ESAT6+ T-cell response are the effector T cell population during early timepoints and the central memory T cell population at later timepoints. The human response is dominated by effector memory T cells. Interestingly, some data suggest that the dose of H56 used in this study may also have contributed to this exaggerated memory T cell response; current thinking will pursue at least a 10-fold lower dose.

A Single Mathematical Model Describes Both Human and NHP T Cell Responses to ESAT6

Statistically, we have shown that there is a difference in NHP and human responses to ESAT6. However, statistical analysis could not answer the following questions: (1) Are the data for both humans and NHPs consistent with the same mechanisms for mounting an immune response? (2) If those mechanisms are the same, can the rates of proliferation and differentiation alone be responsible for the differences we observe in ESAT immunogenicity? These questions require a method that can address the dynamics of priming, proliferation, and differentiation that are intrinsic to the development of an immune response. In Methods, we present a mathematical model that describes T cell priming, proliferation, and differentiation in response to APCs in the blood and LN of primates. Here, we hypothesize that this mathematical model can capture both human and NHP T cell responses to ESAT6; however, it will require the use of different sets of parameter values. In **Figure 4**, experimental data from **Figure 3** were replotted as box and whisker plots (blue–NHP, red–human) and simulation curves are shown by the cloud and median lines (blue and red, respectively).

NHP simulation data recapitulates the variability in the experimental data by capturing the dynamics of the experimental data. In particular, the median simulation line demonstrates how the model captures the general behavior of the data, by traveling through the interquartile range of at least 4 of the 8 timepoints for each subpopulation of T cells. The human simulations capture the clinical data—our maximum and minimum simulations include nearly all of the outlying data points across the subpopulations of T cells. A

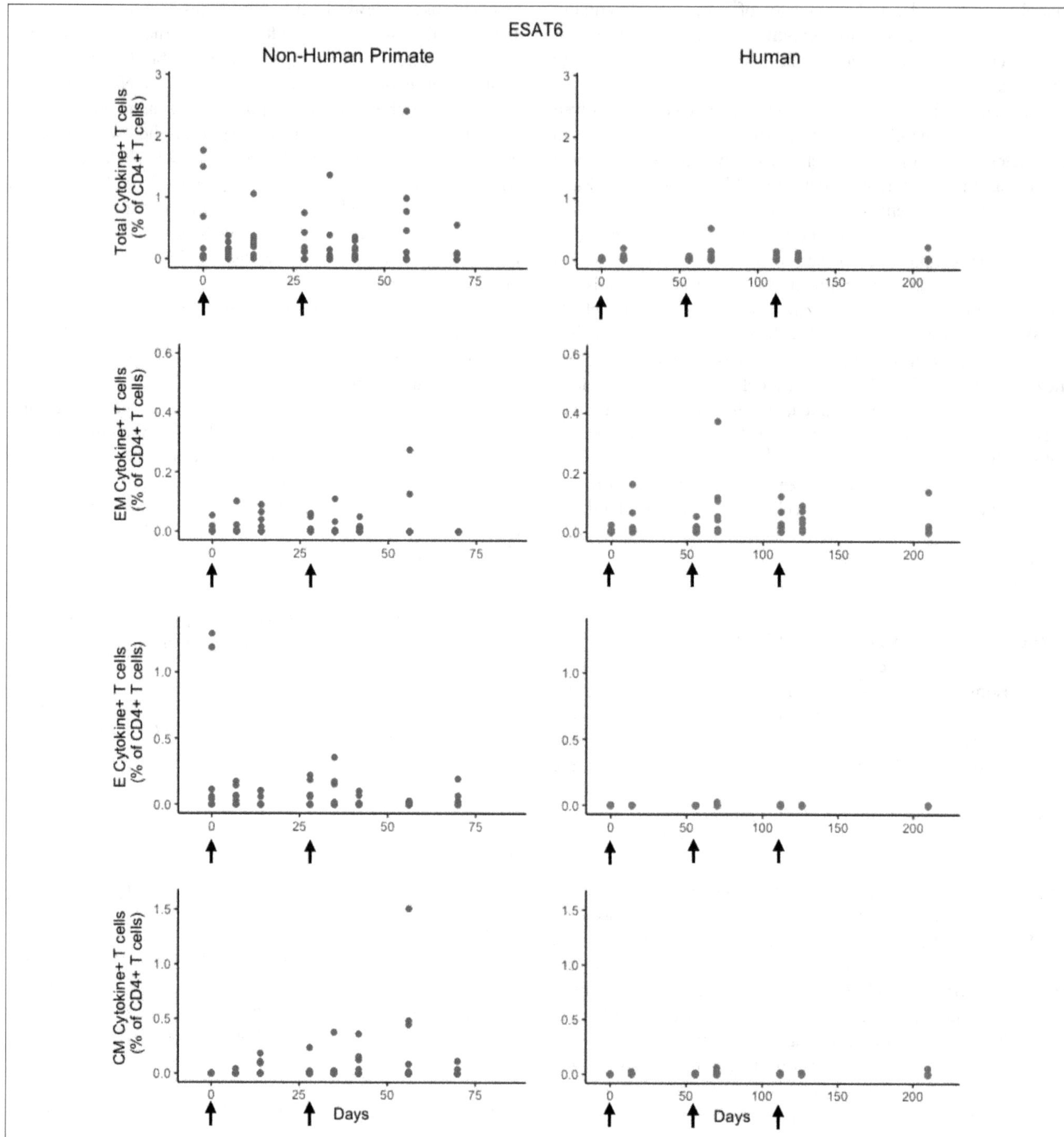

FIGURE 3 | Experimental data show different responses to ESAT6 antigen following H56 vaccination. The percentage of blood CD4+ T cells that respond to ESAT6 by producing cytokines (cytokine+) is divided by the total number of CD4+ T cells in the blood. T cell subtypes are also shown. Each time point shows the responses of all 8 human (red) or all 8 NHPs (blue) subjects. Note that it can be difficult to perceive 8 individual dots–if the subject's responses are similar or the same, as individual dots overlap. For ease of comparison, we have placed both panels of data on the same y-axis. Arrows represent vaccination timepoints.

visual comparison of these parameter ranges is displayed in **Supplementary Materials 2.** Altogether, we demonstrate that our model captures the ESAT6 immunogenicity dataspace of both NHPs and humans—suggesting that the mechanisms of generating a primary immune response are the same for both NHPs and humans.

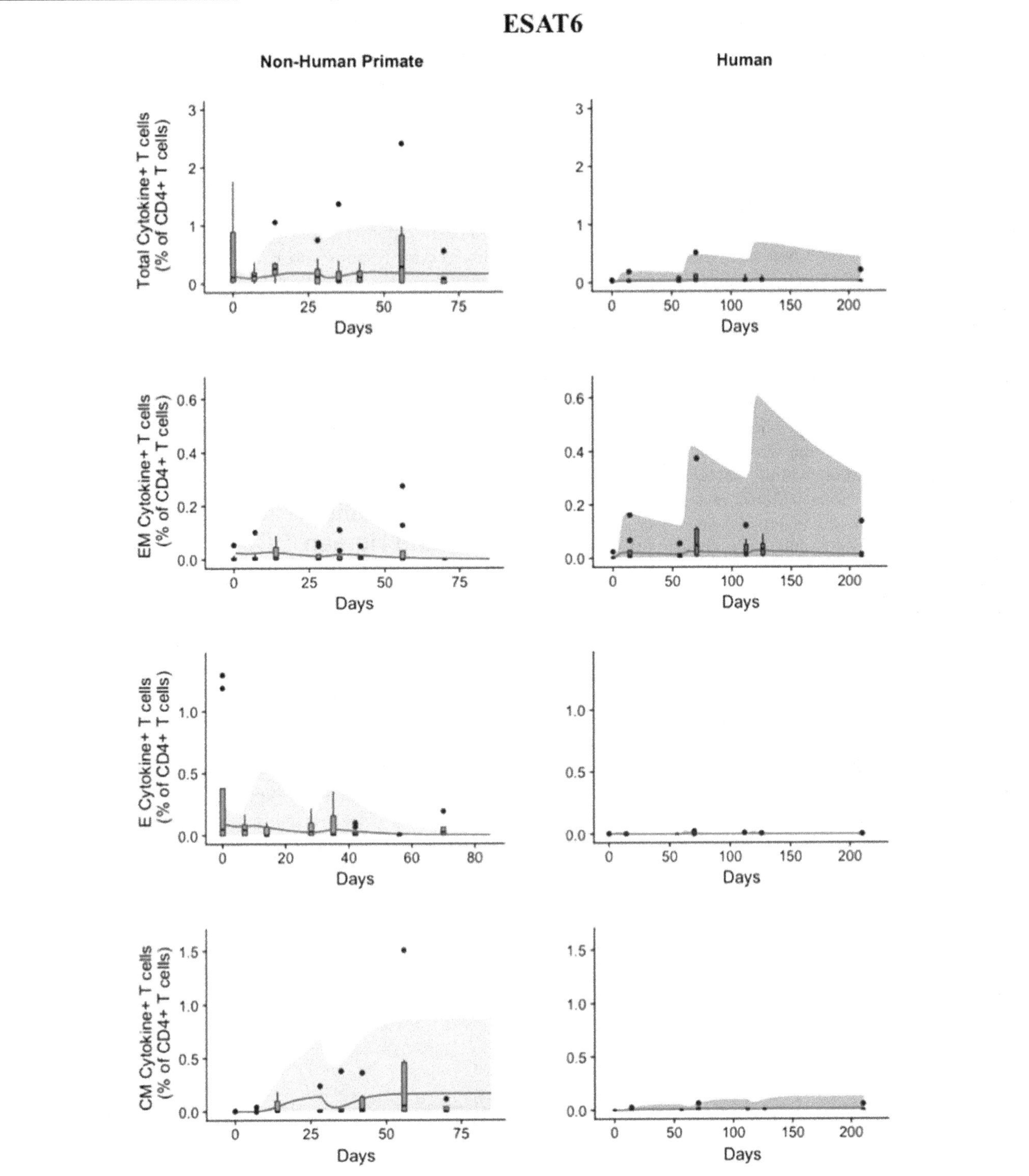

FIGURE 4 | Model captures diverse response of both NHP and Humans to ESAT6 antigen following H56 vaccination. The percentage of blood CD4+ T cells that respond to ESAT6 by producing cytokines (cytokine+) is divided by the total number of CD4+ T cells in the blood. T cell subtypes are also shown. Each time point shows the responses of all 8 human (red) or all 8 NHPs (blue) subjects using a box and whisker plot. These box and whisker plots provided a guide for the boundaries of immunogenicity dataspace. Whiskers were created by extending from the edge of the box to the data point that is the closest, but does not exceed 1.5 times the interquartile range (defined as the distance between the first and third quartiles) from the edge of the box. Any experimental points beyond the edge of the whisker are deemed as outliers and plotted as black points. Simulation data are displayed as a blue or red cloud that outline the min and max of 500 runs for NHP or human calibrations, respectively. The blue or red line represents the median of those simulations. Our goal when calibrating to cell levels in blood of both species was to ensure that *in silico* simulations fell reasonably within these dataspaces, as outlined in the Methods section. Parameter ranges used to generate the simulation curves are shown in **Supplementary Table 1**.

Sensitivity Analysis Reveals Both Similar and Distinct Outcome Drivers Across Species in Response to ESAT6

Having calibrated our model to both ESAT6 human and ESAT6 NHP immunogenicity dataspaces, we next used these two model fits to ask questions about important processes within the CD4+ T cell response. In particular, we wanted to better understand the dual roles of proliferation and differentiation that drive immune response magnitude and timing following vaccination in both species. To investigate these processes, we performed uncertainty and sensitivity analysis on 3 outcomes (ESAT6-specific central memory, effector, and effector memory T cell subtypes) of our model. **Table 1** highlights processes (i.e., parameters) found to be significantly associated with changes in T cell response subpopulations for each species.

For both species, uncertainty and sensitivity analysis support a key role for priming and proliferation within lymph nodes. This is not a novel concept, but rather acts as a proper control for the utility of our model, as it is accepted that priming and proliferation within the lymph node underlies immunogenicity of a vaccine (Moliva et al., 2017). Specifically, uncertainty and sensitivity analysis revealed a crucial role for CD4+ T cell precursor proliferation rates (k4) within the lymph node compartment. The significant, positive association between precursor T cell proliferation rates and 3 different T cell subtypes in the blood represents an inter-compartmental effect–not only does the parameter influence the dynamics within its own compartment (lymph node), it drives the dynamics of the compartment yielding experimentally validated results (blood).

There were also modest differences in the mechanisms driving model fits for NHP and humans, (**Table 1**). For example, only the human dataset showed significant negative correlations between cellular responses in the blood and the half-saturation values of precursor proliferation and differentiation in the lymph node (represented as "likelihood of proliferation and differentiation" in **Table 1**). We predict that humans and NHPs are generally alike in response to ESAT6, but proliferation and differentiation in humans is not quite as easily triggered as proliferation and differentiation in the NHP. This could be in part due to the influence of humans regularly exposed to many and diverse environmental factors.

Humans and Non-human Primates Exhibit Different T-Cell Responses to Ag85B Following H56 Vaccination

While the immunological response between humans and NHPs to the ESAT6 antigen in H56 vaccination can be attributed to intrinsic similarities and differences between species, the response to the Ag85B antigen offers an opportunity to investigate the role of prior BCG vaccination on H56 immunogenicity (**Figure 5**). When we compare magnitude and timing of responses across species, several differences emerge. As observed for responses to ESAT6, the total response of CD4+ Ag85B+ T cells in NHPs is higher and more variable than the response in humans. For example, an *F* test to compare variances for the central memory T cell population at day 14 revealed a significant difference (p = 3.984e-06; variance in NHPs is about 96 times greater than humans). While the magnitude of effector and central memory subpopulation responses were larger in NHPs, it appeared that humans had a larger effector memory subpopulation response.

A Single Mathematical Model Describes NHP and Human T Cell Responses to Ag85B

Using statistical analysis, we have revealed a difference between species in immune response to Ag85B. However, statistical analysis cannot answer the following questions: (1) what is the impact of different BCG timing on H56 response? (2) is the influence of BCG prime on H56 immune response the same for both species—i.e., do the two species possess a similar secondary response to an antigen? To mechanistically understand the role and timing of BCG prime on H56 vaccination, we require a mathematical modeling approach to predict dynamics of the different T cell responses to Ag85B. As with ESAT6, we tested whether our mathematical model can capture the Ag85B immunogenicity dataspace for both NHPs and humans (**Figure 6**). Our simulation data mimic the variability in the NHP experimental data by tracking most outlier points and whiskers. For example, simulations reflect a contraction of the central memory population and follow expected logic—a percentage of central memory cell populations will reactivate and become

TABLE 1 | Parameters with significant PRCCs for ESAT6 immune response outcomes.

ESAT6	Central memory	Effector	Effector memory
NHP	central memory reactivation rate; precursor proliferation and differentiation into central memory cells; APC and precursor death rates	precursor proliferation and differentiation into effector cells; effector, APC, and precursor death rates	precursor proliferation and differentiation into effector cells; APC and precursor death rates
Human	Likelihood of proliferation; precursor proliferation and differentiation to central memory; central memory recruitment; APC, and precursor death rates;	Likelihood of proliferation and differentiation; Naïve T cell recruitment; Precursor proliferation and differentiation to Effector; effector differentiation to effector Memory; effector Lymph efflux; effector, APC, and precursor death rates;	Likelihood of proliferation and differentiation; precursor proliferation; effector memory, APC, and precursor death rates;

One row displays humans, the other displays NHPs. Columns list the 3 model outcomes of interest – ESAT6-specific central memory, effector and effector memory T cell phenotypes. These outcomes were selected for analysis because the model was calibrated to their dataspace. Each table cell contains a general description of significant (i.e., $p < 10^{-3}$) parameters with respect to each output of the model.

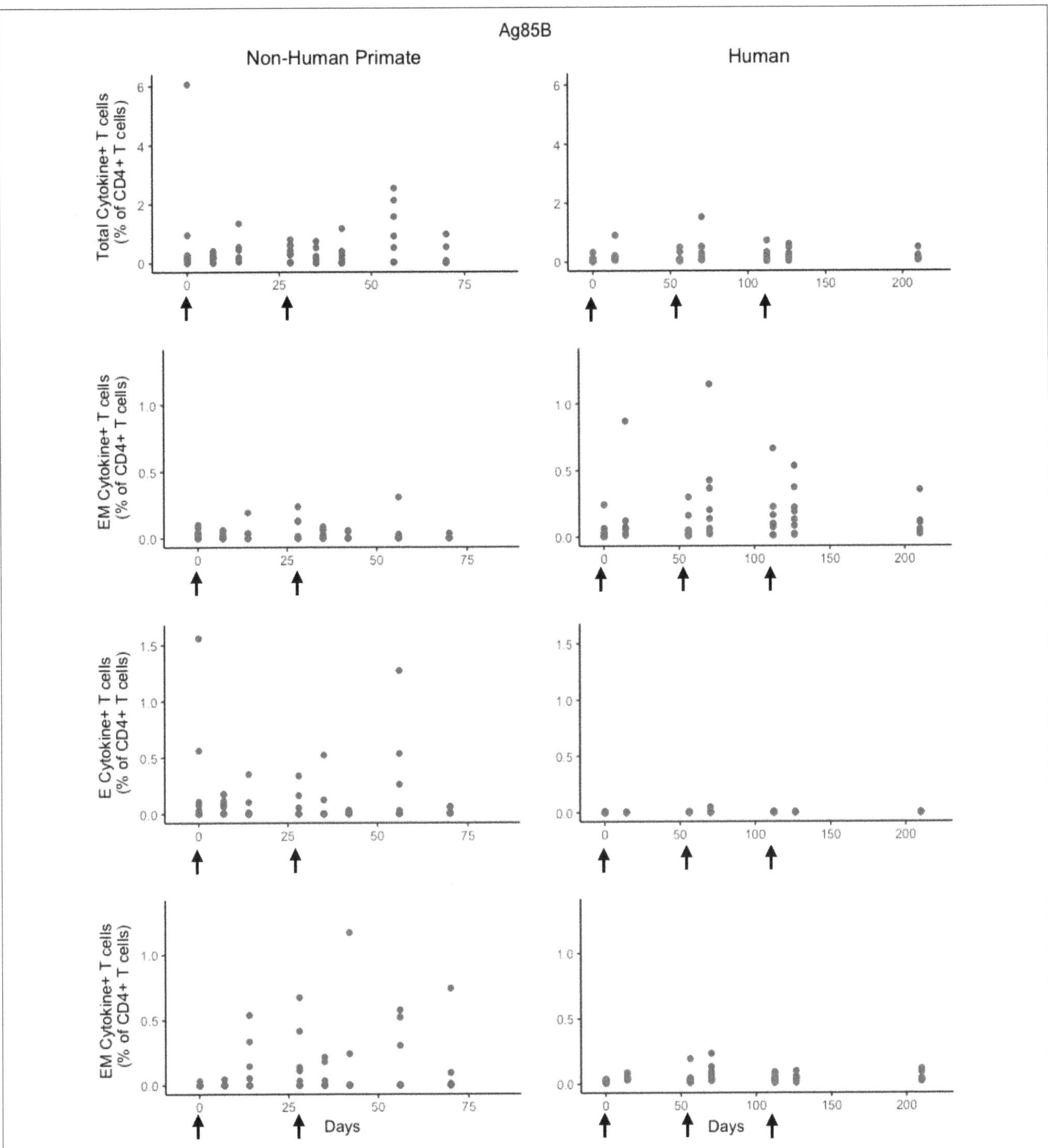

FIGURE 5 | Human and NHP experimental data show different responses to Ag85B antigen following H56 vaccination. The percentage of blood CD4+ T cells that respond to Ag85B by producing cytokines (cytokine+) is divided by the total number of CD4+ T cells in the blood. T cell subtypes are also shown. Each time point shows the responses of all 8 human (red) or all 8 NHPs (blue) subjects (some responses overlap, so it might be difficult to see 8 distinct dots). For comparison, we placed both panels of data on the same y-axis. Arrows represent vaccination timepoints.

precursor T cells in the LN. Thus, the percentage of central memory T cells should contract within blood.

The human simulations also capture the variability of the human dataset as well as the general trends, as shown by the median red line. A visual comparison between the parameter ranges is displayed in **Supplementary Materials 2** using radar charts. Altogether, we show that our mathematical model can capture the Ag85B immunogenicity dataspace of NHPs and humans with species-specific parameter ranges.

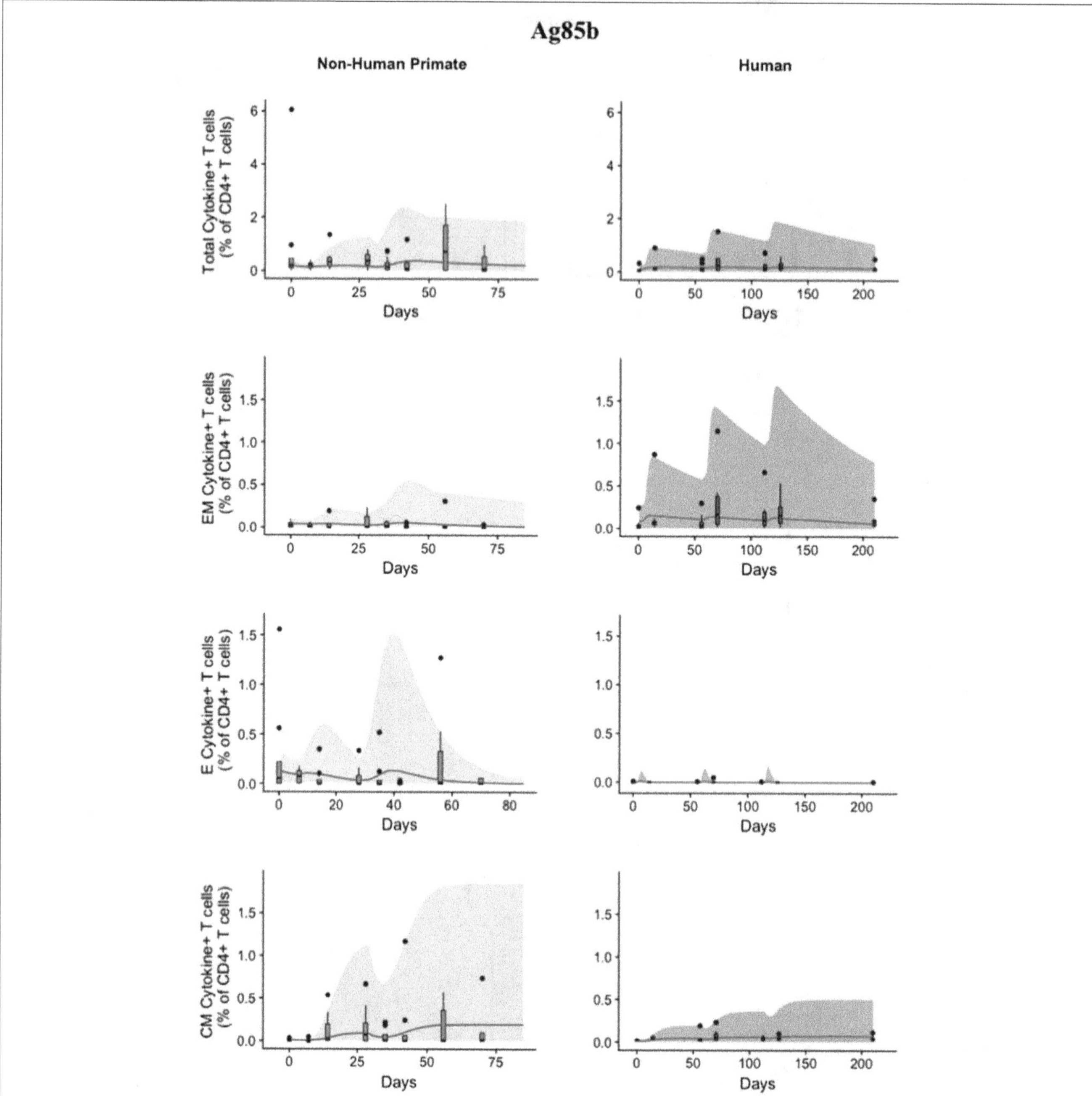

FIGURE 6 | Model can fit diverse responses of both NHP and Humans to Ag85B antigen following H56 vaccination. The percentage of blood CD4+ T cells that respond to Ag85B by producing cytokines (cytokine+) is divided by the total number of CD4+ T cells in the blood. T cell subtypes are also shown. Each time point shows the responses of all 8 human (red) or all 8 NHPs (blue) subjects as a box and whisker plot. Whiskers were created in the same manner as the ESAT6 datasets. Simulation data are displayed as a blue or red cloud that outline the min and max of 500 runs for NHP or human calibrations, respectively. The blue or red line represents the median of those simulations and demonstrates that the model captures the general behavior of the data, by traveling through the interquartile range of at least 4 of the 8 timepoints for each subpopulation of T cells. Exact parameters ranges used to generate the simulation curves for NHP and human CD4+Ag85B+ T cells are shown in **Supplementary Table 1**.

Differences in BCG Timing Between Humans and NHPs Is Captured by Initial Conditions

Throughout our calibration process, we were aware of the potential for the timing of BCG priming events to influence the immune response of each species to Ag85B (as NHPs received BCG vaccination 70 days before H56 vaccination and humans received their BCG vaccination roughly 30 years before the clinical trial began – see Methods and **Figure 1**). Instead of explicitly modeling a BCG vaccination event 70 days or 30 years

TABLE 2 | Initial conditions represent the difference in BCG timing between experimental protocols.

Initial condition of cell type		ESAT6		Ag85b	
		NHP	Human	NHP	Human
	Units	Range of values	Range of values	Range of values	Range of values
Naïve CD4+ specific Blood T cells	cell/mm^3	(0.1,0.25)	(0.07, 0.6)	(0.17,0.37)	(0.04,0.27)
Effector CD4+ specific Blood T cells	cell/mm^3	(0.001,1.5)	0	(0.001,2.5)	0
Central Memory CD4+ specific Blood T cells	cell/mm^3	(0.0015,0.006)	(0.00002, 0.03)	(0.002,0.2)	(0.02,0.3)
Effector Memory CD4+ specific Blood T cells	cell/mm^3	(0.001,0.5)	(0.003, 0.15)	(0.003, 0.9)	(0.0016,2.6)
Naïve CD4+ nonspecific Blood T cells	cell/mm^3	(160,240)	(100,600)	(241,361)	(59,272)
Effector CD4+ nonspecific Blood T cells	cell/mm^3	(200,800)	(530,110)	(445, 670)	(358,875)
Central Memory CD4+ nonspecific Blood T cells	cell/mm^3	(1,3)	(0.009,10)	(1,100)	(10,100)
Effector Memory CD4+ nonspecific Blood T cells	cell/mm^3	(1,150)	(1,22)	(1,300)	(0.3,370)
Naïve CD4+ specific LN T cells	cell count	(91957, 322492)	(8255,111806)	(144500,546200)	(5000,5720)
Precursor CD4+ specific LN T cells	cell count	0	0	(6770, 10150)	0
Effector CD4+ specific LN T cells	cell count	0	0	(22,34)	0
Central Memory CD4+ specific LN T cells	cell count	(1295,7878)	(3.4, 5046)	(2377,285871)	(3132, 59431)
Effector Memory CD4+ specific LN T cells	cell count	0	0	(828,1241)	0
Naïve CD4+ nonspecific LN T cells	cell count	(123430594,355639025)	(11839508, 122029962)	(177300481, 535316901)	(7865162, 53811216)
Central Memory CD4+ nonspecific LN T cells	cell count	(775507,4253381)	(1229, 1895598)	(1219316, 134489106)	(1401106, 19893946)
APC (Prime Vaccination of H56)	cell count	(150,800)	(200,500)	(350,500)	(500,1000)
APC (Boost Vaccination 1 of H56)	cell count	(50, 150)	(200,500)	(250,500)	(400,600)
APC (Boost Vaccination 2 of H56)	cell count	***** *****	(200,500)	***** *****	(400,600)

*The disparity between initial condition values that preceded the NHP response and those corresponding values for the human response represent the impact of prior presentation of Ag85B via BCG on the system. ***** signifies that NHP experimental protocol did not give the NHPs a second boost of H56 vaccination.*

TABLE 3 | Significant PRCCs for Ag85B immune response outcomes.

Ag85B	Central memory	Effector	Effector memory
NHP	central memory reactivation rate; Likelihood of differentiation; precursor proliferation and differentiation into central memory cells; APC and precursor death rates	Likelihood of differentiation; precursor proliferation and differentiation into effector cells; effector, APC, and precursor death rates	precursor proliferation and differentiation into effector cells; APC and precursor death rates
Human	Likelihood of proliferation; precursor proliferation and differentiation into central memory; central memory recruitment rate; APC and precursor death rates	Likelihood of proliferation and differentiation; naïve T cell recruitment; precursor proliferation and differentiation to effector; effector differentiation to effector memory; effector Lymph efflux; effector, APC, and precursor death rates	Likelihood of proliferation; precursor Proliferation; effector memory, APC, and precursor death rates

One row represents humans, the other represents NHPs. Columns list the 3 model outcomes of interest–Ag85B-specific central memory, effector and effector memory T cell phenotypes. These outcomes were selected for analysis because the model was calibrated to their dataspace. Each table cell contains a general description of significant (i.e., $p < 10^{-3}$) parameters with respect to outputs of the model.

prior to H56 vaccination, we varied initial concentrations of memory cell types in the LN and blood as a proxy for these BCG vaccinations. The initial cell concentrations represent the value of memory antigen-specific T cells within the system. That is, these T cells, prior to vaccination with H56, were specific for the Ag85B antigen. The initial condition values that led to the best model fits for both NHP and human T cell response are shown in **Table 2**. Note that the abbreviated time between BCG and H56 vaccinations for NHPs meant that many precursor CD4+ T cells were present in the LN; this population may well have waned in humans who were vaccinated many years (to decades) prior. As a portion of these precursor T cells differentiate into central memory T cells and effector T cells, the BCG vaccination event enabled the model to recapitulate the immunogenicity dataspaces for these two T cell subpopulations and could also explain the larger NHP response to the vaccine.

Sensitivity Analysis Reveals Both Similar and Distinct Outcome Drivers Across Species in Magnitude of T-Cell Responses to Ag85B Antigen

We performed uncertainty and sensitivity analysis on the same 3 model outcomes as the ESAT6 response analysis to identify important processes in CD4+ T cell response to Ag85B in each species. We identified factors, such as CD4+ central memory cell recruitment, to be significantly associated with changes in T cell response subpopulations (**Table 3**). Uncertainty and sensitivity analysis also revealed a crucial role for CD4+

Precursor proliferation and half-saturation rates within the lymph node compartment (**Table 3**).

Modest differences also exist in the mechanisms driving model fits for NHP and human (see **Supplementary Table 1**). In addition to the stark differences in initial conditions (from BCG timing), uncertainty and sensitivity analysis predicts that in NHPs, central memory reactivation rates were significantly associated with the total CD4+Ag85B+ response outcome. The importance of reactivation in the central memory population supports not only the role of BCG memory in this system, but could indirectly explain the late increase in Ag85B+ effector cells around day 56 (as the central memory cells that reactivate become precursor cells that, in turn, can become effector cells). Overall, the human and NHP Ag85B responses differ in values of initial conditions, central memory reactivation, and T cell differentiation. Despite these differences, like the ESAT6 response, we predict that the Ag85B response in NHPs and humans are generally alike–this similarity hints at a general secondary response that is conserved across species.

Secondary Response to Ag85B Antigen Is Characterized by the Upregulation of Differentiation to Central Memory Phenotype

If we consider the T cell response of NHP and humans to ESAT6 as the epitome of each species' primary response to an antigen in vaccination, then we can view the parameter values that recapitulate the Ag85B response (a secondary response to the same antigen) as a BCG-induced modification to the parameter values that captured the ESAT6 response. For NHPs (blue) and humans (red), three parameters (k5, k6, k7) are represented on each axis of the radar charts for ESAT6 and Ag85B (**Figure 7**). Notice that, for each species, the radar charts include the maximum value for each parameter across the ESAT6 and Ag85B response fits. In the ESAT6 radar charts, both NHPs and humans skew toward the differentiation of effector and effector memory T cell phenotypes. As neither species has encountered ESAT6 prior to H56 vaccination, the relatively high rates of differentiation to effector and effector memory T cell phenotypes constitute a primary response that may be conserved across species.

Ag85B is an antigen that was first presented in BCG vaccination; if we compare the dynamics of ESAT6 responses to the dynamics of Ag85B responses, we can predict the BCG-induced modifications to T-cell differentiation during secondary responses to the same antigen. In the Ag85B radar charts, both species' ranges for differentiation to effector and effector memory become relatively smaller than the ranges that fit the ESAT6 response. Further, the ranges for the parameter that captures differentiation to a central memory phenotype grow larger relative to the ranges shown in ESAT6 response. We speculate that this change in response is conserved across species - upon secondary response to the same antigen, both species' precursor T-cell populations upregulate the production of a central memory phenotype during differentiation.

DISCUSSION

In the pursuit of a vaccine that can confer long-term, consistent immunity against TB, H56 is one new vaccine candidate. However, the role of prior BCG vaccination on H56 immunogenicity is unclear. In addition, the differences between NHP–a useful model animal for vaccine studies - and human responses to H56 has not been explicitly characterized. Identifying the influence of BCG on H56 vaccination and characterizing the species-specific responses to H56 will better facilitate our understanding of H56 immunogenicity and could potentially pave the way for more effective therapies. In addition, we strive to elaborate how computational modeling can assist with vaccine development and testing.

In this work, we used a systems biology approach that utilized mathematical modeling to explore both NHP and human response datasets to H56. We calibrated our two-compartment mathematical model to the ESAT6 and Ag85B immunogenicity dataspaces for both NHPs and humans. This calibration allowed us to study pre-exposure vaccination dynamics such as antigen presentation, T cell priming, and differentiation in both the lymph node and blood. Specifically, we utilized antigen specificity to draw our main conclusion: *BCG similarly influences H56 immunogenicity in both NHPs and humans* by upregulating differentiation to the central memory phenotype in the Ag85B-specific CD4+ T cell response. While Lin *et al.* found that H56 boosts the effects of BCG and prevents reactivation of latent infection (Lin et al., 2012), to our knowledge no one has documented the direct impact of prior BCG on H56 immunogenicity.

Using mathematical modeling, we were also able to isolate the impact of BCG timing differences on H56 immunogenicity. We discovered that the narrow window between BCG prime and H56 vaccination in NHPs promotes a larger quantity of antigen-specific cells that reside in the lymph node prior to H56 vaccination. Calibration to the Ag85B immunogenicity dataspace for NHPs revealed a much larger initial number of precursor T cells in the lymph node than the number of initial precursor cells that were required for calibration to the human data. The difference in timing of BCG for the NHP experimental protocol (70 days prior to H56 vaccination) and human experimental protocol (up to decades before H56) explains the necessary differences required in model initial conditions to capture these events. Experimental assessment of vaccines in NHPs preclude the administration of BCG years prior to boosting with a subunit vaccine, due to costs. However, our data indicate that the timing of BCG and booster vaccines strongly influence the subsequent immune responses. Whether this also affects protection conferred by a vaccine remains to be tested.

Using uncertainty and sensitivity analysis, we found that each species' response to H56 vaccination was generally similar. While each species resides in a separate parameter space, the general dynamics dictating the H56 immune response was quite similar. This finding contrasts with previous findings

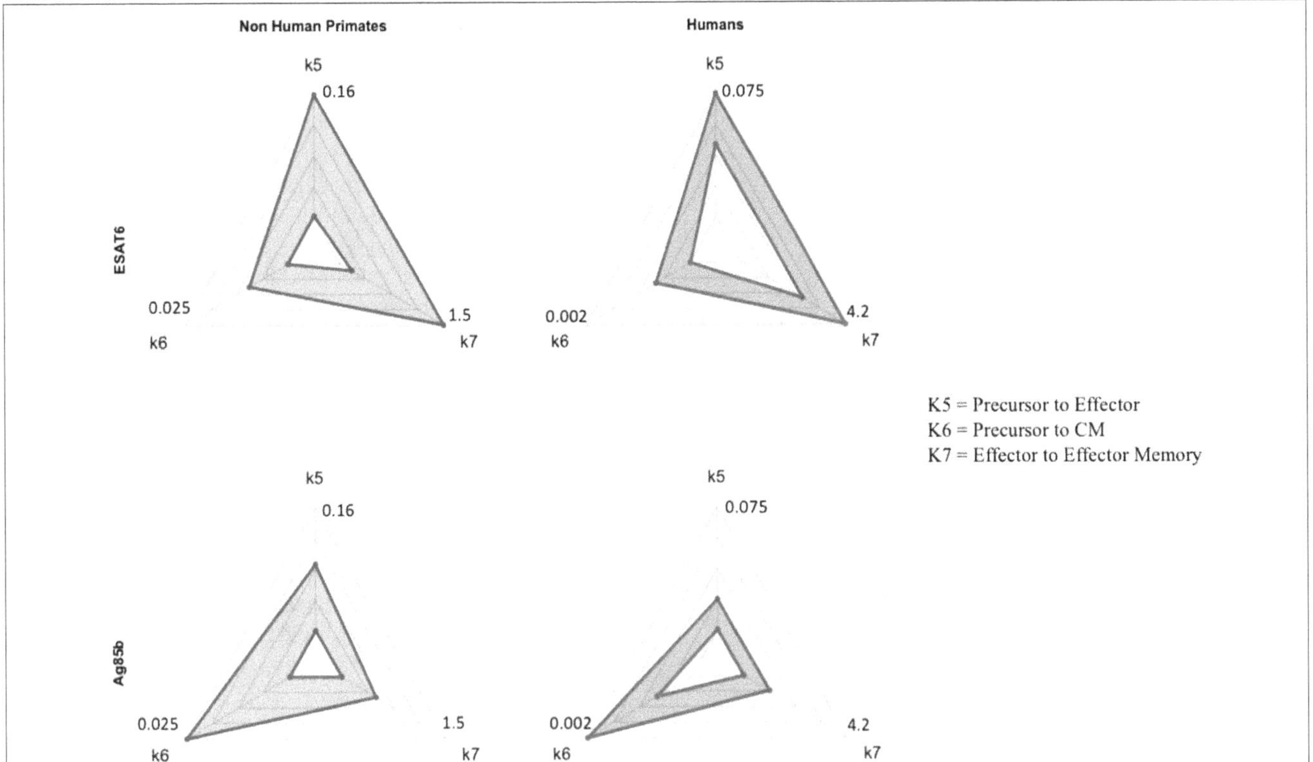

FIGURE 7 | Radar charts reveal impact of immunological memory in response to Ag85B. We display 4 radar charts (see **Supplementary Materials 2** and Methods) that visually represent the parameter space for several key parameters (as identified by PRCC) in model fits for both species and antigens. Each chart includes the maximum value of each parameter (for each species) on the diagrams. The top chart shows the parameter ranges that fit the ESAT6 immunogenicity dataspace. The bottom radar chart displays the parameter ranges that fit the Ag85B immunogenicity dataspace. These parameters were picked as they represent T-cell differentiation rates to central memory (k6), effector (k5), and effector memory (k7) T cell phenotypes. Each parameter space is represented by a blue (NHP) or red (human) band, which represents the min and max parameter value for each model fit. **Supplementary Table 1** shows the numerical values of the parameter ranges. To directly compare the impact of BCG memory on the H56 immune response, we created the Human radar charts with a minimum and maximum for each axis defined by the minimum and maximum parameter value across Human model fits to ESAT6 or Ag85B. We created the NHP radar charts by displaying the parameter ranges within the min and maximum values across NHP model fits to either antigen. Viewers should not compare the charts from left to right, as the human charts display a parameter range that is wholly distinct from that of the non-human primates. For each species, the maximum values for each parameter are displayed at the edges of the radar charts.

that show the immune response of monkeys and humans to SIV or HIV (respectively) differs (Davenport et al., 2004; Yang and Ganusov, 2017), however, like many others in the field of TB research, we conclude that NHPs are a good model for human responses (Kaushal et al., 2012; Scanga and Flynn, 2014; Flynn et al., 2015; Peña and Ho, 2015). However, one consistent difference between NHP and human response were observed. Unlike the NHP response, the humans' central memory, effector, and effector memory T cell phenotypes was significantly negatively correlated with the half-saturation values of proliferation and differentiation in both the ESAT6 and Ag85B immunogenicity dataspaces. As the half-saturation values in our model measure the affinity (or likelihood) of a cell to proliferate or differentiate upon priming, our findings suggest that humans differ from NHPs in the ability of T cells to quickly react to H56 vaccination antigens within lymph nodes. Perhaps presentation of these antigens to T cells is not as effective in humans as it is in NHPs. We indirectly modeled adjuvant impact on vaccination (see Methods); however, a more mechanistic approach may be necessary to elucidate these species-specific differences in antigen uptake and presentation.

Furthermore, uncertainty and sensitivity analysis revealed an intriguing result regarding the human experimental protocol. Throughout our analysis, the number of APCs that entered the system via vaccinations (prime or boost events) was significantly, positively, associated with cellular responses in the blood. However, our analysis also showed that the number of APCs that entered the system as a result of the second boosting event (third H56 vaccination event) for humans did not significantly impact the number of central memory T cells within the blood compartment. This result agrees with the previous finding that 50 ug of H56 is too high of a dose (Luabeya et al., 2015), resulting in large effector responses that may be suboptimal for long-term memory. As one major goal of any vaccination is to provide long lasting immunity in the form of immunological memory, our computational analysis has revealed that the third dose was likely redundant and that optimization of dose using computational predictions could have potentially improved outcomes, especially prior to the clinical trial. In the future our systems biology approach together with virtual clinical trials could help investigate these issues and assist in improving the vaccine pipeline.

One potential limitation of this study is that our current model represents the complex processes of proliferation, differentiation, and reactivation rates as a single parameter with a range of values. We believe this suffices since our goal was to identify the role of BCG in H56 vaccination response across humans and NHPs. However, future investigations into the processes dictating proliferation, differentiation, or reactivation could create a more detailed mathematical model including those details. In fact, the field of T-cell memory and the exact mechanisms of reactivation have been extensively studied (Harrington et al., 2008; MacLeod et al., 2010; Akondy et al., 2017; Youngblood et al., 2017). Conversely, phenomenological modeling has provided insights for T cell expansion (Davenport et al., 2004; Antia et al., 2005; Akondy et al., 2015). Future work could discuss the benefits of mechanistic or phenomenological models when addressing distinct questions about proliferation, differentiation, or reactivation.

In summary, we used a systems biology approach that combined NHP and human datasets with mathematical modeling to better understand the differences between NHP and human immune response to H56 vaccination. Specifically, we showed that each primate species had a similar response to H56, identified the role of BCG timing on H56 vaccination, and discovered that BCG similarly influences H56 immunogenicity in humans and NHPs.

Beyond the scope of this paper, we could have characterized other comparisons between humans and NHPs. For example, future studies could identify the species-specific differences during TB infection, identify the adaptive immune response differences to other antigens, or capture the dissimilarities of each species' innate immune response to adjuvant. Further, future studies could also model the cellular dynamics following H56 vaccination before, during, or after TB infection in an effort to evaluate the potential success of this vaccine candidate. We argue that a systems biology approach that melds mathematical modeling together with experimental and clinical studies has the greatest potential to discover, predict, and evaluate new vaccination strategies that could end the TB epidemic.

AUTHOR CONTRIBUTIONS

LJ, EP, JL, and DK performed mathematical modeling, data analysis. LJ, EP, JL, DK, TS, and JF contributed conception and design of the study. RD and JF prepared and sorted NHP dataset. SS, BK, and TS prepared and sorted the human H56 dataset. All authors contributed to writing and editing of this manuscript.

FUNDING

This research was supported by the following grants: NIH: R01 AI123093, R01 HL110811, U01HL131072.

ACKNOWLEDGMENTS

We are grateful to Dr. Peter Andersen, Statens Serum Institut, for providing the H56 vaccine for the NHP studies. Also, we thank Stephanie Thiede for early efforts on this project and we thank Paul Wolberg for technical support.

SUPPLEMENTARY MATERIAL

Supplementary Figure 1 | Radar charts reveal parameter space differences between species. Each parameter space is represented by a blue (NHP) or red (human) band, which represents the min and max parameter value for each model fit. Each chart displays parameter names around its outside boundary, at each axis. Parameter names are ordered alphabetically starting with 'hs1' and 'ending with xi6'. Points near the center of each axis represent a lower value whereas points near the outer edges of each axis represent larger values. To compare parameter ranges across species, we calculated the minimum and maximum for each axis on the charts as the minimum and maximum value for each parameter across all species and antigen specific fits.

Supplementary Table 1 | Parameter ranges for model fits of the ESAT6 and Ag85B response in humans and NHPs. Parameter names, descriptions, units, and ranges are listed.

Supplementary Table 2 | Parameter names in radar charts. The leftmost column shows the name of each parameter. The rightmost column displays a short description of each parameter.

REFERENCES

Aagaard, C., Hoang, T., Dietrich, J., Cardona, P.-J., Izzo, A., Dolganov, G., et al. (2011). A multistage tuberculosis vaccine that confers efficient protection before and after exposure. *Nat. Med.* 17, 189–194. doi: 10.1038/nm.2285

Agger, E. M. (2016). Novel adjuvant formulations for delivery of anti-tuberculosis vaccine candidates. *Adv. Drug Deliv. Rev.* 102, 73–82. doi: 10.1016/j.addr.2015.11.012

Ahsan, M. J. (2015). Recent advances in the development of vaccines for tuberculosis. *Ther. Adv. Vaccines* 3, 66–75. doi: 10.1177/2051013615593891

Akondy, R. S., Fitch, M., Edupuganti, S., Yang, S., Kissick, H. T., Li, K. W., et al. (2017). Origin and differentiation of human memory CD8 T cells after vaccination. *Nature* 552: 362. doi: 10.1038/nature24633

Akondy, R. S., Johnson, P. L. F., Nakaya, H. I., Edupuganti, S., Mulligan, M. J., Lawson, B., et al. (2015). Initial viral load determines the magnitude of the human CD8 T cell response to yellow fever vaccination. *Proc. Natl. Acad. Sci. U.S.A.* 112, 3050–3055. doi: 10.1073/pnas.1500475112

Andersen, P., and Doherty, T. M. (2005). Opinion: the success and failure of BCG — implications for a novel tuberculosis vaccine. *Nat. Rev. Microbiol.* 3, 656–662. doi: 10.1038/nrmicro1211

Antia, R., Ganusov, V. V., and Ahmed, R. (2005). The role of models in understanding CD8+ T-cell memory. *Nat. Rev. Immunol.* 5, 101–111. doi: 10.1038/nri1550

Betts, J. C., Lukey, P. T., Robb, L. C., McAdam, R. A., and Duncan, K. (2002). Evaluation of a nutrient starvation model of Mycobacterium tuberculosis persistence by gene and protein expression profiling. *Mol. Microbiol.* 43, 717–731. doi: 10.1046/j.1365-2958.2002.02779.x

Brandt, L., Elhay, M., Rosenkrands, I., Lindblad, E. B., and Andersen, P. (2000). ESAT-6 subunit vaccination against Mycobacterium tuberculosis. *Infect. Immun.* 68, 791–795. doi: 10.1128/IAI.68.2.791-795.2000

Colditz, G. A., Berkey, C. S., Mosteller, F., Brewer, T. F., Wilson, M. E., Burdick, E., et al. (1995). The efficacy of bacillus Calmette-Guérin vaccination of newborns and infants in the prevention of tuberculosis: meta-analyses of the published literature. *Pediatrics* 96, 29–35.

Cole, S. T., Brosch, R., Parkhill, J., Garnier, T., Churcher, C., Harris, D., et al. (1998). Deciphering the biology of Mycobacterium tuberculosis from the complete genome sequence. *Nature* 393, 537–544. doi: 10.1038/31159

Davenport, M. P., Ribeiro, R. M., and Perelson, A. S. (2004). Kinetics of virus-specific $CD8^+$ T cells and the control of human immunodeficiency virus infection. *J. Virol.* 78, 10096–10103. doi: 10.1128/JVI.78.18.10096-10103.2004

Evans, T. G., Schrager, L., and Thole, J. (2016). Status of vaccine research and development of vaccines for tuberculosis. *Vaccine* 34, 2911–2914. doi: 10.1016/j.vaccine.2016.02.079

Fine, P. E. M. (1995). Variation in protection by BCG: implications of and for heterologous immunity. *Lancet* 346, 1339–1345. doi: 10.1016/S0140-6736(95)92348-9

Flynn, J. L., Gideon, H. P., Mattila, J. T., and Lin, P. (2015). Immunology studies in non-human primate models of tuberculosis. *Immunol. Rev.* 264, 60–73. doi: 10.1111/imr.12258

Fourie, P. B. (1987). BCG vaccination and the EPI. *South African Med. J.* 72, 323–326.

Ganguly, N., Giang, P. H., Gupta, C., Basu, S. K., Siddiqui, I., Salunke, D. M., et al. (2008). Mycobacterium tuberculosis secretory proteins CFP-10, ESAT-6 and the CFP10:ESAT6 complex inhibit lipopolysaccharide-induced NF-κB transactivation by downregulation of reactive oxidative species (ROS) production. *Immunol. Cell Biol.* 86, 98–106. doi: 10.1038/sj.icb.7100117

Gong, C., Linderman, J. J., and Kirschner, D. (2014). Harnessing the heterogeneity of T cell differentiation fate to fine-tune generation of effector and memory T cells. *Front. Immunol.* 5:57. doi: 10.3389/fimmu.2014.00057

Gonzalo-Asensio, J., Dessislava, M., Carlos, M., and Aguilo, N. (2017). MTBVAC: attenuating the human pathogen of tuberculosis (TB) toward a promising vaccine against the TB Epidemic. *Front. Immunol.* 8:1803. doi: 10.3389/fimmu.2017.01803

Govender, L., Abel, B., Hughes, E. J., Scriba, T. J., Kagina, B. M. N., de Kock, M., et al. (2010). Higher human CD4 T cell response to novel Mycobacterium tuberculosis latency associated antigens Rv2660 and Rv2659 in latent infection compared with tuberculosis disease. *Vaccine* 29, 51–57. doi: 10.1016/j.vaccine.2010.10.022

Harrington, L. E., Janowski, K. M., Oliver, J. R., Zajac, A. J., and Weaver, C. T. (2008). Memory CD4 T cells emerge from effector T-cell progenitors. *Nature* 452, 356. doi: 10.1038/nature06672

Horwitz, M. A., Lee, B. W., Dillon, B. J., and Harth, G. (1995). Protective immunity against tuberculosis induced by vaccination with major extracellular proteins of *Mycobacterium tuberculosis*. *Proc. Natl. Acad. Sci. U.S.A.* 92, 1530–1534. doi: 10.1073/pnas.92.5.1530

Kamath, A. T., Valenti, M. P., Rochat, A. F., Agger, E. M., Lingnau, K., von Gabain, A., et al. (2008). Protective anti-mycobacterial T cell responses through exquisite *in vivo* activation of vaccine-targeted dendritic cells. *Eur. J. Immunol.* 38, 1247–1256. doi: 10.1002/eji.200737889

Kaushal, D., Mehra, S., Didier, P. J., and Lackner, A. A. (2012). The non-human primate model of tuberculosis. *J. Med. Primatol.* 41, 191–201. doi: 10.1111/j.1600-0684.2012.00536.x

Lanckriet, C., Lévy-bruhl, D., Bingono, E., Siopathis, R. M., and Guérin, N. (1995). Efficacy of BCG vaccination of the newborn: evaluation by a follow-up study of contacts in Bangui. *Int. J. Epidemiol.* 24, 1042–1049. doi: 10.1093/ije/24.5.1042

Langermans, J. A. M., Doherty, T. M., Vervenne, R. A. W., Van Der Laan, T., Lyashchenko, K., Greenwald, R., et al. (2005). Protection of macaques against *Mycobacterium tuberculosis* infection by a subunit vaccine based on a fusion protein of antigen 85B and ESAT-6. *Vaccine* 23, 2740–2750. doi: 10.1016/j.vaccine.2004.11.051

Lin, P. L., Dietrich, J., Tan, E., Abalos, R. M., Burgos, J., Bigbee, C., et al. (2012). The multistage vaccine H56 boosts the effects of BCG to protect cynomolgus macaques against active tuberculosis and reactivation of latent Mycobacterium tuberculosis infection. *J. Clin. Invest.* 122, 303–314. doi: 10.1172/JCI46252

Luabeya, A. K. K., Kagina, B. M. N., Tameris, M. D., Geldenhuys, H., Hoff, S. T., Shi, Z., et al. (2015). First-in-human trial of the post-exposure tuberculosis vaccine H56: IC31 in Mycobacterium tuberculosis infected and non-infected healthy adults. *Vaccine* 33, 4130–4140. doi: 10.1016/j.vaccine.2015.06.051

MacLeod, M. K. L., Kappler, J. W., and Marrack, P. (2010). Memory CD4 T cells: generation, reactivation and re-assignment. *Immunology* 130, 10–15. doi: 10.1111/j.1365-2567.2010.03260.x

Marino, S., Gideon, H. P., Gong, C., Mankad, S., McCrone, J. T., Lin, P. L., et al. (2016). Computational and empirical studies predict *Mycobacterium tuberculosis*-specific T cells as a biomarker for infection outcome. *PLoS Comput. Biol.* 12:e1004804. doi: 10.1371/journal.pcbi.1004804

Marino, S., Hogue, I. B., Ray, C. J., and Kirschner, D. E. (2008). A methodology for performing global uncertainty and sensitivity analysis in systems biology. *J. Theor. Biol.* 254, 178–196. doi: 10.1016/j.jtbi.2008.04.011

Marino, S., and Kirschner, D. (2016). A Multi-compartment hybrid computational model predicts key roles for dendritic cells in tuberculosis infection. *Computation* 4, 39. doi: 10.3390/computation4040039

Mittal, S. K., Aggarwal, V., Rastogi, A., and Saini, N. (1996). Does B.C.G. vaccination prevent or postpone the occurrence of tuberculous meningitis? *Indian J. Pediatr.* 63, 659–664.

Moliva, J. I., Turner, J., and Torrelles, J. B. (2017). Immune responses to bacillus Calmette-Guérin vaccination: why do they fail to protect against mycobacterium tuberculosis? *Front. Immunol.* 8:407. doi: 10.3389/fimmu.2017.00407

Mustafa, A. S., Oftung, F., Amoudy, H. A., Madi, N. M., Abal, A. T., Shaban, F., et al. (2000a). Multiple epitopes from the *Mycobacterium tuberculosis* ESAT-6 antigen are recognized by antigen-specific human T cell lines. *Clin. Infect. Dis.* 30(Suppl. 3): S201–S205. doi: 10.1086/313862

Mustafa, A. S., Shaban, F. A., Abal, A. T., Al-Attiyah, R., Wiker, H. G., Lundin, K. E. A., et al. (2000b). Identification and HLA restriction of naturally derived Th1-cell epitopes from the secreted *Mycobacterium tuberculosis* antigen 85B recognized by antigen-specific human CD4+ T-cell lines. *Infect. Immun.* 68, 3933–3940. doi: 10.1128/IAI.68.7.3933-3940.2000

Nakazawa, M. (2017). *fmsb: Functions for Medical Statistics Book with some Demographic Data*. Available online at: https://cran.r-project.org/package=fmsb

Olsen, A. W., Van Pinxteren, L. A. H., Okkels, L. M., Rasmussen, P. B., and Andersen, P. (2001). Protection of mice with a tuberculosis subunit vaccine based on a fusion protein of antigen 85B and ESAT-6. *Infect. Immun.* 69, 2773–2778. doi: 10.1128/IAI.69.5.2773-2778.2001

Olsen, A. W., Williams, A., Okkels, L. M., Hatch, G., and Andersen, P. (2004). Protective effect of a tuberculosis subunit vaccine based on a fusion of antigen 85B and ESAT-6 in the aerosol guinea pig model. *Infect. Immun.* 72, 6148–6150. doi: 10.1128/IAI.72.10.6148-6150.2004

Peña, J. C., and Ho, W. Z. (2015). Monkey models of tuberculosis: lessons learned. *Infect. Immun.* 83, 852–862. doi: 10.1128/IAI.02850-14

Rohde, K. H., Veiga, D. F. T., Caldwell, S., Balázsi, G., and Russell, D. G. (2012). Linking the transcriptional profiles and the physiological states of Mycobacterium tuberculosis during an extended intracellular infection. *PLoS Pathog.* 8:e1002769. doi: 10.1371/journal.ppat.1002769

Ronning, D. R., Klabunde, T., Besra, G. S., Vissa, V. D., Belisle, J. T., and Sacchettini, J. C. (2000). Crystal structure of the secreted form of antigen 85C reveals potential targets for mycobacterial drugs and vaccines. *Nat. Struct. Biol.* 7, 141–146. doi: 10.1038/72413

Scanga, C. A., and Flynn, J. L. (2014). Modeling tuberculosis in nonhuman primates. *Cold Spring Harb. Perspect. Med.* 4:a018564. doi: 10.1101/cshperspect.a018564

Sterne, J. A. C., Rodrigues, L. C., and Guedes, I. N. (1998). Does the efficacy of BCG decline with time since vaccination? *Int. J. Tuberc. Lung Dis.* 2, 200–207

Tameris, M. D., Hatherill, M., Landry, B. S., Scriba, T. J., Snowden, M. A., Lockhart, S., et al. (2013). Safety and efficacy of MVA85A, a new tuberculosis vaccine, in infants previously vaccinated with BCG: a randomised, placebo-controlled phase 2b trial. *Lancet* 381, 1021–1028. doi: 10.1016/S0140-6736(13)60177-4

WHO (2016). *WHO Global Tuberculosis Report 2016*. Geneva: World Health Organization

Wickham, H. (2009). *ggplot2: Elegant Graphics for Data Analysis*. Available online at: http://ggplot2.org

Wickham, H. (2011). The split-apply-combine strategy for data analysis. *J. Stat. Softw.* 40, 1–29. doi: 10.18637/jss.v040.i01

Wickham, H., and Henry, L. (2017). *tidyr: Easily Tidy Data with "spread()" and "gather()" Functions.* Available online at: https://cran.r-project.org/package=tidyr

Wilkinson, R. J., DesJardin, L. E., Islam, N., Gibson, B. M., Andrew Kanost, R., Wilkinson, K. A., et al. (2001). An increase in expression of a Mycobacterium tuberculosis mycolyl transferase gene (fbpB) occurs early after infection of human monocytes. *Mol. Microbiol.* 39, 813–821. doi: 10.1046/j.1365-2958.2001.02280.x

Yang, Y., and Ganusov, V. V. (2017). Defining kinetic properties of HIV-specific CD8+ T-cell responses in acute infection. *bioRxiv[Preprint].* bioRxiv. doi: 10.1101/158683

Youngblood, B., Hale, J. S., Kissick, H. T., Ahn, E., Xu, X., Wieland, A., et al. (2017). Effector CD8 T cells dedifferentiate into long-lived memory cells. *Nature* 552, 404. doi: 10.1038/nature25144

Ziraldo, C., Gong, C., Kirschner, D. E., and Linderman, J. J. (2016). Strategic priming with multiple antigens can yield memory cellphenotypes optimized for infection with mycobacterium tuberculosis: A computational study. *Front. Microbiol.* 6:1477. doi: 10.3389/fmicb.2015.01477

Zodpey, S. P., Shrikhande, S. N., Maldhure, B. R., Vasudeo, N. D., and Kulkarni, S. W. (1998). Effectiveness of Bacillus Calmette Guerin (BCG) vaccination in the prevention of childhood pulmonary tuberculosis : a case control study in Nagpur, India. *Southeast Asian J. Trop. Med. Public Health* 29, 285–288.

14

Kinetics of HIV-Specific CTL Responses Plays a Minimal Role in Determining HIV Escape Dynamics

Yiding Yang[1]* *and Vitaly V. Ganusov*[1,2,3]

[1] *Department of Microbiology, University of Tennessee, Knoxville, TN, United States,* [2] *National Institute for Mathematical and Biological Synthesis, University of Tennessee, Knoxville, TN, United States,* [3] *Department of Mathematics, University of Tennessee, Knoxville, TN, United States*

Correspondence:
Yiding Yang
yyang42@utk.edu

Cytotoxic T lymphocytes (CTLs) have been suggested to play an important role in controlling human immunodeficiency virus (HIV-1 or simply HIV) infection. HIV, due to its high mutation rate, can evade recognition of T cell responses by generating escape variants that cannot be recognized by HIV-specific CTLs. Although HIV escape from CTL responses has been well documented, factors contributing to the timing and the rate of viral escape from T cells have not been fully elucidated. Fitness costs associated with escape and magnitude of the epitope-specific T cell response are generally considered to be the key in determining timing of HIV escape. Several previous analyses generally ignored the kinetics of T cell responses in predicting viral escape by either considering constant or maximal T cell response; several studies also considered escape from different T cell responses to be independent. Here, we focus our analysis on data from two patients from a recent study with relatively frequent measurements of both virus sequences and HIV-specific T cell response to determine impact of CTL kinetics on viral escape. In contrast with our expectation, we found that including temporal dynamics of epitope-specific T cell response did not improve the quality of fit of different models to escape data. We also found that for well-sampled escape data, the estimates of the model parameters including T cell killing efficacy did not strongly depend on the underlying model for escapes: models assuming independent, sequential, or concurrent escapes from multiple CTL responses gave similar estimates for CTL killing efficacy. Interestingly, the model assuming sequential escapes (i.e., escapes occurring along a defined pathway) was unable to accurately describe data on escapes occurring rapidly within a short-time window, suggesting that some of model assumptions must be violated for such escapes. Our results thus suggest that the current sparse measurements of temporal CTL dynamics in blood bear little quantitative information to improve predictions of HIV escape kinetics. More frequent measurements using more sensitive techniques and sampling in secondary lymphoid tissues may allow to better understand whether and how CTL kinetics impacts viral escape.

Keywords: HIV, CTL escape, multiple responses, mathematical model, model fitting, likelihood

---

Abbreviations: CTL, cytotoxic T lymphocyte; HIV, human immunodeficiency virus; SIV, simian immunodeficiency virus.

1. INTRODUCTION

In 2014, the number of people living with human immunodeficiency virus 1 (HIV-1 or simply HIV) was estimated as 36.9 million (1), with roughly 2 million new HIV infections and 1.2 million people dead of HIV-induced diseases (AIDS) (2). Cytotoxic $CD8^+$ T lymphocyte (CTL) responses play an important role in control of virus replication (3, 4) by modulating some important predictors of disease progression (e.g., viral set-point and the rate of $CD4^+$ T cell loss (5)). Generation of HIV-specific $CD8^+$ T cells by vaccination is one of the current approaches in developing HIV vaccines (6, 7). However, HIV is able to generate mutants (termed "CTL escape mutants") that are not recognized by HIV-specific T cells, which may be one of the reasons for failure of T cell based vaccines (8–10). Better understanding of mechanisms of viral escape and principles governing $CD8^+$ T cell responses to HIV may allow us to evaluate *in silico* a potential efficacy of T cell-based HIV vaccines.

Viral escape from CTL responses follows a somewhat predictive pattern with more dominant (larger magnitude) CTL responses leading to earlier viral escape (11, 12). However, not every CTL response elicits an escape and sometimes viral mutations occur in regions predicted to be recognized by CTLs but in the absence of detectable response (13). To understand the timing and kinetics of CTL escape in HIV/SIV infection, mathematical models have been proposed previously on the dynamics of viral escape from a single CTL response (e.g., Ref. (14–20)). These initial models made a strong assumption of independent viral escape—i.e., it was assumed that viruses escaping from different CTL responses do not compete. Recent work, however, suggested presence of clonal interference and genetic hitchhiking among immune escape variants through reconstruction of HIV whole genome haplotypes (21), and similar concurrent CTL escapes were observed in four HIV-infected patients (22). Clonal interference was suggested to impact the estimates of the escape rates (23, 24). Even though several models have been developed to describe the dynamics of escapes from multiple CTL responses (e.g., Ref. (17, 18, 23–26)), many of these studies involved only model simulations and did not use information on the actual kinetics of HIV-specific CTL responses in predicting viral escape.

Here, we explored whether including experimentally measured CTL kinetics improves description of the viral escape data. In doing so, we compared predictions of three alternative models of viral escape from CTL responses such as independent escapes, sequential escapes, and concurrent escapes. In the first model (independent escapes), we assumed that escape from any given CTL response occurs independently of other escapes and directly from the wild-type, i.e., we ignored the effects of clonal interference—in essence assuming high effective population size and/or high recombination rate. Of note, several recent experimental papers also assumed independent escapes (11–13). In the second model (sequential escape), we assumed that escapes from different CTL responses occur along a defined pathway, generally set by the sequences of escape occurrence in the data. This model assumes strong clonal interference, which may arise at low effective population size or when recombination rate is low. Finally, in the third model (concurrent escape), we tracked all escape variants simultaneously, thus allowing for co-existence of multiple escape variants (i.e., escapes could occur along multiple alternative pathways). Interestingly, we found that for well-sampled data on virus evolution, the estimated CTL killing efficacies were independent of the model for viral escape. Some escape data could not be well described by the sequential escape model for biologically reasonable parameters. Furthermore, explicitly taking CTL kinetics into account did not improve the quality of fit of different models to escape data. Our results suggest that CTL kinetics in the blood as it is currently available may bear limited information relevant to improve description of kinetics of HIV escape from CTL responses.

2. MATERIALS AND METHODS

2.1. Experimental Data

Experimental details of patient enrollment and data collection were described in detail previously (12, 13). In short, data from 17 patients in the Center for HIV/AIDS Vaccine Immunology (CHAVI) infected acutely with HIV-1 (subtypes B or C) were analyzed in great detail. All patients were infected with a single transmitted/founder (T/F) virus as determined by the single genome amplification and sequencing (SGA/S), and there were enough samples to accurately quantify CTL response to the whole viral proteome. In each patient, the kinetics of virus-specific CTL ($CD8^+$ T cell) responses were measured using peptide-stimulated IFN-γ ELISPOT assay and/or intracellular cytokine staining (ICS) 6 months after enrollment using peptides matched to the founder virus sequence (12, 13). For CTL responses measured by ELISPOT, the reported magnitude of the response was the number of cells, producing IFN-γ, per 10^6 peripheral blood mononuclear cells (PBMC). Multiple viruses were sequenced by SGA/S, and all sequences were compared at cites coding for CTL epitopes, and changes in the percentage of transmitted (wild-type) sequences were followed over time (12). The dynamics of the HIV-specific CTL responses and viral escape from epitope-specific CTL responses were measured longitudinally. Escape mutants were identified as viral variants with mutations in regions recognized by patient's CTL responses with a reduced (or fully abrogated) production of IFN-γ following T cell stimulation. In many cases, mutation in a single position was responsible for the escape. In our analysis, all viral variants, which did not have the wild-type amino acid in the epitope region, were considered as escape variants.

Review of the virus evolution and CTL dynamics data in all 17 patients revealed some data limitations. In particular, data for many patients lacked adequate temporal resolution to accurately estimate virus escape rates. In the vast majority of viral escape variants, escapes often occurred rapidly between two sequential time points with the frequency of the escape variant jumping from 0 to 1. While previously it was suggested that such data may be modified to provide an estimate of the escape rate (14, 15, 17), such approaches may lead to biased parameter estimates (25). While development of a method for unbiased estimation of escape rate from sparse data was recently proposed (27), for this analysis, we focused on patients CH131 and CH159 in which viral escape rates could potentially be accurately estimated due to sufficiently frequent sampling. While data from these patients were presented before (12), linking of escape and CTL response dynamics was not yet performed.

2.2. Model of Viral Escape from a Single CTL Response

Models describing the dynamics of viral escape from a single cytotoxic T lymphocyte (CTL) response have been developed and adopted by different researchers (e.g., Ref. (14–18)). Here, we start with the basic model formulated earlier (18) and extend it to viral escape dynamics from multiple CTL responses. The model of viral escape from a single CTL response can be extended from the basic viral dynamics model (28) in the following way:

$$\begin{aligned}
\frac{dT(t)}{dt} &= s(T_0 - T(t)) - \beta_w T(t)V_w(t) - \beta_m T(t)V_m(t),\\
\frac{dI_w(t)}{dt} &= \beta_w(1-\mu)T(t)V_w(t) - \delta I_w(t) - kI_w(t),\\
\frac{dI_m(t)}{dt} &= \beta_m T(t)V_m(t) + \beta_w\mu T(t)V_w(t) - \delta I_m(t),\\
\frac{dV_w(t)}{dt} &= p_w I_w(t) - c_v V_w(t),\\
\frac{dV_m(t)}{dt} &= p_m I_m(t) - c_v V_m(t),
\end{aligned} \tag{1}$$

where $T(t)$ is the density of uninfected target cells; $I_w(t)$ and $I_m(t)$ is the density of target cells infected by the wild-type or escape variant viruses, respectively; $V_w(t)$ and $V_m(t)$ is the density of wild-type or escape variant viruses, respectively; s is the turnover rate of uninfected target cells; T_0 is the preinfection level of uninfected target cells; β_w and β_m is infection rate of wild-type or escape variant viruses, respectively; μ is the probability of mutation from wild-type to escape mutant during reverse transcription of viral RNA into proviral DNA; δ is the death rate of infected cells due to viral pathogenicity; k is the killing rate of wild-type virus infected cell due to CTL response; p_w and p_m is the rate at which cells infected by wild-type or escape mutant viruses produce viruses; and c_v is the clearance rate of free viral particles.

In this model (equation (1)), we assume that target cells infected by wild-type ($V_w(t)$) and escape viruses ($V_m(t)$) differ by two factors: viral infectivity (β_w and β_m) and the rate of virus production (p_w and p_m). Given that *in vivo* viral particles are short-lived (29, 30), to a good approximation, we may assume a quasi steady state for the virus particle concentration leading to $V_w^*(t) = \frac{p_w}{c_v}I_w(t)$ and $V_m^*(t) = \frac{p_m}{c_v}I_m(t)$. We define a fitness cost $c = 1 - \frac{\beta_m p_m}{\beta_w p_w}$, where c can be positive or negative. Positive c means true fitness cost of escape mutations, which is escape variant and has a lower replication rate ($\beta_m p_m \leq \beta_w p_w$) (31), and negative c implies fitness advantage of escape virus (31, 32). By straightforward calculation, the system (equation (1)) can be written as

$$\begin{aligned}
\frac{dV_w^*(t)}{dt} &= [(1-\mu)r(t) - \delta - k]V_w^*(t),\\
\frac{dV_m^*(t)}{dt} &= [(1-c)r(t) - \delta]V_m^*(t) + \mu r(t)V_w^*(t)\frac{p_m}{p_w}.
\end{aligned} \tag{2}$$

For convenience, we replace $V_w^*(t)$ and $V_m^*(t)$ by $w(t)$ or $m(t)$, respectively, and assume that the wild-type and escape viruses differ only in the rate of infectivity (that is $\beta_w \geq \beta_m$ and $p_w = p_m$) (13), the system (2) can be simplified as

$$\begin{aligned}
\frac{dw(t)}{dt} &= [(1-\mu)r(t) - \delta - k]w(t),\\
\frac{dm(t)}{dt} &= [(1-c)r(t) - \delta]m(t) + \mu r(t)w(t),
\end{aligned} \tag{3}$$

where $r(t) = \frac{\beta_w p_w}{c_v}T(t)$ is the replication rate of cells infected by wild-type virus, and $c = 1 - \frac{\beta_m}{\beta_w}$ is the cost of the escape mutation defined as a selection coefficient. The frequency of the escape variant in the whole population is given by $f(t) = \frac{m(t)}{w(t)+m(t)}$. This is perhaps the simplest model for a viral escape from a single CTL response. This is denoted as model 1 in the paper.

2.3. Models of Viral Escapes from Multiple CTL Responses

Mathematical model given in equation (3) tracks changes in densities of wild-type virus and a single variant that has escaped recognition from a single epitope-specific CTL response. In acute HIV infection, the virus can escape from recognition of multiple CTL responses, which are specific to several viral epitopes (13, 33). Several models have been developed to describe the dynamics of escapes from multiple CTL responses (e.g., Ref., (17, 18, 26)). Our model is an extension of previous models (17, 18) incorporating mutations from wild-type virus to different viral escapes. In contrast with previous studies, in our analyses, here, we used experimentally measured time courses of different CTL responses (12).

To track the dynamics of viral escape from multiple responses, we assume that there are in total n CTL responses that control viral growth, and virus can potentially escape from all n responses. We use $m_{\mathbf{i}}$ to denote the density of variants where $\mathbf{i}$ is a vector $\mathbf{i} = (i_1, i_2, \ldots, i_n)$ denoting the positions of n epitopes, and we define $i_j = 0$ if there is no mutation in the jth CTL epitope and $i_j = 1$ if there is a mutation leading to an escape from the jth ($1 \leq j \leq n$) CTL response. We denote the set of escape variant as I, which is $\mathbf{i} \in I$. The wild-type variant is then denoted as $(0, 0, \ldots 0)$.

For our analysis, we neglect recombination and backward mutation from mutant to wild-type. We use k_i, c_i, and μ_i to denote killing rate due to ith CTL response, cost of escape mutation from the ith CTL response and mutation rate for the ith epitope, respectively. Due to a small rate of double mutation (34), we assume that escape virus is generated with only one mutation in a single generation. That is, for two escape variants $m_{\mathbf{i}} = m_{(i_1, i_2, \ldots, i_n)}$ and $m_{\mathbf{j}} = m_{(j_1, j_2, \ldots, j_n)}$, we define the mutation rate $M_{\mathbf{i},\mathbf{j}}$ from $m_{\mathbf{i}}$ to $m_{\mathbf{j}}$ as μ_k, if and only if $m_{\mathbf{j}}$ has only one more mutation at position k than $m_{\mathbf{i}}$ and all other positions are exactly same. For example, when there are 3 CTL responses, the mutation rate from $m_{(1,0,0)}$ to $m_{(1,1,0)}$ is μ_2, and the mutation rate from $m_{(0,0,0)}$ to $m_{(1,0,1)}$ is 0. Assuming multiplicative fitness (detailed deviation is given in Section S2 in Supplementary Material), that is, the fitness cost of a variant $\mathbf{i} = (i_1, i_2, \ldots, i_n)$ is $C_{\mathbf{i}} = 1 - \prod_{j=1}^{n}(1 - c_j i_j)$. The death rate of the escape variant $\mathbf{i} = (i_1, i_2, \ldots, i_n)$ due to remaining CTL responses is given by $K_{\mathbf{i}} = \sum_{j=1}^{n} k_j(1 - i_j)$, where we assume that killing of infected cells by different CTL responses is additive.

Similar to equation (3), the dynamics of the wild-type and escape variants are given by

$$\frac{dm_{\mathbf{i}}(t)}{dt} = \left[r(1 - C_{\mathbf{i}}) \left(1 - \sum_{\mathbf{j} \in I} M_{\mathbf{i},\mathbf{j}} \right) - K_{\mathbf{i}} - \delta \right] m_{\mathbf{i}}(t) + \sum_{\mathbf{j} \in I} r(1 - C_{\mathbf{j}}) M_{\mathbf{j},\mathbf{i}} m_{\mathbf{j}}(t), \ \mathbf{i} \in I. \quad (4)$$

We define $M(t) = \sum_{\mathbf{i} \in I} m_{\mathbf{i}}$ as the total density of all variants in the population, and $f_j(t)$ ($j = 1, \ldots, n$) is the fraction of viral variants that have escaped recognition from the jth CTL response. The frequency of a viral variant escaping from the jth response is given by

$$f_j(t) = \sum_{\mathbf{i} \in J} m_{\mathbf{i}}(t)/M(t), \ J = (i_1, \ldots i_j, \ldots, i_n) \text{ with } i_j = 1. \quad (5)$$

Based on previous work (22, 25, 35), we assume that there are two alternative ways to generate escape mutants (**Figure 1**). The first way can be called "sequential" escape (model 2), that is escape mutants are generated sequentially along a defined path from wild-type viruses. This is likely to happen when the effective population size of HIV is small and when the rate of recombination is negligible. The second way can be described as "concurrent" escape (model 3), in which the virus can escape from n CTL responses simultaneously along multiple different pathways. This is likely to happen when the HIV effective population size is large. With n CTL responses, there are n escape variants for "sequential" escape and $2^n - 1$ escape variants for "concurrent" escape in addition to the wild-type variant. For example, with $n = 3$ CTL responses, for "sequential" escape, there are 3 escape variants: $m_{(1,0,0)}$, $m_{(1,1,0)}$, and $m_{(1,1,1)}$ with $m_{(0,0,0)}$ being the wild-type virus. For "concurrent" escape, there are 7 escape variants: $m_{(1,0,0)}$, $m_{(0,1,0)}$, $m_{(0,0,1)}$, $m_{(1,1,0)}$, $m_{(1,0,1)}$, $m_{(0,1,1)}$, and $m_{(1,1,1)}$ with $m_{(0,0,0)}$ being the wild-type virus (**Figure 1**). Detailed equations for both models with $n = 3$ CTL responses can be found in Supplement (Section S2 in Supplementary Material). It is interesting to note that "sequential" escape is a simplification of "concurrent" escape when the effective population size is small. Previous work did not fully resolve whether CTL escapes in HIV infection occur sequentially or concurrently (22, 25); most likely the type of escape varies by patient.

2.4. Models for CTL Response

The killing rate k_i of the CTL response specific to the ith epitope in all three models is composed of two parts: the per-cell killing efficacy of CTLs (k_i') and the number of epitope-specific CTLs (E_i) (16). Previously the killing rates k_i were often set to a constant (e.g., Ref. (16, 18)), or were set to a certain form $k_i' g(E_i(t))$ where $g(E_i(t))$ is a function of epitope-specific CTL responses $E_i(t)$ (e.g., Ref. (24, 36)). With the measured epitope-specific CTL response dynamics (13), we adopted two forms of killing rate: constant k_i (termed as "constant response") or time-dependent killing rate $k_i' E_i(t)$ (termed as "interpolated/fitted response"). We used the "mass-action" killing term to describe effect of CTLs on virus dynamics because it is the simplest form, it involves minimum parameters, and it is supported by some experimental data (37).

Based on the available time course information of epitope-specific T cell response $E_i(t)$, we used the first-order interpolation function (termed as "interpolated response") or the fitted response function (termed as "fitted response") by the T_{on}–T_{off} model (38) to quantify the kinetics of HIV-specific CTL responses. The T_{on}–T_{off} model assumes that the response starts with E_0 epitope-specific CD8$^+$ T cells that become activated at time T_{on}. Activated T cells start proliferating at a rate ρ and reach the peak at time T_{off}. After the peak, epitopes-specific CD8$^+$ T cells decline at a rate α. The dynamics of the CD8$^+$ T cell response $E(t)$ is given thus by the following differential equation:

$$\frac{dE}{dt} = \begin{cases} 0, & \text{if } t < T_{\text{on}}, \\ \rho E, & \text{if } T_{\text{on}} \leq t \leq T_{\text{off}}, \\ -\alpha E, & \text{if } t > T_{\text{off}} \end{cases} \quad (6)$$

with $E(0) = E_0$. Here the "precursor frequency" E_0 is a generalized recruitment parameter, which combines the true precursor frequency and the recruitment rate/time (38, 39). Our recent work showed that this model (equation (6)) reasonably well describes kinetics of HIV-specific CTL responses in acute HIV infection (40). When fitting the model (equation (6)) to experimental data of CTL dynamics, we changed all initial undetected response values from 0 to 1; the latter was the detection limit in the data.

2.5. Statistics

Previously, under the assumption that some mutants are present initially, researchers (e.g., Ref. (16, 36)) fit a logistic model to data on viral escape kinetics by the method of nonlinear least squares (41). In essence, this is a maximum likelihood method, which assumes normally distributed residuals. While this standard statistical method provides reasonable parameter estimates, it assumes equal weights to different data points independently of how many viral sequences were measured at every time point, which is likely to be unrealistic for most experimental studies. Here, we follow the method proposed recently (18) to use binomial distribution (and thus different weights for different measurements/time points) in the likelihood of the model given the escape data. For HIV escape from a single CTL response, the log-likelihood function is given by

$$\mathcal{L} = \sum_{j=1}^{T_i} [a_j \ln(f(t_j)) + (N_j - a_j) \ln(1 - f(t_j))], \quad (7)$$

where a_j is the number of escape variant sequences in a sample of N_j sequences at the sample time t_j, T_i is the number of measured time points for a ith specific viral escape trajectory, and $f(t_j)$ is the predicted frequency of a specific viral escape variant at time t_j. Model parameters were thus found by maximizing the log-likelihood function (equation (7)).

To discriminate between alternative models under different parameter constrains, we used corrected Akaike information criterion (AIC) scores (42). The model fit with the minimum AIC score among tested models was treated as the best model; however, a difference of less than 3 AIC units is generally viewed as not

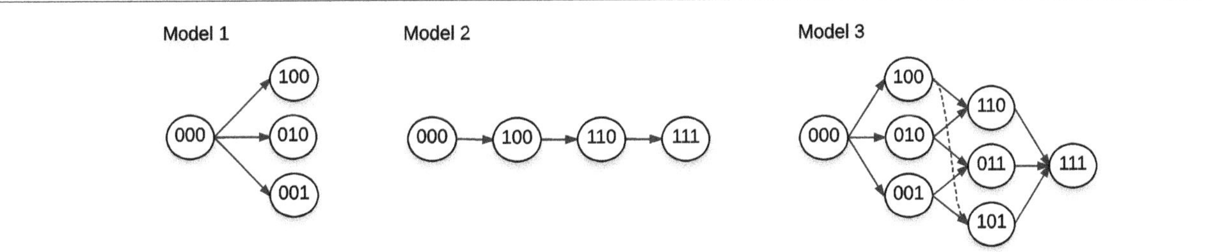

FIGURE 1 | Escape paths for models 1, 2, and 3 with 3 CTL responses. For model 1, there are 3 escape variants: $m_{(1,0,0)}$, $m_{(0,1,0)}$, and $m_{(0,0,1)}$. For model 2, there are also 3 escape variants: $m_{(1,0,0)}$, $m_{(1,1,0)}$, and $m_{(1,1,1)}$. For model 3, there are 7 escape variants: $m_{(1,0,0)}$, $m_{(0,1,0)}$, $m_{(0,0,1)}$, $m_{(1,1,0)}$, $m_{(1,0,1)}$, $m_{(0,1,1)}$, and $m_{(1,1,1)}$. In each case, $m_{(0,0,0)}$ is the wild-type virus.

significant (42). To test the statistical significance of the differences between parameters found by fitting different models, we used a bootstrap approach (43). In this approach, we resampled the data 1,000 times using the `Random` routine in `Mathematica` assuming beta distribution for sequencing data (44), fitted models to bootstrap samples, and recorded all estimated parameters. For the same parameter, we use either paired and unpaired t-test to compare the parameter averages for different models.

Both fitness costs of escape mutations and the killing efficacy of the CTL response determine the kinetics of viral escape from T cells (14–16), and that viral escape (sequence) data in most cases are not sufficient to estimate both rates (16). Therefore, in our analyses, to avoid overfitting, we set fitness cost of escape to 0 $c_i = 0$. In all fits, we assumed that the rate of virus replication $r = 1.5$/day (28).

While multiple models may be able to describe accurately experimental data, some models may do so at biologically unreasonable parameters. For example, estimated rate of mutation at different epitopes may be unrealistically large. Thus, in our analysis, we assume that mutation rates, which are above 10^{-3} are likely to be unrealistic given that currently estimated HIV mutation rate is about 3.2×10^{-5} per bp per generation (34) and size of a CTL epitope is 8–10 amino acids ($3 \times 10 \times 3.2 \times 10^{-5} \approx 10^{-3}$).

To fit the T_{on}–T_{off} model [equation (6)] to experimental data using non-linear least squares, we log-transformed the model predictions and the data.

When interpolating CTL response kinetics, there was often not enough information on the starting point (day 0). In such situations, we set the initial CTL density as 1 (the detection level for this data set) for simplicity. Other starting points (e.g., intersection point of the CTL response axis and the reverse extension line of the interpolation function) were also tested and led to similar results (not shown). This was largely due to the fact that, in our models, CTLs at low densities are not expected to exert large selective pressure on the virus population due to assumed mass-action killing term.

3. RESULTS

3.1. Statistical Model Impacts Estimation of the Escape (Killing) Rate

Given virus evolution data, we may be often interested in quantifying selecting pressures driving specific changes in the virus population. Following HIV-1 infection, the virus escapes from several cytotoxic T lymphocyte (CTL) responses (45), and multiple studies used mathematical models of various levels of complexity to estimate the predicted efficacy at which CTLs recognize and eliminate cells, infected with the wild-type (unescaped) virus (14–18, 25). Many of these previous studies estimated the rate of HIV escape from immunity using nonlinear least squares, which explicitly assumes normal distribution of the deviations between model predictions and data (14–17). However, the assumption of normally distributed residuals is likely to be violated for data when only a handful of viral genomes are sequenced—which is common in many studies involving single genome amplification and sequencing techniques (SGA/S). We have recently proposed to use a likelihood approach, which assumes virus genome sampling to follow a binomial distribution (18). This binomial distribution-based likelihood approach showed to impact the estimates of the CTL killing rate (escape rate can be proportional to the killing rate under an assumption of constant CTL response) when compared to normal distribution-based likelihood approach (least squares) (18). However, this previous comparison was done on data, which were fairly sparse and comparison involved modifications of data to allow for non-zero and non-one frequencies of the escape variant (14, 15), and thus, it remained unclear if estimates of escape rates are truly dependent on the statistical model for better sampled data.

Unfortunately, in our cohort of 17 patients (12), very few patients were sampled frequently enough to observe gradual accumulation of escape variants in the population (i.e., data with two sequential time points with mutant frequency in the range $0 < f < 1$ were rare). For the analysis, we, therefore, used the escape data from two patients, CH131 and CH159, where CTL and HIV sequence measurements were sufficiently frequent to address our modeling questions. We fitted a simple mathematical model describing escape of the virus from a single constant (non-changing) CTL response (equation (3)) to the data from one patient CH159 (**Figure 2**) assuming two different statistical models: with normally distributed residuals (least squares) or binomial distribution-based likelihood (equation (7)). Consistent with our previous observation, we found that the type of statistical model impacts the estimate of the escape rate (k in **Figure 2**) with difference being nearly twofold ($k = 0.27$/day vs. $k = 0.51$/day). It is interesting to note that, visually, the least squares method appear to describe the data better by accurately fitting the points with intermediate frequency of the escape variant in 20–30 days

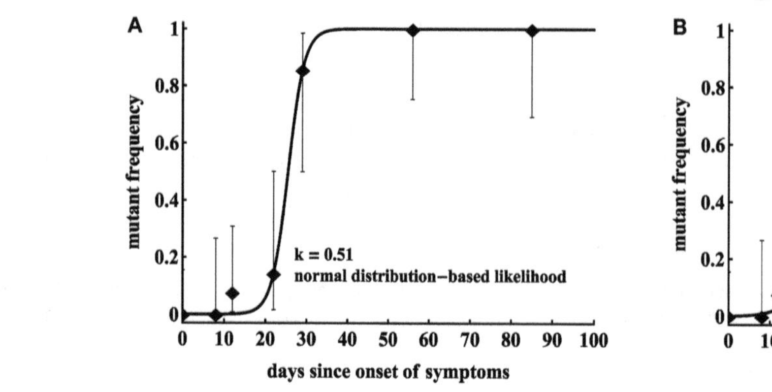

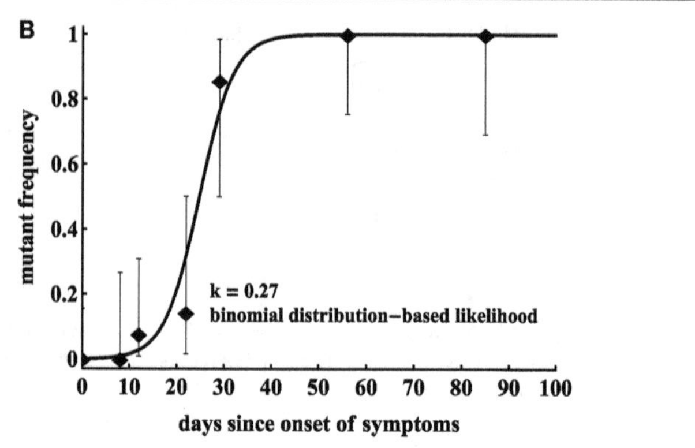

FIGURE 2 | Statistical model has a strong impact on the estimated killing rate. We fit model in equation (7) to the same data for HIV escape in the protein region DREVLIWKFDSSLARRHL of Nef (Nef 177–194) in patient CH159, assuming normal distribution-based likelihood (normally distributed residuals or nonlinear least squares **(A)**) or binomial distribution-based likelihood method **(B)**. Data are shown as dots and bars represent the 95% confidence intervals calculated using beta distribution (Jefferey's intervals (44)). The fitted parameters are $\mu = 7.76 \times 10^{-7}$ and $k = 0.51$ day^{-1} **(A)**, or $\mu = 2.00 \times 10^{-4}$ and $k = 0.27$ day^{-1} **(B)**.

after the symptoms (but missing the another intermediate data point (12, 0.08)). However, this visually better fit is not supported by the statistics: likelihood of the model for these data is -12.64 or -10.53 for normal (**Figure 2A**) or binomial (**Figure 2B**) distribution, respectively (and AIC scores being 31.0 vs. 26.8, respectively). Interestingly, the main difference in the estimated escape rates was driven by just one data point ($(t, f) = (12, 0.08)$); removing this data point from the data led to identical estimates of the escape rate, $k = 0.51$/day, from two statistical models (results not shown). This is not surprising because with this data point removed, the information on escape rate is only coming from two data points when the frequency of the escape variant is intermediate ($0 < f < 1$).

As discussed before, least squares may not allow to estimate escape rates, e.g., in cases when mutant frequency jumps from 0 to 1 between two subsequent time points unless data are modified (14, 15). Similarly, models assuming normally distributed residuals may not be able to fit other types of data, in which frequency of the mutant has an intermediate value ($0 < f < 1$) at one time point only. In particular, in our analysis of another escape in patient CH159 (Rev GRPTEPVPFQLPPLERLC, see **Figure 3**), we could not obtain finite estimates of the escape rate using normally distributed residuals (results not shown). Rather, the model fits tended to describe accurately two data points ($t = 22$ days and $t = 29$ days) and ignore another data point ($t = 56$ days) leading to extremely high predicted escape rates (results not shown). Interestingly, using binomial distribution-based likelihood allowed for an accurate fit of the model to data and the fit compromised between describing early and late data points (**Figure 4A**). The reason for the compromise is that a fit predicting fast escape and nearly 100% escape variant by 56 days since symptoms is highly disfavored by the binomial distribution-based likelihood because some wild-type variants were still present at day 56 (thus, the weight for missing this point by the model fit was very high in binomial distribution-based likelihood but not in the normal distribution-based likelihood). Taken together, these results suggest that the type of the statistical model used to estimate HIV escape rates influences the final estimates. Therefore, many previous studies on HIV escape assuming normally distributed residuals may need to be re-evaluated for the robustness of their conclusions.

3.2. CTL Response Kinetics Do Not Improve Description of the Escape Data

As CTL responses drive HIV escape from epitope-specific T cells, it is expected that the magnitude of the CTL response should naturally impact escape kinetics. Previous studies provided some evidence that the relative magnitude of a given CTL response in the total HIV-specific CTL response early in infection (% immunodominance) predicts the timing of viral escape (11, 12). Immune response was also shown to impact escape of simian immunodeficiency virus (SIV) from T cell responses (19, 46, 47). Immune response magnitude, and as a consequence, the overall CTL killing efficacy is important in determining both timing and speed of viral escape with the rate of viral escape being directly related to the immune response efficacy (16, 17). In contrast, both initial mutant frequency, virus mutation rate, and CTL killing efficacy determine timing of viral escape (17). Whether inclusion of the experimentally measured CTL dynamics impacts ability of mathematical models to accurately describe viral escape data has not been tested.

To test the benefits of using longitudinally measured CTL responses in describing viral escape data, we considered several alternative models for the CTL dynamics and viral escape. Our model 1 describes the dynamics of viral escape from each CTL response independently. Models 2 and 3 describe escape from multiple CTL response that occurs sequentially or concurrently, respectively (see Materials and Methods for more details). CTL dynamics was either considered to be unimportant (i.e., killing rate k_i was set constant over time), or when killing rate was proportional to the experimentally measured CTL frequency ($k_i^{\prime} E_i(t)$), respectively. To describe CTL dynamics, we either used the first order interpolation function or the $T_{\text{on}}-T_{\text{off}}$ model (equation (6) and see Materials and Methods for more detail).

In patient CH159, four CTL responses were detected (**Figure 3B**), and three of these responses were escaped within nearly 4 years of infection. Interestingly, the response specific

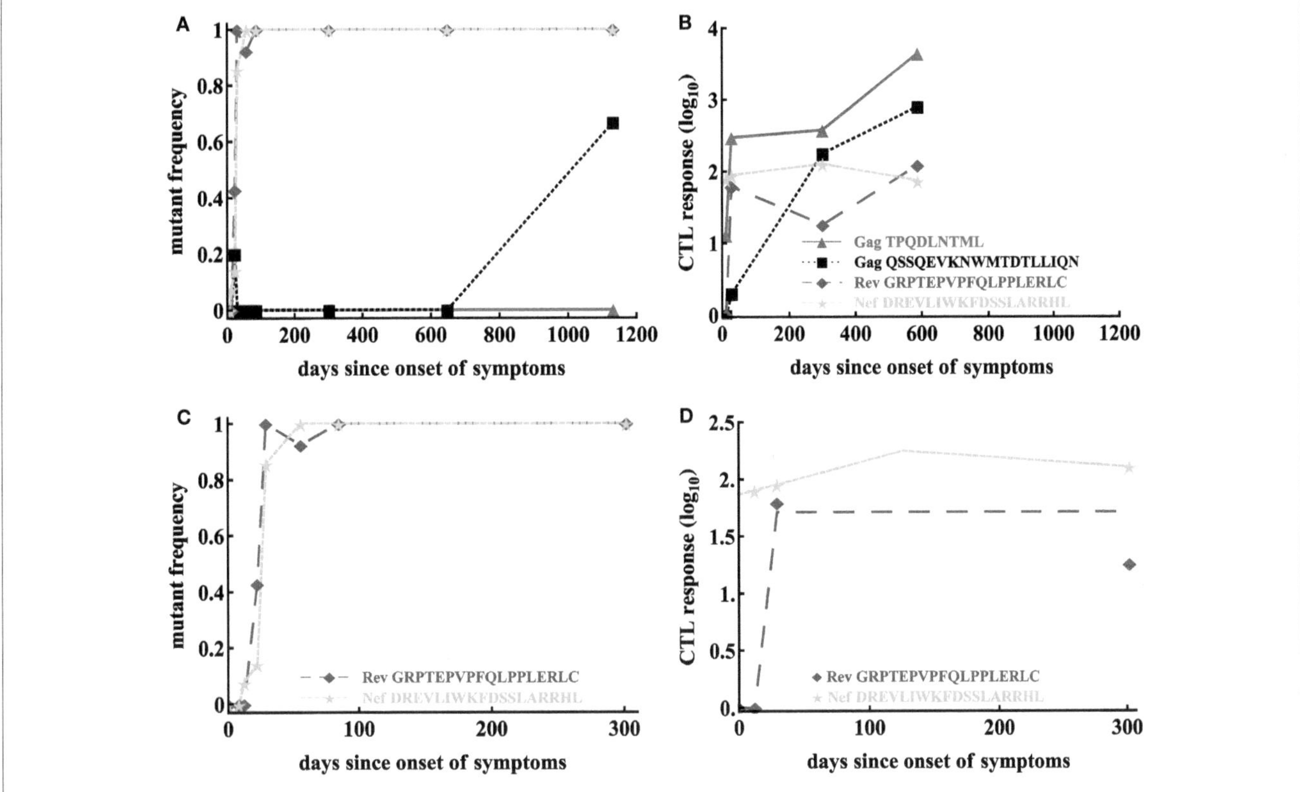

FIGURE 3 | Basic dynamics of CTL response and HIV escape for patient CH159. Data are from a previous publication (12); the data show four CTL responses in the patient **(B)** and frequencies of corresponding escape variants **(A)**. Based on the selection criteria described in the Materials and Methods, we focused our analysis on CTL dynamics and escape in two regions: Rev GRPTEPVPFQLPPLERLC (65–82) and Nef DREVLIWKFDSSLARRHL (177–194) shown for the first 200 days in panels **(C,D)**. Dashed lines in panel **(D)** are the prediction of the T_{on}–T_{off} model to these data with the following estimated parameters for the Rev-specific T cell response: $E_0 = 1$ IFNγ + SFC/10^6 PBMC, $T_{on} = 12$ day, $T_{off} = 29$ day, $\rho = 0.23$ day^{-1}, $\alpha = 1.67 \times 10^{-6}$ day^{-1}; and for the Nef-specific T cell response: $E_0 = 73.59$ IFNγ + SFC/10^6 PBMC, $T_{on} = 0$ day, $T_{off} = 126.05$ day, $\rho = 6.98 \times 10^{-3}$ day^{-1}, $\alpha = 1.86 \times 10^{-3}$ day^{-1}.

to Gag TPQDLNTML was dominant (**Figure 3B**), but the corresponding escape mutant Gag TPQDLNTMLNTVGGHQAA did not appear up to 1,132 days since onset of symptoms (**Figure 3A**).

Patient CH159 had two escape mutants in regions Rev GRPTEPVPFQLPPLERLC (Rev 65–82) and Nef DREVLIWKFDSSLARRHL (Nef 177–194) satisfying our selection criteria (**Figure 3C**). Despite a relative small magnitude of CTL responses specific to Rev65 and Nef177 early in infection (up to 29 days since onset of symptoms), escape mutants appeared early and their frequencies arose rapidly.

We fitted three alternative mathematical models for viral escape and three alternative models for the CTL dynamics to the data on viral escape (**Figure 3C**) using binomial distribution-based likelihood method (see Materials and Methods for more detail). Surprisingly, we found that the models 1 and 3 with a constant immune response described the data with best quality as judged by the AIC (or likelihood). Parameter estimates in the model 1, which assumes independent escape were nearly identical to the parameters in the model 3, which assumed concurrent escape (**Figure 4**; **Table 1**). Importantly, adding experimentally measured CTL response dynamics (as interpolated function or by using parameterized T_{on}–T_{off} model) did not improve the quality of the model fit to escape data (**Table 1**). Even worse, for models 1 and 3, the fits with a fitted response were of lower quality as judged by the large increase in AIC (**Table 1**). Models that included an interpolated CTL response provided better fits than models with a fitted response (**Table 1**).

The exact reasons of why including experimentally measured CTL response dynamics led to worse fits of the escape data are unclear but perhaps rapid change in magnitude of CTL responses in this patient—if response directly impacts killing of infected cells—was simply not reflected in the kinetics of viral escape (**Figures 4D,G**). Specifically, CTL kinetics-driven escape would predict non-monotonic rise in the escape variant frequency, which was not observed in the data, thus, favoring a model with a constant killing rate by CTLs.

Interestingly, the model 2 fits of the data resulted in unphysiologically large estimates for the mutation rate μ_2 (**Table 1**). As we elaborate later (see below), this failure of the model to describe these data stems from the fact that escapes in the data occur nearly at the same time and assuming that escapes are sequential led to an unrealistic mutation rate in the second epitope. This suggests that the observed dynamics of viral escape in patient CH159 is not consistent with sequential escape.

Models 1 and 3 also predicted slightly higher than expected mutation rate μ_1 (bigger than 10^{-3}) for the peptide Rev 65–82. Constraining this parameter to remain $\mu_1 \leq 10^{-3}$ led to fits of

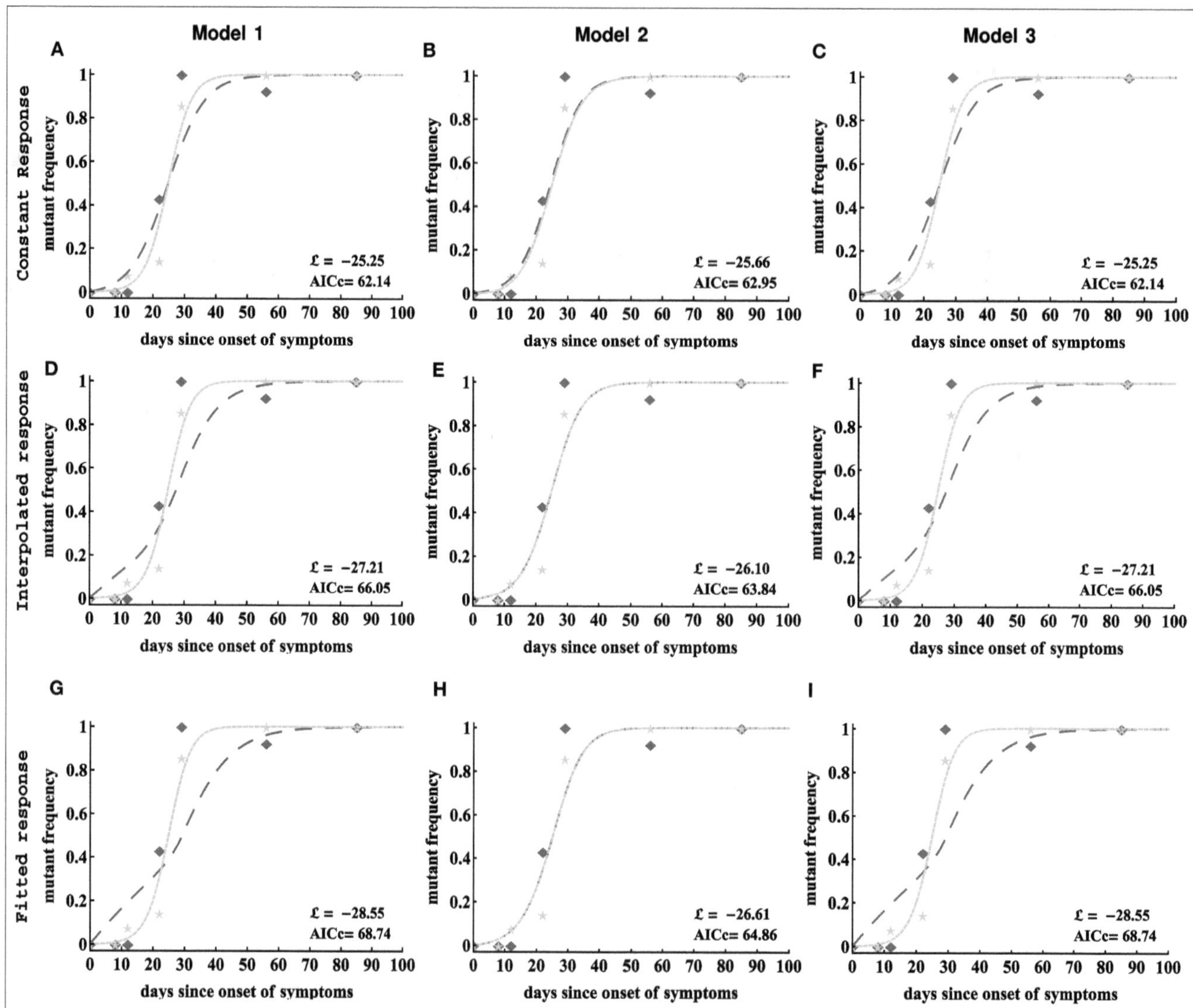

FIGURE 4 | Including CTL response dynamics worsened model fits of HIV escape data in patient CH159. We fitted model 1 (independent escapes, equation (3), panels **(A,D,G)**), model 2 (sequential escape, equation S6 in Supplemental Material, panels **(B,E,H)**), and model 3 (concurrent escape, equation S8 in Supplementary Material, panels **(C,F,I)**) to escape data in patient CH159 with different response inputs (constant, interpolated, or fitted response, see Materials and Methods for more detail). Adding direct time-dependent response (interpolated or fitted response) did not improve the quality of the model fit to data (see **Table 1** for parameter estimates). Model 2 was not able to accurately describe these data for biologically reasonable mutation rates (see **Table 1**).

significantly lower quality (likelihood ratio test, $p < 0.05$). Due to large length of the peptide, the overall mutation rate in this region could indeed be slightly higher than our calculated high bound for the mutation rate (see Materials and Methods for more detail). Furthermore, since peptide Rev 65–82 is the epitope in which first escape occurred, it was possible that the high estimate of the mutation rate could be due to late sampling of viral sequences. In these, data sampling was done after patients were diagnosed with infection; however, viral escape could have started earlier and for escapes starting earlier, it may be possible to describe the data with a lower mutation rate (18, 48).

Therefore, to test whether the timing of the start of the escape influences the estimate of the mutation rate we did the following. We shifted the data for two escapes forward by adding some initial zeroes to data and reverse extended the predicted CTL response curves. Then we refitted models 1 and 3 to the data under the constrain $\mu \leq 10^{-3}$. We found shifting the data did not improve the quality of the model fits as compared to unmodified data when CTL dynamics is explicitly taken into account as interpolated or fitted response (results not shown). However, assuming a constant response allowed to obtain lower, more physiological estimates of the mutation rate. These results suggest that inability of the models, which explicitly incorporate CTL dynamics to explain kinetics of first escape with physiologically reasonable mutation rate is due to late appearance of the CTL response. Indeed, escape can only accumulate when CTL response is present and extending the time window for virus evolution but not having CTL response active will not significantly impact estimates of the mutation rate.

Given our results for one patient, we next sought to investigate whether our conclusions will remain robust when looking at

TABLE 1 | Parameters for the three models fitted to escape data from patient CH159.

	Peptide	Model 1		Model 2		Model 3	
		Mutation rate (μ_i, i = 1, 2)	Killing rate (k_i, i = 1, 2)	Mutation rate (μ_i, i = 1, 2)	Killing rate (k_i, i = 1, 2)	Mutation rate (μ_i, i = 1, 2)	Killing rate (k_i, i = 1, 2)
Constant response	Rev 65–82	*1.68×10^{-3}*	0.17	9.71×10^{-4}	0.20	*1.68×10^{-3}*	0.17
	Nef 177–194	2.02×10^{-4}	0.27	*0.11*	6.29×10^{-12}	2.0×10^{-4}	0.27
		$\mathcal{L}$ = **−25.25**, AICc = **62.14**		$\mathcal{L}$ = −25.66, AICc = 62.95		$\mathcal{L}$ = **−25.25**, AICc = **62.14**	
		Mutation rate (μ_i, i = 1, 2)	Killing rate (k_i', i = 1, 2)	Mutation rate (μ_i, i = 1, 2)	Killing rate (k_i', i = 1, 2)	Mutation rate (μ_i, i = 1, 2)	Killing rate (k_i', i = 1, 2)
Interpolated response	Rev 65–82	*8.88×10^{-3}*	2.12×10^{-3}	*1.64×10^{-3}*	2.03×10^{-10}	*8.88×10^{-3}*	2.12×10^{-3}
	Nef 177–194	4.94×10^{-4}	3.23×10^{-3}	*697.77*	2.32×10^{-3}	4.93×10^{-4}	3.23×10^{-3}
		$\mathcal{L}$ = −27.21, AICc = 66.05		$\mathcal{L}$ = −26. 10, AICc = 63.84		$\mathcal{L}$ = −27. 21, AICc = 66.05	
		Mutation rate (μ_i, i = 1, 2)	Killing rate (k_i', i = 1, 2)	Mutation rate (μ_i, i = 1, 2)	Killing rate (k_i', i = 1, 2)	Mutation rate (μ_i, i = 1, 2)	Killing rate (k_i', i = 1, 2)
Fitted response	Rev 65–82	*1.43×10^{-2}*	1.39×10^{-3}	*1.13×10^{-3}*	8.50×10^{-18}	*1.43×10^{-2}*	1.39×10^{-3}
	Nef 177–194	2.46×10^{-4}	3.25×10^{-3}	*13,004.84*	2.29×10^{-3}	2.47×10^{-4}	3.25×10^{-3}
		$\mathcal{L}$ = −29.68, AICc = 70.99		$\mathcal{L}$ = −26.61, AICc = 64.86		$\mathcal{L}$ = −29.68, AICc = 70.99	

*Fits of the model to data are shown in **Figure 4**. $\mathcal{L}$ and AICc are the log-likelihood and the corrected Akaike information criterion value, respectively. In bold, we show maximum $\mathcal{L}$ and minimum AICc reached by the models 1 and 3 with constant response. There are some unrealistic mutation rates given by model 2 (much bigger than 10^{-3}, highlighted as italic), and models 1 and 3 also led to slightly unrealistic mutation rates at the peptide Rev 65–82 (slightly bigger than 10^{-3}). Units for k_i and k_i' are day^{-1} and μ_i is dimensionless (same for all tables below).*

data from another patient. Patient CH131 had 6 CTL responses, and there was escape from at least 5 of these responses in 2 years since symptoms (**Figure 5**). One escape, Nef EEVGFPVKPQV (Nef 64–74), occurred very early in infection, and two escapes, Env RQGYSPLSFQTLIPNPRG (Env 709–726) and Gag VKVIEEKAFSPEVIPMFT (Gag 156–173), occurred late (**Figure 5**). In this patient, the pattern of escape followed the ranking of immunodominance of CTL responses (12): Nef64-specific CTLs were dominant at symptoms and drove earlier escape, while Env 709- and Gag156-specific CTLs arose later with escapes occurring later in infection (**Figures 5A,B**). However, there were apparently discrepancies such as two escapes in Tat epitopes (Tat DPWNHPGSQPKTACNNCY, that is Tat 9–26 and Tat FQKKGLGISY, that is Tat 38–47) occurred at the same time while CTL responses specific to these different epitopes were of different sizes (**Figures 5A,B**). Because escapes in these two Tat epitopes occurred rapidly and did not have two intermediate measurements of the mutant frequency, our following analysis was only restricted to escapes in three CTL epitopes: Nef64, Env709, Gag156 (**Figures 5C,D**).

We thus fitted 3 different models of viral escape combined with 3 different models for the CTL dynamics to the data on viral escape (**Figure 6**). Importantly, as with the analysis of data from patient CH159, we found that including the data-driven CTL dynamics in the escape models did not improve the quality of the model fit to the escape data (**Table 2**). In contrast with the previous results, though, the assumption of the constant and time-variable killing efficacy (i.e., due to variation in the immune response magnitude) did not strongly impact the quality of the model fit as judged by the AIC or likelihood (**Table 2**). Importantly, however, models 1 and 3 gave nearly identical estimates of the CTL killing efficacy, suggesting that for data with good temporal resolution model estimates of the CTL killing efficacy (or by inference, escape rates) are not strongly dependent on the specific mechanisms used to describe escape (independent vs. concurrent escape). This observation also suggests that exclusion of the data on escape occurring at intermediate times after symptoms in Tat should not influence the accuracy of estimation of the killing rates of CTLs specific to other epitopes in CH131.

Extending the observation made with the patient CH159 data, we found that model assuming sequential escape (model 2) could not accurately describe the dynamics of viral escape for biologically reasonable parameter values specifically for the third escape in Gag156 although this inability was significant only for a constant killing efficacy (**Table 2**). Allowing time-dependent killing efficacy resulted in small yet larger values for the mutation rate than that expected from basic calculations. Forcing the mutation rate μ_3 to be constrained ($\mu_3 \leq 10^{-3}$) significantly reduced the quality of the model fit to data (likelihood ratio test, $p \ll 0.001$). Furthermore, estimates for the CTL killing efficacy differed between model 2 and models 1 and 3 suggesting that model choice (sequential vs. concurrent) may indeed influence estimates of the killing efficacy.

3.3. No Difference in Predicted Killing Efficacy of CTLs, Specific to Different Epitopes

Our analyses, so far, demonstrated that several different mathematical models were capable of accurately describing the escape data, but this ability was dependent on the specific pathway of how escape mutants were generated and the assumption on whether data-driven CTL dynamics was included in the model. In cases, when a model was able to accurately describe the data, we generally observed different estimates for the parameters for HIV escape in different epitopes; for example, for the data in patient CH131 estimated CTL killing rate in the model 1 (independent escapes) with interpolated response different nearly 100-fold between k_1' and k_3' (**Table 2**). Knowing which immune responses may be more efficient on a per cell basis in killing virus-infected cells may be beneficial for inducing such responses by vaccination. We, therefore, investigated how robust these differences in estimated per capita killing rates are. For that, we fitted mathematical models assuming equal killing efficacies to the data on escape.

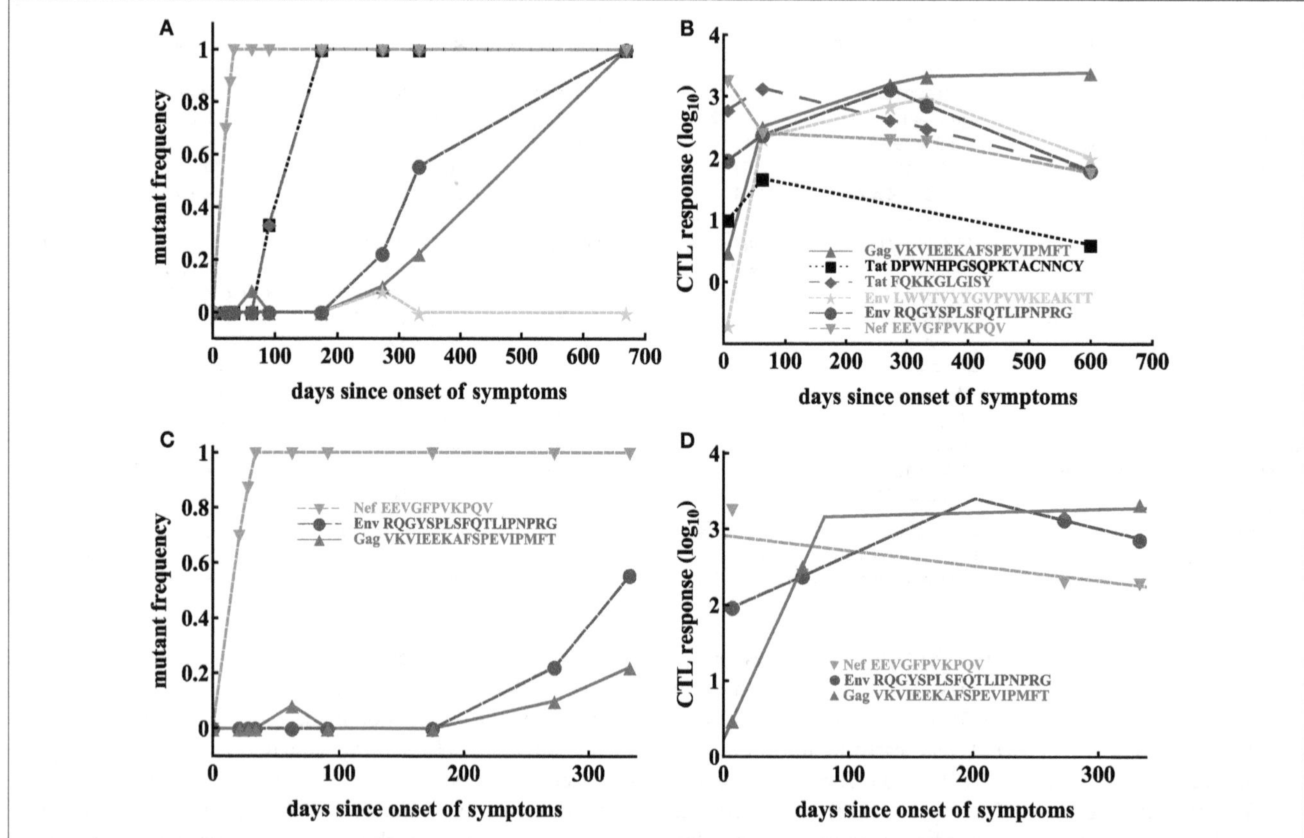

FIGURE 5 | Basic dynamics of CTL response and HIV escape in patient CH131. Patient CH131 had 6 CTL responses **(B)** and 5 responses were escaped by 700 days since infection **(A)**. Based on our selection criteria (see Materials and Methods), we focused our analysis on escape in three epitopes: Nef 64–74, Env 709–726, and Gag 156–173 **(C)** with the corresponding CTL dynamics **(D)**. Dashed lines in panel **(D)** denote fits of the T_{on}–T_{off} model (equation (6)) to these data resulting in the following estimates for the model parameters for Nef-specific T cell responses: $E_0 = 808.59$ IFNγ + SFC/10^6 PBMC, $\alpha = 4.55 \times 10^{-3}$ day^{-1}; for Env-specific T cell responses: $E_0 = 82.97$ IFNγ + SFC/10^6 PBMC, $T_{on} = 0$ day, $T_{off} = 202.02$ day, $\rho = 0.017$ day^{-1}, $\alpha = 9.23 \times 10^{-3}$ day^{-1}; for Gag-specific T cell responses: $E_0 = 1.67$ IFNγ + SFC/10^6 PBMC, $T_{on} = 0$ day, $T_{off} = 80.76$ day, $\rho = 0.084$ day^{-1}, $\alpha = -1.04 \times 10^{-3}$ day^{-1}.

As expected, reducing the number of fitted parameters led to fits of lower quality (as judged by the log-likelihood); however, this reduction in complexity of the model was favored by the AIC and in most cases by the likelihood ratio test (Tables S2 and S4 in Supplementary Material). Visually, the reduction in the quality of the model fit to data was also relatively small (Figures S2 and S4 in Supplementary Material). Thus, for these data, we found no strong evidence in the difference in the estimated per capita killing efficacy of the CTL response specific to different viral epitopes.

3.4. Identifying Conditions When the Model 2 (Sequential Escapes) Fails

In analysis of data from both patients, we found that model 2, describing sequential escape from CTL responses, was not able to accurately describe experimental data for biologically reasonable parameter values; these model fits predicted extremely high mutation rates (e.g., see **Tables 1** and **2**). Additional analyses demonstrated that fitting the models with constrained mutation rates, $\mu_i \leq 10^{-3}$ led to fits of significantly lower quality (based on increased AIC, results not shown).

A closer look at the experimental data for which model 2 provided unreasonably high mutation rates revealed that the trajectories of two subsequent escapes in the model 2 were too close to each other, which naturally required a high mutation rate from one variant to another. Therefore, only when trajectories are separated in time mutation rate μ_2 is expected to be biologically reasonable. Indeed, by simulating virus dynamics using model for sequential escapes by varying model parameters, we found that CTL killing rate has the major impact on the time delay between two escapes (**Figure 7**). This analysis thus suggested that for the model 2 (sequential escape) to be consistent with the data, escapes from 2 responses must be separated in time by about 20–50 days.

4. DISCUSSION

CTL responses play a major role in HIV within-host evolution (45, 49). Recent studies suggested that a relative magnitude of the CTL response (relative immunodominance) plays an important role in determining the time of viral escape from T cell responses (11, 12). These previous studies, however, only utilized a maximum value of the CTL response early in infection, in general, within 50 days since the onset of symptoms, and thus impact of the kinetics of CTL response on the rate of virus escape remained undetermined. Furthermore, the pathways of HIV escape from CTL responses were not fully resolved as escapes occurring sequentially and

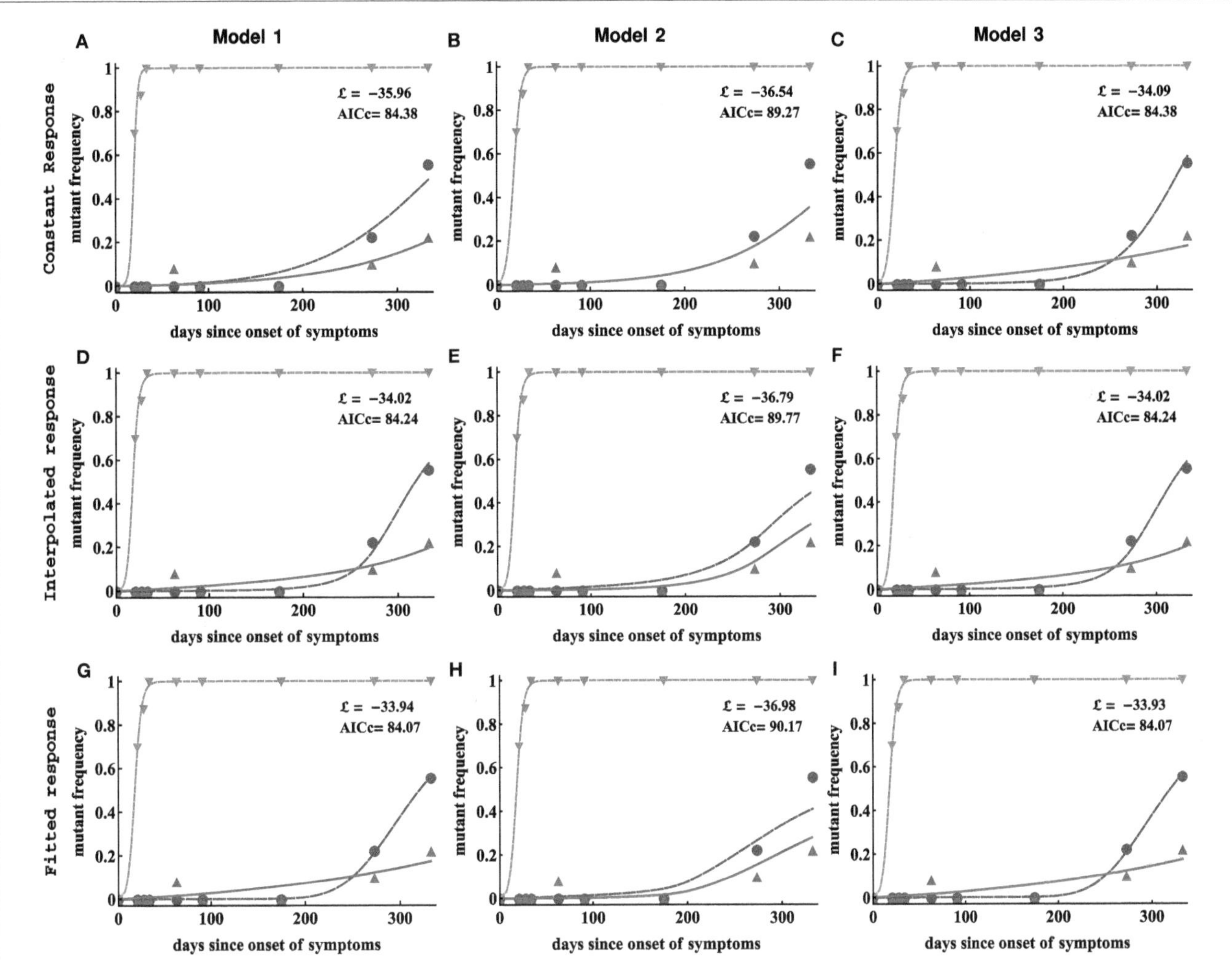

FIGURE 6 | Including CTL response dynamics did not improve model fits of HIV escape data in patient CH131. We fitted model 1 (independent escapes, panels **(A,D,G)**), model 2 (sequential escape, panels **(B,E,H)**), and model 3 (concurrent escape, panels **(C,F,I)**) to escape data in patient CH131 with different CTL response inputs (constant, interpolated, or fitted response). Adding data-derived time-dependent CTL response (interpolated or fitted response) does not improve the fitting results in most cases (**Table 2**). Notably, model 2 was unable to accurately describe late escape for biologically reasonable mutation rate μ_3. Model parameters providing the best fit are given in **Table 2**.

concurrently have been proposed (21, 22, 25), and several previous studies assumed that escapes occur independently from each other (14, 15, 17). Here, by using experimental data on evolution of HIV sequences from acute infection into chronic phase and temporally resolved dynamics of HIV-specific CTL responses, we tested the hypothesis that CTL dynamics plays an important role in virus escape.

Perhaps, in contrast with our initial expectations (e.g., due to Ref. (11, 50)), we found that including experimentally measured dynamics of epitope-specific CTL responses did not lead to a better description of the kinetics of viral escape from T cells (e.g., in patient CH131, **Table 2**), or even reduced the quality of the model for viral escape fit to data (e.g., in patient CH159, **Table 1**). This was not because we assumed that killing of virus-infected cells was dependent on the absolute magnitude of epitope-specific CTL responses; assuming frequency-dependent killing, that is, when killing of infected cells expressing ith epitope was given by $k_i E_i(t) / \sum_{j=1}^{n} E_j(t)$ $(1 \leq i \leq n)$, led to similar conclusions (results not shown). Because previous work suggested that kinetics of escape was independent of the specific mechanism of how CTLs suppress wild-type virus (e.g., killing of infected cells or virus production by infected cells) (16), we did not investigate non-lytic control of HIV by T cells. It is interesting that the lack of correlation between the rate of viral escape and CTL response magnitude was highlighted previously (17).

Reasons of why a model with time-variable CTL response did not describe experimental data better than a model with a constant response remain unclear but several hypotheses could be generated. First, frequency of sampling of the viral sequences may not be high enough to detect change in the speed at which mutant viruses accumulate in the population. Indeed, in mathematical models, CTL dynamics has a direct impact on the rate of escape (e.g., see equation (3)), and the observed changes in CTL densities may not be reflected in escape data if measurements are infrequent. Second, virus sequence data could simply be noisy. Because only handful of viral sequences were analyzed by the SGA/S, measurements of frequencies of viral variants have in general large expected error (e.g., **Figure 2**). Third, CTL dynamics

TABLE 2 | Parameters estimated by fitting different models of viral escape to escape data in patient CH131 assuming constant killing rates k_i (panels A–C), or time-varying killing rates due to interpolated CTL response (panels D–E) or CTL response in the T_{on}–T_{off} model (panels G–I).

	Peptide	Model 1		Model 2		Model 3	
		Mutation rate ($\mu_i, i=1, 2, 3$)	Killing rate ($k_i, i=1, 2, 3$)	Mutation rate ($\mu_i, i=1, 2, 3$)	Killing rate ($k_i, i=1, 2, 3$)	Mutation rate ($\mu_i, i=1, 2, 3$)	Killing rate ($k_i, i=1, 2, 3$)
Constant response	Nef 64–74	*1.75×10^{-3}*	0.25	*1.72×10^{-3}*	0.25	*1.78×10^{-3}*	0.25
	Env 709–726	1.03×10^{-7}	0.031	3.18×10^{-5}	5.45×10^{-3}	9.91×10^{-7}	0.031
	Gag 156–173	1.49×10^{-4}	5.16×10^{-3}	*433,780.63*	0.010	1.49×10^{-4}	5.19×10^{-3}
		$\mathcal{L} = -34.09$, $AICc = 84.38$		$\mathcal{L} = -36.54$, $AICc = 89.27$		$\mathcal{L} = -34.09$, $AICc = 84.38$	
		Mutation rate ($\mu_i, i=1, 2, 3$)	Killing rate ($k'_i, i=1, 2, 3$)	Mutation rate ($\mu_i, i=1, 2, 3$)	Killing rate ($k'_i, i=1, 2, 3$)	Mutation rate ($\mu_i, i=1, 2, 3$)	Killing rate ($k'_i, i=1, 2, 3$)
Interpolated response	Nef 64–74	4.33×10^{-4}	1.97×10^{-4}	3.95×10^{-4}	2.00×10^{-4}	4.30×10^{-4}	1.96×10^{-4}
	Env 709–726	7.07×10^{-6}	3.01×10^{-5}	8.76×10^{-5}	1.56×10^{-5}	7.17×10^{-6}	3.00×10^{-5}
	Gag 156–173	1.56×10^{-4}	4.59×10^{-6}	*3.33×10^{-3}*	7.48×10^{-14}	1.55×10^{-4}	4.61×10^{-6}
		$\mathcal{L} = -34.02$, $AICc = 84.24$		$\mathcal{L} = -36.79$, $AICc = 89.77$		$\mathcal{L} = -34.02$, $AICc = 84.24$	
		Mutation rate ($\mu_i, i=1, 2, 3$)	Killing rate ($k'_i, i=1, 2, 3$)	Mutation rate ($\mu_i, i=1, 2, 3$)	Killing rate ($k'_i, i=1, 2, 3$)	Mutation rate ($\mu_i, i=1, 2, 3$)	Killing rate ($k'_i, i=1, 2, 3$)
Fitted response	Nef 64–74	*3.25×10^{-3}*	3.38×10^{-4}	*2.99×10^{-3}*	3.46×10^{-4}	*3.16×10^{-3}*	3.41×10^{-4}
	Env 709–726	1.38×10^{-6}	2.59×10^{-5}	8.90×10^{-5}	1.05×10^{-5}	1.12×10^{-6}	2.66×10^{-5}
	Gag 156–173	1.73×10^{-4}	2.82×10^{-6}	*3.41×10^{-3}*	6.90×10^{-14}	1.73×10^{-4}	2.83×10^{-6}
		$\mathcal{L} = \mathbf{-33.94}$, $AICc = \mathbf{84.07}$		$\mathcal{L} = -36.98$, AICc $= 90.17$		$\mathcal{L} = \mathbf{-33.94}$, $AICc = \mathbf{84.07}$	

Alternative models assume independent escape (model 1, panels A, D, and G), sequential escape (model 2, panels B, E, and H), or concurrent escape (model 3, panels C, F, and I). Fits of models 1 and 3 gave very close parameter values, but there were some unrealistic parameter values (italicized in the table) from fits of the model 2. $\mathcal{L}$ and AICc give the log-likelihood score and the correlated Akaike information criterion value, respectively. Models 1 and 3 fit almost equally with three types of response inputs and the lowest $\mathcal{L}$ and AICc are shown in bold.

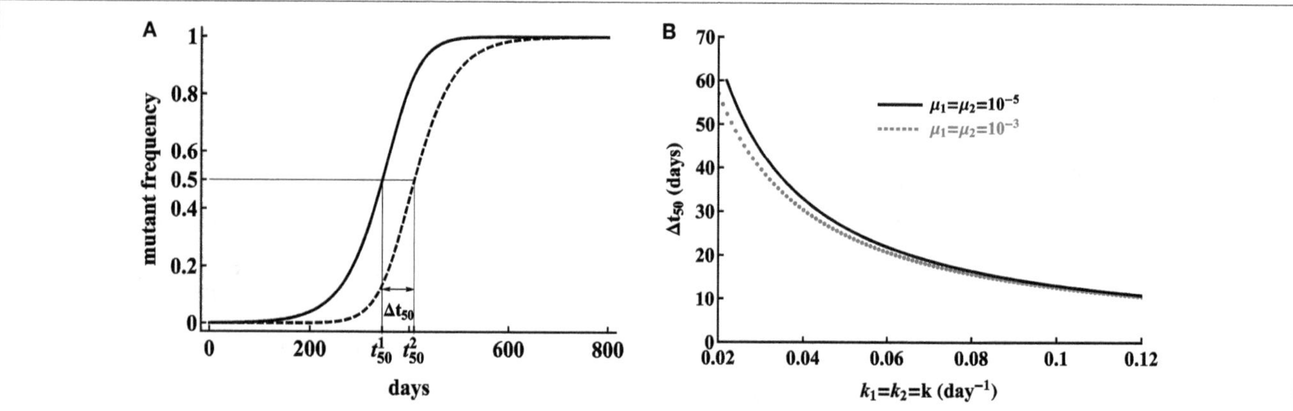

FIGURE 7 | Model, assuming sequential escape (model 2), can be consistent with escape data when the trajectories for two sequential viral escape are separated in time. We illustrate that separation of trajectories by $\Delta t_{50} = 409.8 - 344.2 \simeq 66$ days is sufficient for the mutation rate to be realistically small **(A)**. Here, t^i_{50} is the time by which the *i*th variant reaches 50% of the viral population, so, $\Delta t_{50} = t^2_{50} - t^1_{50}$. Parameters used in simulations are $\mu_1 = \mu_2 = 10^{-5A}$, $k_1 = k_2 = 0.02\,\text{day}^{-1A}$, $r = 1.5\,\text{day}^{-1}$, $\delta = 1\,\text{day}^{-1}$. The distance between trajectories needed for small predicted mutation rates is reduced for higher CTL killing rates **(B)** and the time is only weakly dependent on the mutation rate assumed in simulations.

in the blood may not reflect CTL dynamics in tissues such as secondary lymphoid organs (lymph nodes and spleen). While it is well known that T cells recirculate in the body (51), how quickly CTLs in the tissues migrate into the blood and then back to the tissues during HIV infection is not known. Finally, it is possible that the measured CTL responses were not the drivers of escape. While the ability of CTLs to recognize the wild-type virus and inability of the same CTLs to recognize mutant viruses is generally interpreted as evidence that these CTLs drove viral escape, such observations are correlational in nature, and thus cannot fully establish the causality of escape, at least in humans.

Our results may be interpreted as contradictory to several previous studies that found a strong correlation between the time of viral escape (time when an escape variant reaches frequency of 50% in the viral population) and a relative magnitude of CTL response (relative or "vertical" immunodominance) (11, 12). However, our studies are not directly compatible because this previous work focused on the timing of escape while we primarily focused on the rate of viral escape. These two parameters are differently impacted by the CTL response (17) and may have different clinical importance. In our simple mathematical model (e.g., equation (3)), CTL response magnitude is expected to directly impact the rate at which an escape mutant accumulates in the population, independently of when this escape may occur. In contrast, timing of viral escape also depends on the mutation rate. Biologically, however, timing of escape may be more important than the rate because it may be more beneficial to the patient if viral escape occurs 5 years after infection but rapidly as compared to slow escape in just 1 year. This conjecture clearly depends on the premise that HIV escapes from CTL responses are detrimental to patients.

In our analysis, we generally found that for well sampled data, the pathway of generation of escape mutants played a minor role in predicting overall CTL killing efficacy; assuming escapes that occur independently (model 1) or concurrently (model 3) gave nearly identical estimates of the CTL killing efficacy (e.g., **Tables 1** and **2**). In contrast, the model assuming sequential escape (model 2) often failed to accurately explain experimental data; this was due to some escapes co-occurring at nearly the same time, which obviously violated the model assumption of sequential escape. This inability of the sequential escape model to describe the data may be the result of the way we compared models to data: by using deterministic model approach and by ignoring recombination. Using deterministic model may be justified because, in acute infection, the effective population size of HIV may be sufficiently large and ignoring recombination may again be appropriate because very few cells in HIV infection are generally infected by 2 or more viruses (52, 53). However, further work is needed to demonstrate whether our conclusions regarding inability of sequential escape model to accurately explain some escape data is due to some of the assumptions made in the model by running stochastic simulations and by allowing some degree of recombination.

Many of our model fits predicted a high mutation rate for the first epitope to be escaped by the virus (e.g., **Table 2**). This model prediction could not be changed by shifting the experimental data to allow for more time to generate escape mutant; in part, this test failed because in the absence of epitope-specific T cells escape variants accumulate rather slowly mainly driven by mutations. It may indicate that immune pressure on the virus population starts much earlier than it is reflected in the blood, echoing our concerns of whether CTL dynamics in the blood is an accurate reflection of T cell response in lymphoid tissues. Currently, it is believed that lymphoid tissues and not the blood are the major places of interactions between the virus and CTLs (50, 54).

Our analysis further highlights the importance of choosing the appropriate statistical model for the analysis of the escape data–assuming normally distributed residuals, and therefore, using least squares approach, may not be appropriate for some escape data with very few sequences analyzed. Importantly, we confirm that the type of statistical model has an impact on the estimate of the escape rate (18).

We found that experimental data on HIV escape can be explained well if we assume identical per capital killing efficacy of CTLs, specific to different viral epitopes. This suggests that individual per capita killing rates not accurately estimated from these data. While it is possible that this result was the consequence of assuming additive killing of virus-infected cells by different CTL responses, we currently do not have any *in vivo* data to support more complex killing terms.

Overall, analyses of data from two patients suggested that models assuming independent escape of HIV from different CTL responses (model 1) or models assuming concurrent escape from multiple CTL responses (model 3) fit the data well and provide very similar (often nearly identical) estimates for the killing efficacy of CTL response. Thus, for well sampled data, assumption of independent escapes may be sufficient to accurately estimate HIV escape rates. Also, the model with data-driven time-dependent CTL response (interpolated or fitted response input) did not improve the quality of the model fit to data, so, at present, it appears to be unnecessary to incorporate the experimentally measured CTL response dynamics in the model describing viral escapes. Yet, because our results were found only for two patients, whether similar conclusions will be reached in other studies/patients remains to be determined. Our analysis nevertheless demonstrates how mathematical modeling may help to quantify HIV evolution in presence of CTL responses and to highlight potential limitations with experimental measurements.

AUTHOR CONTRIBUTIONS

YY and VG designed the study, contributed to analysis, interpolation of data, and simulation results, and wrote the paper. YY performed the simulations.

ACKNOWLEDGMENTS

The authors would like to thank Dr. Nilu Goonetilleke and the Center for HIV/AIDS Vaccine Immunology (CHAVI) for data access.

FUNDING

This work was supported by the American Heart Association (AHA: 13SDG16960053) grant to VG and in part by the National Institutes of Health (NIH: R01-GM118553) grant to VG. Funding for open access to this research was provided by University of Tennessee's Open Publishing Support Fund.

REFERENCES

WHO. *Global Health Observatory (GHO) Data*. Geneva: WHO (2016).

WHO. *Global HIV and AIDS Statistics*. Geneva: WHO (2016).

Borrow P, Lewicki H, Hahn BH, Shaw GM, Oldstone MB. Virus-specific $CD8^+$ cytotoxic T-lymphocyte activity associated with control of viremia in primary human immunodeficiency virus type 1 infection. *J Virol* (1994) 68(9):6103–10.

Ndhlovu ZM, Kamya P, Mewalal N, Klverpris HN, Nkosi T, Pretorius K, et al. Magnitude and kinetics of CD8$^+$ T cell activation during hyperacute HIV infection impact viral set point. *Immunity* (2015) 43(3):591–604. doi:10.1016/j. immuni.2015.08.012

Streeck H, Jolin JS, Qi Y, Yassine-Diab B, Johnson RC, Kwon DS, et al. Human immunodeficiency virus type 1-specific CD8$^+$ T-cell responses during primary infection are major determinants of the viral set point and loss of CD4$^+$ T cells. *J Virol* (2009) 83(15):7641–8. doi:10.1128/jvi.00182-09

Hansen SG, Ford JC, Lewis MS, Ventura AB, Hughes CM, Coyne-Johnson L, et al. Profound early control of highly pathogenic SIV by an effector memory T-cell vaccine. *Nature* (2011) 473(7348):523–7. doi:10.1038/nature10003

Walker BD, Ahmed R, Plotkin S. Moving ahead an HIV vaccine: use both arms to beat HIV. *Nat Med* (2011) 17(10):1194–5. doi:10.1038/nm.2529

Barouch DH, Kunstman J, Kuroda MJ, Schmitz JE, Santra S, Peyerl FW, et al. Eventual AIDS vaccine failure in a rhesus monkey by viral escape from cytotoxic T lymphocytes. *Nature* (2002) 415(6869):335–9. doi:10.1038/415335a

Goulder PJR, Watkins DI. HIV and SIV CTL escape: implications for vaccine design. *Nat Rev Immunol* (2004) 4(8):630–40. doi:10.1038/nri1417

Rolland M, Tovanabutra S, Decamp AC, Frahm N, Gilbert PB, Sanders-Buell E, et al. Genetic impact of vaccination on breakthrough HIV-1 sequences from the STEP trial. *Nat Med* (2011) 17(3):366–71. doi:10.1038/nm.2316

Barton JP, Goonetilleke N, Butler TC, Walker BD, McMichael AJ, Chakraborty AK. Relative rate and location of intra-host HIV evolution to evade cellular immunity are predictable. *Nat Commun* (2016) 7:11660. doi:10.1038/ncomms11660

Liu MK, Hawkins N, Ritchie AJ, Ganusov VV, Whale V, Brackenridge S, et al. Vertical T cell immunodominance and epitope entropy determine HIV-1 escape. *J Clin Invest* (2013) 123(1):380–93. doi:10.1172/JCI65330

Goonetilleke N, Liu MK, Salazar-Gonzalez JF, Ferrari G, Giorgi E, Ganusov VV, et al. The first T cell response to transmitted/founder virus contributes to the control of acute viremia in HIV-1 infection. *J Exp Med* (2009) 206(6):1253–72. doi:10.1084/jem.20090365

Asquith B, Edwards CTT, Lipsitch M, McLean AR. Inefficient cytotoxic T lymphocyte-mediated killing of HIV-1-infected cells in vivo. *PLoS Biol* (2006) 4(4):e90. doi:10.1371/journal.pbio.0040090

Fernandez CS, Stratov I, Rose RD, Walsh K, Dale CJ, Smith MZ, et al. Rapid viral escape at an immunodominant simian-human immunodeficiency virus cytotoxic T-lymphocyte epitope exacts a dramatic fitness cost. *J Virol* (2005) 79(9):5721–31. doi:10.1128/jvi.79.9.5721-5731.2005

Ganusov VV, De Boer RJ. Estimating costs and benefits of CTL escape mutations in SIV/HIV infection. *PLoS Comput Biol* (2006) 2(3):e24. doi:10.1371/journal.pcbi.0020024

Ganusov VV, Goonetilleke N, Liu MKP, Ferrari G, Shaw GM, McMichael AJ, et al. Fitness costs and diversity of the cytotoxic t lymphocyte (CTL) response determine the rate of CTL escape during acute and chronic phases of HIV infection. *J Virol* (2011) 85(20):10518–28. doi:10.1128/jvi.00655-11

Ganusov VV, Neher RA, Perelson AS. Mathematical modeling of escape of HIV from cytotoxic T lymphocyte responses. *J Stat Mech* (2013) 2013(01):01010. doi:10.1088/1742-5468/2013/01/p01010

Mandl JN, Regoes RR, Garber DA, Feinberg MB. Estimating the effectiveness of simian immunodeficiency virus-specific CD8$^+$ T cells from the dynamics of viral immune escape. *J Virol* (2007) 81(21):11982–91. doi:10.1128/jvi.00946-07

Petravic J, Loh L, Kent SJ, Davenport MP. Cd4$^+$ target cell availability determines the dynamics of immune escape and reversion in vivo. *J Virol* (2008) 82(8):4091–101. doi:10.1128/jvi.02552-07

Pandit A, De Boer RJ. Reliable reconstruction of HIV-1 whole genome haplotypes reveals clonal interference and genetic hitchhiking among immune escape variants. *Retrovirology* (2014) 11(1):56. doi:10.1186/1742-4690-11-56

Leviyang S, Ganusov VV. Broad CTL response in early HIV infection drives multiple concurrent CTL escapes. *PLoS Comput Biol* (2015) 11(10):e1004492. doi:10.1371/journal.pcbi.1004492

Garcia V, Feldman MW, Regoes RR. Investigating the consequences of interference between multiple CD8+ T cell escape mutations in early HIV infection. *PLoS Comput Biol* (2016) 12(2):e1004721. doi:10.1371/journal.pcbi.1004721

Garcia V, Regoes RR. The effect of interference on the CD8$^+$ T cell escape rates in HIV. *Front Immunol* (2015) 5:661. doi:10.3389/fimmu.2014.00661

Kessinger TA, Perelson AS, Neher RA. Inferring HIV escape rates from multi-locus genotype data. *Front Immunol* (2013) 4:252. doi:10.3389/fimmu.2013.00252

Van Deutekom HWM, Wijnker G, De Boer RJ. The rate of immune escape vanishes when multiple immune responses control an HIV infection. *J Immunol* (2013) 191(6):3277–86. doi:10.4049/jimmunol.1300962

Ganusov VV. Time intervals in sequence sampling, not data modifications, have a major impact on estimates of HIV escape rates. *bioRxiv* (2017). doi:10.1101/ 221812

Perelson AS. Modelling viral and immune system dynamics. *Nat Rev Immunol* (2002) 2(1):28–36. doi:10.1038/nri700

Perelson AS, Neumann AU, Markowitz M, Leonard JM, Ho DD. HIV-1 dynamics in vivo: virion clearance rate, infected cell life-span, and viral generation time. *Science* (1996) 271(5255):1582–6. doi:10.1126/science.271.5255.1582

Ramratnam B, Bonhoeffer S, Binley J, Hurley A, Zhang L, Mittler JE, et al. Rapid production and clearance of HIV-1 and hepatitis C virus assessed by large volume plasma apheresis. *Lancet* (1999) 354(9192):1782–5. doi:10.1016/s0140- 6736(99)02035-8

Song H, Pavlicek JW, Cai F, Bhattacharya T, Li H, Iyer SS, et al. Impact of immune escape mutations on HIV-1 fitness in the context of the cognate transmitted/founder genome. *Retrovirology* (2012) 9(1):89. doi:10.1186/1742- 4690-9-89

Wright JK, Brumme ZL, Carlson JM, Heckerman D, Kadie CM, Brumme CJ, et al. Gag-protease-mediated replication capacity in HIV-1 subtype c chronic infection: associations with HLA type and clinical parameters. *J Virol* (2010) 84(20):10820–31. doi:10.1128/jvi.01084-10

Turnbull EL, Wong M, Wang S, Wei X, Jones NA, Conrod KE, et al. Kinetics of expansion of epitope-specific T cell responses during primary HIV-1 infection. *J Immunol* (2009) 182(11):7131–45. doi:10.4049/jimmunol.0803658

Mansky LM, Temin HM. Lower in vivo mutation rate of human immunodeficiency virus type 1 than that predicted from the fidelity of purified reverse transcriptase. *J Virol* (1995) 69(8):5087–94.

Leviyang S. Computational inference methods for selective sweeps arising in acute HIV infection. *Genetics* (2013) 194(3):737–52. doi:10.1534/genetics.113. 150862

Althaus CL, De Boer RJ. Dynamics of immune escape during HIV/SIV infection. *PLoS Comput Biol* (2008) 4(7):e1000103. doi:10.1371/journal.pcbi. 1000103

Ganusov VV, Barber DL, De Boer RJ. Killing of targets by CD8$^+$ T cells in the mouse spleen follows the law of mass action. *PLoS One* (2011) 6(1):e15959. doi:10.1371/journal.pone.0015959

De Boer RJ, Oprea M, Antia R, Murali-Krishna K, Ahmed R, Perelson AS. Recruitment times, proliferation, and apoptosis rates during the CD8$^+$ T-cell response to lymphocytic choriomeningitis virus. *J Virol* (2001) 75(22):10663–9. doi:10.1128/jvi.75.22.10663-10669.2001

De Boer RJ, Homann D, Perelson AS. Different dynamics of CD4$^+$ and CD8$^+$ T cell responses during and after acute lymphocytic choriomeningitis virus infection. *J Immunol* (2003) 171:3928–35. doi:10.4049/jimmunol.171.8.3928

Yang YD, Ganusov VV. Defining kinetic properties of HIV-specific CD8$^+$ T-cell responses in acute infection. *bioRxiv* (2017). doi:10.1101/158683

Bates DM, Watts DG. *Nonlinear Regression Analysis and Its Applications*. New York: Wiley (1988).

Burnham KP, Anderson DR. *Model Selection and Multimodel Inference: A Practical Information-Theoretic Approach*. New York: Springer (2002).

Efron B, Tibshirani R. *An Introduction to the Bootstrap*. New York: Chapman & Hall (1993).

Brown L, Cai T, DasGupta A, Agresti A, Coull B, Casella G, et al. Interval estimation for a binomial proportion. *Stat Sci* (2001) 16(2):101–33. doi:10.1214/ ss/1009213285

McMichael AJ, Borrow P, Tomaras GD, Goonetilleke N, Haynes BF. The immune response during acute HIV-1 infection: clues for vaccine development. *Nat Rev Immunol* (2010) 10(1):11–23. doi:10.1038/nri2674

Love TMT, Thurston SW, Keefer MC, Dewhurst S, Lee HY. Mathematical modeling of ultradeep sequencing data reveals that acute CD8$^+$ T-lymphocyte responses exert strong selective pressure in simian immunodeficiency virus- infected macaques but still fail to clear founder epitope sequences. *J Virol* (2010) 84(11):5802–14. doi:10.1128/JVI.00117-10

Martyushev AP, Petravic J, Grimm AJ, Alinejad-Rokny H, Gooneratne SL, Reece JC, et al. Epitope-specific CD8+ T cell kinetics rather than viral vari- ability determine the timing of immune escape in simian immunodeficiency virus infection. *J Immunol* (2015) 194(9):4112–21. doi:10.4049/jimmunol. 1400793

Kijak GH, Sanders-Buell E, Chenine A-L, Eller MA, Goonetilleke N, Thomas R, et al. Rare HIV-1 transmitted/founder lineages identified by deep viral sequencing contribute to rapid shifts in dominant quasispecies during acute and early infection. *PLoS Pathog* (2017) 13:e1006510. doi:10.1371/journal.ppat. 1006510

McMichael AJ, Phillips RE. Escape of human immunodeficiency virus from immune control. *Annu Rev Immunol* (1997) 15:271–96. doi:10.1146/annurev. immunol.15.1.271

Li Q, Skinner PJ, Ha SJ, Duan L, Mattila TL, Hage A, et al. Visualizing antigen-specific and infected cells in situ predicts outcomes in early viral infection. *Science* (2009) 323(5922):1726–9. doi:10.1126/science.1168676

Ganusov VV, Auerbach J. Mathematical modeling reveals kinetics of lymphocyte recirculation in the whole organism. *PLoS Comput Biol* (2014) 10:e1003586. doi:10.1371/journal.pcbi.1003586

Josefsson L, King MS, Makitalo B, Brännström J, Shao W, Maldarelli F, et al. Majority of $CD4^+$ T cells from peripheral blood of HIV-1-infected individuals contain only one HIV DNA molecule. *Proc Natl Acad Sci U S A* (2011) 108(27):11199–204. doi:10.1073/pnas.1107729108

Haase AT. Population biology of HIV-1 infection: viral and $CD4^+$ T cell demographics and dynamics in lymphatic tissues. *Annu Rev Immunol* (1999) 17:625–56. doi:10.1146/annurev.immunol.17.1.625

15

Dimensionality of Motion and Binding Valency Govern Receptor–Ligand Kinetics as Revealed by Agent-Based Modeling

Teresa Lehnert[1,2] *and Marc Thilo Figge*[1,2,3]*

[1] *Research Group Applied Systems Biology, Leibniz Institute of Natural Product Research and Infection Biology – Hans Knöll Institute (HKI), Jena, Germany,* [2] *Center for Sepsis Control and Care (CSCC), Jena University Hospital, Jena, Germany,* [3] *Faculty of Biology and Pharmacy, Friedrich Schiller University Jena, Jena, Germany*

Correspondence:
Marc Thilo Figge
thilo.figge@leibniz-hki.de

Mathematical modeling and computer simulations have become an integral part of modern biological research. The strength of theoretical approaches is in the simplification of complex biological systems. We here consider the general problem of receptor–ligand binding in the context of antibody–antigen binding. On the one hand, we establish a quantitative mapping between macroscopic binding rates of a deterministic differential equation model and their microscopic equivalents as obtained from simulating the spatiotemporal binding kinetics by stochastic agent-based models. On the other hand, we investigate the impact of various properties of B cell-derived receptors—such as their dimensionality of motion, morphology, and binding valency—on the receptor–ligand binding kinetics. To this end, we implemented an algorithm that simulates antigen binding by B cell-derived receptors with a Y-shaped morphology that can move in different dimensionalities, i.e., either as membrane-anchored receptors or as soluble receptors. The mapping of the macroscopic and microscopic binding rates allowed us to quantitatively compare different agent-based model variants for the different types of B cell-derived receptors. Our results indicate that the dimensionality of motion governs the binding kinetics and that this predominant impact is quantitatively compensated by the bivalency of these receptors.

Keywords: agent-based model, ordinary differential equations, antibody–antigen binding, receptor–ligand interaction, dimensionality of motion, binding valency

1. INTRODUCTION

In recent decades, computational biology has developed into an autonomous scientific discipline that has become indispensable for contemporary biological research. Major contributions of computational biology comprise: (i) directing studies by providing insights that cannot otherwise be obtained in wet-lab experiments, (ii) advancing biological research toward a quantitative science through large-scale computations, and (iii) generating experimentally testable hypotheses through simulations of mathematical models.

The strength of mathematical modeling is actually in the simplification of complex processes by focusing on the most relevant aspects of a system. The art of modeling is in the appropriate choice of a mathematical approach that describes all existing experimental data and still can make relevant predictions. At this point a reasonable compromise has to be made between the level of system complexity that is transferred into the mathematical model and the feasibility of simulations with regard to computational resources.

Models based on ordinary differential equations (ODE) are presumably most frequently applied in biological research, even though this modeling approach is only valid if the system under consideration consists of large amounts of constituents, e.g., molecules, that are homogeneously distributed or well stirred in some spatial environment (1). This is because ODE models do not explicitly account for any spatial aspects of a system and changes in system variables, e.g., concentrations of molecules, are consequently described by functions of time that are continuous and deterministic. However, these assumptions, which may be typically appropriate for chemical systems, are for biological systems at best applicable from a macroscopic point of view. In these macroscopic models the biological processes are characterized by two specific types of parameters, which are referred to as *rates* or *reaction rates*. Rates characterize unimolecular processes that occur spontaneously and have unit 1/time. Reactions involving two types of molecules, i.e., bimolecular processes, are characterized by reaction rates with unit 1/(concentration × time). Typical experimental assays to determine these macroscopic rates for uni- and bimolecular processes are the adhesion frequency assay and the surface plasmon resonance assay (2). The advantage of ODE models is that they are based on a minimal set of parameters and can be formulated with relative ease (1, 3), which makes them belonging to the so-called simple modeling approaches (4). Deterministic ODE models may be extended to account for the stochasticity of chemical reactions in solution. Various numerical schemes have been introduced by Gillespie to sample the underlying master equation for the probability to find the system in a particular state at a given time (5). These are referred to as the *direct method* (6) and the *first reaction method* (7) and were later advanced for computational speed-up with the *next reaction method* by Gibson and Bruck (8). Albeit more detailed than deterministic ODE models, all these approaches have in common that a macroscopic viewpoint on the system is taken.

In contrast, agent-based models (ABMs), which belong to the so-called detailed modeling approaches (4), consider biological systems from a microscopic viewpoint by taking details of their individual constituents in space and time into account. A system's constituents, e.g., molecules and/or cells, are represented by agents in the model and their motion in a specific spatial environment as well as their stochastic interactions with other agents are monitored in the simulations. In this microscopic modeling approach, all reactions are performed with a specific probability per time-step. This implies that not only the rates for unimolecular processes are measured in unit 1/time, but also the reaction rates for bimolecular processes, because the microscopic reactions are between two single molecules and not between concentrations of molecules as is the case for macroscopic ODE models. The microscopic rates for molecular interactions could be experimentally measured using thermal fluctuation assays (2). However, the level of detail represented by ABM comes at the price of a relatively large number of model parameters, which may be unknown and/or even inaccessible to experiment (1, 9), and simulations of ABM are typically associated with a high computational load (10, 11).

In this study, we focus on specific receptor–ligand (RL) binding, i.e., antibody–antigen binding as a central part of the adaptive immune response, and model this process in a comparative fashion by ODE models and by ABM. Binding between receptors and ligands represents an essential process in the immune system by which important information is transferred. For example, in the process termed *opsonization*, pathogen-derived antigens can be neutralized and labeled by antibodies for removal from the organism. Antibodies are soluble molecules that play a key role in the humoral response of adaptive immunity (12), because they can bind antigens with high affinity and can provide life-long protection against specific antigens. Of interest, antibodies do also exist as membrane-anchored molecules on B lymphocytes and are then referred to as B cell receptors (BCR). Binding of cognate antigen by BCR activates naïve B cells in lymphoid organs, such as spleen and lymph node (13), and this may initiate a germinal center (GC) reaction for antibody affinity maturation (12). During a GC reaction, B cells are proliferating and mutating their BCR followed by the selection of B cells with BCR that have high affinities to presented antigens. B cells with BCR that successfully accomplished the selection procedure differentiate into plasma cells that produce large amounts of these BCR as soluble antibodies. The GC reaction has been the subject of various interdisciplinary studies combining experimental and theoretical investigations (5, 14–17). In particular, it could be shown that the GC reaction is not only initiated by antigen binding to BCR on B cells, but that its termination is as well regulated by the high-affinity antibodies produced in soluble form (18). Taken together, antibodies represent a prime example for this study because of three reasons: (i) they exist as soluble as well as membrane-anchored receptors, (ii) they have a peculiar Y-shaped morphology that raises the question on its impact on RL binding as compared to spherically shaped receptors, and (iii) they have two binding sites and can bind antigen mono- or bivalently. The computational biology approach that is pursued in this study allows investigating the relative importance of receptor morphology, binding valency and dimensionality of motion that depends on receptors being soluble or membrane anchored on a cell. Applying different modeling approaches, e.g., ODE models and ABM, in a comparative fashion enables a quantitative mapping of the macroscopic and microscopic viewpoint on RL binding dynamics.

2. MATERIALS AND METHODS

2.1. Microscopic Modeling of Receptor–Ligand Binding

Agent-based models (ABMs) are widely used in computational biology to simulate processes at the microscopic scale (9–11, 19). The individual constituents of the biological system under consideration are represented as agents that can move in a defined spatial environment and can interact with each other according to specific rules. We studied receptor–ligand (RL) binding and, in particular, the impact of specific receptor properties on the dynamics of the binding process. While ligands were modeled as molecules in solution with spherical shape, we considered receptors with different morphologies, i.e., being either spherically shaped (O) or Y-shaped (Y), and in settings with different dimensionality of motion, i.e., receptors in solution (SOL) or membrane anchored (MEM) on the surface of a cell. The four combinations of receptor properties are depicted in **Figures 1** and **2**, and give rise to four different ABM variants. These are denoted by their receptor properties, respectively, as O-SOL (see **Figures 1A** and **2A**), O-MEM (see **Figures 1B** and **2B**), Y-SOL (see **Figures 1C** and **2C**), and Y-MEM (see **Figures 1D** and **2D**). Simulations of the different ABM variants are shown in Videos S1–S5 in Supplementary Material. While in what follows we describe the general setup of the ABM, a detailed overview of the model parameters and of their corresponding values is provided in the Table S1 in Supplementary Material.

2.1.1. Model System

In this study, we considered the model system of a B cell with Y-shaped B cell receptors (BCR), because these receptors do as well exist in a soluble form as antibodies. In the ABM, BCR with their *Fab*-fragments as binding sites are represented by a cylindrical stem with two cylindrical arms and spherical binding regions at the distal sides, which are hereafter referred to as *binding spheres*. A schematic representation of the BCR in soluble and membrane-anchored form is shown, respectively, in **Figure 2C** for ABM variant Y-SOL and in **Figure 2D** for ABM variant Y-MEM. The binding spheres on top of each arm represent the active binding sites of the BCR, whose surface areas are estimated from the size of *Fv*-regions, i.e., the variable parts of the BCR *Fab*-arms. Thus, the binding spheres implicitly account for the attractive short-range interactions between the binding sites of receptors and ligands (20–23). For the reason of comparison between BCR and spherically shaped receptors, we set the values of binding radii such that the effective area of all binding spheres are of comparable size, as can be inferred from the relative receptor sizes in **Figures 2A,B** for ABM variants O-SOL and O-MEM, respectively. For the same reason, when comparing Y-shaped and spherically shaped receptors, we impose the condition that receptors can only bind one ligand at a time. In addition, we also compared Y-shaped receptors that can bind mono- and bivalently.

2.1.2. Molecular Diffusion and Interaction

Receptors and ligands perform diffusive motion in the ABM. The corresponding diffusion coefficients can vary by orders of magnitude for soluble and membrane-anchored receptors. Diffusion coefficients were estimated based on the Stokes-Einstein equation (24) and the values for the corresponding ABM variants (see Table S1 in Supplementary Material) were calculated as outlined in Supplementary Material. In this study, we aim to investigate the impact of the dimensionality of motion for different receptor morphologies during the process of RL binding. In the ABM, molecules with diffusion coefficient D move per time step Δt

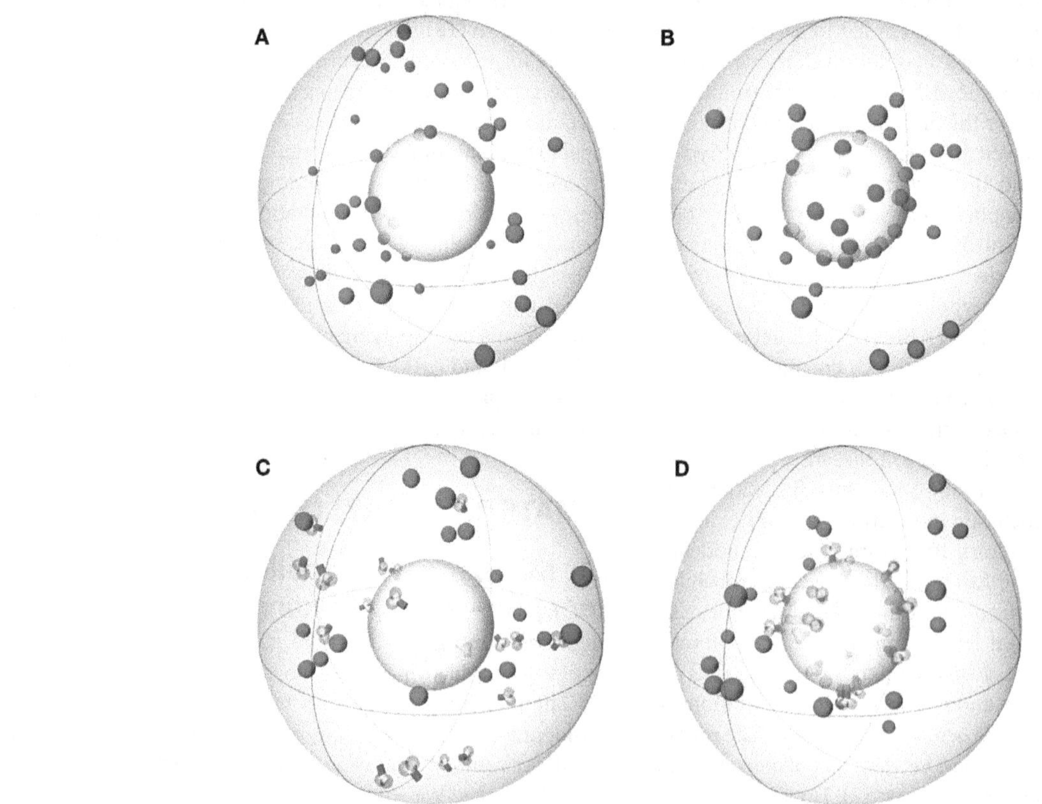

FIGURE 1 | Schemes of ABM variants for receptor–ligand binding. The ABM variants are composed of the same spherical environment (large gray sphere) containing a spherical cell (small gray sphere) at the center. Ligands (orange) are always soluble, whereas receptors (blue) are studied in the variants: spherical receptor morphology in **(A)** soluble (O-SOL) or **(B)** membrane-anchored (O-MEM) form and Y-shaped receptor morphology in **(C)** soluble (Y-SOL) or **(D)** membrane-anchored (Y-MEM) form.

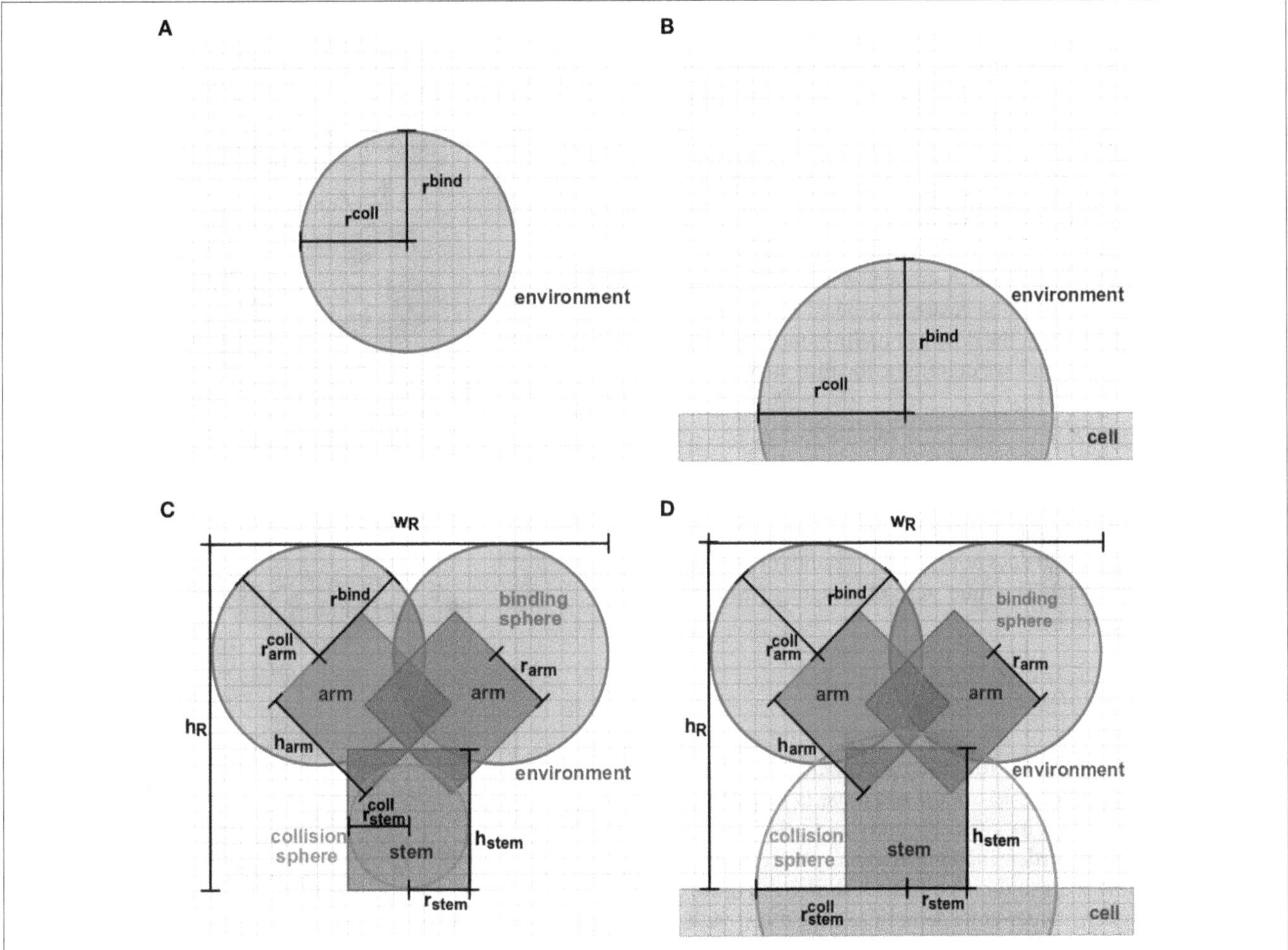

FIGURE 2 | Detailed representation of receptor morphologies. Two-dimensional projection of three-dimensional receptors in ABM variants **(A)** O-SOL, **(B)** O-MEM, **(C)** Y-SOL, and **(D)** Y-MEM. Each receptor consists of binding spheres and collision spheres that may be overlapping in position and size. Ligands can bind by encountering a receptor's binding sphere but are prohibited to penetrate receptors by the collision spheres. Details on the parameter values are provided in Table S1 in Supplementary Material.

the specific distance $\Delta s = \sqrt{2dD\Delta t}$ in a direction of the d-dimensional space that is chosen from a uniformly random distribution. This motion involves also a random rotation of Y-shaped receptors around their two axes in a spherically uniform fashion.

Two types of interaction processes are possible in the ABM: binding of receptor and ligand to form a molecular complex and dissociation of such a complex into individual receptor and ligand. The latter process occurs with rate k_{off}^{micro} and translates into the probability $p_{off}^{micro} = k_{off}^{micro}\Delta t$ that a complex dissociates during one time step Δt. In this study, we set the microscopic and macroscopic dissociation rates to be equal, i.e., $k_{off}^{micro} = k_{off}^{macro}$. As analyzed in detail in Supplementary Material, this approach is valid for typical parameter values of antibody–antigen dissociation rates, implying that dissociation and rebinding are relatively rare processes. On the other hand, binding of diffusing receptor and ligand requires that these molecules first encounter each other in the spatial environment. Then, upon contact of the ligand with the respective binding sphere of a receptor, binding occurs with probability $p_{on}^{micro} = k_{on}^{micro}\Delta t$, where k_{on}^{micro} denotes the microscopic binding rate with unit s^{-1}. Note, that this rate is conceptually different from the macroscopic reaction rate k_{on}^{macro} with unit $\mu m^3 s^{-1}$, because the latter incorporates the process of encounter of molecules in a spatially homogeneous system by their concentrations. In this study, we establish a relation between k_{on}^{micro} and k_{on}^{macro} by mapping the microscopic and macroscopic RL binding kinetics onto each other.

2.1.3. Implementation and Simulation

We implemented the ABM in a spherical environment with the cell positioned at its center and for reasons of comparison this was the same in all four ABM variants. The boundary condition at the outer boundary of the environment was chosen to be random-periodic for molecule motion, i.e., a molecule leaving the system at one point was entering the system at another random position of this boundary, where the newly added molecule was given an entirely new identity. At the inner boundary of the cell surface, reflecting boundary conditions were imposed. By applying these realistic boundary conditions, we ensure that the number of molecules in the system is constant during the simulation time.

For a highly realistic implementation of RL binding dynamics, a continuous space representation was used and combined with the neighbor-list method (25, 26) to speed up the detection of interaction partners in this off-lattice approach. Molecules in motion may approach each other and become overlapping. We implemented a push-back procedure, such that the overlap by the moving molecule was reduced to a point contact with the other molecule. Thus, we imposed the condition that molecules cannot penetrate each other and this choice impacts on the effective reaction volume between the molecules.

For reasons of comparison between the different ABM variants, we use the same time step Δt in each simulation, such that changes in the simulation results can be clearly attributed to differences in the receptor morphology, the dimensionality of motion and/or binding valency. To this end, we determine the time step

$$\Delta t = \min\left(\min\left(k_{off}^{micro\,-1}, k_{on}^{micro\,-1}\right), \min(\Delta t_R, \Delta t_L)\right), \quad (1)$$

from the smallest considered rate of binding (k_{on}^{micro}) and dissociation (k_{off}^{micro}) as well as the smallest time step associated with a diffusion step in space that does not exceed the radius of receptors (Δs_R) and ligands (Δs_L). The time steps of receptors (Δt_R) and ligands (Δt_L) are given by

$$\Delta t_{R,L} = \frac{\Delta s_{R,L}^2}{2d\,D_{R,L}}. \quad (2)$$

The simulation algorithm for RL binding dynamics is based on random selection dynamics (5). Each molecule is updated per time step with regard to its diffusion and interaction that are performed in random order applying the acceptance-rejection method (27). A flowchart of the algorithm is shown in **Figure 3**. For the model system under consideration, i.e., a B cell with a number of BCR in the order 10^5 and an equal amount of ligands, simulation run times would exceed all limits. In fact, it can be estimated that the ratio of the typical simulation time over the simulated real time becomes as large as 10^9. Therefore, since the size of the time step is determined by the accurate resolution of molecular motion and interaction, we down-scale the number of molecules and decrease the system size while keeping the molecular concentration constant. The details of the down-scaling procedure are described in Supplementary Material and the associated values are summarized in Table S2 in Supplementary Material. All simulations were performed after down-scaling the number of molecules by a factor $s = 10^{-2}$, i.e., reducing the B cell size by a factor 10 and the number of BCR to the order 10^3.

The ABM framework was implemented in the object-oriented programming language C++.

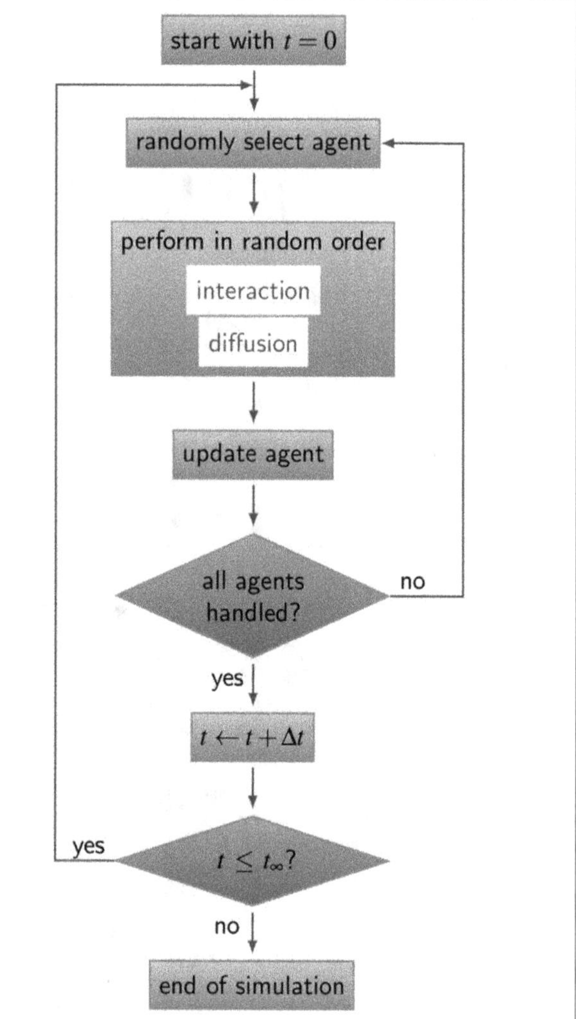

FIGURE 3 | Flow chart of the ABM simulation algorithm for receptor–ligand binding kinetics. The gray boxes represent operations and are connected by directive arrows depicting the sequence of the ABM simulation algorithm. In each time step Δt, all agents perform diffusive motion and undergo interactions with other agents in random order until simulation time t_∞ is reached. Simulations of all ABM variants are shown in Videos S1–S5 in Supplementary Material.

2.2. Macroscopic Modeling of Receptor–Ligand Binding

Modeling RL binding from a macroscopic point of view can be done in a straightforward fashion using ordinary differential equations (ODE). This approach is appropriate to describe chemical processes where reaction partners occur in large amounts and are homogeneously distributed in the spatial environment. Consequently, ODE models represent time-dependent changes of molecule concentrations in a continuous and deterministic fashion. We considered the binding of receptors (R) and ligands (L) to form a molecular complex (C) as well as their unbinding:

$$R + L \underset{k_{off}^{macro}}{\overset{k_{on}^{macro}}{\rightleftarrows}} C. \quad (3)$$

Here, k_{on}^{macro} is the reaction rate for binding, k_{off}^{macro} is the dissociation rate and the corresponding association constant K_a is defined by their ratio: $K_a = k_{on}^{macro}/k_{off}^{macro}$.

The reaction equation (3) was then translated into the coupled system of ODE:

$$\frac{dR}{dt} = -k_{on}^{macro}RL + k_{off}^{macro}C, \quad (4)$$

$$\frac{dL}{dt} = -k_{on}^{macro}RL + k_{off}^{macro}C, \quad (5)$$

$$\frac{dC}{dt} = +k_{on}^{macro}RL - k_{off}^{macro}C. \quad (6)$$

Assuming that initially no molecular complexes exist, $C\ (t=0)=0$, it follows from the relations $R(t)=R(0)-C(t)$ and $L(t)=L(0)-C(t)$ that it is sufficient to solve the non-linear equation for $C(t)$:

$$\frac{dC}{dt} = \alpha C^2 - \beta C + \gamma, \tag{7}$$

where we defined the constants

$$\alpha = k_{on}^{macro}, \tag{8}$$

$$\beta = k_{off}^{macro} + k_{on}^{macro}[R(0) + L(0)], \tag{9}$$

$$\gamma = k_{on}^{macro}\, R(0)L(0). \tag{10}$$

The ODE for $C(t)$ can be solved by the separation of variables and yields the analytical solution:

$$C(t) = C_-\, C_+ \frac{1 - e^{\alpha(C_+ - C_-)t}}{C_- - C_+\, e^{\alpha(C_+ - C_-)t}} \tag{11}$$

with

$$C_\pm = \frac{\beta}{2\alpha} \pm \sqrt{\frac{\beta^2}{4\alpha^2} - \frac{\gamma}{\alpha}}. \tag{12}$$

Note that the concentration $C(t)$ is associated with the number of receptor–ligand (RL) complexes in the microscopic model (see Materials and Methods section 2.1.2).

2.3. Mapping Microscopic and Macroscopic Binding Kinetics

A relation between the macroscopic and microscopic viewpoint on the binding kinetics of receptors and ligands can be established *via* the corresponding reaction rates for RL binding k_{on}^{macro} and k_{on}^{micro}. Given the concentration of molecular complexes C(t) (see equation (11)), we fit this analytical solution from macroscopic binding kinetics to the numerical results of simulations obtained from ABM at the microscopic level. This yields the desired relation $k_{on}^{macro}(k_{on}^{micro})$ that can be compared for different ABM variants.

The fitting procedure was performed within the open source programming language R (28). We used the function *nls*() that returns optimal parameter values of non-linear model equations by least-squares fitting. In particular, we used the fitting algorithm option "port" that refers to the adaptive non-linear least-squares algorithm NL2SOL (29) provided by the Port library. The algorithm adaptively switches between the Gauss-Newton method and an augmented Hessian approximation (30).

In practice, we applied the fitting procedure in two different respects: (i) The macroscopic binding rate k_{on}^{macro} in equation (11) was estimated from fitting to the data points obtained from numerical simulations with the ABM over time. (ii) The values determined for k_{on}^{macro} were used as data points to fit the optimal parameter values of the Hill equation $k_{on}^{macro}(k_{on}^{micro})$ (see equation (13)) in order to map the microscopic and macroscopic binding kinetics.

3. RESULTS

In this section, we present our simulation results on receptor–ligand (RL) binding by comparing the dynamics of individual receptors and ligands at the microscopic level with the population kinetics at the macroscopic level. The population kinetics can be straightforwardly described by a coupled system of ordinary differential equations (ODE), whereas agent-based models (ABM) resolve spatial structures of receptors and ligands and account for the dimensionality of the spatial environment in which these molecules diffuse and interact. In particular, we study monovalent receptors with different morphologies, i.e., being either spherically shaped (O) or Y-shaped (Y), and in settings with different dimensionality of motion, i.e., in solution (SOL) or membrane anchored (MEM). While ligands are throughout considered as being in solution and as having spherical shape, the four combinations of receptor properties give rise to four different ABM variants that are denoted by their receptor properties, respectively, as O-SOL, O-MEM, Y-SOL, and Y-MEM. These are schematically depicted in **Figure 1** and the differences between receptors are shown in **Figure 2.** In addition, videos of simulations for the different ABM variants with monovalent receptors are provided in Videos S1-S5 in Supplementary Material, where Videos S1-S4 represent down-scaled systems with factor $s=10^{-2}$, while Video S5 shows a simulation of ABM variant Y-MEM with $s=1$. A flow chart of the simulation algorithm is provided in **Figure 3** and details on the implementation of the ABM and on the model parameters are given in the Materials and Methods section.

3.1. Binding Kinetics for Different Receptor Properties Qualitatively Comparable

The binding kinetics at the macroscopic level, which can be determined from the analytical solution of the ODE model (see Materials and Methods section), was observed to be in qualitative agreement with the simulation results of all four ABM variants with monovalent receptors at the microscopic level. This can be seen from the ABM simulation results in **Figure 4,** where the microscopic rate for RL dissociation was fixed at $k_{off}^{micro} = 0.1\,s^{-1}$, while the microscopic rate for RL binding was set to $k_{on}^{micro} = 10^6\,s^{-1}$ (**Figure 4A**) and $k_{on}^{micro} = 10^7\,s^{-1}$ (**Figure 4B**). Note that we provide the concentration of molecular complexes in units $1/\mu m^3$ to enable the comparison of the binding dynamics simulated by ODE and ABM variants with soluble and membrane-anchored receptors. Since the initial numbers of receptors and ligands as well as the system volumes are identical in all models and simulations, we basically perform a comparison with regard to the number of complexes in each system. In general, we observed that the impact of the stochasticity on RL binding dynamics in the ABM is small, e.g., the relative standard deviation in the number of RL complexes was found to be around 1% for equilibrated systems (see the thickness of curves in pale colors in **Figure 4**). This is due to the large number of molecules in each simulation, such that five repetitions—involving in total the simulation of 10^4 molecules—yielded vanishingly small standard deviations.

We generally found a decrease in the concentration of free receptors and ligands with time, which was naturally associated with an increase in the concentration of RL complexes. This

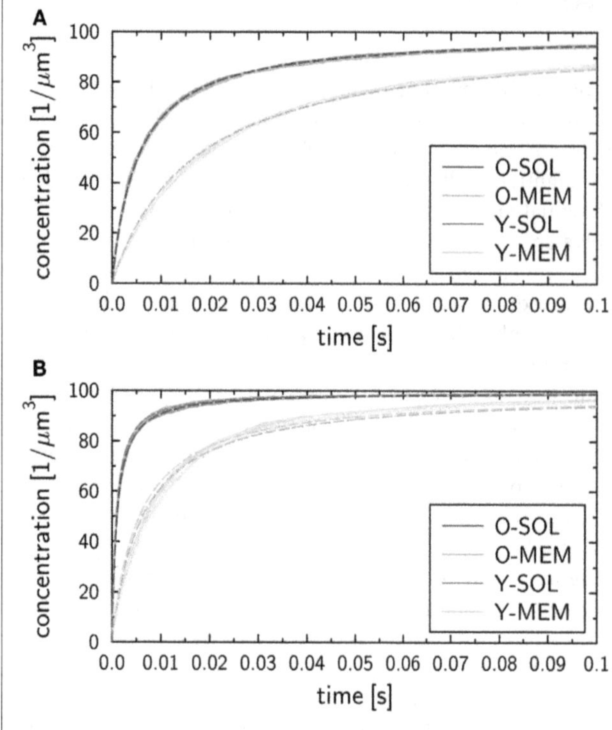

FIGURE 4 | Receptor–ligand binding kinetics for the four ABM variants. Time-dependent concentration of RL complexes with monovalent receptors as obtained from simulations of all four ABM variants with dissociation rate $k_{off}^{micro} = 0.1\ s^{-1}$ and binding rate **(A)** $k_{on}^{micro} = 10^6\ s^{-1}$ or **(B)** $k_{on}^{micro} = 10^7\ s^{-1}$. Dark and pale lines in different colors represent, respectively, mean values and standard deviations of five simulation runs per ABM variant. Dashed lines indicate the corresponding ODE models after fitting the macroscopic reaction rate k_{on}^{macro}.

observation was robust against variations in the receptor properties, i.e., all four ABM variants—O-SOL, O-MEM, Y-SOL, and Y-MEM—showed the same qualitative behavior. Thus, the qualitative agreement with the macroscopic binding kinetics based on the ODE was not limited to the ABM variant O-SOL as its direct microscopic counterpart. Therefore, in what follows, the analytical ODE solution can be used to fit the simulation results of all four ABM variants and to characterize them by their quantitative differences in the macroscopic binding rate k_{on}^{macro}. Note that this is the only free model parameter, since the dissociation of RL complexes occurs spontaneously at both the microscopic and macroscopic level implying that the corresponding rates are identical: $k_{off}^{macro} = k_{off}^{micro}$. Arguments for this relation between macroscopic and microscopic dissociation rates are provided based on the analysis in Supplementary Material.

3.2. Receptor Properties Have Quantitative Impact on Binding Kinetics

At the quantitative level, we observed differences in the binding kinetics depending on the receptor properties as well as on the microscopic binding rate k_{on}^{micro}. As could be expected, formation of RL complexes occurred slower for smaller $k_{on}^{micro} = 10^6\ s^{-1}$ (**Figure 4A**) than for larger $k_{on}^{micro} = 10^7\ s^{-1}$ (**Figure 4B**). Moreover, for a fixed value k_{on}^{micro}, the ABM variants with monovalent receptors in solution—O-SOL (red lines) and Y-SOL (blue lines)—exhibited quantitative agreement in the binding kinetics. While for the corresponding ABM variants with membrane-anchored receptors—O-MEM (orange lines) and Y-MEM (green lines)—this quantitative agreement was also observed, a quantitative difference in the binding kinetics between receptors in solution and membrane-anchored receptors was clearly visible (see **Figure 4**).

Using the analytical ODE solution of the binding kinetics, we fitted the simulation results of all four ABM variants to characterize them by their quantitative differences in the macroscopic binding rate k_{on}^{macro}. The fitted curves are shown in **Figure 4** and yielded for $k_{on}^{micro} = 10^6\ s^{-1}$ (**Figure 4A**) the values $k_{on}^{macro} \approx 1.9\mu m^3\ s^{-1}$ for the ABM variants O-SOL and Y-SOL and $k_{on}^{macro} \approx 0.6\ \mu m^3\ s^{-1}$ for the ABM variants O-MEM and Y-MEM. For $k_{on}^{micro} = 10^7\ s^{-1}$ (**Figure 4B**), we obtained the values $k_{on}^{macro} \approx 10.5\ \mu m^3\ s^{-1}$ for the ABM variants O-SOL and Y-SOL and $k_{on}^{macro} \approx 1.7\mu m^3\ s^{-1}$ for the ABM variants O-MEM and Y-MEM. It should be noted that the goodness of the fit, which was evaluated by the error of least squares fitting, was comparable for all simulations with microscopic binding rates in the range $10^4\ s^{-1} \leq k_{on}^{micro} \leq 10^6\ s^{-1}$. Even though for $k_{on}^{micro} > 10^6$ the error of least squares fitting for ABM variants with membrane-anchored receptors can be up to two orders of magnitude larger than for those with receptors in solution (see Figure S1 in Supplementary Material), all fitted curves still represented a fair representation of the simulation results (see **Figure 4B**).

These results were the first indication that the receptor morphology plays a relatively minor role in the binding kinetics compared to the dimensionality of motion of receptors, i.e., whether receptors diffuse in three-dimensional solution or on the surface of a cell. To further analyze these findings, we decided to establish a detailed quantitative mapping between the macroscopic and microscopic binding rates.

3.3. Quantitative Mapping of the Macroscopic and Microscopic Binding Rates Reveals Impact of Dimensionality of Motion

We performed numerical simulations to quantify the difference in monovalent RL binding as a function of receptor properties. All four ABM variants were applied using the fixed dissociation rate $k_{off}^{micro} = k_{off}^{macro} = 0.1\ s^{-1}$ and varying the microscopic binding rate in the range $10^4\ s^{-1} \leq k_{on}^{micro} \leq 2.5 \times 10^7\ s^{-1}$. The corresponding macroscopic binding rate k_{on}^{macro} was determined for each numerical experiment from the best fit of the analytical solution of the ODE model to the simulation result of the ABM. The resulting function $k_{on}^{macro}(k_{on}^{micro})$ is shown in **Figure 5** for each ABM variant. The steady state concentrations of complexes and receptors obtained by fitting the ODE kinetics to the dynamics of the four various ABM variants are summarized in Tables S3–S6 in Supplementary Material.

As expected from our previous considerations, the quantitative difference between morphologies of monovalent receptors is negligible compared to the dimensionality of motion, i.e., whether receptors were diffusing in solution or within the membrane on the surface of a cell. Moreover, the numerical results $k_{on}^{macro}(k_{on}^{micro})$ in **Figure 5** resemble Hill functions,

$$k_{on}^{macro}\left(k_{on}^{micro}\right) = \frac{a\, k_{on}^{micro}}{b + k_{on}^{micro}}, \quad (13)$$

with parameters a and b that are specific for given receptor properties. Here, a denotes the upper limit for the macroscopic binding rate, $k_{on}^{macro}(k_{on}^{micro} \gg b) \to a$, and b is a constant that determines the slope of the Hill function, $k_{on}^{macro}(k_{on}^{micro} \ll b) \to (a/b)k_{on}^{micro}$, while at intermediate value $k_{on}^{micro} = b$ the Hill function attains half of its maximal value: $k_{on}^{macro}(k_{on}^{micro} = b) = a/2$. The two parameters can be determined from a fit to the numerical simulations and the resulting curves are shown in **Figure 5** as solid lines. The corresponding values are summarized in Table S7 in Supplementary Material for the four ABM variants.

The observed functional dependence of k_{on}^{macro} on k_{on}^{micro} is in agreement with theoretical considerations by Collins and Kimball on binding reactions of diffusing receptors and ligands in three spatial dimensions (31–33). They arrived at the expression

$$k_{on}^{macro}(\kappa) = \frac{k_s\, \kappa}{k_s + \kappa}, \quad (14)$$

where $k_s = 4\pi(r_L + r_R)(D_L + D_R)$ denotes the diffusion-controlled reaction rate that was previously introduced by Von Smoluchowski (34) and that depends on the radii of receptor (r_R) and ligand (r_L) as well as on the diffusion coefficients of receptor (D_R) and ligand (D_L). This rate refers to the frequency at which diffusing receptors and ligands come into contact, i.e., have the distance $r_R + r_L$. Furthermore, κ denotes the intrinsic reaction rate, $\kappa = V_r\, k_{on}^{micro}$, which is directly related to the microscopic binding rate k_{on}^{micro} and the reaction volume $V_r = (4/3)\pi(r_L + r_R)^3$ (35, 36). Combining equations (13) and (14) yields the following relationships:

$$a = k_s, \quad (15)$$

$$b = \frac{k_s}{V_r}. \quad (16)$$

It should be stressed that this correspondence can strictly speaking only be applied to monovalent receptors with spherical morphology and to RL binding in three-dimensional solution with receptor and ligand being allowed to penetrate each other. In other words, equations (15) and (16) could only be expected to hold for the ABM variant O-SOL, however, even this scenario is different from the theoretical considerations in that molecules are not allowed to penetrate each other in our ABM. In the ABM, we generally do not allow for molecular penetration in RL interactions, which reduces their possible overlap to a point contact. The implementation of push-back collisions between molecules effectively reduces the reaction volume V_r, i.e., we set $V_r \to f_r V_r$ with scaling factor $f_r \leq 1$. This parameter will only affect the slope of the Hill function, while it was observed in **Figure 5** that the upper limit of the macroscopic binding rate, k_s, does as well depend on the receptor properties. To account for these observations, we set $k_s \to f_s k_s$ with scaling factor f_s. It then follows that f_r and f_s can be computed from the equations

$$f_s = \frac{a}{k_s}, \quad (17)$$

$$f_r = \frac{f_s\, k_s}{b\, V_r} \quad (18)$$

in terms of the two fitting parameters a and b (see Table S7 in Supplementary Material). The resulting scaling factors are summarized in Table S8 in Supplementary Material.

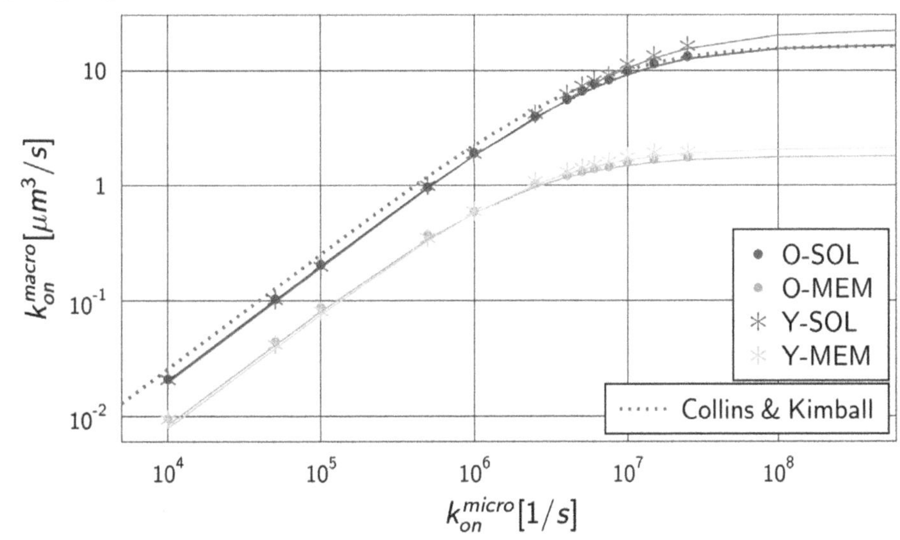

FIGURE 5 | Mapping of microscopic and macroscopic binding rates for different ABM variants. Simulation of all four ABM variants for varying k_{on}^{micro} and the fitted reaction rate k_{on}^{macro} of the ODE models. Solid lines represent Hill functions with parameters fitted to the data points $k_{on}^{macro}(k_{on}^{micro})$. Results for ABM variants are similar for the same dimensionality of motion for receptors, i.e., either in solution (O-SOL, Y-SOL) or membrane anchored (O-MEM, Y-MEM), but are distinct for ABM variants with soluble and membrane-anchored receptors. The dotted line represents the binding rate as determined by Collins and Kimball (see equation (14)) that is, as expected, comparable to the simulation result for ABM variant O-SOL.

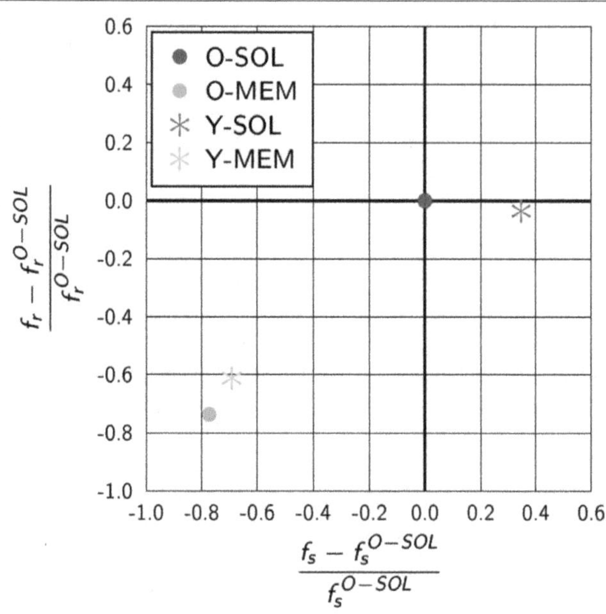

FIGURE 6 | Quantitative difference in the scaling factors of ABM variants relative to O-SOL. The scaling factors f_s and f_r are calculated from equations (17) and (18) for parameters specific to the considered ABM variant. ABM variant O-SOL resembles the conditions of the theoretical considerations by Collins and Kimball (31–33) most of all. Scaling factors of ABM variants with membrane-anchored receptors that are either spherically shaped (O-MEM) or Y-shaped (Y-MEM) exhibit similar but clear differences to ABM variant O-SOL, whereas ABM variant Y-SOL is most similar to O-SOL.

As could be expected, for the ABM variant O-SOL we found the scaling factor $f_s^{O-SOL} = 1.02$ to be close to 1, implying that the upper limit for the macroscopic binding rate as predicted by Collins and Kimball was quantitatively recovered (31–33). Regarding the increase of k_{on}^{macro} as a function of k_{on}^{micro}, we found the difference in the underlying assumptions on RL interactions to be reflected by a decrease in the reaction volume V_r with scaling factor $f_r^{O-SOL} = 0.79$.

We compared the scaling factors for the other ABM variants and present the results relative to ABM variant O-SOL in **Figure 6**. The scaling factor f_r^{Y-SOL} of ABM variant Y-SOL was found to be similar to f_r^{O-SOL} with a relative decrease of only 4%, whereas this scaling factor for the ABM variants with membrane-anchored receptors, i.e., f_r^{O-MEM} and f_r^{Y-MEM}, was decreased by 74 and 61%, respectively. Furthermore, as shown in **Figure 6**, the scaling factors f_s^{O-MEM} and f_s^{Y-MEM} for membrane-anchored receptors were found to be decreased from f_s^{O-SOL} by 77 and 69%, respectively, indicating a significant change in the upper limit of the macroscopic binding rate. On the other hand, this scaling factor was always somewhat higher for membrane-anchored receptors, i.e., ABM variants O-MEM and Y-MEM, compared to their respective counterparts with soluble receptors.

We checked the dependency of the mapping between macroscopic and microscopic binding rates (see **Figure 5**) as well as the scaling factors f_s and f_r (see **Figure 6**) on the down-scaling factor s of the simulated ABM variants. It was generally observed that simulations for soluble receptors were not affected by the system down-scaling, whereas in simulations for membrane-anchored receptors increasing the down-scaling factor s resulted into lower values for k_{on}^{macro} as a function of k_{on}^{micro}. This implies that the difference between ABM variants with soluble and membrane-anchored receptors as observed in **Figure 5** as well as the distances between the respective scaling factors in **Figure 6** represents a lower limit.

Since the diffusion coefficients of receptors in the soluble ($D_R = 90\ \mu m^2\ s^{-1}$) and membrane-anchored ($D_R = 0.05\ \mu m^2\ s^{-1}$) variant differed by orders of magnitude, we checked whether differences in the upper limit of the macroscopic binding rate were indeed merely a consequence of the dimensionality of motion rather than of the magnitude of the diffusion coefficient itself. This was done by running simulations with interchanged diffusion coefficients, i.e., ABM variant O-SOL with $D_R = 0.05\ \mu m^2\ s^{-1}$ and ABM variant O-MEM with $D_R = 90\ \mu m^2\ s^{-1}$. However, even this dramatic modification of diffusion coefficients did not eliminate the significant difference in the dependence of k_{on}^{macro} on k_{on}^{micro} between the ABM variants (see Figures S2 and S3 in Supplementary Material).

Taken together, our quantitative analysis of monovalent RL binding kinetics revealed the impact of receptor properties on the macroscopic binding rate and by that on the association constant of the RL binding. It was shown that the diffusion coefficients of receptors and their morphology have minor effects, whereas the strongest impact was due to the dimensionality of motion. Compared to soluble receptors in three dimensions, RL binding kinetics of membrane-anchored receptors on a cellular surface were retarded and could not achieve comparably high association constants. In what follows, we consider the impact of the binding valency by taking into account that the Y-shaped receptors can bind a ligand at each receptor arm.

3.4. Binding Valency Reduces Differences in the Binding Kinetics of BCR and Antibodies

To investigate the influence of the receptor binding valency on the binding kinetics for monovalent receptors (see **Figure 5**), we modified ABM variants Y-MEM and Y-SOL as to allow for bivalent binding of the Y-shaped receptors, i.e., a ligand can bind at each of the two receptor arms. Thus, in these ABM variants the term complex refers to receptors that are bound to either one or two ligands. The simulations were performed with varied binding rate k_{on}^{micro} between 5×10^6 and $2.5 \times 10^7\ s^{-1}$. The temporal course of the binding kinetics for simulations of the bivalent and monovalent ABM variants is shown in **Figure 7**. The simulations of $k_{on}^{micro} = 1 \times 10^7\ s^{-1}$ exhibit the typical relations between the binding kinetics of the ABM variants. As could be expected, both ABM variants with bivalent receptors showed a faster binding kinetics and also reached higher association constants than their monovalent counterparts. In **Figure 8**, we show the relative difference in receptor-bound ligands for ABM variant Y-MEM relative to ABM variant Y-SOL and for different values of k_{on}^{micro}. This difference is significantly smaller (down to 72%) for bivalent receptors compared to monovalent receptors, and in the limit of long times this difference vanishes only for bivalent but not for monovalent receptors. These results indicate that the binding valency makes a clear difference for RL binding: In the case of monovalent receptors, the dimensionality of motion induces a

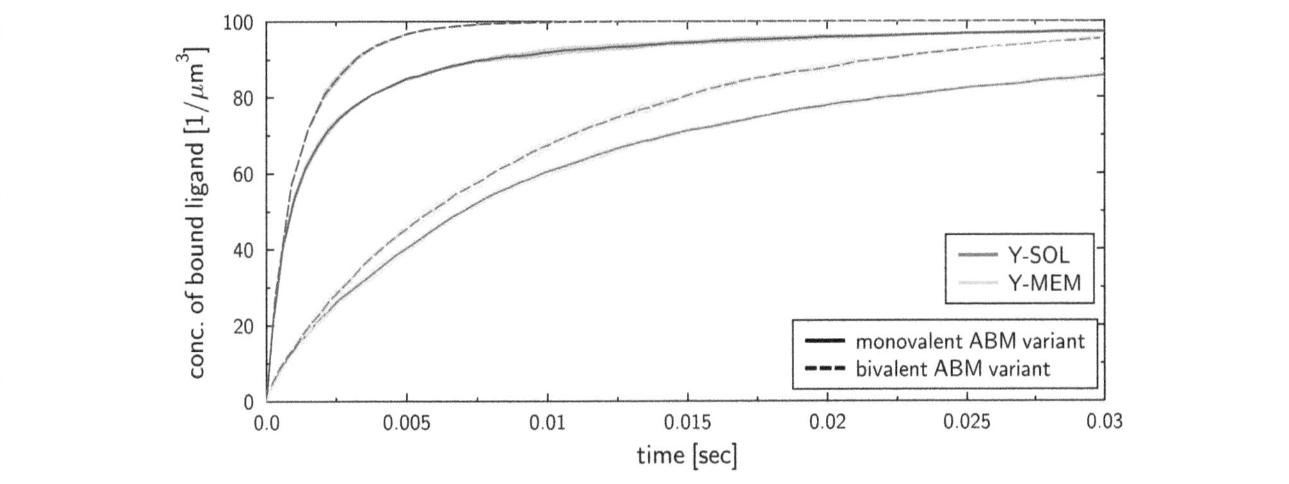

FIGURE 7 | Kinetics of bound ligands for Y-MEM and Y-SOL ABM variants with either monovalent or bivalent receptors. Time-dependent concentration of bound ligands for ABM variants Y-MEM and Y-SOL for models with either monovalent receptors or bivalent receptors. All models were simulated with dissociation rate $k_{off}^{micro} = 0.1\ s^{-1}$ and binding rate $k_{on}^{micro} = 10^7\ s^{-1}$. Dark and pale lines in different colors represent, respectively, mean values and standard deviations of five simulation runs per ABM variant.

significant difference in the binding kinetics, whereas this difference is largely compensated by the bivalency of receptors. Thus, it turns out that membrane-anchored BCR and soluble antibodies do reach comparable association constants for bivalent receptors.

In order to investigate whether these observations are caused by the effectively twofold number of binding sites for the bivalent receptors, we performed simulations with ABM variants that have twice as much monovalent receptors than the so far applied physiological number of receptors (N_p^R). The binding kinetics of ABM variants with $N^R = 2 \times N_p^R$ monovalent receptors turned out to be even faster as the binding kinetics of bivalent ABM variants with $N^R = N_p^R$ (see Figure S4 in Supplementary Material). Additionally, the relative differences between binding kinetics of ABM variants with soluble and membrane-bound receptors vanishes with increasing time, and this occurs slightly faster as for ABM variants with bivalent receptors (see Figure S5 in Supplementary Material). These results indicate that comparable association constants of membrane anchored and soluble receptors can be observed for systems with higher amounts of binding sites at receptors.

4. DISCUSSION

The focus of this study on receptor–ligand (RL) binding was twofold. Firstly, we established a quantitative mapping between macroscopic binding rates of an ordinary differential equation (ODE) model and their microscopic equivalents as obtained from simulating the spatiotemporal binding kinetics by agent-based models (ABM). Secondly, we investigated the impact of various properties of B cell-derived receptors—such as their dimensionality of motion, morphology and binding valency—on the RL binding kinetics.

Regarding the quantitative mapping of binding rates, we recovered for fixed dissociation rates $k_{off}^{micro} = k_{off}^{macro} = 0.1\ s^{-1}$ the non-linear relationship between the binding rates k_{on}^{macro} and k_{on}^{micro}. This resembles a Hill-type function (see **Figure 5**), which is in line with theoretical predictions by Collins and Kimball (31–33). Scanning k_{on}^{micro} over more than four orders of magnitude, we obtained upper limiting values for k_{on}^{macro} in the range 10^0–$10^1\ \mu m^3\ s^{-1}$, which corresponds to 10^8–$10^9\ M^{-1}\ s^{-1}$ using Avogadro's number. For $k_{off}^{macro} = 0.1\ s^{-1}$, the resulting association constant is $K_a = 10^{10}\ M^{-1}$. This is in agreement with experimentally measured values for BCR-antigen binding, where typical values up to $K_a = 10^{10}\ M^{-1}$ are reached (37, 38), which is a strong indication for our ABM variants to be realistic and quantitative to-scale representations of RL binding.

The ABM variants were implemented in three-dimensional representations of continuous space and RL binding was simulated by the random selection method (5). We implemented different ABM variants where binding of spherical ligands occurs either with soluble receptors or with membrane-anchored receptors. The receptors are either spherically shaped or Y-shaped and can be mono- or bivalent. We simulated RL binding in identical environments to allow for quantitative comparisons of the different scenarios. In particular, we considered the Y-shaped and bivalent antibodies in solution and the B cell receptors (BCR) as their membrane-anchored counterparts on a spherical cell to be an appropriate example. In previous work on BCR binding, ABM implementations typically involved simplifications with regard to the spatial representation, i.e., using a planar cell surface and imposing a spatial grid for molecule diffusion (39, 40) and have been applied to simulate the immunological synapse involving B cells (41–45) or T cells (46, 47). Besides this work on immune cell receptor–ligand interaction, there exist software packages for the simulation of various type, such as Smoldyn (48) and MCell (49, 50). Even though these simulators represent molecular diffusion in lattice-free continuous space, they lack features that are essential in the present study. For example, Smoldyn represents molecules in a point-like fashion (48, 51–53), while MCell does only allow to determine an upper limit of the simulation time step Δt (54) implying that simulations with different model systems may differ in the time step Δt. Therefore, we did not consider these simulators suitable for the investigation of morphological

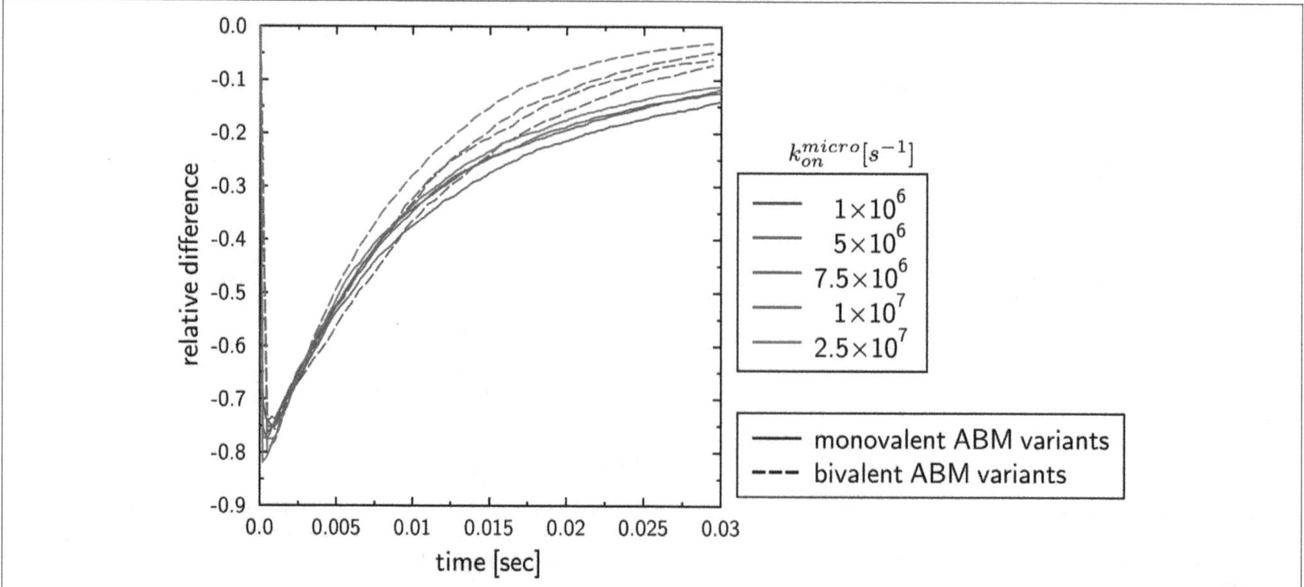

FIGURE 8 | Relative differences between ABM variants Y-MEM and Y-SOL with either monovalent or bivalent receptors. Temporal evolution of the relative differences of bound ligands between ABM variants Y-MEM and Y-SOL for models with either monovalent receptors (monovalent ABM variant) or bivalent receptors (bivalent ABM variant). The colors refer to ABM variants with varying binding rates K_{on}^{micro}.

aspects of receptors and for comparing models at the microscopic and macroscopic scale. Moreover, the RL binding of soluble and membrane-anchored receptors was previously also investigated by non-spatial ODE models (55, 56). These two-step ODE models comprise the process of encounter formation by molecule diffusion and the reaction process itself, so that molecular parameters, like diffusion constant and size, could also be incorporated. However, several simplifications were made, such as the derivation of the binding rate of membrane-bound receptors from cell–ligand interaction rate, which turned out to be not applicable in general (55, 56).

To study the impact of various receptor properties on RL binding kinetics, we compared scenarios that differ in the dimensionality of motion, morphology and binding valency of receptors. These receptor properties were investigated since they are characteristic for B cell-derived receptors that play a key role in the adaptive immune response. Interestingly, the RL binding kinetics for monovalent Y-shaped receptors was observed to be quantitatively comparable to that of spherical receptors (see **Figure 5**), i.e., the difference in the morphology of monovalent receptors did not reveal a substantial impact. In contrast, the dimensionality of motion for BCR compared to soluble antibodies did reveal a clear difference in the binding kinetics, i.e., the association constants were found to be significantly lower for membrane-anchored receptors compared to soluble receptors (see **Figure 5**). Furthermore, our results show that the diffusion constant of receptors, which is much smaller for membrane-anchored molecules as for soluble molecules, does not strongly influence the observed differences in the binding kinetics. This suggest that the difference in the association constants for soluble and membrane-anchored monovalent receptors originate from the difference in the dimensionality of motion. However, this difference was largely compensated by taking into account that BCR and soluble antibodies are bivalent (see **Figure 8**), i.e., the relative difference in the binding kinetics of membrane-anchored and soluble receptors vanished only in the case of bivalent receptors. It is generally known that the bivalency of BCR supports cross-linking in the binding to multivalent ligands. However, the current findings suggest that the bivalency of BCR does also compensate the difference in the association constant that exist for monovalent receptors between the soluble and membrane-anchored variants.

In the future, the extensibility of the current simulation framework can be exploited to study more complex scenarios. For example, antigens may be represented by multivalent ligands that do not only allow for cross-linking of BCR but also binding to coreceptors required for B cell activation. This enables to study the important process of BCR clustering on the cell surface (57–59) that has also been the subject of theoretical investigations (39, 40, 60, 61). We envisage that such studies will strongly benefit from an image-based systems biology approach, for example, as applied by Mech et al. (62) and conceptionally reviewed by Medyukhina et al. (63). Recently, we took the first steps toward an image-based investigation of B cell activation that requires the concerted action of various receptors and ligands (64). Based on these data, our ABM can be extended by various agent types with specific properties to predict prerequisites for experimentally observed molecular patterns. Moreover, the ABM variants could be modified to represent various receptor properties of different antibody isotypes and/or subclasses, which would allow investigating the impact of specific receptor properties on the RL binding kinetics. Based on this modification, the impact of naturally occurring antibody complexes, such as IgA dimers and IgM pentamers, could be investigated. Furthermore, extending the ABM to represent arbitrarily shaped cells that are brought in close contact, it can be used to simulate the molecular patterns during synapse formation involving B cells, T cells as well as phagocytes (65–68).

This would enable to investigate the impact of the dimensionality of motion of ligands that is reported to be an important parameter for regulating B cell activation and signaling (69).

AUTHOR CONTRIBUTIONS

TL and MF conceived and designed the study, evaluated and analyzed the results, and wrote the manuscript and critically revised it. MF contributed materials and computational resources. TL processed the data, implemented, and applied the computational algorithm.

ACKNOWLEDGMENTS

We acknowledge support by Bertram Vogel regarding the initial implementation of the agent-based model.

FUNDING

This work was financially supported by the Center for Sepsis Control and Care (CSCC) (Project Quantim to MTF, FKZ 01EO1502) that is funded by the Federal Ministry for Education and Research (BMBF) and by the CRC/TR124 FungiNet (Project B4 to MTF) that is funded by the Deutsche Forschungsgemeinschaft (DFG).

SUPPLEMENTARY MATERIAL

VIDEO S1 | Simulation of down-scaled scaled O-SOL ABM variant. ABM simulation with monovalent receptors (blue objects) that are spherically shaped and move in solution by performing three-dimensional diffusion. Upon contact between receptors and ligands (red objects) these may bind and form RL complexes (green objects) depending on the binding rate $k_{on}^{micro} = 2.5 \times 10^7\ s^{-1}$. The system is down-scaled with factor s = 0.01 (see Supplementary Material) and values of model parameters are provided in Tables S1 and S2 in Supplementary Material. The video is composed of 15 frames s^{-1} and the simulation time between two consecutive frames is 6.8×10^{-8} s. A high-resolution video is available for download from https://asbdata.hki-jena.de/LehnertFigge2017_FrontImmun/.

VIDEO S2 | Simulation of down-scaled O-MEM ABM variant. ABM simulation with monovalent receptors (blue objects) that are spherically shaped and move in the cell membrane by performing two-dimensional diffusion. Upon contact between receptors and ligands (red objects) these may bind and form RL-complexes (green objects) depending on the binding rate $k_{on}^{micro} = 2.5 \times 10^7\ s^{-1}$. The system is down-scaled with factor s = 0.01 (see Supplementary Material) and values of model parameters are provided in Tables S1 and S2 in Supplementary Material. The video is composed of 15 frames s^{-1} and the simulation time between two consecutive frames is 6.8×10^{-8} s. A high-resolution video is available for download from https://asbdata.hki-jena.de/LehnertFigge2017_FrontImmun/.

VIDEO S3 | Simulation of down-scaled Y-SOL ABM variant. ABM simulation with monovalent receptors (blue objects) that are Y-shaped and move in solution by performing three-dimensional diffusion. Upon contact between receptors and ligands (red objects) these may bind and form RL-complexes (green objects) depending on the binding rate $k_{on}^{micro} = 2.5 \times 10^7\ s^{-1}$. The system is down-scaled with factor s = 0.01 (see Supplementary Material) and values of model parameters are provided in Table S1 in Supplementary Material and Supplementary Material. The video is composed of 15 frames s^{-1} and the simulation time between two consecutive frames is 6.8×10^{-8} s. A high-resolution video is available for download from https://asbdata.hki-jena.de/LehnertFigge2017_FrontImmun/.

VIDEO S4 | Simulation of down-scaled Y-MEM ABM variant. ABM simulation with monovalent receptors (blue objects) that are Y-shaped and move in the cell membrane by performing two-dimensional diffusion. Upon contact between receptors and ligands (red objects) these may bind and form RL-complexes (green objects) depending on the binding rate $k_{on}^{micro} = 2.5 \times 10^7\ s^{-1}$. The system is down-scaled with factor s = 0.01 (see Supplementary Material) and values of model parameters are provided in Tables S1 and S2 in Supplementary Material. The video is composed of 15 frames s^{-1} and the simulation time between two consecutive frames is 6.8×10^{-8} s. A high-resolution video is available for download from https://asbdata.hki-jena.de/LehnertFigge2017_FrontImmun/.

VIDEO S5 | Simulation of Y-MEM ABM variant. ABM simulation with monovalent receptors (blue objects) that are Y-shaped and move in the cell membrane by performing two-dimensional diffusion. Upon contact between receptors and ligands (red objects) these may bind and form RL-complexes (green objects) depending on the binding rate $k_{on}^{micro} = 2.5 \times 10^7\ s^{-1}$. The system is down-scaled with factor s = 0.01 (see Supplementary Material) and values of model parameters are provided in Table S1 in Supplementary Material. The video is composed of 15 frames s^{-1} and the simulation time between two consecutive frames is 6.8×10^{-8} s. A high-resolution video is available for download from https://asbdata.hki-jena.de/LehnertFigge2017_FrontImmun/.

REFERENCES

Resat H, Petzold L, Pettigrew MF. Kinetic modeling of biological systems. *Methods Mol Biol* (2009) 541:311–35. doi:10.1007/978-1-59745- 243-4_14

Faro J, Castro M, Molina-París C. A unifying mathematical framework for experimental TCR-pMHC kinetic constants. *Sci Rep* (2017) 7:46741. doi:10.1038/srep46741

Andrews SS, Arkin AP. Simulating cell biology. *Curr Biol* (2006) 16(14):R523–7. doi:10.1016/j.cub.2006.06.048

Goldstein B, Faeder JR, Hlavacek WS. Mathematical and computational models of immune-receptor signalling. *Nat Rev Immunol* (2004) 4(6):445–56. doi:10.1038/nri1374

Figge MT. Stochastic discrete event simulation of germinal center reactions. *Phys Rev E Stat Nonlin Soft Matter Phys* (2005) 71(5):051907. doi:10.1103/PhysRevE.71.051907

Gillespie DT. Exact stochastic simulation of coupled chemical reactions. *J Phys Chem* (1977) 81(25):2340–61. doi:10.1021/j100540a008

Gillespie DT. A general method for numerically simulating the stochastic time evolution of coupled chemical reactions. *J Comput Phys* (1976) 22:403–34. doi:10.1016/0021-9991(76)90041-3

Gibson MA, Bruck J. Efficient exact stochastic simulation of chemical systems with many species and many channels. *J Phys Chem A* (2000) 104(9):1876–89. doi:10.1021/jp993732q

Yu JS, Bagheri N. Multi-class and multi-scale models of complex biological phe- nomena. *Curr Opin Biotechnol* (2016) 39:167–73. doi:10.1016/j.copbio.2016.04. 002

Bonabeau E. Agent-based methods and techniques for simulating human systems. *Proc Natl Acad Sci U S A* (2002) 99(10):7280–7. doi:10.1073/pnas.082080899

Takahashi K, Vel Arjunan SN, Tomita M. Space in systems biology of signaling pathways – towards intracellular molecular crowding in silico. *FEBS Lett* (2005) 579(8):1783–8. doi:10.1016/j.febslet.2005.01.072

Liu W, Meckel T, Tolar P, Sohn HW, Pierce SK. Antigen affinity discrimination is an intrinsic function of the B cell receptor. *J Exp Med* (2010) 207(5):1095–111. doi:10.1084/jem.20092123

Coico R, Sunshine G. *Immunology: A Short Course*. 7th ed. Oxford, UK: John Wiley & Sons Ltd (2015).

Figge MT, Garin A, Gunzer M, Kosco-Vilbois M, Toellner K-M, Meyer-Hermann M. Deriving a germinal center lymphocyte migration model from two-photon data. *J Exp Med* (2008) 205(13):3019–29. doi:10.1084/jem. 20081160

Meyer-Hermann M, Figge MT, Toellner KM. Germinal centres seen through the mathematical eye: B-cell models on the catwalk. *Trends Immunol* (2009) 30(4):157–64. doi:10.1016/j.it.2009.01.005

Garin A, Meyer-Hermann M, Contie M, Figge MT, Buatois V, Gunzer M, et al. Toll-like receptor 4 signaling by follicular dendritic cells is pivotal for germinal center onset and affinity maturation. *Immunity* (2010) 33(1):84–95. doi:10.1016/j.immuni.2010.07.005

Raychaudhuri S. The problem of antigen affinity discrimination in B-cell immunology. *ISRN Biomath* (2013) 2013:1–18. doi:10.1155/2013/845918

Zhang Y, Meyer-Hermann M, George LA, Figge MT, Khan M, Goodall M, et al. Germinal center B cells govern their own fate via antibody feedback. *J Exp Med* (2013) 210(3):457–64. doi:10.1084/jem.20120150

Horn F, Heinekamp T, Kniemeyer O, Pollmächer J, Valiante V, Brakhage AA. Systems biology of fungal infection. *Front Microbiol* (2012) 3:108. doi:10.3389/ fmicb.2012.00108

Zhang C, Chen J, DeLisi C. Protein-protein recognition: exploring the energy funnels near the binding sites. *Proteins* (1999) 34(2):255–67. doi:10.1002/ (SICI) 1097-0134(19990201)34:2<255::AID-PROT10>3.0.CO;2-O

Tsai C-J, Kumar S, Ma B, Nussinov R. Folding funnels, binding funnels, and protein function. *Protein Sci* (1999) 8(6):1181–90. doi:10.1110/ps.8.6.1181

Northrup SH, Erickson HP. Kinetics of protein-protein association explained by Brownian dynamics computer simulation. *Proc Natl Acad Sci U S A* (1992) 89:3338–42.

Tovchigrechko A, Vakser IA. How common is the funnel-like energy landscape in protein-protein interactions? *Protein Sci* (2001) 10(8):1572–83. doi:10.1110/ ps.8701

Einstein A. Über die von der molekularkinetischen Theorie der Wärme geforderte Bewegung von in ruhenden Flüssigkeiten suspendierten Teilchen. *Macromol Symp* (1905) 322(8):549–60.

Lehnert T, Timme S, Pollmächer J, Hünniger K, Kurzai O, Figge MT. Bottom-up modeling approach for the quantitative estimation of parameters in pathogen- host interactions. *Front Microbiol* (2015) 6:608. doi:10.3389/ fmicb.2015.00608

Rapaport DC. *The Art of Molecular Dynamics Simulation*. New York, NY, USA: Cambridge University Press (2004).

Press W, Teukolsky S, Vetterling W, Flannery B, Ziegel E, Press W, et al. *Numerical Recipes: The Art of Scientific Computing*. 3rd ed. New York: Cambridge University Press (2007).

Ihaka R, Gentleman R. *R: A Language for Data Analysis and Graphics*. *J Comput Graph Stat* (1996) 5(3):299–14. doi:10.2307/1390807

Dennis JE, Gay DM, Welsch RE. Algorithm 573: NL2SOL – an adaptive nonlin- ear least-squares algorithm [E4]. *ACM Trans Math Software* (1981) 7(3):369–83. doi:10.1145/355958.355966

Butcher J, Jackiewicz Z, Mittelmann H. A nonlinear optimization approach to the construction of general linear methods of high order. *J Comput Appl Math* (1997) 81(97):181–96. doi:10.1016/S0377-0427(97)00039-3

Collins FC, Kimball GE. Diffusion-controlled reaction rates. *J Colloid Sci* (1949) 4(4):425–37. doi:10.1016/0095-8522(49)90023-9

Collins FC, Kimball GE. Diffusion-controlled reactions in liquid solutions. *Indus Eng Chem* (1949) 41:2551–3. doi:10.1021/ie50479a040

Shoup D, Szabo A. Role of diffusion in ligand binding to macromolecules and cell-bound receptors. *Biophys J* (1982) 40(1):33–9. doi:10.1016/S0006-3495(82) 84455-X

Von Smoluchowski M. Versuch einer mathematischen Theorie der Koagulationskinetik. *Phys Chem* (1917) 92(1912):156.

Klann MT, Lapin A, Reuss M. Agent-based simulation of reactions in the crowded and structured intracellular environment: influence of mobility and location of the reactants. *BMC Syst Biol* (2011) 5(1):71. doi:10.1186/1752-0509- 5-71

Klann MT, Koeppl H. Spatial simulations in systems biology: from molecules to cells. *Int J Mol Sci* (2012) 13(12):7798–827. doi:10.3390/ijms13067798

Batista FD, Neuberger MS. Affinity dependence of the B cell response to antigen: a threshold, a ceiling, and the importance of off-rate. *Immunity* (1998) 8(6):751–9. doi:10.1016/S1074-7613(00)80580-4

Carrasco YR, Fleire SJ, Cameron T, Dustin ML, Batista FD. LFA-1/ICAM-1 interaction lowers the threshold of B cell activation by facilitating B cell adhesion and synapse formation. *Immunity* (2004) 20(5):589–99. doi:10.1016/ S1074-7613(04)00105-0

Reddy S, Tsourkas PK, Raychaudhuri S. Monte Carlo study of B-cell receptor clustering mediated by antigen crosslinking and directed transport. *Cell Mol Immunol* (2011) 8(3):255–64. doi:10.1038/cmi.2011.3

Reddy S, Chilukuri S, Raychaudhuri S. The network of receptors characterize B cell receptor micro- and macroclustering in a Monte Carlo model. *J Phys Chem B* (2010) 114(1):487–94. doi:10.1021/jp9079074

Tsourkas PK, Baumgarth N, Simon SI, Raychaudhuri S. Mechanisms of B- cell synapse formation predicted by Monte Carlo simulation. *Biophys J* (2007) 92(12):4196–208. doi:10.1529/biophysj.106.094995

Tsourkas PK, Longo ML, Raychaudhuri S. Monte Carlo study of single molecule diffusion can elucidate the mechanism of B cell synapse formation. *Biophys J* (2008) 95(3):1118–25. doi:10.1529/biophysj.107.122564

Tsourkas PK, Raychaudhuri S. Modeling of B cell synapse formation by Monte Carlo simulation shows that directed transport of receptor molecules is a potential formation mechanism. *Cell Mol Bioeng* (2010) 3(3):256–68. doi:10. 1007/s12195-010-0123-1

Tsourkas PK, Liu W, Das SC, Pierce SK, Raychaudhuri S. Discrimination of membrane antigen affinity by B cells requires dominance of kinetic proofread- ing over serial engagement. *Cell Mol Immunol* (2012) 9(1):62–74. doi:10.1038/ cmi.2011.29

Tsourkas PK, Somkanya CD, Yu-Yang P, Liu W, Pierce SK, Raychaudhuri S. Formation of BCR oligomers provides a mechanism for B cell affinity discrim- ination. *J Theor Biol* (2012) 307:174–82. doi:10.1016/j. jtbi.2012.05.008

Figge MT, Meyer-Hermann M. Geometrically repatterned immunological synapses uncover formation mechanisms. *PLoS Comput Biol* (2006) 2(11):e171. doi:10.1371/journal.pcbi.0020171

Figge MT, Meyer-Hermann M. Modeling receptor-ligand binding kinetics in immunological synapse formation. *Eur Phys J D* (2009) 51(1):153–60. doi:10. 1140/epjd/e2008-00087-1

Andrews SS, Bray D. Stochastic simulation of chemical reactions with spatial resolution and single molecule detail. *Phys Biol* (2004) 1(3–4):137–51. doi:10. 1088/1478-3967/1/3/001

Stiles JR, Van Helden D, Bartol TM, Salpeter EE, Salpeter MM. Miniature endplate current rise times less than 100 microseconds from improved dual recordings can be modeled with passive acetylcholine diffusion from a synaptic vesicle. *Proc Natl Acad Sci U S A* (1996) 93(12):5747–52. doi:10.1073/pnas.93. 12.5747

Kerr RA, Bartol TM, Kaminsky B, Dittrich M, Chang J-CJ, Baden SB, et al. Fast Monte Carlo simulation methods for biological reaction-diffusion systems in solution and on surfaces. *SIAM J Sci Comput* (2008) 30(6):3126. doi:10.1137/ 070692017

Andrews SS. Spatial and stochastic cellular modeling with the Smoldyn simulator. *Methods Mol Biol* (2012) 804(1):519–42. doi:10.1007/978-1-61779- 361-5_26

Andrews SS. Serial rebinding of ligands to clustered receptors as exemplified by bacterial chemotaxis. *Phys Biol* (2005) 2(2):111–22. doi:10.1088/1478-3975/2/ 2/004

Andrews SS, Addy NJ, Brent R, Arkin AP. Detailed simulations of cell biol- ogy with Smoldyn 2.1. *PLoS Comput Biol* (2010) 6(3):e1000705. doi:10.1371/ journal.pcbi.1000705

Burrage K, Burrage PM, Leier A, Marquez-Lago T, Nicolau DV Jr. Stochastic simulation of spatial modelling of dynamic processes in a living cell. In: Koeppl H, Densmore D, Setti M, Di Bernardo M, editor. *Design and Analysis of Biomolecular Circuits*. New York: Springer (2011). p. 43–62.

Berg HC, Purcell EM. Physics of chemoreception. *Biophys J* (1977) 20(2):193–219. doi:10.1016/S0006-3495(77)85544-6

DeLisi C. The effect of cell size and receptor density on ligand-receptor reaction rate constants. *Mol Immunol* (1981) 18(6):507–11. doi:10.1016/0161-5890(81) 90128-0

Maity PC, Yang J, Klaesener K, Reth M. The nanoscale organization of the B lymphocyte membrane. *Biochim Biophys Acta* (2015) 1853(4):830–40. doi:10. 1016/j.bbamcr.2014.11.010

Yang J, Reth M. Oligomeric organization of the B-cell antigen receptor on resting cells. *Nature* (2010) 467(7314):465–9. doi:10.1038/nature09357

Yang J, Reth M. The dissociation activation model of B cell antigen recep- tor triggering. *FEBS Lett* (2010) 584(24):4872–7. doi:10.1016/j.febslet.2010.09. 045

Perelson AS, DeLisi C. Receptor clustering on a cell surface. I. The- ory of receptor cross-linking by ligands bearing two chemically identical functional groups. *Math Biosci* (1980) 48:71–110. doi:10.1016/0025-5564(80) 90017-6

Perelson AS, Weisbuch G. Immunology for physicists. *Rev Mod Phys* (1997) 69(4):1219–67. doi:10.1103/RevModPhys.69.1219

Mech F, Wilson D, Lehnert T, Hube B, Thilo Figge M. Epithelial invasion outcompetes hypha development during *Candida albicans* infection as revealed by an image-based systems biology approach. *Cytometry A* (2014) 85(2):126–39. doi:10.1002/cyto.a.22418

Medyukhina A, Timme S, Mokhtari Z, Figge MT. Image-based systems biology of infection. *Cytometry A* (2015) 87(6):462–70. doi:10.1002/cyto.a. 22638

Buhlmann D, Eberhardt HU, Medyukhina A, Prodinger WM, Figge MT, Zipfel PF, et al. FHR3 blocks C3d-mediated coactivation of human B cells. *J Immunol* (2016) 197(2):620–9. doi:10.4049/jimmunol.1600053

Dustin ML. Signaling at neuro/immune synapses. *J Clin Invest* (2012) 122(4):1149–55. doi:10.1172/JCI58705

Batista FD, Iber D, Neuberger MS. B cells acquire antigen from target cells after synapse formation. *Nature* (2001) 411(6836):489–94. doi:10.1038/35078099

Weikl TR, Lipowsky R. Pattern formation during T-cell adhesion. *Biophys J* (2004) 87(6):3665–78. doi:10.1529/biophysj.104.045609

Ketchum C, Miller H, Song W, Upadhyaya A. Ligand mobility regulates B cell receptor clustering and signaling activation. *Biophys J* (2014) 106(1):26–36. doi:10.1016/j.bpj.2013.10.043

16

A Population Dynamics Model for Clonal Diversity in a Germinal Center

Assaf Amitai[1,2,3], *Luka Mesin*[4], *Gabriel D. Victora*[4], *Mehran Kardar*[5] *and Arup K. Chakraborty*[1,2,3,6*]

[1] Chemical Engineering, Massachusetts Institute of Technology, Cambridge, MA, United States, [2] Institute for Medical Engineering and Science, Massachusetts Institute of Technology, Cambridge, MA, United States, [3] Ragon Institute of MGH, MIT and Harvard, Cambridge, MA, United States, [4] Laboratory of Lymphocyte Dynamics, Rockefeller University, New York, NY, United States, [5] Physics, Massachusetts Institute of Technology, Cambridge, MA, United States, [6] Biological Engineering and Chemistry, Massachusetts Institute of Technology, Cambridge, MA, United States

Correspondence:
Arup K. Chakraborty
arupc@mit.edu

Germinal centers (GCs) are micro-domains where B cells mature to develop high affinity antibodies. Inside a GC, B cells compete for antigen and T cell help, and the successful ones continue to evolve. New experimental results suggest that, under identical conditions, a wide spectrum of clonal diversity is observed in different GCs, and high affinity B cells are not always the ones selected. We use a birth, death and mutation model to study clonal competition in a GC over time. We find that, like all evolutionary processes, diversity loss is inherently stochastic. We study two selection mechanisms, birth-limited and death limited selection. While death limited selection maintains diversity and allows for slow clonal homogenization as affinity increases, birth limited selection results in more rapid takeover of successful clones. Finally, we qualitatively compare our model to experimental observations of clonal selection in mice.

Keywords: germinal center reaction, population dynamics, modeling and simulations, clonal evolution, affinity maturation

INTRODUCTION

Upon natural infection or vaccination, antibodies develop in domains within secondary lymphoid organs called germinal centers (GC), which appear shortly after infection (Victora and Nussenzweig, 2012). B cells with some threshold affinity for the antigen can seed GCs and, with help from several other types of immune cells, undergo affinity maturation (AM) (Eisen and Siskind, 1964), which is an evolutionary process of mutation, competition and proliferation, that ultimately generates high affinity antibodies.

At the initial stage of the GC reaction (GCR), naïve B cells are recruited. During AM, the AID protein induces random mutations in the gene coding for the BCR at a high rate (Muramatsu et al., 2000). A GC is not histologically uniform but divided roughly into two areas: a dark zone (DZ) and a light zone (LZ). After proliferating and mutating in the DZ, B cells migrate to the LZ, where they consume antigen displayed on the surface of follicular dendritic cells, and display antigen-derived peptide-MHC complexes on their surface. These B cells then compete for limiting amounts of T follicular helper cells (TfhCs). Following a proliferation signal from TfhCs (Rolf et al., 2010), the majority of B cells migrate back to the DZ, while a few differentiate in to antibody-producing plasma cells and memory cells (Oprea and Perelson, 1997). Iterative cycles of such hypermutation and selection result in both an increase in B cell affinity over time, and the loss of B cell clones in the competition process, such that a few successful clones are thought to remain at the end of the GCR

(Jacob et al., 1993). After roughly 2 weeks, although this time can vary significantly, the process stops and the GC collapses.

The number of founding clones of a GC was traditionally thought to be between 1 and 6 (Kroese et al., 1987; Liu et al., 1991; Jacob et al., 1993). However, a recent study has shown that the initial number of clones is much higher, of the order of 50–200 initial clones, and that the clonal number variability after 3 weeks remains high (Tas et al., 2016). The experimental system uses the "brainbow" allele for multicolor fate mapping to permanently tag individual B cells and their progeny with different combinations of fluorescent proteins (Livet et al., 2007), resulting in up to 10 different colors. Thus, a number of distinct observable sub-clonal lineages emerge when a cell belonging to a certain clone chooses a color. The sub-clonal lineages are observed at different time points of the GCR (Tas et al., 2016). This method underestimates the number of clones in very diverse GCs (Tas et al., 2016) as not all clones choose a color, and multiple clones can choose the same color. Since recombination occurs after the initial clone has proliferated, multiple colors may represent the same clone. However, the method provides a high throughput estimate of GC clonality. Moreover, GC clonal diversity was also estimated by sequencing B cells, which allows for exact reconstruction of the lineages, and both methods point to the same qualitative behavior. Surprisingly, it was found that while clonal diversity is lost with time, the number of remaining clones varied significantly between GCs, even ones from the same lymph node that shared many clones.

AM has been modeled extensively over the last 30 years (Brink, 2007; Chan et al., 2013), dating back to the seminal work of Perelson et al., showing that cycling of B cells between the DZ and the LZ is optimal for affinity gain (Kepler and Perelson, 1993; Oprea and Perelson, 1997). Meyer-Hermann et al. (2012) developed very detailed simulations capbable of reproducing the dynamics and interactions of individual B and T cells within a GC. More recently, several computational studies (Chaudhury et al., 2014; Luo and Perelson, 2015; Wang et al., 2015; Shaffer et al., 2016) have investigated the effect of different immunization strategies with multiple variant antigens on the development of cross-reactive antibodies. Many of these models assume that selection is done by eliminating cells with low affinity BCR (Figge, 2005; Zhang and Shakhnovich, 2010). However, new evidence suggests that the extent of B cell proliferation in the DZ is proportional to the strength of the signal the B cell has received in the LZ (Victora et al., 2010; Gitlin et al., 2014, 2015) which can lead to rapid expansion of the progeny of a selected cell. We denote these two scenarios "death-limited" and "birth-limited" selection respectively. Since there is a minimum threshold for any response, and proliferation is related to BCR affinity, we suggest that both are needed to explain AM. We use here tools from population dynamics and stochastic processes to show that the AM process and clonal selection can be understood in terms of stochastic clonal competition, leading to an inherently probabilistic selection of fitter clones.

We estimate numerically clonal loss (*homogenization*) in a GC and show that the magnitude by which affinity changes per single mutation is the determinant factor in explaining clonal homogenization rate. Because clonal selection is a stochastic process, we show that clonal diversity has a large variability between different GCs. While we do not include spatial resolution of B cell LZ-DZ migration (Figge et al., 2008), recycling of antibodies (Zhang et al., 2013), the model captures qualitatively the essence of clonal selection with effective rates of birth, death and mutation. We suggest that the basic aspects of clonal diversity in the GC can be captured using simple population dynamics models.

MODEL DESCRIPTION

AM as a Birth-Death-Mutation Process

We model B cell proliferation and death during the GCR using a birth-death (BD) process (Renshaw, 1991). AID mutates the gene encoding for the BCR (Muramatsu et al., 2000) and as a consequence, affinity for the antigen changes. The resulting increase (or decrease) in affinity translates to a higher (lower) fitness of the B cell. Regarding the stochastic variation of BCR in affinity space as a form of diffusion, the model resembles a "birth-death-diffusion process" (Adke and Moyal, 1963).

Growth Phase

In the first days following immunization, while the GC is still coalescing, B cells proliferate without competition, creating a pool of cells on which AM may operate. Few or no mutations are introduced to the BCR sequence at this early stage. We start from a simple birth/death (BD) process using an agent-based model. Each cell is associated with a birth rate λ and a death rate μ (see **Figure 1A**). We assume that a GCR starts with M different clones and the system evolves for a period of 6 days, which we denote by T_{growth} (Jacob et al., 1991; see **Figure 1B**).

During the growth phase, the probability distribution $P_{n_i}(t)$ of the number of cells n_i that belong to clone i evolves in time according to the master equation (Bailey, 1990):

$$\begin{aligned}\frac{\partial P_{n_i}(t)}{\partial t} &= \lambda_{n-1}P_{n_i-1}(t) + \mu_{n+1}P_{n_i+1}(t)\\ &\quad - (\lambda_n + \mu_n)P_{n_i}(t) \quad \text{for } n_i = 1,..,\infty,\\ \frac{\partial P_{0_i}(t)}{\partial t} &= \mu_1 P_{1_i}(t),\end{aligned} \tag{1}$$

where (in the absence of interactions): $\lambda_n = n\lambda$ and $\mu_n = n\mu$ and P_{0_i} is the probability of extinction of clone i. The average number of cells $\langle n_i \rangle$ in clone i, after time t is given by (Bailey, 1990).

$$\langle n_i(t) \rangle = n_i(t=0)e^{(\lambda-\mu)t}. \tag{2}$$

The time dependent extinction probability of a clone is

$$p_{0_i}(t) = \frac{\mu(e^{(\lambda-\mu)t} - 1)}{\lambda e^{(\lambda-\mu)t} - \mu}, \tag{3}$$

and the size distribution of a clone lineage is

$$p_{n_i}(t) = (1 - p_0)(1 - \lambda p_0/\mu)(\lambda p_0/\mu)^{n_i} \text{ for } n_i \geq 1. \tag{4}$$

Both equations are the solution of Equation (1). After T_{growth}, there is a supply of cells on which AM can work, while some

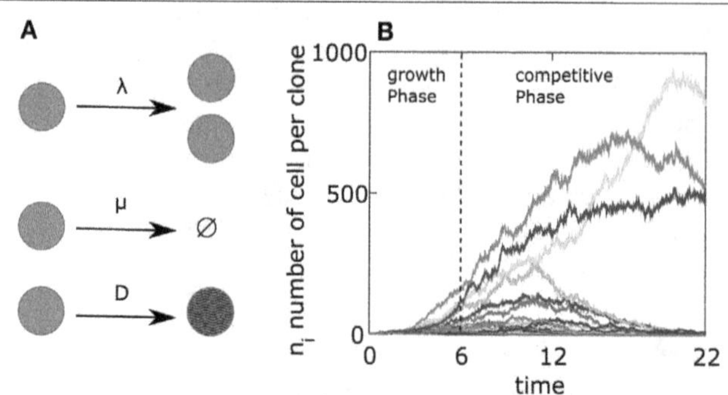

FIGURE 1 | Germinal Center reaction as a birth-death-mutation process. **(A)** Schematics representation of the agent based model. Each cell has a birth rate (λ), a death rate (μ). Upon division the BCR affinity changes according to Equation (9) with a constant D. **(B)** Example of a single simulation. The free growth phase lasts for 6 days, followed by a competitive phase lasting 16 days. Each colored curve represents a different clone. The parameters used in the simulation are detailed in **Table 1** but with $D = 0.01$.

TABLE 1 | Values of the parameters used in the simulation presented in **Figure 2A**.

Parameters	Value
Number of initial clones: M	50
Basal death rate μ_0	1 day^{-1}
Birth rate λ_0	1.5 day^{-1}
Germinal center capacity N	2,000
Diffusion coefficient D	0.001
Initial affinity w_0	1.5
Growth phase T_{growth}	6 days
Competitive phase T_{comp}	16 days

clones disappear. This distribution function is the starting point for the competitive phase of the GCR.

For our parameter choices (see **Table 1**), which represents a GC development, the average lineage size of a clone at the end of the growth phase (6 days) is $\langle n_i(6\text{ days})\rangle = 20$ cells, the total number of surviving cells is $\langle N(6\text{ days})\rangle = 1000$ cells, while $p_0(6\text{ days}) \approx 2/3$ corresponding to an average of $50 \times 1/3 \approx 17$ surviving clones. This number is lower than the number of surviving clones in Tas et al. (2016) which was 50–200 but as we are interested in the qualitative behavior of the system, we choose a smaller number to facilitate the numerical calculations.

Competition Phase

After day 6, B cells survival depends on TfhC signals that are a shared resource. Indeed, it has been shown (Victora et al., 2010; Gitlin et al., 2015) that TfhCs have a role in regulating the duration of cell cycle in B cells during AM and controlling their behavior in the GC. To mimic B cell competition over the limited resource of TfhCs, we used the stochastic logistic growth process (Nåsell, 2001), which constrains the B cell population size. The death rate decreases with the population size, from a basal rate of μ_0, to roughly the birth rate λ_0 for a mature population:

$$\mu(\mathbf{n}) = \left(\mu_0 + (\lambda_0 - \mu_0)\frac{\sum_{i=1}^{M} n_i}{N}\right), \tag{5}$$

where N is the population capacity. Here $\mathbf{n} = (n_1, n_2, ..., n_M)$ is the vector of cell number n_i for the M lineages. The competitive phase continues for a period (T_{comp}), which we take to be 16 days (Tas et al., 2016). The total number of cells in the GC grows gradually until reaching the capacity N, where it remains approximately fixed.

Birth Limited Selection

Occasionally, B cells undergo a proliferative burst that is proportional to the amount of presented antigen and thus to the BCR affinity (Victora et al., 2010; Gitlin et al., 2015). B cells move then to the DZ, remain there and divide multiple times (4–6) before going back to the LZ to go through another round of selection (Gitlin et al., 2014, 2015; Tas et al., 2016). We model this process as an increase in the birth rate (see Supplementary Information "Heterozygosity of a Moran process"). Since cell-cycle is modified (shortened) in this process, we take the birth rate of cell i as

$$\lambda_i = \lambda_0 \frac{w_i}{\langle w\rangle_{Population}}, \tag{6}$$

where w_i is the affinity of cell i, $\langle w\rangle_{Population}$ is the mean affinity of the population and λ_0 is the basal birth rate. Indeed, the average birthrate of B cell clones in a GC, was found to be similar (Anderson et al., 2009) in B cell clones with different affinities. The normalization serves to keep the average population birth rate constant at λ_0. Since the clone birth rate λ_i is related to the clone affinity w_i, we designate this scenario "*birth limited selection.*".

Death Limited Selection

During the GCR, cells with poor affinity do not receive a survival signal from T helper cells because they do not display a sufficient amount of peptide-MHC molecules. Previous studies model this process by noting that the probability of a B cell being able to successfully compete with other B cells that have internalized antigen and receive T cell help, grows monotonically with the affinity of its BCR for antigen (Zhang and Shakhnovich, 2010; Wang et al., 2015), with surviving cells proliferating at approximately the same rate (Batista and Neuberger, 1998). Additionally, it was found (Anderson et al., 2009) that on average, B cell clones with different affinities differ in their death rate, where the low affinity clone dies at a higher rate than ones with intermediate affinity. Such a scenario is considered "*death limited selection*" in our scheme with a death rate μ that depends inversely on the affinity. To study the consequences of such a selection mechanism, we constructed the following model

$$\begin{aligned} \mu_i^n &= \mu_i(w_i) + (\lambda - \langle\mu\rangle_{population})\frac{\sum_i n_i}{N}, \\ \mu_i &= A\exp(-\alpha w_i), \end{aligned} \tag{7}$$

where α is a constant, μ_i is the death rate of a cell with affinity w_i and μ_i^n is the GC-size dependent death rate keeping the population size fixed. Thus, higher affinity is related to a lower death rate.

We also examine a model where the birthrate is normalized over the population and as a result, the average of affinity dependent element of death rate, is constant.

$$\mu_i^n = \mu_0 \frac{\mu_i(w_i)}{\langle \mu \rangle_{population}} + (\lambda - \mu_0) \frac{\sum_i n_i}{N}. \tag{8}$$

Affinty Change following BCR Mutation

During AM B cells mutate their BCR encoding genes. The effect of a single mutation on fitness in models of Wright-Fisher-like selection is often taken to be small (Park and Krug, 2007; Hallatschek, 2011; Goyal et al., 2012; Tas et al., 2016), which allows analytical treatment of the population dynamics as a diffusion problem. In this spirit, we modeled the effect of mutation as a change in the affinity upon cell division, where one of the daughter cells has the parent affinity and for the other daughter:

$$w_{\text{daughter}} = w_{parent} + \text{N}(0, \sqrt{2D}), \tag{9}$$

where N is a normal distribution with zero mean and standard deviation of $\sqrt{2D}$, with D akin to an effective diffusion coefficient determining the magnitude of affinity change. Within this model, affinity can increase or decrease with equal probability at every division.

RESULTS

We performed numerical simulations of our model where we started with 50 different clones all having the same initial affinity ($w_0 = 1.5$) and progressed the reaction in a GC with capacity $N = 2,000$, which is the characteristic size of GCs in mice (Jacob et al., 1991). We track the fraction of the GC occupied by the different clonal lineages and observe a gradual homogenization of clonal diversity (**Figure 2A**). We qualitatively compare our results to *in vivo* measurements of clonal diversity, where we track the clones and their respective lineages. In the experiment, each initial clone is colored during the formation of the GC with a specific color by the recombination of the confetti allele. Subsequently, the subclonal lineage has the same color (the details of the experiment are explained in the introduction). Using two-photon microscopy, the size of subclonal lineages formed by the descendants of a cell that is permanently fluorescently labeled is measured (**Figure 2B**). We observe that with time, fewer clones survive in a GC. Additionally, the fraction of the GC occupied by the most dominant clone has a large variability. A similar behavior is observed experimentally as the fraction of the dominant sub-clonal lineage increase over time. The variability of this fraction across different GCs increases as well (**Figure 2B**; Tas et al., 2016). By sequencing the BCR region of B cells, the linages of the clones could be reconstructed. From these lineages we estimated the fraction of GC occupied by the dominant clone (Figure S1) and found that it is qualitatively similar to the results obtained with the coloring technique.

Diversity Loss Depends on the Rate of Affinity Increase

At the end of the growth phase we are left with 17.2 clones on average, consistent with the stochastic simulations (**Figure 2C**). At this point, the size of remaining lineages has a large variability according to Equation (4). We find that changing the "diffusion coefficient" D has a strong impact on the homogenization rate (**Figure 2D**). For larger values of D, fewer clones survive to be part of a mature GC (**Figures 2C,D**). The participation ratio, which is the probability that two randomly chosen B cells belong to the same clone, also suggests rapid loss of diversity for large value of D (Figure S2). Surprisingly, we find that the variability of different GC realizations increases with time (**Figures 2A,E**). Naturally, at long times diversity is lost and only a few clones are left, and the variation in the fraction of the most dominant clones decreases (**Figure 2E**). Thus, the highest number of possible outcomes, in clonal variability, occurs at an intermediate time, which for high values of D, happens at day 11 of the competitive phase.

The case of a GCR without mutation was also studied experimentally, in a setting in which multiple clones all having the same BCR seeded the GC and the AID gene was genetically deleted (Tas et al., 2016). Interestingly, even with no changes in affinity, there is a gradual and slow homogenization (**Figure 2B**, empty circles). To study this scenario, we performed numerical simulations in the absence of mutation ($D = 0$) and saw a gradual take over by the dominant clone (**Figures 2C–E**), as seen experimentally. As all clones have the same affinity, clonal loss and homogenization in this case is due to random drift (Renshaw, 1991). To gain intuition regarding the selection and fixation process, we recall known results for a case where the population size is fixed, corresponding to a Wright-Fisher process (Bailey, 1990). When affinity differences between the clones are neglected and a starting group of M clones all occupy the same fraction of the population size, the mean time to fixation of a single clone is given by $\tau_{\text{fixation}} = 2(M-1)\log(M/M-1)$. With non-uniform initial numbers of clones, the probability of a clone to fix is equal to its initial fraction in the population (Bailey, 1990), which in our model is the probability distribution at the end of the growth phase (Equation 4).

GC Clonal Diversity Negatively Correlates with Affinity

A clone whose affinity is relatively higher than that of the other clones in the GC has a better chance of being selected and becoming dominant (Equation 6). Since all clones had the same initial affinity, during the first few days of the competitive phase the affinity distribution of the population relaxes from a delta function ($\delta(w - w_0)$) (**Figure 3A**). A GC reaches its capacity only a few days after the beginning of the competitive stage (Figure S3A). Before that, diversity loss continues at the same rate of the growth phase and is D independent (**Figure 2C**). Beyond a certain threshold, the homogenization rate is independent of the birth-rate (Figure S3B).

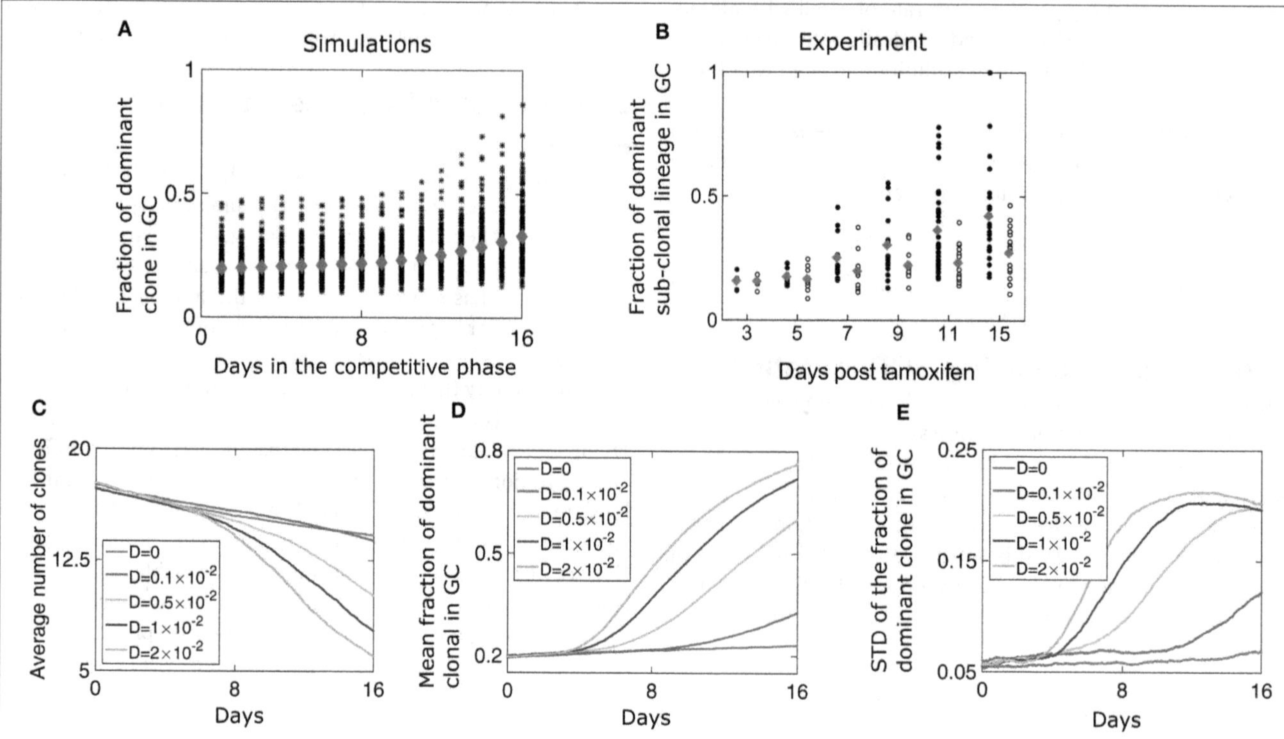

FIGURE 2 | Loss of diversity in a GC. **(A)** The fraction of the GC of size $N = 2000$ occupied by the most dominant clone during the competitive phase. Red diamonds are the mean of 200 independent runs while each black asterisk is the result of a single simulation. The parameters of the simulation are listed in **Table 1**. **(B)** Fraction of a GC occupied by the dominant sub-clonal lineage, which adopts a unique color upon Tamoxifen-induced recombination (adopted from Tas et al., 2016, **Figure 3F**). Tamoxifen triggers recombination of one or both Confetti alleles in individual GC B cells, independently of clonal origin. Mice were immunized with chicken gamma globulin at day-5, and GC where B cells participate in the AM process were extracted and analyzed (black circles). Each circle represents one GC. In the control experiment (white circles) all B cells had the same BCR and SHM was prevented by the absence of a functional AID allele. **Clonal size distribution in a GC. (C)** Mean number of surviving clones representing loss of clonal diversity during the competitive phase of the GC reaction. The average **(D)** and standard deviation **(E)** of the fraction of the GC of size occupied by the most dominant clone lineage during the competitive phase, for different values of D. The simulation started with $M = 50$ at day 0 of the growth phase that lasted 6 days. The parameters used are detailed in **Table 1**. The results represent 200 independent simulations.

At later times, the affinity distribution moves as a traveling wave (Tsimring et al., 1996; Hallatschek, 2011; **Figure 3A**), as fitter strains at the higher end of the affinity distribution function constitute the moving edge while the cells on the other end die. The velocity of the affinity wave depends on D (Cohen et al., 2005; **Figure 3B**) and since affinity changes upon cell division, it depends also on λ (Figure S3D). As expected for a traveling wave solution, the average affinity grows linearly with time. During this period in the GCR, since the affinity of all clones change due to the same stochastic process, a clone which after a single mutation has an affinity larger than the mean, is likely to outperform the other clones. Such deviations from the mean affinity, are governed by large jumps, which are related to the value of D.

To study if loss of clonal diversity in a GC is the result of homogenizing selection toward high affinity clones, we computed the correlation between the number of surviving clones in a GC and the average affinity of the most dominant clone at the end of the selection phase (**Figure 3C**). On day 16, the affinity of the dominant clone is a good proxy for the average affinity in the population. Interestingly, while we observe a weak negative correlation ($r = -0.53$), many GCs maintained diversity in spite of having high affinity clones.

We can consider the width of the affinity distribution of a GC population to be a proxy for its clonal diversity. It was shown that the ratio of the mean affinity to its standard deviation (STD) grows during AM when the amount of antigen used in the immunization was relatively low (Kang et al., 2015). Indeed, the STD of a stochastic variable grows with time (Schuss, 2009), while the growth of the average affinity is evidence of selection (Desai and Fisher, 2007). When the mean grows faster than the STD it is a sign of strong selection. We estimated this ratio from our simulations. Initially, as the affinity distribution spreads from a delta function and before the GC reaches its capacity, the ratio decays, but following the initial relaxation phase, the mean affinity increases faster than the spread of the distribution (**Figure 3D**). Thus, our system operates in the strong selection limit as in the experimental system studied in Kang et al. (2015).

Dependence of the Final Number of Cells on the Initial Growth Phase

To what extent does the initial growth phase determine the later state of the GCR? We define the state of a GC as the vector of proportions of clonal lineages at time t; $n(t)$ =

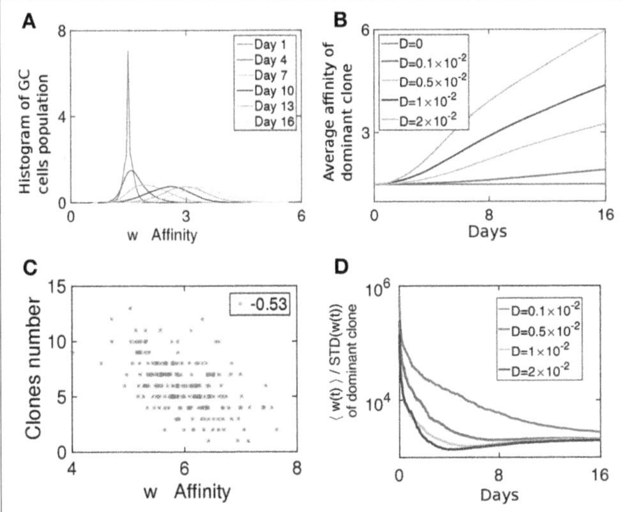

FIGURE 3 | Fitness growth during the competitive phase. **(A)** Affinity distribution of a GC cell population at different days of the competitive phase. Affinity gradually increases as a traveling wave phenomena. The simulation was performed with $D = 0.005$. **(B)** Mean affinity as a function of time for the most dominant clone. Similar parameters were used as in **Figures 2C–E**. **(C)** Scatter plot of the number of clones in a GC vs. the affinity of the most dominant clone. **(D)** The ratio of the mean affinity of a GC population and its standard deviation.

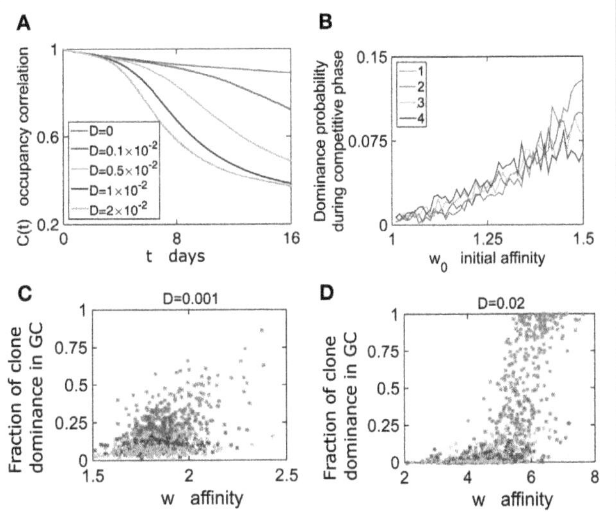

FIGURE 4 | GC content depends on the initial conditions. **(A)** Following growth phase of 6 days, we estimate the occupancy correlation $C(t)$ Equation (10) during the competitive phase. **(B)** The dominance probability depending on the initial affinity w_0. In the growth phase all cells proliferate with the same rate λ_0. w_0 determines the birth rate in the competitive phase according to Equation (6) ($D = 0.02$). **(C,D)** The dominance probability is shown for the most dominant clone (blue), second dominance (red), third (yellow) fourth dominance (purple), and fifth (green).

$(n_1(t), n_2(t), ..., n_M(t))/N_{tot}(t)$. The correlation with the initial state of the GC is quantified by

$$C(t) = \frac{1}{N_{tot}(t)} \sum_i n_i(T_{growth}) n_i(T_{growth} + t), \qquad (10)$$

and is observed to decay with time (**Figure 4A**). The initial fractions of clones change when stochastic increases or decreases in the affinity of cells give relative advantages or disadvantages to particular clones (Equations 6, 9). Thus, for larger values of D, C decays faster. Similarly, the decay rate of correlations is inversely proportional to the basal birth rate (Figure S3C) and to N, since the fixation probability of a species in a population is inversely proportional to population size (Desai and Fisher, 2007) (data not shown). This result raises the question of whether a GC effectively filters the best clones, as the system has a finite probability to be "stuck" in an unfavorable state.

To further explore the relation between clonal competition and affinity we performed numerical simulations where each B cell of the M initial ones had different initial affinity w_0. Following growth, we studied clonal dominance in the competitive phase. Interestingly, while the clone with the highest initial affinity ($w_0 = 1.5$) had the highest probability of becoming the dominant clone, the clone with $w_0 = 1.25$ still had a chance of becoming dominant (**Figure 4B**). This exemplifies the stochastic nature of the selection process. The effect of the initial affinity w_0 in determining the second, third and fourth dominant clone is smaller (**Figure 4B**).

We addressed the relation between affinity and dominance by estimating the correlation between the average clonal affinity and the fraction occupied by the first to fifth dominant clones. Interestingly, we see that often clones with high affinity compose a small fraction of the GC at the end of the GCR (**Figure 4C**). We also see that this depends on the value of D, and for a larger value the positive correlation between dominance and affinity is stronger (**Figure 4D**).

Death Limited Selection

To study the effect of a death-limited model on the progression of the GCR we preform stochastic simulations using an affinity-dependent death rate (Equation 7). The GC population's affinity continues to increase throughout the simulation (**Figures 5A,B**). We assume that clones with higher affinity have a smaller probability of dying, as they are likely to receive a survival signal from the TfhCs. Thus, in our death-limited model, affinity increase results in decrease of the death rate (Equation 7). Thus, we observe a gradual decrease of the death rate distribution of the cell population (**Figure 5C**). We found two homogenization regimes (**Figure 5D**). While the GC has not yet reached its capacity and death rate distribution of the cell population relaxes from a delta function, which was the initial condition ($w(t = 0) = \delta(w - w_0)$), to steady state, homogenization is slow. Indeed, for $D = 0$ the homogenization rate remains constant. In this case, diversity loss is related to random drift only. At later times, homogenization occurs at a fixed rate, dependent on D (**Figure 5D**). The exponential relation between affinity and death rate in this death-limited selection model acts to modulate large affinity jumps. Thus, homogenization occurs at a slower rate than that of the birth-limited model we studied in the previous section.

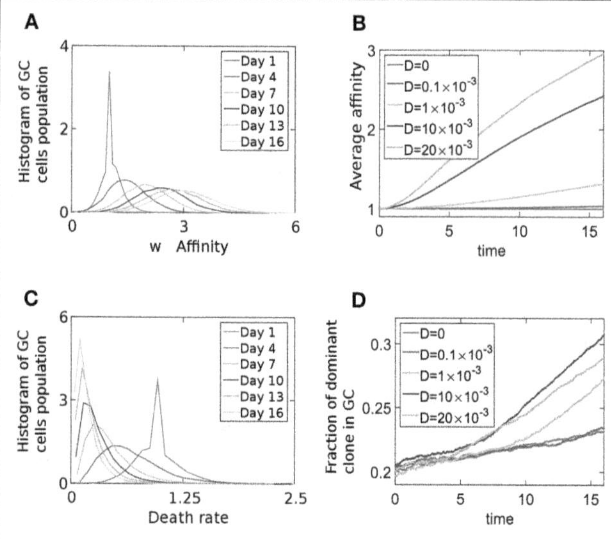

FIGURE 5 | Death limited selection of B cells. **(A)** Affinity distribution of a GC cell population at different times of the competitive phase in the death-limited model Equation (7). The parameters used were: $N = 2000, D = 0.01$, $\lambda_0 = 1.5\ \text{day}^{-1}, \alpha = 1, A = exp(1)\ \text{day}^{-1}, w_0 = 1$. **(B)** Average affinity of dominant clone in the death-limited model. **(C)** The death rate distribution corresponding to **(A)**. **(D)** The fraction of the GC occupied by the most dominant clone.

To investigate if the difference between the death and birth limit selection model is due to normalization of the birth-rate (Equation 6), we performed simulations where the death rate of cell i was given by Equation (8). When the average affinity dependent death rate remains μ_0, the homogenization rate increases (Figure S4) with respect to the un-normalized case, but still remains slower than that for the birth-limited model. There are experimental evidences that the average birthrate is constant in the GC, independent of the affinity of B cells (Anderson et al., 2009). However, such is not the case for death limited selection, since no survival signal is given to B cells by T cells when no Ag is captured. This presumably will occur when the affinity is small. Thus, it is likely that a dependence of death rate and affinity (Equation 7) exists in the GC.

DISCUSSION

In this study, motivated by recent experimental results, which allowed imaging of AM in GCs over time, we explored simple models to understand the observed phenomenology of clonal selection. The main experimental observation is that clonal selection and homogenization is heterogeneous in a GC population. It appears that the selection of B cell clones, while correlated to the BCR affinity, is probabilistic and lower affinity cells are often selected for proliferation.

We find large variability in the fraction of a GC occupied by different clone lineages. Since selection is a stochastic process, GCs have varying resulting clonal fractions starting from the same founding clone composition. Interestingly, this variability reaches a maximum at intermediate times during the GCR, before decreasing. Our numerical simulations show that the relevant parameter determining homogenization dynamics is the magnitude of affinity modification per single mutation. A large single-mutation change in affinity allows a cell to gain fitness advantage in the population. We find that a fast increase in affinity leads to rapid diversity loss.

Clonal competition can be understood using classical concepts in population dynamics. When the selection pressure is very strong, the fittest variant will survive, that is, the cell with the highest affinity BCR. However, when selection is weaker or when variants compete for different resources, multiple clones or variants can co-exist. The first case is called selective sweep, where one clone dominates over the population (Desai and Fisher, 2007). Alternatively, when selection forces are weaker or mutation rate is fast, clonal interference (Desai and Fisher, 2007) is apparent, where at any time, several clones can coexist. While the first case would result in a relatively homogeneous GC, the second one would appear as a dynamically heterogeneous GC. Interestingly, it appears that both phenomena are possible in different GCs, even ones residing in the same lymph node that have similar initial clonal populations (Tas et al., 2016). This suggests that the GCR lives close to the transition line between the two limiting cases and can stochastically converge in a manner that may depend on the initial conditions, or on fluctuations in the different parameters. We hypothesize that the proliferation boost given to a high affinity (or lucky) B cell can result in a selective sweep. This can presumably occur at any stage of the GC reaction, when a B cell with high affinity manages to capture a lot of Ag and receives multiple proliferation signals from TfhCs leading to multiple divisions in the DZ.

The selection mechanisms we have studied (birth-limited vs. death-limited) result in different homogenization rates and affinities. B cells divide multiple times in the DZ before going back to the LZ. We have shown in the SI that this selection mechanism is equivalent to having a birth rate which is proportional to affinity. This progeny will replace other cells in the GC, thus diversity loss is accelerated. In death-limited selection however, cells with poor affinity are removed one by one. Thus, as a rule, diversity loss in death-limited selection is slower than that of a birth-limited one. For medium and low affinity clones, it was found (Anderson et al., 2009) that they will have approximately the same proliferation rate, while the death depends on the affinity. This could reduce the rate of death-limited selection at later times in the GC, when affinity is higher.

The GCR likely uses these two approaches intermittently. When the fitness landscape of an antibody is very rugged, an optimization algorithm (Bornholdt, 1998) to find a local or global maximum is not effective, as each mutation is likely to greatly decrease the cell fitness. It is possible that the GCR has evolved an approach to use death-limited selection in the LZ as the basal mechanism that would not lead to rapid clonal expansion and GC takeover by a single clone. The second, a birth-rate affinity-dependent selection mechanism, gives a strong proliferation boost to a very successful clone, or to ones that due to random fluctuations managed to capture a large quantity of Ag. Such events may be rarer than death-limited selection, allowing a clone to take over the GC. Thus, diversity is kept as long as no clone distinguishes itself.

We model here selection as a stochastic process using a simple population dynamics model, leading to the gradual homogenization and the variability in GC state. Current experimental results can be recapitulated qualitatively by our coarse-grained model (**Figure 2**). This suggests that the features we consider are sufficient to recapitulate the qualitative experimental observations regarding diversity loss. Of course, quantitative detailed predictions would require more detailed models including Ag recycling, model of Ag concentration dynamics over time (Tam et al., 2016), explicit description of B-T cells interactions (Meyer-Hermann et al., 2012) can explain the termination of a GCR and interaction between separated GCs in the same lymph node (Figge et al., 2008). Our model could be extended to study complex affinity landscapes and describe AM for multiple antigens and epitopes. It would be interesting to estimate in a high-throughput manner the spectrum of affinities for an antigen and measure the respective selection. Such data could be used to infer the affinity-selection mechanism in a GC.

AUTHOR CONTRIBUTIONS

AA, AC, MK, LM, and GV conceived and designed the *in silico* studies; AA performed *in silico* studies. LM and GV performed experiments. AA, MK, AC, LM, and GV wrote the paper.

FUNDING

Financial support for this work was provided by a grant from the Ragon Institute of MGH, MIT, & Harvard (AC, AA). MK acknowledges support from NSF grant no. DMR-1708280. GV acknowledges support from NIH grant R01 AI119006.

REFERENCES

Adke, S., and Moyal, J. (1963). A birth, death, and diffusion process. *J. Math. Anal. Appl.* 7, 209–224. doi: 10.1016/0022-247X(63)90048-9

Anderson, S. M., Khalil, A., Uduman, M., Hershberg, U., Louzoun, Y., Haberman, A. M., et al. (2009). Taking advantage: high-affinity B cells in the germinal center have lower death rates, but similar rates of division, compared to low-affinity cells. *J. Immunol.* 183, 7314–7325. doi: 10.4049/jimmunol.0902452

Bailey, N. T. J. (1990). *The Elements of Stochastic Processes with Applications to the Natural Sciences*. New York, NY: Wiley.

Batista, F. D., and Neuberger, M. S. (1998). Affinity dependence of the B cell response to antigen: A threshold, a ceiling, and the importance of off-rate. *Immunity* 8, 751–759. doi: 10.1016/S1074-7613(00)80580-4

Bornholdt, S. (1998). Genetic algorithm dynamics on a rugged landscape. *Phys. Rev.* 57, 3853–3860. doi: 10.1103/PhysRevE.57.3853

Brink, R. (2007). Germinal-center B cells in the zone. *Immunity* 26, 552–554. doi: 10.1016/j.immuni.2007.05.002

Chan, C., Billard, M., Ramirez, S. A., Schmidl, H., Monson, E., and Kepler, T. B. (2013). A model for migratory B cell oscillations from receptor down-regulation induced by external chemokine fields. *Bull. Math. Biol.* 75, 185–205. doi: 10.1007/s11538-012-9799-9

Chaudhury, S., Reifman, J., and Wallqvist, A. (2014). Simulation of B cell affinity maturation explains enhanced antibody cross-reactivity induced by the polyvalent malaria vaccine AMA1. *J. Immunol.* 193, 2073–2086. doi: 10.4049/jimmunol.1401054

Cohen, E., Kessler, D. A., and Levine, H. (2005). Front propagation up a reaction rate gradient. *Phys. Rev.* 72, 1–11. doi: 10.1103/PhysRevE.72.066126

Desai, M. M., and Fisher, D. S. (2007). Beneficial mutation-selection balance and the effect of linkage on positive selection. *Genetics* 176, 1759–1798. doi: 10.1534/genetics.106.067678

Eisen, H. N., and Siskind, G. W. (1964). Variations in affinities of antibodies during the immune response. *Biochemistry* 3, 996–1008.

Figge, M. T. (2005). Stochastic discrete event simulation of germinal center reactions. *Phys. Rev.* 71, 1–15. doi: 10.1103/PhysRevE.71.051907

Figge, M. T., Garin, A., Gunzer, M., Kosco-Vilbois, M., Toellner, K.-M., and Meyer-Hermann, M. (2008). Deriving a germinal center lymphocyte migration model from two-photon data. *J. Exp. Med.* 205, 3019–3029. doi: 10.1084/jem.20081160

Gitlin, A. D., Mayer, C. T., Oliveira, T. Y., Shulman, Z., Jones, M. J., Koren, A., et al. (2015). T cell help controls the speed of the cell cycle in germinal center B cells. *Science* 349, 643–646. doi: 10.1126/science.aac4919

Gitlin, A. D., Shulman, Z., and Nussenzweig, M. C. (2014). Clonal selection in the germinal centre by regulated proliferation and hypermutation. *Nature* 509, 637–640. doi: 10.1038/nature13300

Goyal, S., Balick, D. J., Jerison, E. R., Neher, R. A., Shraiman, B. I., and Desai, M. M. (2012). Dynamic mutation-selection balance as an evolutionary attractor. *Genetics* 191, 1309–1319. doi: 10.1534/genetics.112.141291

Hallatschek, O. (2011). The noisy edge of traveling waves. *Proc. Natl. Acad. Sci. U.S.A.* 108, 1783–1787. doi: 10.1073/pnas.1013529108

Jacob, J., Kassir, R., and Kelsoe, G. (1991). In situ studies of the primary immune response to (4-hydroxy-3-nitrophenyl) acetyl. I. The architecture and dynamics of responding cell populations. *J. Exp. Med.* 173, 1165. doi: 10.1084/jem.176.3.679

Jacob, J., Przylepa, J., Miller, C., and Kelsoe, G. (1993). *In situ* studies of the primary immune response to (4-hydroxy-3-nitrophenyl)acetyl. III. The kinetics of V region mutation and selection in germinal center B cells. *J. Exp. Med.* 178, 1293–1307. doi: 10.1084/jem.178.4.1293

Kang, M., Eisen, T. J., Eisen, E. A., Chakraborty, A. K., and Eisen, H. N. (2015). Affinity inequality among serum antibodies that originate in lymphoid germinal centers. *PLoS ONE* 10:e0139222. doi: 10.1371/journal.pone.0139222

Kepler, T. B., and Perelson, A. S. (1993). Cyclic re-entry of germinal center B cells and the efficiency of affinity maturation. *Immunol. Today* 14, 412–415. doi: 10.1016/0167-5699(93)90145-B

Kroese, F. G., Wubbena, A. S., Seijen, H. G., and Nieuwenhuis, P. (1987). Germinal centers develop oligoclonally. *Eur. J. Immunol.* 17, 1069–1072. doi: 10.1002/eji.1830170726

Liu, Y. J., Zhang, J., Lane, P. J., Chan, E. Y., and MacLennan, I. C. (1991). Sites of specific B cell activation in primary and secondary responses to T cell-dependent and T cell-independent antigens. *Eur. J. Immunol.* 21, 2951–2962. doi: 10.1002/eji.1830211209

Livet, J., Weissman, T. A., Kang, H., Draft, R. W., Lu, J., Bennis, R. A., et al. Lichtman, J. W. (2007). Transgenic strategies for combinatorial expression of fluorescent proteins in the nervous system. *Nature* 450, 56–62. doi: 10.1038/nature06293

Luo, S., and Perelson, A. S. (2015). Competitive exclusion by autologous antibodies can prevent broad HIV-1 antibodies from arising. *Proc. Natl. Acad. Sci. U.S.A.* 112, 11654–11659. doi: 10.1073/pnas.1505207112

Meyer-Hermann, M., Mohr, E., Pelletier, N., Zhang, Y., Victora, G. D., and Toellner, K. M. (2012). A theory of germinal center b cell selection, division, and exit. *Cell Rep.* 2, 162–174. doi: 10.1016/j.celrep.2012.05.010

Muramatsu, M., Kinoshita, K., Fagarasan, S., Yamada, S., Shinkai, Y., and Honjo, T. (2000). Class switch recombination and hypermutation require Activation-Induced Cytidine Deaminase (AID), a Potential RNA Editing Enzyme. *Cell* 102, 553–563. doi: 10.1016/S0092-8674(00)00078-7

Nåsell, I. (2001). Extinction and quasi-stationarity in the Verhulst logistic model. *J. Theor. Biol.* 211, 11–27. doi: 10.1006/jtbi.2001.2328

Neher, R. A., Vucelja, M., Mezard, M., and Shraiman, B. I. (2013). Emergence of clones in sexual populations. *J. Stat. Mech. Theory Exp.* 2013, P01008. doi: 10.1088/1742-5468/2013/01/P01008

Oprea, M., and Perelson, A. S. (1997). Somatic mutation leads to efficient affinity maturation when centrocytes recycle back to centroblasts. *J. Immunol* 158, 5155–5162.

Park, S.-C., and Krug, J. (2007). Clonal interference in large populations. *Proc. Natl. Acad. Sci. U.S.A.* 104, 18135–18140. doi: 10.1073/pnas.0705778104

Renshaw, E. (1991). *Modelling Biological Populations in Space and Time.* Cambridge, UK: Cambridge University Press.

Rolf, J., Bell, S. E., Kovesdi, D., Janas M. L., Soond, D. R., Webb, L. M., et al. (2010). Phosphoinositide 3-kinase activity in T cells regulates the magnitude of the germinal center reaction. *J. Immunol.* 185, 4042–4052. doi: 10.4049/jimmunol.1001730

Schuss, Z. (2009). *Diffusion and Stochastic Processes. An Analytical Approach.* New York, NY: Springer-Verlag.

Shaffer, J. S., Moore, P. L., Kardar, M., and Chakraborty, A. K. (2016). Optimal immunization cocktails can promote induction of broadly neutralizing Abs against highly mutable pathogens. *Proc. Natl. Acad. Sci. U.S.A.* 113, E7039–E7048. doi: 10.1073/pnas.1614940113

Tam, H. H., Melo, M. B., Kang, M., Pelet, J. M., Ruda, V. M., Foley, M. H., et al. (2016). Sustained antigen availability during germinal center initiation enhances antibody responses to vaccination *Proc. Natl. Acad. Sci. U.S.A.* 113, E6639–E6648. doi: 10.1073/pnas.1606050113

Tas, J. M. J., Mesin, L., Pasqual, G., Targ, S., Jacobsen, J. T., Mano, Y. M., et al. (2016). Visualizing antibody affinity maturation in germinal centers. *Science* 58, 7250–7257. doi: 10.1126/science.aad3439

Tsimring, L. S., Levine, H., and Kessler, D. A. (1996). RNA virus evolution via a fitness-space model. *Phys. Rev. Lett.* 76, 4440–4443. doi: 10.1103/PhysRevLett.76.4440

Victora, G. D., and Nussenzweig, M. C. (2012). Germinal centers. *Annu. Rev. Immunol.* 30, 429–457. doi: 10.1146/annurev-immunol-020711-075032

Victora, G. D., Schwickert, T. A., Fooksman, D. R., Kamphorst, A. O., Meyer-Hermann, M., Dustin, M. L., et al. (2010). Germinal center dynamics revealed by multiphoton microscopy with a photoactivatable fluorescent reporter. *Cell* 143, 592–605. doi: 10.1016/j.cell.2010.10.032

Wang, S., Mata-Fink, J., Kriegsman, B., Hanson, M., Irvine, D. J., Eisen, H. N., et al. (2015). Manipulating the selection forces during affinity maturation to generate cross-reactive HIV antibodies. *Cell* 160, 785–797. doi: 10.1016/j.cell.2015.01.027

Zhang, J., and Shakhnovich, E. I. (2010). Optimality of mutation and selection in germinal centers. *PLoS Comput. Biol.* 6:e1000800. doi: 10.1371/journal.pcbi.1000800

Zhang, Y., Meyer-Hermann, M., George, L. A., Figge, M. T., Khan, M., Goodall, M., et al. (2013). Germinal center B cells govern their own fate via antibody feedback. *J. Exp. Med.* 210, 457–464. doi: 10.1084/jem.20120150

17

Quantitative Simulations Predict Treatment Strategies against Fungal Infections in Virtual Neutropenic Patients

*Sandra Timme[1,2], Teresa Lehnert[1,3], Maria T. E. Prauße[1,2], Kerstin Hünniger[4,5], Ines Leonhardt[3,4], Oliver Kurzai[3,4,5] and Marc Thilo Figge[1,2,3]**

[1] Research Group Applied Systems Biology, Leibniz Institute for Natural Product Research and Infection Biology—Hans Knöll Institute, Jena, Germany, [2] Faculty of Biological Sciences, Friedrich Schiller University Jena, Jena, Germany, [3] Center for Sepsis Control and Care (CSCC), Jena University Hospital, Jena, Germany, [4] Fungal Septomics, Septomics Research Center, Leibniz Institute for Natural Product Research and Infection Biology—Hans Knöll Institute, Friedrich Schiller University, Jena, Germany, [5] Institute for Hygiene and Microbiology, University of Würzburg, Würzburg, Germany

***Correspondence:**
Marc Thilo Figge
thilo.figge@leibniz-hki.de

The condition of neutropenia, i.e., a reduced absolute neutrophil count in blood, constitutes a major risk factor for severe infections in the affected patients. *Candida albicans* and *Candida glabrata* are opportunistic pathogens and the most prevalent fungal species in the human microbiota. In immunocompromised patients, they can become pathogenic and cause infections with high mortality rates. In this study, we use a previously established approach that combines experiments and computational models to investigate the innate immune response during blood stream infections with the two fungal pathogens *C. albicans* and *C. glabrata.* First, we determine immune-reaction rates and migration parameters under healthy conditions. Based on these findings, we simulate virtual patients and investigate the impact of neutropenic conditions on the infection outcome with the respective pathogen. Furthermore, we perform *in silico* treatments of these virtual patients by simulating a medical treatment that enhances neutrophil activity in terms of phagocytosis and migration. We quantify the infection outcome by comparing the response to the two fungal pathogens relative to non-neutropenic individuals. The analysis reveals that these fungal infections in neutropenic patients can be successfully cleared by cytokine treatment of the remaining neutrophils; and that this treatment is more effective for *C. glabrata* than for *C. albicans*.

Keywords: fungal infections, neutropenia, treatment strategies, bottom-up modeling approach, computer simulations

INTRODUCTION

The human immune system protects the body against various environmental cues, such as microorganisms. It covers mechanisms on different levels ranging from physical barriers, like the skin and mucosal surfaces, down to cellular and molecular components of the innate and adaptive immune system (1). However, congenital or acquired diseases as well as medical treatments may impair proper functioning of the immune system, which can result in the loss of its protective ability. Neutrophils constitute the highest fraction of blood leukocytes, as they make up over 70% of all blood leukocytes (2). Since they can migrate to sites of infection and clear the organism from pathogens, they constitute an important part of the immune system.

Candida spp. cause 5–15% of all bloodstream infections and are associated with high mortality rates of 30–40% (3). A significant proportion (>50%, depending on the study setting) of the human population is colonized with *Candida* spp. The most prevalent species are *Candida albicans* and *Candida glabrata* that are both human commensals and reside predominantly on the human skin and mucosal surfaces (4–6). *C. albicans* is a morphotype-switching yeast, which in its commensal state exhibits the typical yeast form, while it forms hyphae when switching to its pathogenic state (7, 8). By contrast, *C. glabrata* does not form hyphae, neither in the commensal nor in the pathogenic state and is smaller than *C. albicans* (4, 9). In healthy people, both species usually stay in their commensal state. However, in immunocompromised patients, these human-pathogenic fungi can switch to their pathogenic state and cause superficial as well as systemic infections that are associated with high mortality rates.

To investigate host–pathogen interactions between the human innate immune system and these fungal pathogens, we applied a systems biology approach, where wet-lab experiments were combined with virtual infection models (10–13). Such virtual infection models have the great advantage of allowing for the identification and quantification of essential parameters that govern the biological system under consideration. This also makes them a powerful tool for hypothesis generation and uncovering new mechanisms, which consequently allows for minimizing the amount of animal experiments (14). Depending on the purpose, such *in silico* models can be built with different modeling techniques, such as *differential equations*, *state-based models* (SBMs) or spatial modeling techniques such as *cellular automata*, *cellular Potts models* or *agent-based models* (ABMs) (15). In a previous systems biology study, we established a human whole-blood infection assay (16), where blood was taken from healthy volunteers and infected with *C. albicans* cells. Then, subpopulations of alive, killed and extracellular fungal cells as well as fungal cells phagocytosed by monocytes and neutrophils were measured by association assays and survival assays. Based on these experimental data, we implemented an SBM that allowed for the quantification of immune-reaction rates, such as phagocytosis and killing rates, by fitting the simulated kinetics to the experimental data. In a subsequent study, we developed a bottom-up modeling approach that enabled not only quantification of immune-reaction rates but also the investigation of spatial aspects (17). Since the SBM simulates the temporal but not the spatial dynamics, we also developed an ABM that was based on a previous ABM implementation (18, 19). We combined both models in a bottom-up modeling approach (17): the SBM was used to determine non-spatial rates that were afterward transformed and used in the ABM to fit migration parameters of immune cells in human whole blood. We found that the *in silico* infection outcome for *C. albicans* was sensitive to changes in the diffusion coefficient of neutrophils, whereas that of monocytes had only minor impact on the system dynamics. This result reflected the more prominent role of neutrophils over monocytes in fighting *C. albicans* infection of human whole blood. Furthermore, immune dysregulation was investigated using the ABM, and the results showed that a reduced diffusion coefficient for neutrophils resembled conditions of neutropenia (17). This important observation is the main motivation of the present study, because it suggests how neutropenic patients may be treated to cope with bloodstream infections. Thus, increasing neutrophil activation in terms of phagocytic activity as well as migration strength is hypothesized to have the potential of balancing neutropenic conditions and clearance of infection. Based on this reasoning, we address infections in human whole blood by *C. albicans* and *C. glabrata* under neutropenic conditions in this study.

Diseases or medical treatments can evoke a reduced absolute neutrophil count (ANC) in blood and result into a condition called *neutropenia*. Neutropenia may result from congenital or acquired impairments, where the latter case is more frequent. A reduced ANC may arise due to a disturbed development of neutrophils in the bone marrow, a disturbed migration to the blood stream or a rapid consumption during an infection (20). In anti-cancer chemotherapy, neutropenia is the most abundant disorder of the immune system due to the relatively short life-span of these terminally differentiated cells (21). Neutropenia emerges in different degrees of severity that are classified by the *Severe Chronic Neutropenia International Registry* (SCNIR) (20). The SCNIR distinguishes three degrees of severity: mild neutropenia with an ANC of 1,000–1,500 neutrophils/μl, moderate neutropenia with an ANC of 500–1,000 neutrophils/μl and severe neutropenia with an ANC of <500 neutrophils/μl. In this study, we focus on neutropenia treatment by stimulation and activation of present neutrophils by inflammatory cytokines and quantitatively investigate the impact on fungal infections by computer simulations. Thus, we aim to investigate a possible treatment strategy where the neutrophil activity is increased by a higher diffusion coefficient and/or phagocytosis rate. For this purpose, we apply the previously established protocol for whole-blood infection assays and perform the bottom-up modeling approach for the two human-pathogenic fungi. As is schematically shown in **Figure 1**, we first determine quantitative values for the immune-reaction rates as well as for diffusion coefficients of monocytes and neutrophils as the key immune cells of innate immunity in whole blood. Furthermore, we use this modeling approach to simulate neutropenia *in silico* and compare effects on the infection outcome between the different pathogens. To evaluate a possible treatment strategy, we simulate virtual neutropenic patients (VNP) with different degrees of severity and increase stepwise the phagocytosis rate and/or the diffusion coefficient of neutrophils to classify the infection outcome. Taken together, we could show that the increase of the phagocytosis rate and/or the migration parameter of neutrophils generally allowed balancing neutropenic conditions and clearance of infection. Furthermore, we predict that *C. albicans* compared with *C. glabrata* always requires stronger increases in the phagocytosis rate and the diffusion coefficient for the same conditions of neutropenia.

MATERIALS AND METHODS

Ethics Statement

This study was conducted according to the principles expressed in the Declaration of Helsinki. All protocols were approved by the Ethics Committee of the University Hospital Jena (permit number: 273-12/09). Written informed consent was obtained from all blood donors.

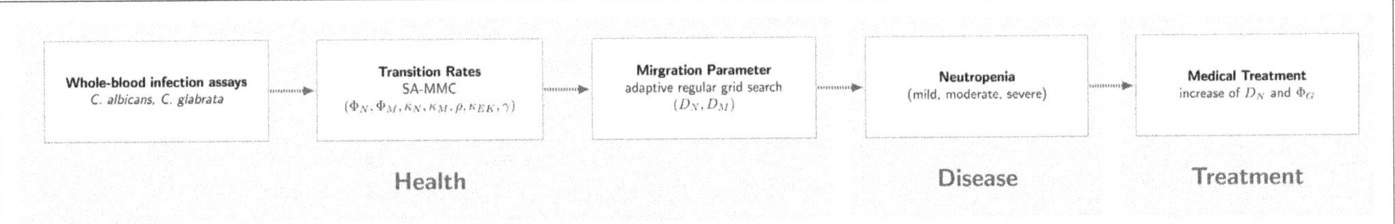

FIGURE 1 | Workflow for studying neutropenia *in silico*. First, whole-blood infection assays with *Candida albicans* and *Candida glabrata* were performed in wet lab. Second, non-spatial immune-reaction rates were fitted using the state-based model. Third, the agent-based model (ABM) was used to estimate migration parameters for neutrophils and monocytes. Based on the fitted non-spatial immune-reaction rates and the fitted migration parameters, virtual neutropenic patients were simulated in the ABM by gradually reducing the neutrophil count. Eventually, a medical treatment of the virtual patients was simulated by increasing the diffusion coefficient and/or the phagocytosis rate of neutrophils.

Fungal Strains and Culture

GFP expressing *C. albicans* strain [constructed as described in Ref. (16)] was grown in liquid yeast extract–peptone–dextrose (YPD) medium at 30°C. *C. glabrata* expressing GFP (22) was incubated at 37°C in YPD. In preparation for the whole-blood assay, both strains were reseeded after overnight culture in YPD medium and grown at 30 and 37°C, respectively, until they reached the mid-log-phase and finally harvested in HBSS until use.

Whole-Blood Infection Assay

Human peripheral blood from healthy individuals was infected with either of the two fungi *C. albicans* and *C. glabrata*, respectively. The assay was performed as described previously (16). In short, 1×10^6 *Candida* cells were added per ml of anti-coagulated blood and incubated at 37°C with gentle rotation for time points indicated. Following the incubation, cells were maintained at 4°C and analyzed immediately *via* flow cytometry. Flow cytometry gating strategy to investigate the distribution of fungal cells in human blood was performed as previously described (16) using FlowJo 7.6.4 software. Survival of fungal cells was determined in a plating assay by analysis of recovered colony-forming units after plating appropriate dilutions of all time points on YPD agar plates.

Bottom-Up Modeling Approach

We established a bottom-up modeling approach for simulation and fitting of whole-blood infection assays in a previous study (17). This bottom-up modeling approach incorporates models with increasing complexity that build on one another, where each model focuses on different aspects of the infection process.

SBM—Immune-Reaction Rates

First, we applied the SBM to quantify and characterize immune-reaction rates for discrete entities of pathogens and innate immune cells. Therefore, the populations of innate immune cells, i.e., neutrophils and monocytes, as well as the pathogens were modeled by different states in the SBM. For the comparison with experimentally measured cell populations, we identified five combined units that are composed of specific states. The states representing extracellular cells are combined in the combined unit P_E that is given by the following equation:

$$P_E \equiv P_{AE} + P_{KE} + P_{AIE} + P_{KIE}, \quad (1)$$

where the states P_{AE} and P_{KE} represent extracellular cells that are alive and killed, respectively. The states P_{AIE} and P_{KIE} describe pathogens that are either alive and evading the immune response or killed and evading the immune response. Pathogens that are in extracellular space and either alive (P_{AE}) or killed (P_{KE}) can be phagocytosed by two different immune cells, i.e., neutrophils (N) and monocytes (M). The combined unit P_N comprises pathogens that are phagocytosed by neutrophils and is given by the following equation:

$$P_N \equiv \sum_{i \geq 0} \sum_{j \geq 0} (i + j) N_{i,j}. \quad (2)$$

Similarly, pathogens that are phagocytosed by monocytes are combined in P_M that is given by the following equation:

$$P_M \equiv \sum_{i \geq 0} \sum_{j \geq 0} (i + j) M_{i,j}. \quad (3)$$

In Eqs 2 and 3, the indices i and j refer to the immune cell state that is defined by the number of internalized alive and killed pathogens, respectively.

Furthermore, the states representing alive and killed pathogens are combined in P_K and P_A, respectively, that are defined by the following equations:

$$P_K \equiv P_{KE} + P_{KIE} + \sum_{i \geq 0} \sum_{j \geq 0} (M_{i,j} + N_{i,j}) j, \quad (4)$$

$$P_A \equiv P_{AE} + P_{AIE} + \sum_{i \geq 0} \sum_{j \geq 0} (M_{i,j} + N_{i,j}) i. \quad (5)$$

The total number of pathogens is given by $P \equiv P_E + P_N + P_M$ or $P \equiv P_K + P_A$.

Transitions between these states are characterized by so-called *transition rates* and allow for dynamic state changes over time. The SBM of whole-blood infection comprises seven different transition rates that are given by the phagocytosis rate ϕ_M of monocytes, the phagocytosis rate ϕ_N of neutrophils, the intracellular killing rates κ_M and κ_N of both monocytes and neutrophils, the transition rates γ and $\bar{\kappa}_{EK}$, which define the extracellular killing by antimicrobial peptides, and the spontaneous immune evasion rate ρ. Note that, in the previous study by Lehnert et al. (17), a distinction between first and subsequent phagocytosis events by neutrophils was made, where the first phagocytosis event was assumed to activate the neutrophils and induce granulation. Since this fact is not experimentally validated for whole-blood infection with *C. glabrata*, we here did not distinguish between these two processes and used only one transition rate (ϕ_N) referring to both first and subsequent phagocytosis events. To determine *a priori* unknown transitions rates, the *in silico* data were fitted to the experimental data by applying the method of *Simulated Annealing* based on the *Metropolis Monte Carlo* scheme (SA-MMC). For a more detailed description of the model and the parameter estimation method, we refer to Hünniger et al. (16) and Lehnert et al. (17).

ABM—Immune Cell Migration

The ABM is based on a previous ABM implementation (18, 19) and was already used in the previous study by Ref. (17). In contrast to the SBM, it allows studying spatial aspects, such as immune cell migration, in whole-blood infection assays. The ABM simulates all cell types, i.e., pathogens as well as immune cells, as individual spherical objects that are referred to as *agents*. All agents migrate, act and interact in a rule-based fashion within a spatially continuous, three-dimensional environment that represents 1 µl of blood.

Furthermore, the ABM was fitted to the experimental data to determine diffusion coefficients of neutrophils (D_N) and monocytes (D_M). This was done by the bottom-up modeling approach, where the previously determined transition rates from the SBM were used in the ABM. However, space-dependent rates, like phagocytosis rates, had to be adequately transformed (17). Regarding the fitting procedure, we used an *adaptive regular grid search* that scans the parameter space within reasonable ranges and uses a more fine-grained grid in regions with relatively small least squares errors (LSEs).

Simulation Workflow

The work flow of this study, comparing wet-lab and *in silico* experiments with different models is displayed in **Figure 1**. First, we performed whole-blood infection assays for the two fungal pathogens *C. albicans* and *C. glabrata*. Afterward, we applied for each of the two pathogens the following steps. The results from association and survival assays were used to fit the model parameters of the SBM to these data. The transition rates of the fit with the lowest LSE were then appropriately transformed and fed into the ABM. Subsequently, the grid search in the parameter space was applied to fit the ABM to the experimental data and, in this way, to estimate the diffusion coefficients of neutrophils and monocytes. The determined transition rates and migration parameters form the basis for all following investigations on neutropenia and possible treatment strategies in virtual patients with varying degree of neutropenia. In the following, each step of this work flow is described in more detail.

Infection in Virtual Patients With Normal Neutrophil Counts

For the quantification of the immune response against the human-pathogenic fungi *C. albicans* and *C. glabrata* with normal neutrophil counts, we first determined the transition rates by fitting the SBM to the corresponding data from whole-blood experiments. These rates were used in the ABM and diffusion coefficients for neutrophils D_N and monocytes D_M were determined by fitting the ABM to the experimental data.

Infection in Virtual Patients Under Neutropenic Condition

To examine the immune response of virtual patients under conditions of neutropenia, we performed simulations with the immune-reaction rates and migration parameters that were identified under non-neutropenic conditions and gradually decreased the number of neutrophils. Subsequently, we compared the infection outcome at 4 h post infection for varying degrees of severity of neutropenia.

Patterns and Classification of Simulations

Since the health of a patient is critically determined by the amount of killed pathogens P_K as well as by the amount of alive and immune-evasive pathogens P_{AIE}, we used these measures to characterize the infection outcome for the virtual patients.

We distinguish four different cases C for the infection outcome: an infection outcome corresponding to non-neutropenic immune conditions as well as the infection outcome under mild, moderate or severe neutropenia, i.e., $C = \{\text{non-neutropenic, mild, moderate, severe}\}$. To discriminate these classes, we calculated the patterns $\psi = (\mu(P_K) \pm \sigma(P_K), \mu(P_{AE}) \pm \sigma(P_{AE}), \mu(P_{AIE}) \pm \sigma(P_{AIE}))$ at the transition between consecutive degrees of neutropenia severity, in terms of the mean and SD. This resulted in the three patterns $\psi = \{\psi^{nm}, \psi^{mm}, \psi^{ms}\}$ at the transitions between two neutropenia severity levels: non-neutropenic–mild (nm), mild–moderate (mm), and moderate–severe (ms). For the classification of a particular simulation, we calculated the class of the values P_K^{sim} and P_{AIE}^{sim} at 4 h post infection. Then, we classified each of the three values of $v(P_K) = (\mu(P_K) + \sigma(P_K), \mu(P_K), \mu(P_K) - \sigma(P_K))$ and $v(P_{AIE}) = (\mu(P_{AIE}) + \sigma(P_{AIE}), \mu(P_{AIE}), \mu(P_{AIE}) - \sigma(P_{AIE}))$ separately. Thus, for each of the three values v_i, we set:

$$C(v_i(P_K)) = \begin{cases} \mu(P_K^{nm}) - \sigma(P_K^{nm}) \leq v_i \leq 1, & C = \text{non-neutropenic} \\ \mu(P_K^{mm}) - \sigma(P_K^{mm}) \leq v_i \leq \mu(P_K^{nm}) + \sigma(P_K^{nm}), & C = \text{mild} \\ \mu(P_K^{ms}) - \sigma(P_K^{ms}) \leq v_i \leq \mu(P_K^{mm}) + \sigma(P_K^{mm}), & C = \text{moderate} \\ 0 \leq v_i \leq \mu(P_K^{ms}) + \sigma(P_K^{ms}), & C = \text{severe} \end{cases} \quad (6)$$

$$C(v_i(P_{AIE})) = \begin{cases} 0 \leq v_i < \mu(P_{AIE}^{nm}) + \sigma(P_{AIE}^{nm}), & C = \text{non-neutropenic} \\ \mu(P_{AIE}^{nm}) - \sigma(P_{AIE}^{nm}) \leq v_i \leq \mu(P_{AIE}^{mm}) + \sigma(P_{AIE}^{mm}), & C = \text{mild} \\ \mu(P_{AIE}^{mm}) - \sigma(P_{AIE}^{mm}) \leq v_i \leq \mu(P_{AIE}^{ms}) + \sigma(P_{AIE}^{ms}), & C = \text{moderate} \\ \mu(P_{AIE}^{ms}) - \sigma(P_{AIE}^{ms}) \leq v_i < 1, & C = \text{severe} \end{cases} \quad (7)$$

The simulation's infection outcome C is then assigned to the class that received the highest number of votes from the nine values of $v_i(P_K)$ and $v_i(P_{AIE})$.

In Silico Treatment of Neutropenia and Identification of Optimal Treatment Strategies

After the simulation of VNP, we simulated the medical treatment of these patients. Therefore, we selected virtual patients with certain degrees of severity of neutropenia. These are the number of neutrophils that are specific for a transition between two degrees of severity as well as the number of neutrophils between these transitions. Therefore, we simulate the following five VNP that are characterized by specific ANC: VNP-1 with 1,250 neutrophils/µl, VNP-2 with 1,000 neutrophils/µl, VNP-3 with 750 neutrophils/µl, VNP-4 with 500 neutrophils/µl, VNP-5 with 250 neutrophils/µl. Thus, the ANC of these VNP corresponds to a decrease in neutrophil number from the standard value by VNP-1: 75%, VNP-2: 80%, VNP-3: 85%, VNP-4: 90%, and VNP-5: 95%. Since the treatment with different drugs might improve the phagocytic activity and/or the migration parameter of neutrophils, we performed simulations with the ABM where the phagocytosis rate of neutrophils ϕ_N as well as their diffusion coefficient D_N was increased. In the following, we refer to these parameters that are affected by the treatment as ϕ_N^T and D_N^T.

For the sake of comparability of both values, we increased both values in a stepwise fashion. The increase of these values lead to an improvement in the infection outcome. For example, a virtual patient with moderate neutropenia and a simulated treatment might attain an infection outcome that corresponded to that of a patient with mild neutropenia or even to an infection outcome for an individual with a non-neutropenic immune status. Therefore, after simulating with a certain parameter set (ϕ_N^T, D_N^T) we classified the simulation outcome as described earlier.

The stepwise increase of the parameters was continued until a parameter configuration was found with an infection outcome for non-neutropenic individuals. For quantification of the improvement of the infection outcome, we fitted an exponential function $f_{\phi_N} = 1 + a \cdot e^{-b \cdot f_{D_N}}$ at the transitions between two consecutive degrees of neutropenia severity. Here, the factors f_{ϕ_N} and f_{D_N} are given by $f_{\phi_N} = \phi_N^T/\phi_N^{min}$ and $f_{D_N} = D_N^T/D_N^{min}$, and denote the ratios between the treatment parameter values (ϕ_N^T, D_N^T) and the parameter values (ϕ_N^{min}, D_N^{min}) obtained from minimizing the LSE under non-neutropenic conditions.

RESULTS

Whole-Blood Infection Assays Differ for *C. albicans* and *C. glabrata*

In this study, we performed human whole-blood infection assays with *C. glabrata* and compared the measured data with experimental measurements for *C. albicans* by applying a previously established protocol (16). The kinetics of pathogens associated with either neutrophils or monocytes can be seen in **Figures 2A,B**, respectively. In case of *C. glabrata*, 81.0 ± 8.1% cells were associated with neutrophils, which is similar to *C. albicans* with 82.3 ± 7%. However, the experimental data show different kinetics for the two species, since *C. glabrata* is phagocytosed by neutrophils in a shorter time. By contrast, the association with monocytes is higher for *C. glabrata* with 10.1 ± 2.7%, while only 2.7 ± 1.9% *C. albicans* cells were associated with monocytes 4 h post infection. Due to the phagocytosis of the pathogens by the immune cells, 4 h post infection, 8.9 ± 7.5% cells remained extracellular for *C. glabrata* and 15.0 ± 5.8% for *C. albicans* (see **Figure 2C**). The remaining extracellular cells are referred to as *immune-evasive* cells, as already introduced in previous studies (16, 17). Furthermore, 1.3 ± 1.5% *C. glabrata* cells remained extracellular and alive 4 h post infection (see **Figure 2D**), which is lower compared with *C. albicans* with 6.5 ± 4.2%. In comparison with

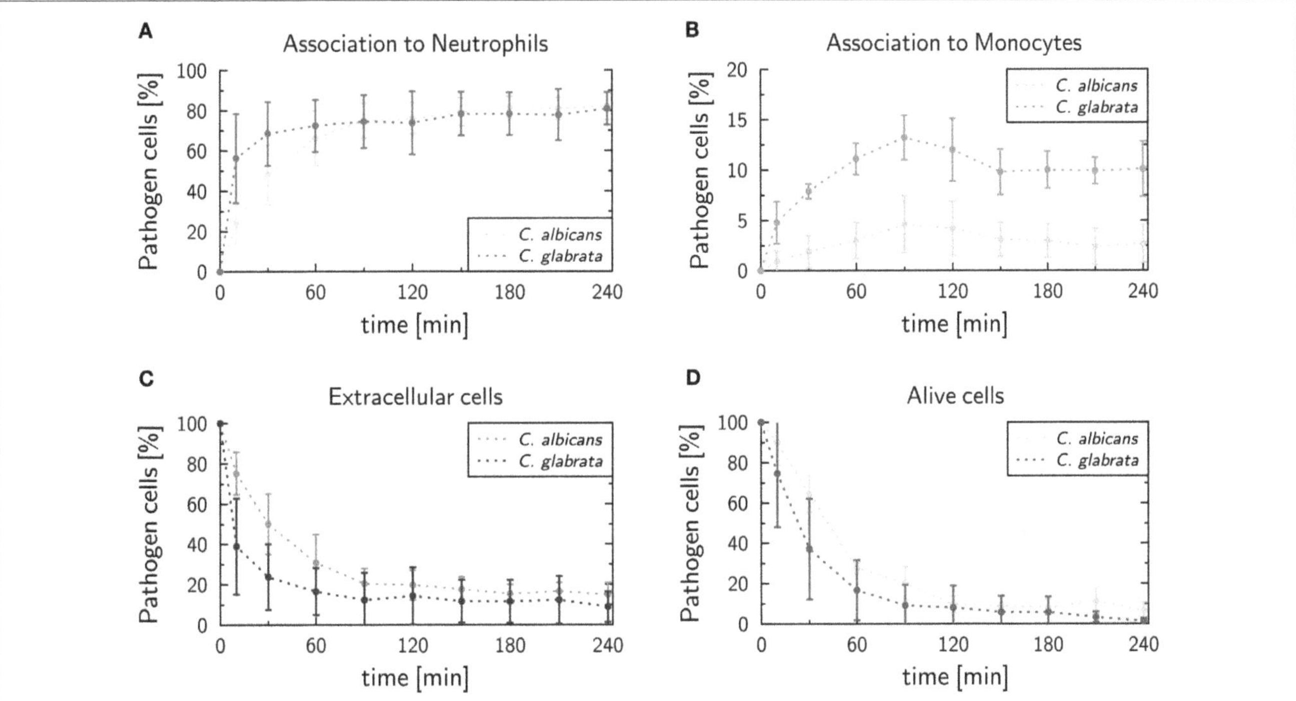

FIGURE 2 | Experimental data of whole-blood infection assays for *Candida albicans* (light color) and *Candida glabrata* (dark color), respectively. After incubation populations of extracellular cells **(A)**, alive cells **(B)**, as well as pathogens phagocytosed by either neutrophils **(C)** or monocytes **(D)**, were measured by flow cytometry and plating assays.

C. albicans, the decrease in alive *C. glabrata* cells mainly occurred during the first 2 h of the experiment exhibiting a much faster kinetics than for *C. albicans*.

Quantification of Immune-Reaction Rates Reveals Differences Between Pathogens

To quantify infection scenarios for the two pathogens, immune-reaction rates of the SBM were estimated by fitting to the experimental data as done previously for *C. albicans* in human whole blood (17). As explained in detail in Section "Material and Methods," this was done by computing the so-called *combined units*, which are combinations of different pathogen states and were directly accessible in experiment. In terms of these combined units, we evaluated the quality of a simulation by calculating the LSE between the experimental data and the *in silico* data. To determine the immune-reaction rates representing the best fit to the experimental data, i.e., that are associated with the lowest LSE, we applied the method of *Simulated Annealing* based on the *Metropolis Monte Carlo* scheme. The resulting immune-reaction rates from the fitting procedure where used to simulate the infection with the pathogens in 1 ml of blood, containing 5×10^6 neutrophils, 5×10^5 monocytes, and 1×10^6 cells, and are shown in **Figure 3** and in Table S1 in Supplementary Material.

The values of immune-reaction rates for *C. albicans* infection of whole blood are in line with our previous results (17). The reaction rate values for *C. glabrata* infection mostly differ in comparison to reaction rates for *C. albicans* infection (see **Figure 3**). The phagocytosis rate of neutrophils in the infection scenario with *C. glabrata* is $\phi_N = 10.11 \times 10^{-2}\ \text{min}^{-1}$, which is 3.5 times higher than for *C. albicans* infection. The phagocytosis rate for monocytes is with $\phi_M = 13.69 \times 10^{-2}\ \text{min}^{-1}$ an order of magnitude higher than in the case of *C. albicans* infection. These higher phagocytosis rates arise due to the faster kinetics measured for *C. glabrata* in the experimental data (see **Figure 2**). Furthermore, the order in the magnitude of phagocytosis rates is reversed in comparison to *C. albicans* infection, because for *C. glabrata* the phagocytosis rate of monocytes is 1.4 times higher than that for neutrophils. The killing rate of neutrophils is for *C. glabrata* $\kappa_N = 6.98 \times 10^{-2}\ \text{min}^{-1}$, which is only slightly higher than for *C. albicans* infection. Furthermore, differences between the fungal pathogens are again observed in the killing rate for monocytes, which is 1.5 times higher for *C. glabrata* with $\kappa_M = 3.22 \times 10^{-2}\ \text{min}^{-1}$ compared with *C. albicans*. As was previously observed for *C. albicans* (16, 17), also *C. glabrata* was found to evade the immune response and to remain even hours post infection alive and non-phagocytosed in human whole blood (**Figures 2C,D**). The rate for fungal cells becoming evasive against the immune response is for both pathogens comparably low, i.e., $\rho = 1.173 \times 10^{-2}\ \text{min}^{-1}$ for *C. glabrata* and $\rho = 0.439 \times 10^{-2}\ \text{min}^{-1}$ for *C. albicans*. A comparison of both rates that define the extracellular killing by antimicrobial peptides ($\kappa_{EK}(t)$) showed that the value of $\bar{\kappa}_{EK}$ is similar for both pathogens (see Table S1 in Supplementary Material) and γ is 2.5 times larger for infection scenarios with *C. glabrata* ($\gamma = 5.39 \times 10^{-2}\ \text{min}^{-1}$).

The time-resolved kinetics of the fits with the lowest LSE for the two fungal pathogens can be seen in Figures S1 and S2 in Supplementary Material, where the thickness of the simulation curves reflect random variations within the SDs of the immune-reaction rates. For both pathogens, the SBM adequately resembled the experimental data. Since the SBM neglects all spatial aspects of the infection scenarios, we performed a bottom-up modeling approach by combining the SBM with the ABM (17).

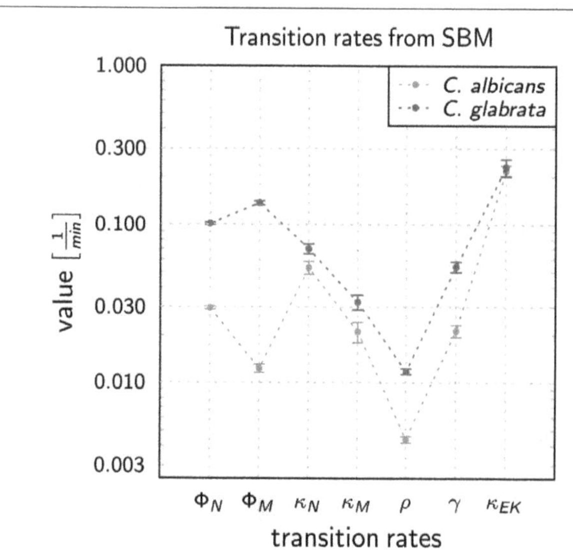

FIGURE 3 | Transition rates obtained from the calibration of the state-based model (SBM) to experimental data of the whole-blood infection assay for *Candida albicans* (blue) and *Candida glabrata* (pink), respectively. The values are compared for the phagocytosis rate for neutrophils (ϕ_N), and by monocytes (ϕ_M), killing rate for neutrophils (κ_N) and monocytes (κ_M), the rate at which the pathogens can evade the immune response with regard to phagocytosis and/or killing (ρ) as well as the rates that define the extracellular killing, i.e., γ and $\bar{\kappa}_{EK}$. Error bars correspond to SDs.

Migration Parameters of Phagocytes in Response to Various Pathogens Differ Quantitatively

To determine the migration parameters of neutrophils and monocytes in whole-blood infection scenarios with the respective pathogens, we used the experimentally measured data as well as the fitted immune-reaction rates from the SBM to perform stochastic spatiotemporal simulations by the ABM in 1 µl of blood. As a result of this bottom-up modeling approach for whole-blood infection assays, we obtained the diffusion coefficients of the immune cells in response to *C. albicans*. This can be seen in **Figure 4A**, where the best solution, i.e., the parameter configuration of (D_N, D_M) that resulted in the smallest LSE, was identified to be $(D_N^{min}, D_M^{min}) = (425\ \mu m^2/\text{min},\ 175\ \mu m^2/\text{min})$. In line with our earlier findings (17), for *C. albicans* the LSE was sensitive for variations in D_N but not for variations in D_M. The range of D_M that still lead to comparably low LSE values spans from approximately 100 µm²/min up to 500 µm²/min, whereas the range with comparably low LSE for D_N was limited to 400–425 µm²/min. As shown in Figure S3 in Supplementary Material, the fitting results are in excellent agreement with the experimental data, and the stochasticity of the *in silico* experiments still give rise to low SDs in the simulation curves, as can be inferred from the thickness of the curves representing 30 runs.

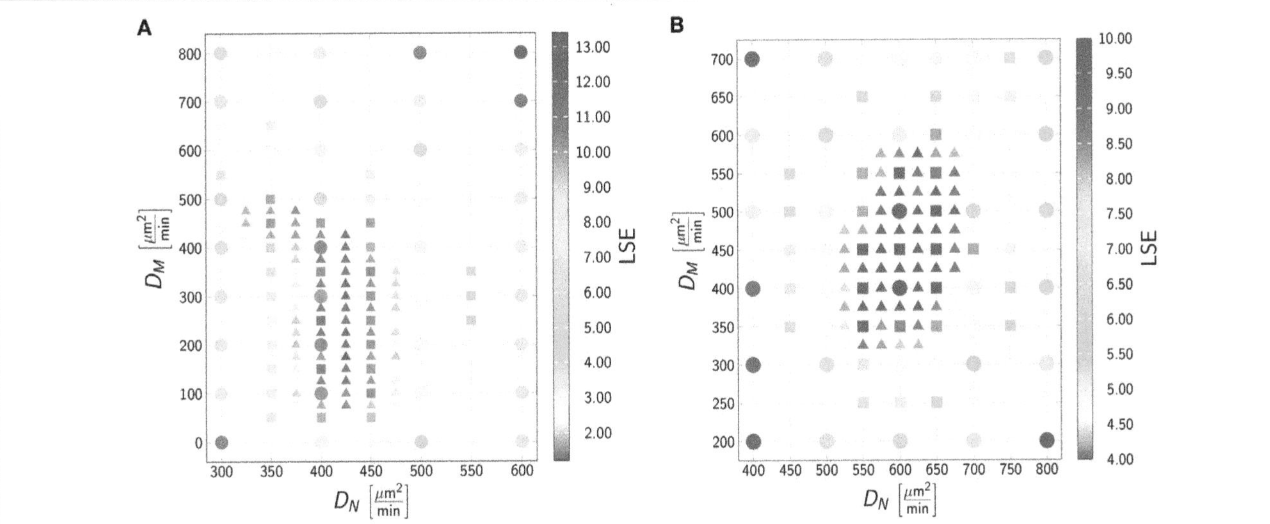

FIGURE 4 | Result of the agent-based model (ABM) parameter estimation for whole-blood infection assays with *Candida albicans* **(A)** and *Candida glabrata* **(B)**. Adaptive regular grid search was applied to fit the ABM to the experimental data and diffusion coefficients for neutrophils (D_N) and monocytes (D_M) were determined. At each grid point 1 µl blood was simulated, and 30 realizations for each parameter configuration were performed. Three different refinement levels were performed: simulations of the first level are represented as dots, simulations of the second level are represented as squares, and simulations of the third level are represented as triangles. The best fit to the experimental data was found at (D_N^{min}, D_M^{min}) = (425 µm^2/min, 175 µm^2/min) for *C. albicans* and at (D_N^{min}, D_M^{min}) = (600 µm^2/min, 425 µm^2/min) for *C. glabrata*.

The best fit of the simulation curves to the experimental data of whole-blood infection assays for *C. glabrata* was achieved for diffusion coefficients for neutrophils and monocytes with values (D_N^{min}, D_M^{min}) = (600 µm^2/min, 425 µm^2/min) (see **Figure 4**). We note that the range in which the diffusion coefficient of monocytes can vary for comparable LSE values was found to be much more restricted than in the case of *C. albicans*, i.e., this range for D_M was from 350 µm^2/min up to 575 µm^2/min for fitting results with comparable LSE. However, in the case of *C. glabrata*, neutrophils were not found to be restricted to the small range of only ±12 µm^2/min as for *C. albicans*, but could vary in a range of ± 80 µm^2/min. As can be seen in Figure S4 in Supplementary Material, the experimentally determined kinetics of the infection scenario with *C. glabrata* is in excellent agreement with the simulation curves of the ABM.

Immune Response in Virtual Patients With Neutropenia Is Strongly Pathogen Dependent

Our previous considerations reveal that immune cells exhibit a qualitatively and quantitatively different response against *C. albicans* and *C. glabrata* in human whole-blood infection assays. Comparing *C. glabrata* to *C. albicans* infection, this is reflected by (i) increased phagocytosis rates and (ii) increased diffusion coefficients by factors of 1.4 and 2.4, respectively, for neutrophils and monocytes. In line with our previous work on the comparison between *C. glabrata* with *C. albicans* by live-cell imaging of phagocytosis assays (23–26), these quantitative differences are accompanied with the qualitative variation in the immune response that involves much stronger monocyte activation in the case of *C. glabrata*. Nevertheless, a prominent role is played by neutrophils that are quantitatively prevalent in cell number and qualitatively important in differently directing the immune response against these fungal pathogens (23).

To investigate the impact of neutropenia on the infection outcome with a specific pathogen, we simulated VNP using the ABM. Here, the optimal immune-reaction rates and diffusion coefficients were used as previously determined for normal ANC values. In the virtual patients, we stepwise decreased the number of neutrophils to resemble different degrees of severity of neutropenia and simulated the early immune response during 4 h post infection. The contributions of the combined units—such as killed, phagocytosed and immune-evasive *Candida* cells at 4 h post infection—are shown in **Figure 5**.

The phagocytosis by neutrophils is for both pathogens quite similar. For mild neutropenia the phagocytosis by neutrophils ranges for both fungal pathogens between ~40 and 50%, for mild neutropenia between ~25 and 40%, and is below ~25% for severe neutropenia. Interestingly, despite these similarities, the infection outcomes for the two pathogens under the condition of neutropenia are predicted to be remarkably different. As shown in **Figure 5A**, a stronger impact on the infection outcome can be observed for *C. albicans*, where in the scenario of severe neutropenia the number of killed fungal cells achieves only 10–45%. By contrast, killing of *C. glabrata* in severe neutropenia is more efficient, and the fraction of dead cells ranges between 45 and 60% of total fungal cells (see **Figure 5B**).

This difference is governed by the behavior of monocytes in response to the two fungal pathogens. Higher phagocytosis rates in case of *C. glabrata* compared with *C. albicans* enable monocytes to partially compensate for the loss of neutrophils under conditions of neutropenia. This compensatory effect is relatively low for *C. albicans*, where the fraction of cells that were phagocytosed by monocytes increased from 3% for normal ANC to only 12% under the condition of severe neutropenia (see **Figure 5A**). For

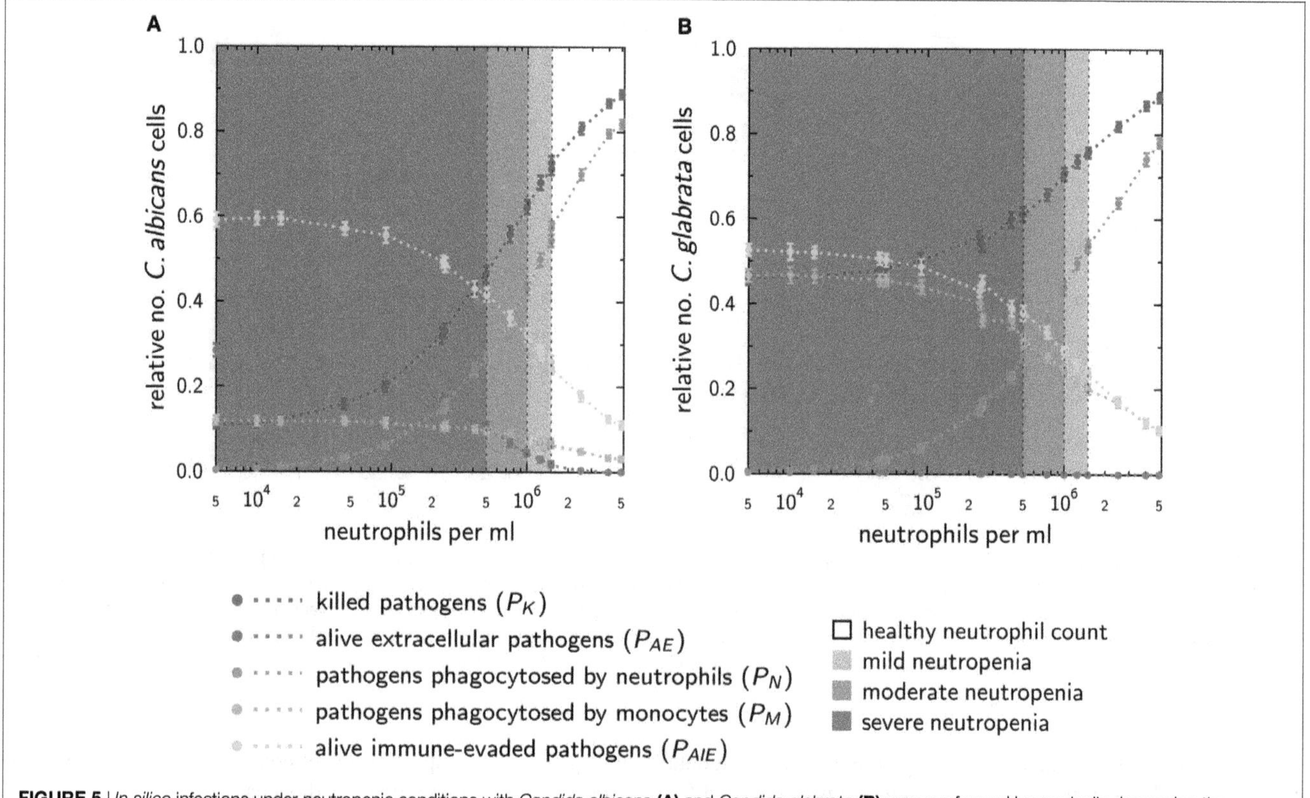

FIGURE 5 | *In silico* infections under neutropenic conditions with *Candida albicans* **(A)** and *Candida glabrata* **(B)** were performed by gradually decreasing the absolute neutrophil count in the agent-based model. Plots show the fraction of killed cells (red), alive and extracellular cells (green), phagocytosed cells by neutrophils (blue), and monocytes (yellow) as well as (alive) cells that are able to evade the immune system (turquoise) at 4 h post infection.

C. glabrata, this increase in monocyte phagocytosis rose from 10 to 46% of the *C. glabrata* cells (see **Figure 5B**). Furthermore, the infection outcome is also characterized by the number of cells that are able to evade the immune response. Immune evasion is more pronounced for *C. albicans*, where also for normal ANC 15% of all fungal cells are able to evade the immune response (see **Figure 5A**). However, with stronger degrees of neutropenia the fraction of these cells even increases to about 60%. In the case of *C. glabrata*, only 10% of the cells can evade the immune response for normal ANC, while this fraction rises up to 50% under conditions of severe neutropenia (see **Figure 5B**). As explained in Section "Materials and Methods," the infection outcome is mainly characterized by the fraction of killed as well as the fraction of alive and immune-evasive *Candida* cells. Therefore, we assigned the values of P_K and P_{AIE} at the boundaries to pattern that characterize the different degrees of severity of neutropenia (see Table S2 in Supplementary Material). Subsequently, with the help of these patterns, we were able to classify simulations of medical treatments in neutropenic patients.

Simulation of Medical Treatment for VNP

After we simulated the infection with the pathogens *C. albicans* and *C. glabrata* in VNP, we selected five types of VNP with different severity degrees of neutropenia for *in silico* treatment. The VNP-1 is characterized by an ANC of 1,250 neutrophils/μl representing patients with mild neutropenia. At the transition between mild and moderate, the ANC is 1,000 neutrophils/μl, and the corresponding VNP is referred to as VNP-2. Similarly, we defined VNP-3, VNP-4 and VNP-5 that are characterized, respectively, by ANC of 750 neutrophils/μl (moderate neutropenia), 500 neutrophils/μl (transition between moderate and severe neutropenia), and 250 neutrophils/μl (severe neutropenia). The *in silico* treatment involves the increase of neutrophil activation in terms of their phagocytosis rate and/or diffusion coefficient to quantitatively investigate its impact on the reduced numbers of neutrophils in these patients. Thus, increasing the phagocytosis rate and/or diffusion coefficient of neutrophils in a stepwise fashion, we simulated the infection with either of the two pathogens *C. albicans* and *C. glabrata* under neutropenic conditions. Afterward, the infection outcome of the simulation was classified according to the previously determined pattern (see Patterns and Classification of Simulations). To find a formal description of the increase of neutrophil phagocytosis rate and diffusion coefficient required for reaching the infection outcome for non-neutropenic individuals, we fitted an exponential function of the form $f_{\phi_N} = 1 + a \cdot e^{-b \cdot f_{D_N}}$ at the transition where the non-neutropenic infection outcome is reached. Here, the factors f_{ϕ_N} and f_{D_N} are defined as $f_{\phi_N} = \phi_N^T/\phi_N^{min}$ and $f_{D_N} = D_N^T/D_N^{min}$, where ϕ_N^T and D_N^T denote parameters that are affected by the treatment, and ϕ_N^{min} and D_N^{min} refer to the parameter values obtained by minimizing the LSE under non-neutropenic conditions. We varied ϕ_N^T and D_N^T over one order of magnitude, i.e., $f_{\phi_N}, f_{D_N} \in [1, 10]$, and plotted the resulting curves for each type of VNP in Figure S5 in Supplementary Material for the fitting parameters a and b as provided in Table S3 in Supplementary Material.

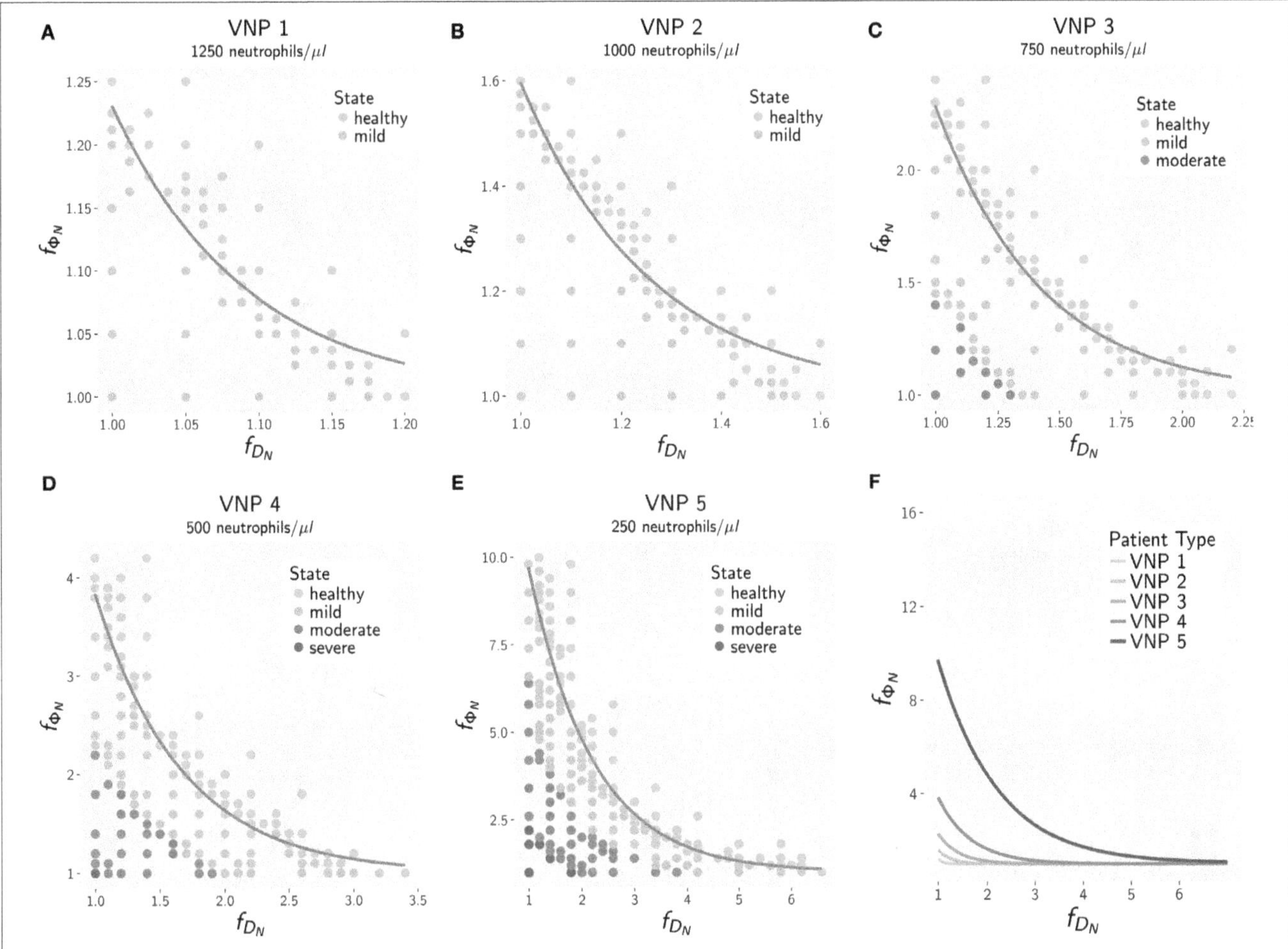

FIGURE 6 | *In silico* treatment of virtual neutropenic patients (VNP) infected with *Candida albicans* was simulated using the agent-based model. Stepwise increase of phagocytosis rate and diffusion coefficient of neutrophils was performed for VNP with various severity degrees of neutropenia: VNP1–5: 1,250 **(A)**, 1,000 **(B)**, 750 **(C)**, 500 **(D)**, and 250 **(E)** neutrophils/μl. Simulated points are classified according to the previously determined patterns: green points show a non-neutropenic infection outcome, yellow points show an infection outcome comparable to a mild neutropenia, orange points show an infection outcome comparable to a moderate neutropenia, and red points show an infection outcome comparable to a severe neutropenia. Solid lines depict the fitted exponential function $f_{\Phi_N} = 1 + a \cdot e^{-b \cdot f_{D_N}}$ at the transition to the non-neutropenic infection outcome. For comparison the fitted curves for the five VNP with their severity degrees of neutropenia are shown in panel **(F)**.

The results for the *in silico* treatment of VNP with *C. albicans* and *C. glabrata* infection are shown in detail in **Figures 6** and 7, respectively. Performing more than 4×10^4 simulations, we generally found that all VNP do reach the infection outcome of non-neutropenic patients by increasing neutrophil activation in terms of phagocytosis rate and/or diffusion coefficient. As could be expected, the required increase in neutrophil activation depends on the severity degree of neutropenia in VNP. For VNP with severe neutropenia (VNP-5), reaching the infection outcome of non-neutropenic patients would require relatively high values for ϕ_N^T with $f_{\phi_N} > 10$, whereas the treatment was always successful for D_N^T with $f_{D_N} \ll 10$. To compare the two fungal pathogens with each other, we first fixed either $\phi_N^T = \phi_N^{min}$ ($f_{\phi_N} = 1$) or $D_N^T = D_N^{min}$ ($f_{D_N} = 1$) and varied only one parameter, respectively, D_N^T or ϕ_N^T. As can be seen in **Figure 8A**, for both fungal pathogens increasing the diffusion coefficient yields the infection outcome of non-neutropenic patients at smaller factors than increasing the phagocytosis rate, i.e., $f_{D_N} < f_{\phi_N}$. Interestingly, increasing only the neutrophil diffusion, the *in silico* treatment was found to be more effective for *C. glabrata*, whereas it turned out to be more effective for *C. albicans* if only the phagocytosis rate was increased. The combined impact of increasing ϕ_N^T and D_N^T yielded a pair ($f_{\phi_N}^*, f_{D_N}^*$) of optimal values with minimal distance from ($f_{\phi_N} = 1, f_{D_N} = 1$) where the infection outcome of non-neutropenic patients was reached. The results are shown in **Figure 8B**, where the comparison between *C. albicans* and *C. glabrata* predicts that $f_{\phi_N}^* < f_{D_N}^*$ for the optimal *in silico* treatment, i.e., the required relative increase of the diffusion coefficient is larger than that for the phagocytosis rate. Moreover, the optimal *in silico* treatment was reached for factors ($f_{\phi_N}^*, f_{D_N}^*$) with lower values for all VNP in the case of *C. glabrata*.

DISCUSSION

In this study, we investigated bloodstream infections with the fungal pathogens *C. albicans* and *C. glabrata* in human whole

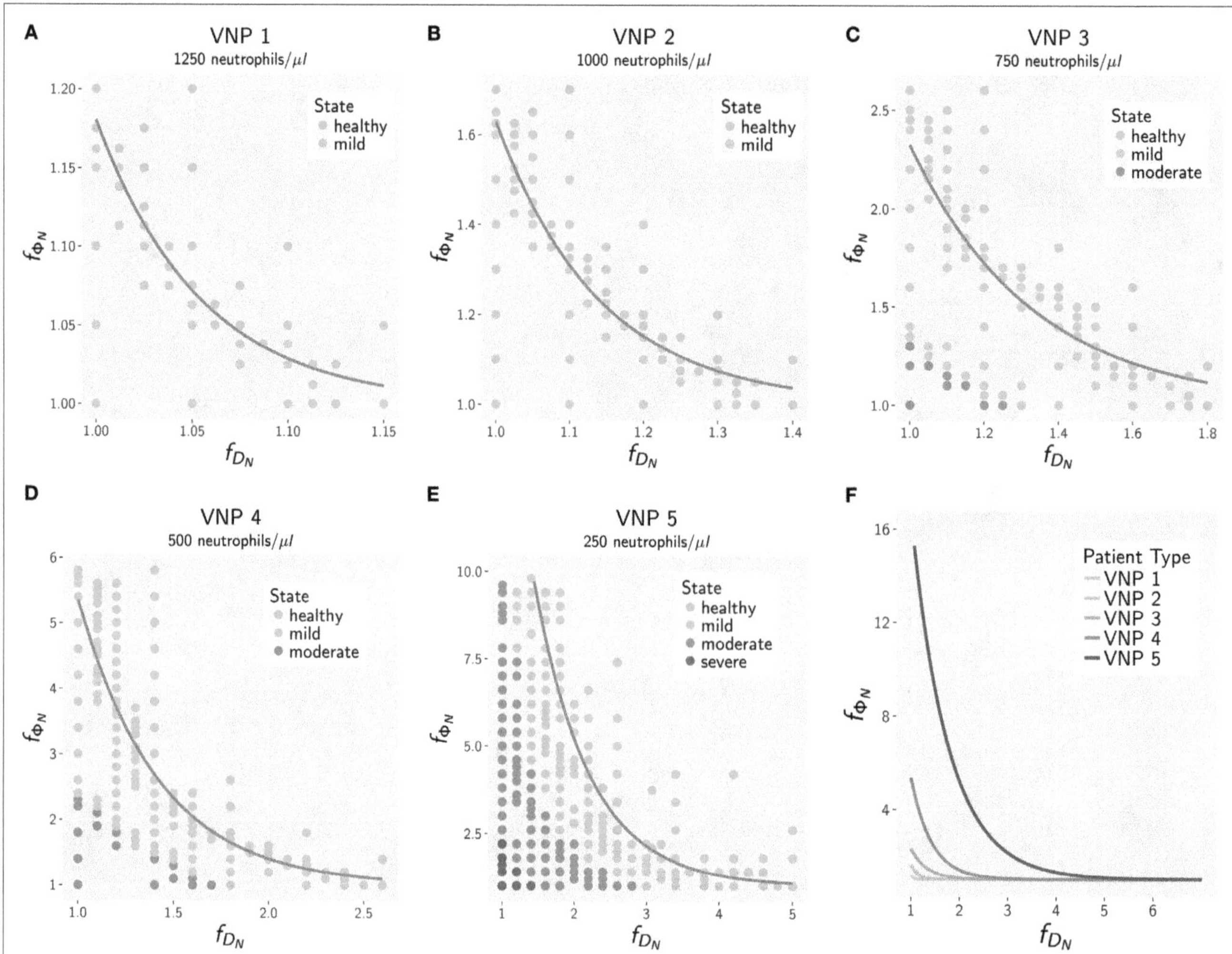

FIGURE 7 | *In silico* treatment of virtual neutropenic patients (VNP) infected with *Candida glabrata* was simulated using the agent-based model. Stepwise increase of phagocytosis rate and diffusion coefficient of neutrophils was performed for VNP with various severity degrees of neutropenia: VNP1–5: 1,250 **(A)**, 1,000 **(B)**, 750 **(C)**, 500 **(D)**, and 250 **(E)** neutrophils/μl. Simulated points are classified according to the previously determined patterns: green points show a non-neutropenic infection outcome, yellow points show an infection outcome comparable to a mild neutropenia, orange points show an infection outcome comparable to a moderate neutropenia, and red points show an infection outcome comparable to a severe neutropenia. Solid lines depict the fitted exponential function $f_{\Phi_N} = 1 + a \cdot e^{-b \cdot f_{D_N}}$ at the transition to the non-neutropenic infection outcome. For comparison, the fitted curves for the five VNP with their severity degrees of neutropenia are shown in panel **(F)**.

blood. Special focus was put on the infection scenario under neutropenic conditions as well as possible treatment strategies. These conditions are clinically relevant as it is well established that neutropenia promotes dissemination of *Candida* spp. during bloodstream infection and impairs prognosis. We used a previously established bottom-up modeling approach that combines different mathematical modeling approaches of increasing complexity based on wet-lab experiments (17). To investigate infection by different fungal pathogens, we first performed whole-blood infection assays using blood of healthy individuals. In the past, these whole-blood infection models have already been successfully applied to analyze the early immune response to clinically relevant pathogens (27–29) and to identify their virulence factors (30, 31). Furthermore, the influence of genetic polymorphisms on the immune response have been tested (32, 33) as well as potential therapeutic approaches and vaccine efficacy (34–38). In this study, we applied this experimental modeling approach to investigate early immune responses to the two *Candida* spp. in blood. The resulting experimental data showed that the immune response followed a faster kinetics for *C. glabrata* than for *C. albicans*, which is reflected by an earlier phagocytosis of this pathogen. In line with our previous studies (16, 17, 23), monocytes were found to contribute more to the immune response against *C. glabrata* compared with *C. albicans*.

The system behavior was quantified by estimating values for immune-reaction rates, such as phagocytosis and killing rates, based on fitting a SBM to the experimentally measured data (17). As expected from the observed difference in the kinetics of the immune response between *C. albicans* and *C. glabrata*, we found that the phagocytosis rates were orders of magnitude higher for *C. glabrata* with monocytes reaching the highest values (see Table S2 in Supplementary Material). Thus, for *C. glabrata* the

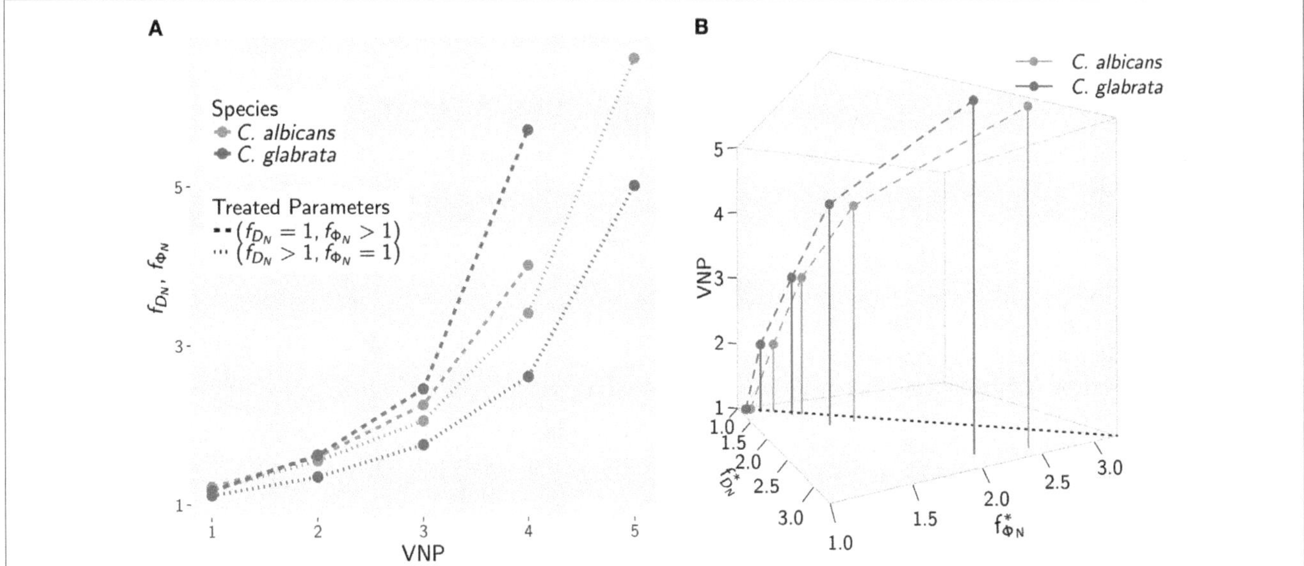

FIGURE 8 | The increase in neutrophil activation required to reach the infection outcome of non-neutropenic patients depends on the severity degree of neutropenia in VNP. **(A)** Comparison of *Candida albicans* (blue) and *Candida glabrata* (pink) infection for various VNP in terms of the factors f_{D_N} and f_{Φ_N} keeping either $f_{\Phi_N} = 1$ or $f_{D_N} = 1$ fixed. **(B)** The same as in panel **(A)** allowing both factors to vary to attain the optimal values ($f^*_{\Phi_N}, f^*_{D_N}$) with minimal distance from ($f_{\Phi_N} = 1, f_{D_N} = 1$) at which the infection outcome of non-neutropenic patients is reached.

phagocytosis rate for monocytes is higher than for neutrophils and this relation is inverted for *C. albicans*. Applying a bottom-up modeling approach (17), we used an ABM to estimate migration parameters for neutrophils and monocytes in response to the two fungal species. For *C. glabrata* these migration parameter were higher than for *C. albicans*. As previously shown for *C. albicans* the outcome of the immune response was restricted to a narrow regime of migration parameters for the neutrophils (17), whereas these migration parameters in the case of *C. glabrata* infections could vary over a significantly wider range to fit the experimental data. This is another indication for the observable fact that monocytes play a more important role in the defense against *C. glabrata* compared with *C. albicans* (23, 39).

Since fungal infections by *Candida* spp. are a major risk for immunocompromised patients, we extended the computer simulations for normal ANC by numerically studying infection scenarios in virtual patients with different severity degrees of neutropenia. Due to the pronounced importance of neutrophils in the immune response against *C. albicans*, these computer simulations predicted a strong negative impact on the infection outcome for VNP depending on the severity degree of neutropenia. Although the impact of neutropenia on the infection outcome during *C. glabrata* infection was not as strong as for *C. albicans*, the immune response was still to a large extent impaired. For example, this was observed by the prediction that the fraction of killed pathogens at 4 h post infection decreased from around 90% for both species under normal ANC to about 50 and 10% for *C. glabrata* and *C. albicans* for severe neutropenic conditions, respectively. Moreover, at 4 h post infection, a fraction of 30% *C. albicans* cells are still alive and extracellular in human blood that could contribute to the dissemination to other body parts in real patients. While the fraction of alive and extracellular *C. glabrata* cells is negligible at 4 h post infection, a large fraction of about 50% is phagocytosed by monocytes including a few percent of fungal cells that are still alive and may disseminate by eventually escaping from the monocytes. These data again point toward different virulence traits in the two *Candida* spp. (40).

The bottom-up modeling approach for the simulation of infection scenarios under neutropenic conditions was established to simulate the effects of medical treatments. To date there exist three different ways to approach neutropenia in the clinical setting, which comprise (i) the stimulation and activation of remaining neutrophils by medical treatment of the patient, (ii) the internal stimulation of neutrophil maturation and release from the bone marrow by medication of patients with *granulocyte colony-stimulating factor* (G-CSF), and (iii) the transfusion of G-CSF/steroid mobilized neutrophils from a donor. The latter treatment of healthy donors leads to a vast increase of peripheral blood neutrophils (41–44), which are subsequently extracted from the donor by leukapheresis and administered to the patient to increase the ANC in blood. This therapy shows higher rates of patient survival in the context of bacterial infections (43), whereas improvement in patient survival was not consistently observed for fungal infections (45–47). In particular, Gazendam et al. (48) show that the G-CSF/dexamethasone stimulation of donor neutrophils leads to a change in their granular content, which impairs the fungal killing capacity with regard to *C. albicans*. The cytokine treatment with G-CSF to trigger the neutrophil release from the bone marrow in patients is mainly applied in congenital neutropenia and causes a significant increase of the ANC in blood (49, 50). Before effective drugs were available, children with congenital neutropenia typically died in their first year of life due to bacterial and fungal infections (51, 52). The G-CSF treatment makes use of the emergency mobilization of neutrophils in response to an inflammatory signal and the secretion of chemokines leading to neutrophil migration into blood vessels (53). However, patients can be also *low-responders* or even *non-responders* exhibiting reduced effects of G-CSF (49, 54). Finally, instead of increasing the circulating number of neutrophils, the option to medically treat neutropenia by inflammatory cytokines, such as *interferon* γ and *tumor necrosis factor* α, yields a modulation of the immune response by the stimulation and activation of neutrophils in blood (41, 44). Both cytokines have been reported to enhance the neutrophil response against fungi, e.g., *Candida* spp. (55), *Aspergillus* spp. (56), and *Cryptococcus* spp. (57).

In this study, we focused on investigating the treatment of neutropenic patients by inflammatory cytokines to quantify the possibility of balancing neutropenic conditions and clearance of infection. The simulations of this *in silico* treatment revealed that an increase of the phagocytosis rate and/or the migration parameter of neutrophils generally improved the infection outcome. For both *Candida* spp. under investigation, conditions of mild neutropenia can be compensated resembling an infection outcome of non-neutropenic individuals by an increase in either the phagocytosis rate or the diffusion coefficient, or a combination of both, by less than 25% percent. The computer simulations allowed us to rigorously quantify the relative change in these parameters needed for any severity level of neutropenia. In the case of severe neutropenia, medical treatments would need to increase these parameters by at least 250% for the phagocytosis rate and at least 300% for the diffusion coefficient to reach infection outcomes in VNP comparable to individuals with normal ANC. It should be noted that the modulation of parameters has to be combined, because even a 10-fold increase of the phagocytosis rate alone would not recover the infection outcome of non-neutropenic individuals. Thus, the quantitative simulation of *in silico* treatments generates concrete predictions regarding the relative impact that treatments with inflammatory cytokines are required to exert on these two parameters. Moreover, our numerical experiments predict that *C. albicans* compared with *C. glabrata* always requires stronger increases in the phagocytosis rate and the diffusion coefficient for the same conditions of neutropenia.

Clearly, the underlying model assumptions (such as spatial homogeneity and absence of external forces) cannot be 1:1 translated into the *in vivo* situation—neither in small vessels nor in tissue. Despite this, several predictions resulting from the model could be confirmed *in vivo* or are in line with clinical findings (16). For this study, this also applies to the observations that (i) neutropenia may result in poor prognosis and a higher ratio of disseminated candidiasis [e.g., Ref. (58, 59)] and (ii) monocytes play a more important role in *C. glabrata* infection (23). Even though clinical studies will ultimately be required to validate our hypotheses, the first step would be to test these treatment strategies in whole-blood infection assays and our simulations for VNP can be used for this testing.

Our study may be extended in different ways. For example, computer simulations for various pathogens, such as *Staphylococcus* spp. and *Streptococcus* spp., which were shown to cause bacteremia and sepsis under conditions of neutropenia, could be performed (52, 60). Moreover, treatment strategies that lead to an increased ANC in neutropenic patients, like the transfusion therapy as well as the G-CSF treatment, could be simulated and compared with the cytokine treatment considered in this study. Furthermore, the bottom-up approach provides the possibility to investigate the impact of other immune disorders on the infection outcome with the pathogens under consideration. Moreover, the generated predictions of this study could be examined in future wet-lab experiments. Therefore, whole-blood infection assays with *C. albicans* or *C. glabrata* in human blood with reduced ANC could be performed. Such neutropenic blood samples could be taken from patients with neutropenia, where it should be considered that primary diseases of the patient may affect the experimental results. Another possibility may be to generate neutropenic blood samples in the wet lab by a controlled reduction of the neutrophil number. However, this poses a high challenge, since the remaining blood constituents will be affected by side effects that cannot be well controlled. Investigating such host–pathogen interactions by combining wet-lab and dry-lab studies is in the spirit of system biology. This approach provides a powerful tool to investigate biological systems in a qualitative as well as quantitative fashion and enables hypothesis generation in dry-lab as well as hypothesis testing in wet-lab studies.

AUTHOR CONTRIBUTIONS

ST and MTF conceived and designed this study. MTF and OK provided computational resources and materials, respectively. Data processing, implementation, and application of the computational algorithm were done by ST, TL, MP, and MTF. Experiments were performed by KH and IL. ST, TL, MP, KH, IL, OK, and MTF evaluated and analyzed the results of this study; drafted the manuscript and revised it critically for important intellectual content and final approval of the version to be published; and agreed to be accountable for all aspects of the work in ensuring that questions related to the accuracy or integrity of any part of the work are appropriately investigated and resolved.

FUNDING

This work was financially supported by the Deutsche Forschungsgemeinschaft (DFG) through the excellence graduate school Jena School for Microbial Communication (JSMC), the CRC/TR124 FungiNet (project B4 to MTF and project C3 to OK), and the Center for Sepsis Control and Care (CSCC) (Project Quantim, FKZ 01EO1502 to MTF and OK) that is funded by the Federal Ministry for Education and Research (BMBF).

REFERENCES

Murphy KP, Janeway C, Travers P, Walport M. *Janeway's Immunobiology*. 7th ed. New York, London: Garland Science (2008)

Schwartzberg LS. Neutropenia: etiology and pathogenesis. *Clin Cornerstone* (2006) 8:S5–11. doi:10.1016/S1098-3597(06)80053-0

Duggan S, Leonhardt I, Hünniger K, Kurzai O. Host response to *Candida albicans* bloodstream infection and sepsis. *Virulence* (2015) 6:316–26. doi:10. 4161/21505594.2014.988096

Fidel PL Jr, Vazquez JA, Sobel JD. Candida glabrata: review of epidemiology, pathogenesis, and clinical disease with comparison to *C. albicans*. Clin Micro- biol Rev (1999) 12:80–96.

Sardi JC, Scorzoni L, Bernardi T, Fusco-Almeida AM, Mendes Giannini MJ. *Candida* species: current epidemiology, pathogenicity, biofilm formation, nat- ural antifungal products and new therapeutic options. *J Med Microbiol* (2013) 62:10–24. doi:10.1099/jmm.0.045054-0

Orasch C, Marchetti O, Garbino J, Schrenzel J, Zimmerli S, Mühlethaler K, et al. *Candida* species distribution and antifungal susceptibility testing according to European Committee on Antimicrobial Susceptibility Testing and new vs. old Clinical and Laboratory Standards Institute clinical breakpoints: a 6-year prospective candidaemia survey from the fungal infection network of Switzer- land. *Clin Microbiol Infect* (2014) 20:698–705. doi:10.1111/1469-0691.12440

Mayer FL, Wilson D, Hube B, Article M. *Candida albicans* pathogenicity mech-anisms. *Clin Infect Dis* (2002) 48105:119–28. doi:10.4161/viru.22913

Calderone RA, Clancy CJ, editors. *Candida and Candidiasis*. 2nd ed. Washing-ton, DC: ASM Press (2002).

Rodrigues CF, Silva S, Henriques M. *Candida glabrata*: a review of its features and resistance. *Eur J Clin Microbiol Infect Dis* (2014) 33:673–88. doi:10.1007/s10096-013-2009-3

Kitano H. Systems biology: a brief overview. *Science* (2002) 295:1662–4. doi:10. 1126/science.1069492

Aderem A. Systems biology: its practice and challenges. *Cell* (2005) 121:511–3. doi:10.1016/j.cell.2005.04.020

Bruggeman FJ, Westerhoff HV. The nature of systems biology. *Trends Microbiol* (2007) 15:45–50. doi:10.1016/j.tim.2006.11.003

Germain RN, Meier-Schellersheim M, Nita-Lazar A, Fraser IDC. Systems biol- ogy in immunology: a computational modeling perspective. *Annu Rev Immunol* (2011) 29:527–85. doi:10.1146/annurev-immunol-030409-101317

Horn F, Heinekamp T, Kniemeyer O, Pollmächer J, Valiante V, Brakhage AA. Systems biology of fungal infection. *Front Microbiol* (2012) 3:108. doi:10.3389/ fmicb.2012.00108

Medyukhina A, Timme S, Mokhtari Z, Figge MT. Image-based systems biology of infection. *Cytometry A* (2015) 87:462–70. doi:10.1002/cyto.a.22638

Hünniger K, Lehnert T, Bieber K, Martin R, Figge MT, Kurzai O. A virtual infection model quantifies innate effector mechanisms and *Candida albicans* immune escape in human blood. *PLoS Comput Biol* (2014) 10:e1003479. doi: 10.1371/journal.pcbi.1003479

Lehnert T, Timme S, Pollmächer J, Hünniger K, Kurzai O, Figge MT. Bottom-up modeling approach for the quantitative estimation of parameters in pathogen- host interactions. *Front Microbiol* (2015) 6:608. doi:10.3389/fmicb.2015.00608

Pollmächer J, Figge MT. Agent-based model of human alveoli predicts chemo-tactic signaling by epithelial cells during early *Aspergillus fumigatus* infection. *PLoS One* (2014) 9:e111630. doi:10.1371/journal.pone.0111630

Pollmächer J, Figge MT. Deciphering chemokine properties by a hybrid agent-based model of *Aspergillus fumigatus* infection in human alveoli. *Front Microbiol* (2015) 6:503. doi:10.3389/fmicb.2015.00503

Dale DC, Cottle TE, Fier CJ, Bolyard AA, Bonilla MA, Boxer LA, et al. Severe chronic neutropenia: treatment and follow-up of patients in the Severe Chronic Neutropenia International Registry. *Am J Hematol* (2003) 72:82–93. doi:10. 1002/ajh.10255

Crawford J, Dale DC, Lyman GH. Chemotherapy-induced neutropenia. *Cancer* (2004) 100:228–37. doi:10.1002/cncr.11882

Seider K, Brunke S, Schild L, Jablonowski N, Wilson D, Majer O, et al. The fac- ultative intracellular pathogen *Candida glabrata* subverts macrophage cytokine production and phagolysosome maturation. *J Immunol* (2011) 187:3072–86. doi:10.4049/jimmunol.1003730

Duggan S, Essig F, Hünniger K, Mokhtari Z, Bauer L, Lehnert T, et al. Neu-trophil activation by *Candida glabrata* but not *Candida albicans* promotes fungal uptake by monocytes. *Cell Microbiol* (2015) 17:1259–76. doi:10.1111/cmi.12443

Essig F, Hünniger K, Dietrich S, Figge MT, Kurzai O. Human neutrophils dump *Candida glabrata* after intracellular killing. *Fungal Genet Biol* (2015) 84:37–40. doi:10.1016/j.fgb.2015.09.008

Brandes S, Mokhtari Z, Essig F, Hünniger K, Kurzai O, Figge MT. Automated segmentation and tracking of non-rigid objects in time-lapse microscopy videos of polymorphonuclear neutrophils. *Med Image Anal* (2015) 20(1):34–51. doi:10. 1016/j.media.2014.10.002

Brandes S, Dietrich S, Hünniger K, Kurzai O, Figge MT. Migration and inter- action tracking for quantitative analysis of phagocyte-pathogen confrontation assays. *Med Image Anal* (2017) 36:172–83. doi:10.1016/j. media.2016.11.007

Tena GN, Young DB, Eley B, Henderson H, Nicol MP, Levin M, et al. Failure to control growth of mycobacteria in blood from children infected with human immunodeficiency virus and its relationship to T cell function. *J Infect Dis* (2003) 187:1544–51. doi:10.1086/374799

Silva D, Ponte CGG, Hacker MA, Antas PRZ. A whole blood assay as a simple, broad assessment of cytokines and chemokines to evaluate human immune responses to *Mycobacterium tuberculosis* antigens. *Acta Trop* (2013) 127:75–81. doi:10.1016/j.actatropica.2013.04.002

Urrutia A, Duffy D, Rouilly V, Posseme C, Djebali R, Illanes G, et al. Stan-dardized whole-blood transcriptional profiling enables the deconvolution of complex induced immune responses. *Cell Rep* (2016) 16:2777–91. doi:10.1016/ j.celrep.2016.08.011

Echenique-Rivera H, Muzzi A, Del Tordello E, Seib KL, Francois P, Rappuoli R, et al. Transcriptome analysis of *Neisseria meningitidis* in human whole blood and mutagenesis studies identify virulence factors involved in blood survival. *PLoS Pathog* (2011) 7:e1002027. doi:10.1371/journal.ppat.1002027

Van Der Maten E, De Jonge MI, De Groot R, Van Der Flier M, Langereis JD. A versatile assay to determine bacterial and host factors contributing to opsonophagocytotic killing in hirudin-anticoagulated whole blood. *Sci Rep* (2017) 7:3–12. doi:10.1038/srep42137

Lin J, Yao YM, Yu Y, Chai JK, Huang ZH, Dong N, et al. Effects of CD14-159 C/T polymorphism on CD14 expression and the balance between proinflam- matory and anti-inflammatory cytokines in whole blood culture. *Shock* (2007) 28:148–53. doi:10.1097/SHK.0b013e3180341d35

Duffy D, Rouilly V, Libri V, Hasan M, Beitz B, David M, et al. Functional anal- ysis via standardized whole-blood stimulation systems defines the boundaries of a healthy immune response to complex stimuli. *Immunity* (2014) 40:436–50. doi:10.1016/j.immuni.2014.03.002

Deslouches B, Islam K, Craigo JK, Paranjape SM, Montelaro RC, Mietzner TA. Activity of the de novo engineered antimicrobial peptide WLBU2 against *Pseudomonas aeruginosa* in human serum and whole blood: implications for systemic applications. *Antimicrob Agents Chemother* (2005) 49:3208–16. doi:10. 1128/AAC.49.8.3208-3216.2005

Jemmett K, Macagno A, Molteni M, Heckels JE, Rossetti C, Christodoulides M. A cyanobacterial lipopolysaccharide antagonist inhibits cytokine production induced by *Neisseria meningitidis* in a human whole-blood model of septicemia. *Infect Immun* (2008) 76:3156–63. doi:10.1128/IAI.00110-08

Li M, Xue J, Liu J, Kuang D, Gu Y, Lin S. Efficacy of cytokine removal by plasmodia filtration using a selective plasma separator: in vitro sepsis model. *Ther Apher Dial* (2011) 15:98–104. doi:10.1111/j.1744-9987.2010.00850.x

Plested JS, Welsch JA, Granoff DM. Ex vivo model of meningococcal bacteremia using human blood for measuring vaccine-induced serum passive protective activity. *Clin Vaccine Immunol* (2009) 16:785–91. doi:10.1128/CVI.00007-09

Sprong T, Brandtzaeg P, Fung M, Pharo AM, Høiby EA, Michaelsen TE, et al. Inhibition of C5a-induced inflammation with preserved C5b-9-mediated bactericidal activity in a human whole blood model of meningococcal sepsis. *Blood* (2003) 102:3702–10. doi:10.1182/blood-2003-03-0703

Jacobsen ID, Brunke S, Seider K, Schwarzmüller T, Firon A, D'Enfért C, et al. *Candida glabrata* persistence in mice does not depend on host immunosuppres- sion and is unaffected by fungal amino acid auxotrophy. *Infect Immun* (2010) 78:1066–77. doi:10.1128/IAI.01244-09

Brunke S, Hube B. Two unlike cousins: *Candida albicans* and *C. glabrata* infection strategies. *Cell Microbiol* (2013) 15:701–8. doi:10.1111/cmi.12091

Posch W, Steger M, Wilflingseder D, Lass-Flörl C. Promising immunotherapy against fungal diseases. *Expert Opin Biol Ther* (2017) 17:861–70. doi:10.1080/14712598.2017.1322576

Marfin AA, Price TH. Granulocyte transfusion therapy. *J Intensive Care Med* (2015) 30:79–88. doi:10.1177/0885066613498045

Einsele H, Northoff H, Neumeister B. Granulocyte transfusion. *Vox Sang* (2004) 87:205–8. doi:10.1111/j.1741-6892.2004.00483.x

Armstrong-James D, Brown GD, Netea MG, Zelante T, Gresnigt MS, van de Veerdonk FL, et al. Immunotherapeutic approaches to treatment of fungal diseases. *Lancet Infect Dis* (2017) 17(12):e393–402. doi:10.1016/S1473-3099(17) 30442-5

Strauss RG. Clinical perspectives of granulocyte transfusions: efficacy to date. *J Clin Apher* (1995) 10:114–8. doi:10.1002/jca.2920100303

Bhatia S, McCullough J, Perry EH, Clay M, Ramsay NK, Neglia JP. Granulo- cyte transfusions: efficacy in treating fungal infections in neutropenic patients following bone marrow transplantation. *Transfusion* (1994) 34:226–32. doi:10. 1046/j.1537-2995.1994.34394196620.x

Safdar A, Hanna HA, Boktour M, Kontoyiannis DP, Hachem R, Lichtiger B, et al. Impact of high-dose granulocyte transfusions in patients with cancer with candidemia: retrospective case-control analysis of 491 episodes of *Candida* species bloodstream infections. *Cancer* (2004) 101:2859–65. doi:10.1002/cncr. 20710

Gazendam RP, van de Geer A, van Hamme JL, Tool ATJ, van Rees DJ, Aarts CEM, et al. Impaired killing of *Candida albicans* by granulocytes mobilized for transfusion purposes: a role for granule components. *Haematologica* (2016) 101:587–96. doi:10.3324/haematol.2015.136630

Fioredda F, Calvillo M, Bonanomi S, Coliva T, Tucci F, Farruggia P, et al. Congenital and acquired neutropenias consensus guidelines on therapy and follow-up in childhood from the Neutropenia Committee of the Marrow Fail- ure Syndrome Group of the AIEOP (Associazione Italiana Emato-Oncologia Pediatrica). *Am J Hematol* (2012) 87:235–8. doi:10.1002/ajh.22225

Palmblad J, Papadaki HA, Eliopoulos G. Acute and chronic neutropenias. What is new? *J Intern Med* (2001) 250:476–91. doi:10.1046/j.1365-2796.2001.00915.x

Zeidler C, Boxer L, Dale DC, Freedman MH, Kinsey S, Welte K. Management of Kostmann syndrome in the G-CSF era. *Br J Haematol.* (2000) 109:490–5. doi:10.1046/j.1365-2141.2000.02064.x

Newburger PE. Disorders of neutrophil number and function. *Hematology Am Soc Hematol Educ Program* (2006) 2006:104–10. doi:10.1182/asheducation-2006.1.104

Köhler A, De Filippo K, Hasenberg M, van den Brandt C, Nye E, Hosking MP, et al. G-CSF-mediated thrombopoietin release triggers neutrophil motility and mobilization from bone marrow via induction of Cxcr2 ligands. *Blood* (2011) 117:4349–57. doi:10.1182/blood-2010-09-308387

Berliner N, Horwitz M, Loughran TP. Congenital and acquired neutrope- nia. *Hematol Am Soc Hematol Educ Progr* (2004) 2004:63–79. doi:10.1182/asheducation-2004.1.63

Kullberg BJ, t Wout JW, Hoogstraten C, van Furth R. Recombinant interferon-gamma enhances resistance to acute disseminated *Candida albicans* infection in mice. *J Infect Dis* (1993) 168:436–43. doi:10.1093/infdis/168.2.436

Nagai H, Guo J, Choi H, Kurup V. Interferon-gamma and tumor necrosis factor- alpha protect mice from invasive aspergillosis. *J Infect Dis* (1995) 172:1554–60. doi:10.1093/infdis/172.6.1554

Clemons KV, Lutz JE, Stevens DA. Efficacy of recombinant gamma interferon for treatment of systemic cryptococcosis in SCID mice. *Society* (2001) 45:686–9. doi:10.1128/AAC.45.3.686

Dutta A, Palazzi DL. *Candida* non-albicans versus *Candida albicans* fungemia in the non-neonatal pediatric population. *Pediatr Infect Dis J* (2011) 30:664–8. doi:10.1097/INF.0b013e318213da0f

Delaloye J, Calandra T. Invasive candidiasis as a cause of sepsis in the critically ill patient. *Virulence* (2014) 5:154–62. doi:10.4161/viru.26187

Donadieu J, Fenneteau O, Beaupain B, Mahlaoui N, Chantelot CB. Congenital neutropenia: diagnosis, molecular bases and patient management. *Orphanet J Rare Dis* (2011) 6:26. doi:10.1186/1750-1172-6-26

18

An Ontology Systems Approach on Human Brain Expression and Metaproteomics

Adolfo Flores Saiffe Farías[1], *Adriana P. Mendizabal*[2] *and J. Alejandro Morales*[1*]

[1] Computer Sciences Department, University of Guadalara, Guadalajara, Mexico, [2] Pharmacobiology Department, University of Guadalajara, Guadalajara, Mexico

Correspondence:
J. Alejandro Morales
jalejandro.morales@academicos.udg.mx

Research in the last decade has shown growing evidence of the gut microbiota influence on brain physiology. While many mechanisms of this influence have been proposed in animal models, most studies in humans are the result of a pathology–dysbiosis association and very few have related the presence of certain taxa with brain substructures or molecular pathways. In this paper, we associated the functional ontologies in the differential expression of brain substructures from the Allen Brain Atlas database, with those of the metaproteome from the Human Microbiome Project. Our results showed several coherent clustered ontologies where many taxa could influence brain expression and physiology. A detailed analysis of psychobiotics showed specific slim ontologies functionally associated with substructures in the basal ganglia and cerebellar cortex. Some of the most relevant slim ontology groups are related to *Ion transport*, *Membrane potential*, *Synapse*, *DNA and RNA metabolism*, and *Antigen processing*, while the most relevant neuropathology found was Parkinson disease. In some of these cases, new hypothetical gut microbiota-brain interaction pathways are proposed.

Keywords: gene ontology, microbiota-gut-brain axis, brain structures, brain physiology, metaproteome, gene silencing, ion channel, Parkinson disease

1. INTRODUCTION

Recently, strong evidence has related the gut microbiota with almost all of the host physiology, including the brain, behavior and cognition. Experiments with both, manipulation of the gut microbiota in stress and germ–free animals, have disclosed a bidirectional communication system between the gut microbiota and the central nervous system: the microbiota-gut-brain axis (MGBa) (Dinan and Cryan, 2016, 2017). The gut microbiome handles hundreds of thousands of different proteins and metabolites, some of which are neuroactive components, and thus can communicate with the host brain, via the peripheral nervous system or through the Blood-Brain Barrier, affecting various molecular pathways (Wall et al., 2014; Dinan and Cryan, 2017). Growing evidence in humans strongly suggests that these microbial neuroactive components not only play an essential role in regulating synaptic circuit activation and neurodevelopment, but they can influence the host's emotions, behavior and cognition (Borre et al., 2014; Rea et al., 2016; Sarkar et al., 2016; Foster et al., 2017). These studies have also revealed that dysbioses, the gut micorbiota alterations or insults, promotes brain-associated diseases and disorders like Parkinson's disease (PD), anxiety and many others (Dinan and Cryan, 2017; Wiley et al., 2017).

Most of the human dysbiosis-associated neurological conditions are the result of statistical approaches using behavioral or cognitive variables, this is due to the complications of performing molecular studies in viable human brains. Although a few communication mechanisms have been suggested within the MGBa (e.g., the metabolism of tryptophan and gastrointestinal hormones microbiota dependent, and the interaction of microbiota dependent signaling molecules to the vagus nerve Wiley et al., 2017), many of them are still unknown. Thus, the complex mechanisms underlying cognition and behavior remain largely uncharacterized.

Here we hypothesize that gut taxa could be coherently associated with regions of the human brain by using functional annotations to provide a conceptual framework of putative influence mechanisms of the microbiota with the brain. We designed an *in silico* pipeline based on metaproteome (the set of microbiotal proteins) and brain expression data processed by sequence alignment tools and Gene Ontology (GO) functional groups, or slims. To our knowledge, this is the first study where whole metaproteome is functionally associated to differential expression patterns in brain regions using a blind systems approach.

2. RESULTS

2.1. Data Curation

We obtained 92 non-redundant metaproteome datasets: one per taxon at the genus level. All protein sequences from each dataset were PSI-blasted against the Human Protein Reference Sequences (RefSeq-prot). The resulting non-redundant Blast hits in each taxon were enriched with functional gene ontologies (GOs). Statistically non-significant GOs were filtered-out. Table S1 contains the number of metaproteins, their hits to the RefSeq-prot and their ontologies found per taxon.

The RNA-seq data from the Allen Brain Atlas, containing 22,318 genes, was filtered (detailed in the section 5) and resulted in 16,242 genes (72.78%). **Figure 1A** shows the leading log2-fold-change Euclidean distances between samples by substructure abbreviation (see **Table 1**), where some substructures are separated from the rest by their differential expression patterns **Figure 1B**. Table S2 contains the log2 difference between the mean counts per million (CPM) from all samples with the CPM of each sample, the *F*-value, *p*-value and Bonferroni's false discovery rate of testing for differential expression between samples. We selected the genes differentially expressed, according to the mean expression from all samples. Expressed genes by brain substructure were enriched with functional GOs, and only the statistically significant were preserved. Table S3 contains both, the number of differentially expressed genes and GOs found in enrichment per brain substructure.

We found 4,599 taxa-to-brain substructure (T2BS) common GOs (see Table S4). From these 108 were unique GOs, 92 taxa and six brain substructures. **Figures 2A,B** show the Sorensen–Dice coefficient of the GOs and genes found in each taxon vs. each substructure respectively. To test if the number of proteins found by Blast and subsequently the number of matching GOs are biased by the number of metaproteins per taxon, we performed a Pearson's correlation between the latter. The resulting value of −0.55 indicates that there is no direct correlation between the number of metaproteins per taxon and the number of GOs (see Figure S1).

2.2. GO Slims

We grouped the 108 unique GOs found, by calculating their semantic similarity (see section 5) among all of them. We applied hierarchical clustering (see Figure S2) to the distances and manually grouped them into coherent clusters with similar function, resulting in a total of 14 slims (see

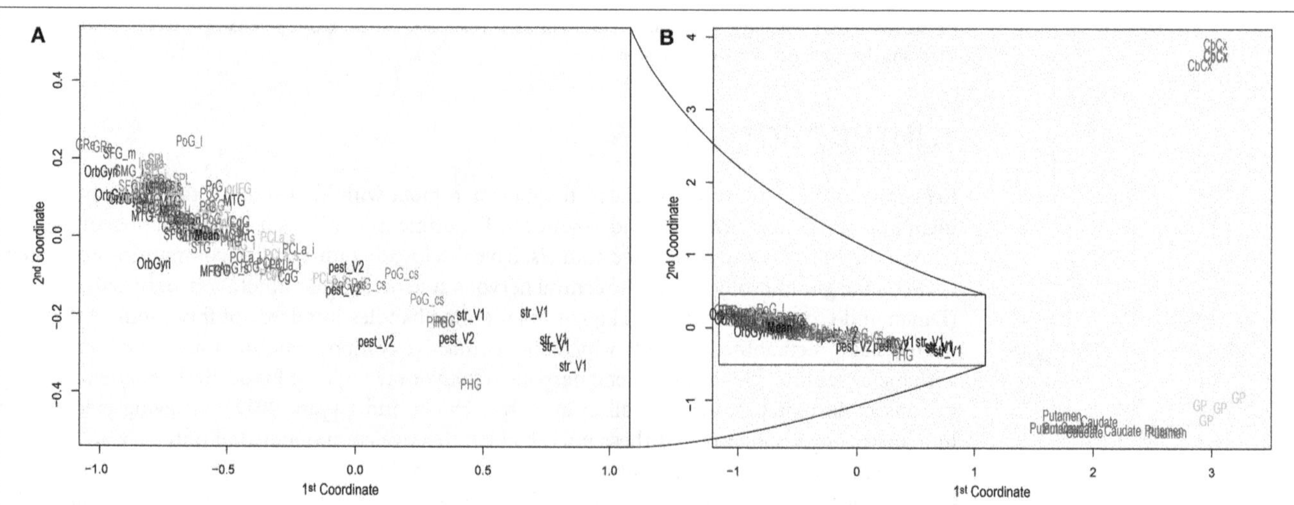

FIGURE 1 | Principal Component Analysis of brain distances obtained using the 500 most informative genes among substructures. The two principal components or coordinates are plotted on the x- and y-axis. The entire component space **(A)** zooms the region of higher density, while **(B)** depicts all substructures, showing the clear separation of a few substructures from the rest. Acronym-to-name relations are presented in **Table 1**.

TABLE 1 | Brain substructure name and their abbreviations.

Abbreviation	Substructure	Abbreviation	Substructure
AnG_i	Angular gyrus inferior	AnG_s	Angular gyrus superior
Caudate	Body of the caudate nucleus	CbCx	Cerebellar cortex
CgG	Cingulate gyrus	FuG_i	Fusiform gyrus lateral
GP	Globus pallidus	GRe	Gyrus rectus
Insula	Long insular gyri	ITG	Inferior temporal gyrus
MFG	Middle frontal gyrus	MTG	Middle temporal gyrus
OrbGyri	Lateral orbital gyrus	orIFG	Inferior frontal gyrus orbital part
PCLa_i	Paracentral lobule anterior inferior	PCLa_s	Paracentral lobule anterior superior
Pcu	Precuneus	pest_V2	Cuneus peristriate
PHG	Parahippocampal gyrus	PoG_cs	Post-central gyrus central sulcus
PoG_l	Post-central gyrus_lateral	PrG	Pre-central gyrus
Putame	Putamen	SFG_l	Superior_frontal gyrus lateral
SFG_m	Superior frontal gyrus medial	SMG_i	Supramarginal gyrus inferior
SPL	Superior parietal lobule	STG	Superior temporal gyrus
str_V1	Lingual gyrus striate		

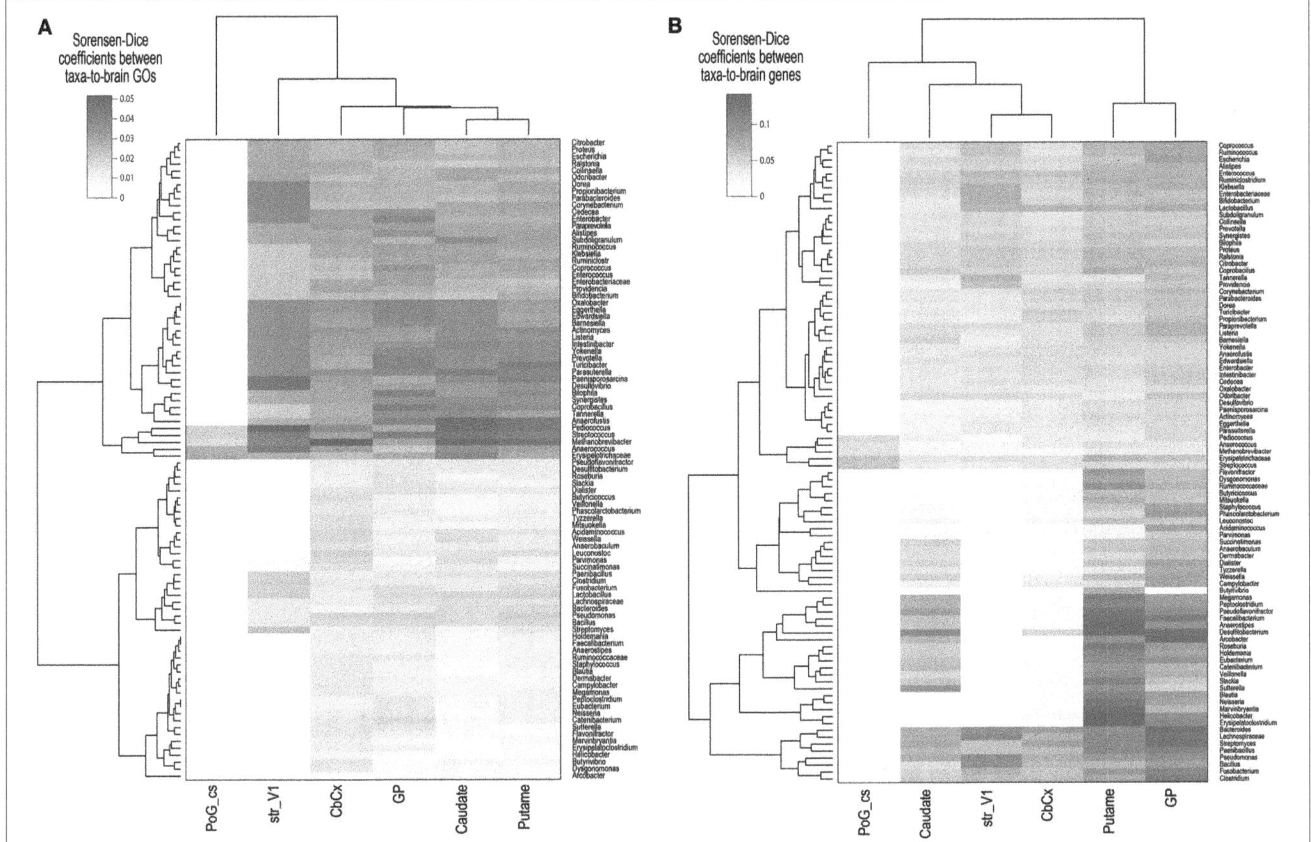

FIGURE 2 | Sorensen–Dice (SD) coefficients heatmap of **(A)** common Gene Ontologies (GOs) and **(B)** genes across brain substructures and taxa. SD coefficient rage values are zero to one, where zero means completely dissimilar and one means identical sets. Acronym–to–name relations are presented in **Table 1**.

Tables S4, S5). The ontological maps for each slim can be found at Figure S3.

Figure 3 shows the number of common GOs between taxon and brain substructure, colored by slims. We can observe that the most frequent slim is *Ion transport*, followed by *Protein metabolism* and *DNA and RNA metabolism*. Also, the Globus pallidus is the substructure where more associations were found, followed by the Cerebellar cortex. **Table 2** shows the GOs, taxa, and brain substructures count per slim.

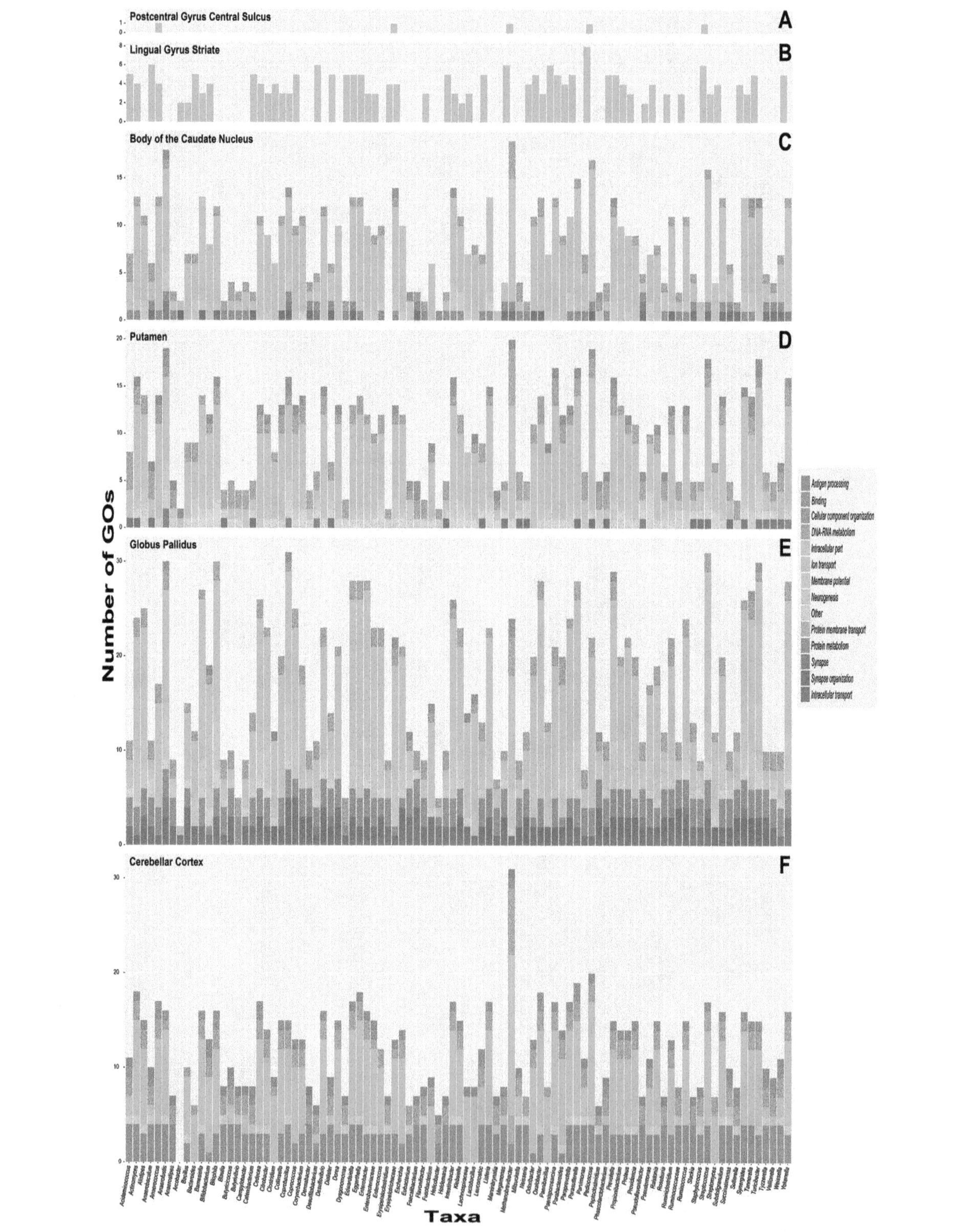

FIGURE 3 | Stacked bar graphs with the quantity of common taxa-to-brain substruture Gene ontology labels on the y-axis and color-coded slims. The x-axis has each of the 92 different genre analyzed. Each graph represent brain substructures **(A)** Postcentral gyrus central sulcus, **(B)** Lingual gyrus striate, **(C)** Body of the caudate nucleus, **(D)** Putamen, **(E)** Globus pallidus and **(F)** Cerebellar cortex.

TABLE 2 | Substructures and counts of GOs and taxa by slim.

Slim	GOs	Taxa	Substructure
Ion transport	30	85	GP, Caudate, CbCx, Putame, str_V1, PoG_cs
Membrane potential	6	86	Caudate, GP, Putame
Protein membrane transport	3	1	CbCx
Synapse	6	9	Caudate, GP, Putame
Synapse organization	3	27	GP
Transport (others)	7	89	Caudate, GP, Putame
Antigen processing	2	2	CbCx
Binding	4	85	CbCx, Putame, GP
Cellular component organization	4	31	CbCx, Caudate, GP, Putame
DNA and RNA metabolism	15	90	CbCx, Caudate, GP, Putame
Intracellular part	10	28	Caudate, CbCx, Putame, str_V1
Neurogenesis	2	28	Caudate, GP, Putame
Other	10	89	CbCx, Caudate, GP, Putame
Protein metabolism	6	84	CbCx, Caudate, GP

3. DISCUSSION

The comorbidity between dysbiosis and cognitive or behavioral impairment has sparked a race to understand the mechanisms of these associations. Since then, researchers have glimpsed the influence of microbiota in behavior and cognition, and several interaction pathways have been proposed via the Blood Brain Barrier or the vagus nerve, involving neuropeptides (Holzer and Farzi, 2014), inflammatory molecular signaling (Rook et al., 2014), hormones (Rehfeld, 2014), microRNAs (miRNAs) (Hoban et al., 2017a), among others (Wall et al., 2014). In our study, the correlation between the brain proteins and the metaproteome into functional ontologies supports these observations.

Advances in sequencing technology have paved the way for the creation of reference databases in many fields of research. The Human Microbiome Project has consistently sequenced the microbiota from different body parts and created the Reference Genome Database body part-specific. On the other side, the Allen Brain Atlas organization has performed RNA-seq (quadruplicate at least) of 29 different brain substructures in two post-mortem subjects. Despite this sampling being biased (due to post-mortem) and underpowered, it enabled us to perform this work as a "test drive." Our aim was not to prove a direct link between gene expression levels in the brain and the presence of specific taxa but to strengthen the evidence of known MGBa mechanisms as well as to uncover putative new avenues of research in the axis.

The analysis pipeline, being a data-driven approach, is prone to false positives. Thus we have used multiple-comparisons correction methods, to increase the proportion of true positives (at the expense of false negatives, though). From the 29 substructures, only six of them were found to have common GO annotations with those associated with microbiota. These six substructures (Cerebellar Cortex, Globus pallidus, Putamen, Body of the caudate nucleus, Lingual gyrus striate and Postcentral gyrus central sulcus) appear distant from the rest (**Figure 1**), which means that they have different and broader expression patterns than most of the substructures and will have more significant enriched GOs (see Table S3).

The tremendous complexity of the human brain has limited the approaches to the MGBa. Most of such studies measure behavioral responses involving different types of memory or stress, while only a few associate cognition or behavior with specific brain regions, circuits, pathways, and taxa. Assuming that cognitive function is associated with structural micro-connectivity and specific gene expression patterns (across cell types) regulating input and output signals, this work is based on the paradigm that cognition is the result of communication patterns that emerge from the interaction of specialized brain substructures connected in certain circuitry across several molecular pathways. Our methodology is designed to find common T2BS functional annotations, based on differential expression of brain structures and the taxa metaproteome, assuming that portions of the latter are expressed under certain conditions.

Given that we cannot assume that homology of a metaprotein with a human brain gene is only associated due to its similarity, we have turned to a differential functional approach. Gene enrichment method is used here to find groups of genes overrepresented with a similar function. Such gene-function association allows us to perform more robust T2BS associations.

The resulting common GOs clustered naturally according to their semantic distances in the ontology map. With these, we performed *a posteriori* design of GO slims that coherently clustered similar GO annotations. These slims enabled us to analyze and discuss our results by functionally coherent groups.

3.1. Pyschobiotic and Slim Selection

Psychobiotics are microorganisms that have a positive influence on the mental health when ingested in adequate amounts (Dinan and Cryan, 2017). Several bacteria have been proposed as such, and we have selected those genera with consistent evidence of mental health influence or neurotransmitter-producing capabilities.

There is evidence of *Actinomyces*, *Bifidobacterium*, and *Faecalibacterium* having positive effects on anxiety and/or depression (Messaoudi et al., 2011; Jiang et al., 2015; Kelly et al., 2016; Zheng et al., 2016) and *Bacteroides*, *Prevotella*, and *Lactobacillus* in autism spectrum disorder. *Bifidobacterium* ameliorates the hypothalamic-pituitary-adrenal system under stress in germ-free mice (Sudo et al., 2004). Tillisch *et al.* tested a healthy women population found that increased abundance of *Prevotella* showed differential response to negatively valenced images and greater white matter connectivity in limbic–cortical–striatal–pallidal–thalamic circuitry, and smaller hippocampal volume in comparison with the *Bacteroides*-high group. The *Prevotella*-high group was also found to have higher connectivity in the temporal lobe (Tillisch et al., 2017). Sheperjans et al. conducted a case–control study of 72 subjects with Parkinson's disease and found reduced *Prevotella* in the feces of case–subjects, and the abundance of *Enterobacteriaceae* correlated with postural instability and gait difficulty (Scheperjans et al., 2015). We have also considered as psychobiotics those microorganisms able to produce neurotransmitters like *Bacillus, Bifidobacterium, Escherichia, Enterococcus, Lactobacillus, Staphilococcus*, and *Streptococcus* (Horiuchi et al., 2003; Bravo et al., 2011; Barrett et al., 2012; Lyte, 2014; Wall et al., 2014; Desbonnet et al., 2015; Dinan and Cryan, 2017). For example, Bravo et al., in 2011 studied mice with a *Lactobacillus* treatment and found altered expression of GABA receptors, vagous nerve-dependent, in cortical regions, hippocampus, amygdala and *locus coerulus* and reduced anxiety and depression-related behavior (Bravo et al., 2011). Based on the evidence here discussed, we have tagged the mentioned bacteria as psychobiotics.

We have selected the slims that could be conceptually directly related to brain activity or the cognition: *Synapse, DNA and RNA metabolism, Protein metabolism, Membrane potential* and *Ion transport*. These slims contained 541 GOs associating T2BS. **Figure 4** shows these relationships. Specific discussion of the putative role of psychobiotics (and other microorganisms) within the slims can be found below.

3.2. Gut Microbiota and Brain Cells Membranes

Behavior and cognition are intrinsically dependent on the communication within the brain, that is electrical impulses and synapses. The flow of electrical impulses is given by the efficient ion movement across the neuron cell membranes through voltage-gated ion channels. Deficiencies in voltage-gated ion channels and synapses have been related to several mental and movement disorders (Baldessarini, 1996; Yogeeswari et al., 2004; Sullivan et al., 2012; Imbrici et al., 2013; Vitaliti et al., 2014; Mourre et al., 2017; Reig-Viader et al., in press; Roeper, 2017). For example, epilepsy (Devergnas et al., 2012; Carecchio and Mencacci, 2017) and PD (Mourre et al., 2017) are associated with the basal ganglia, while ataxia has been observed with ion channel dysfunction in the cerebellum (Waszkielewicz et al., 2013).

On the other hand, gut dysbioses have been previously associated to most of these conditions (Parracho et al., 2005; MacFabe et al., 2011; Rook et al., 2014; Maqsood and Stone,

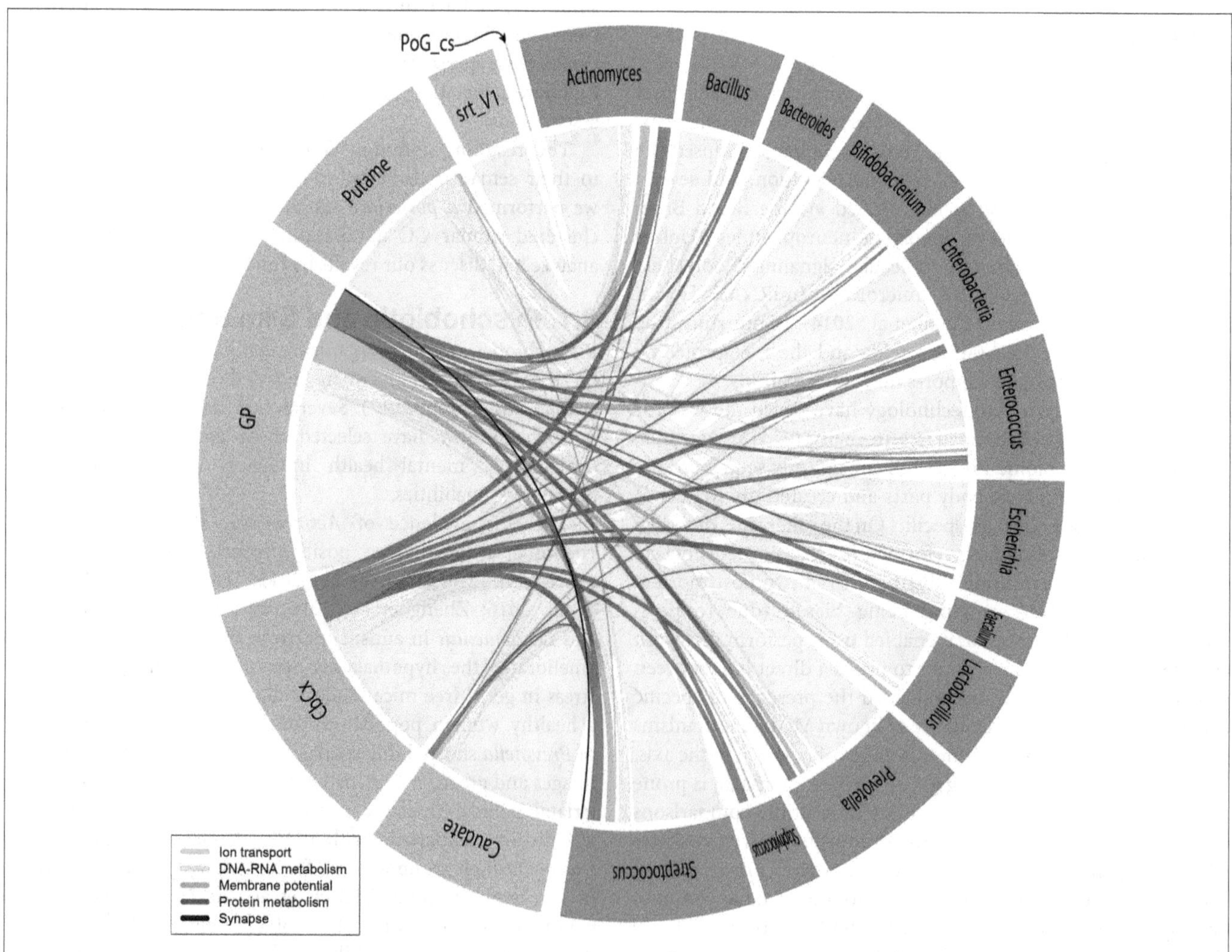

FIGURE 4 | Psychobiotic–brain relationships represented by a colored edge corresponding to the slims of interest as indicated in the caption. Pink–colored circle fractions correspond to brain sub-structure (Abbreviation) and blue–gray–colored circle fractions correspond to the following psychobiotics: *Actinomyces, Bacillus, Bacteroides, Bifidobacterium, Enterobacteriaceae, Enterococcus, Escherichia, Faecalibacterium, Lactobacillus, Prevotella, Staphylococcus*, and *Streptococcus*.

2016). Sudo et al., and Neufeld et al. reported a decreased expression of subunits of the NMDA receptor (a glutamate and ion channel protein) in both, cortex and hippocampus (Sudo et al., 2004), and in central amygdala in GF-mice (Neufeld et al., 2011). This suggests possible mechanisms of microbiota–mediated synapses and ion channel regulation.

We report a high density of functional associations related to electrical impulses and synapse communication (see Figure S3, slims *Ion transport*, *Membrane potential*, *Protein membrane transport*, *Synapse*, *Synapse organization*, and *Transport* (*others*)). We have found four ontologies (GO:0005249, GO:0005267, GO:0022843, and GO:0034705) present in more than 50% of the T2BS relations (see Figure S3 and Table S4). Surprisingly these four are part of the *Ion transport* slim, which is related to ion voltage-gated channel activities (see Table S5). Also, more than half of all of the T2BS GO relations are associated by the *Ion transport* slim, especially at the Globus pallidus, Putamen and the Body of the Caudate nucleus (substructures of the basal ganglia), Cerebellum cortex and Striate. Our findings strongly support the hypothesis of the influence of the metaproteome with mental and movement–related neurological disorders by the direct or indirect interaction with ion channels (slim *Ion transport*) and regulation of membrane potential (slim *Membrane potential*).

We have found 89 taxa that putatively influence the basal ganglia at the level of neurotransmitter transport and other chemicals (see the *Transport (others)* ontology map in Figure S3). Also, we have found 27 taxa that could influence the structural organization of synapse at the Globus pallidus (see the *Synapse organization* ontology map in Figure S3). Our results agree with the evidence of microbiota influencing neurotransmitter receptors, like the serotonin receptor 1A (5HT1A) (Sudo et al., 2004) and GABA receptors via the vagus nerve (Bravo et al., 2011), and the altered neurotransmitter levels found in the striatum of GF–mice (Diaz Heijtz et al., 2011).

Other approaches suggest that the gut microbiota can influence synapse function and neurogenesis by influencing the brain-derived neurotrophic factor (BDNF), a key regulator on neurogenesis and synapses (Sudo et al., 2004; Bercik et al., 2011). In this context, we found nine taxa within the *Synapse* slim and 28 taxa within the *Neurogenesis* slim, both associated with the basal ganglia.

By selecting the taxa and slims mentioned in the psychobiotics analysis, we observed that the seven most abundant GOs (all within the *Ion transport* slim), represent 64% of the T2BSs, and 76% of those, are associated with the potassium ion channels (see **Figure 4**). Also, the Globus Pallidus (34%) was found to share most of mentions followed by the cerebellar cortex, the putamen and the caudate. These results suggest that psychobiotics could influence voltage-gated channels, especially those involved with potassium channels in the basal ganglia. As discussed above, there is evidence of movement disorders associated with basal ganglia and ion channels (Devergnas et al., 2012; Carecchio and Mencacci, 2017; Mourre et al., 2017) and with psychobiotic dysbioses (Scheperjans et al., 2015; Hill-Burns et al., 2017; Li et al., 2017). Also, we have found other GO labels within the slims of *Membrane potential* and *Synapse* which suggests that psychobiotics also play a role in the action potential and synaptic membrane.

3.3. Gene Expression of the Host Brain and the Influence of Gut Microbiota

Cognition and behavior disorders are also associated with gene expression processes and their highly complex regulatory mechanisms, which involve miRNAs (a product of splicing) and epigenomic regulatory marks (e.g., DNA methylation, histone modifications, non-coding RNAs). The slim of *DNA and RNA metabolism*, which contains 12.3% of the total T2BS, associates 90 taxa with four brain substructures (see **Table 2**) through 15 GO terms (GO:0016072, GO:0006399, GO:0006364, GO:0008033, GO:0009451, GO:0004518, GO:0006402, GO:0000375, GO:0000398, GO:0000184, GO:0019083, GO:0071013, GO:0000956, GO:0006353, GO:0016570). Suggesting that the microbiome is capable of regulating host's nucleic acid metabolism via the spliceosome, catabolic processing the RNA, histone modification, RNA modification, rRNA and tRNA processing or nuclease activity based on the GO terms found (see Figure S3 and Table S4).

Methanobrevibacter, the most abundant archaea in the human gut, appears in mentions of the spliceosome (GO:0000398, GO:0000375, and GO:0071013) in the Globus pallidus, Putamen, Body of the Caudate nucleus and Cerebellar cortex. The spliceosome is the machinery that regulates transcript RNA splicing, into various RNA functional products, including mRNAs and miRNAs. Hasler et al. found evidence of the microbiota influencing host-gene expression and RNA splicing in host-mucosal cells (Häsler et al., 2016), which suggest the involvement of miRNAs in regulatory mechanisms. These are known to have a role in neuropsychiatric disorders (Alural et al., 2017), anxiety-like behaviors (Hoban et al., 2017b) and movement disorders (Tan et al., 2013). Increased miRNAs have been reported in GF–mice at amygdala and prefrontal cortex (Hoban et al., 2017a) and in the striatum (putamen and caudate) (Diaz Heijtz et al., 2011) as well as in post-mortem humans with PD compared to healthy controls (Nair and Ge, 2016).

There is also evidence of the microbiome influence on the host's epigenomics, which is known to influence gene expression, in the context of patho-epigenomics (Bierne, 2017), infection (Hamon and Cossart, 2008; Eskandarian et al., 2013), depression (Tsankova et al., 2006) and drug addiction (Renthal et al., 2007). We have found that *Paenisporosarcina* could influence the epigenetics of the putamen by modifying its histones (GO:0016570) (see Figure S3 and Table S4). Histone deacetylase activity in mice has been observed during stress and depression in the hippocampus (Tsankova et al., 2006) and nucleus accumbens (Renthal et al., 2007). There is growing evidence of microbiota influencing epigenetic changes outside brain tissue (Bierne, 2017) and some mechanisms have been described (Hamon and Cossart, 2008; Eskandarian et al., 2013). Recent evidence has shown dysbiosis associated with epigenetic alterations in cognitive conditions and diseases like autism (Loke et al., 2015), PD (Coppedè, 2012), and many others (Alam et al., 2017).

Eighty two taxa (including the 10 psychobiotics) presented mentions in the cerebral cortex and putamen through the

RNA modification/editing ontology (GO:0009451, see Figure S3 and Table S4). It has been found that an epitranscriptomic modification, N^6-methyladenosine (m6A), is highly enriched in miRNAs targets in the mouse brain, and it has an important role in neurodevelopment (Wahlstedt et al., 2009; Meyer et al., 2012). RNA editing has been found to be a key regulator of ion channels in the mouse (Seeburg et al., 2001). As discussed above, these regions could have implications for movement disorders. However, we have not found relevant literature directly associating the MGBa to epitranscriptomics.

Within the *DNA and RNA metabolism* slim, we have found three GOs related to mRNA catabolism (GO:0006402, GO:0000956, and GO:0000184) that associates *Methanobrevibacter* with the cerebellar cortex and the putamen (see Table S4). One of these GOs, labeled "nuclear-transcribed mRNA catabolic process, non-sense-mediated decay" refers to the degradation of mRNAs with a premature stop codon, a process that prevents the translation of potentially harmful proteins (Hentze and Kulozik, 1999). This result suggests a novel microbiota-mediated mechanism of mRNAs cleavage, affecting the expression levels in the brain.

3.4. Gut Microbiota Influencing Brain Immune System

Strong and consistent evidence has emerged on the association between the host's immune system and the microbiota, which is given by inflammatory mediators. Persistent states of inflammation are also associated with several neurological conditions like depression and anxiety. Evidence shows that inflammatory responses during pregnancy increase the risk of neurodevelopmental conditions like autism spectrum disorders and schizophrenia (Rook et al., 2014).

Dermabacter and *Methanobrevibacter* resulted mentioned with the cerebellar cortex by the *Antigen processing* slim (see Table S4). Within this slim, we can find two ontologies associated with the process in which the Major Histocompatibility Complex class I (MHC-I) interacts with a peptide antigen presented in its cell wall (GO:0002474) by the Transporter associated with antigen processing (TAP) pathway (GO:0002479) (see Table S5 and Figure S3). This pathway mediates the translocation of cytosolic peptides into the endoplasmic reticulum that bind to the MHC-I.

Consistent with our results, neuronal expression of MHC-I has been reported in the cerebellum (Letellier et al., 2008; Shatz, 2009). Evidence shows that MHC-I could limit motor learning in the cerebellum, have implications in long-term depression (McConnell et al., 2009) and be associated with the visual system's development and maintenance in marmoset monkeys (Ribic et al., 2011). The expression of this complex is involved in the synaptic plasticity regulation during neurodevelopment (Goddard et al., 2007) and axonal regeneration following injury (Wu et al., 2011). Also, there is evidence of its involvement in neuronal diseases (Pereira and Simmons, 1999; Friese and Fugger, 2005; Chevalier et al., 2011; Kim et al., 2013; Prabowo et al., 2013; Cebrian et al., 2014). A study performed by Mulder et al. showed that low microbiota (hygienic) environment could increase gut expression of MHC-I and other chemokines compared to "natural" environmental acquired microbiota in piglets (Mulder et al., 2009). Our study implicates the microbiota diversity with the expression of MHC-I.

3.5. Parkinson's Disease

We have found multiple associations with PD (and other motor disorders) through ion channel deficiencies (Mourre et al., 2017; Roeper, 2017), miRNAs (Tan et al., 2013; Nair and Ge, 2016), epigenetic alterations (Coppedè, 2012) and alterations in MHC-I (Cebrian et al., 2014); some of them associating the same cerebral structures like the ones we have found. Our results are particularly interesting given that some of the latter hypothesis of PD etiology has previously involved the microbiota as a relevant and mechanistic factor (Parashar and Udayabanu, 2017).

Gut microbiota have been found altered in subjects with PD, and evidence strongly suggests that it could cause PD through different mechanisms. Reduced organisms found in fecal samples of subjects with PD are *Blautia*, *Coprococcus*, and *Roseburia* (Keshavarzian et al., 2015) and the psychobiotic *Prevotella* (Scheperjans et al., 2015). Hill-Burns et al., recently reported altered abundances of the psychobiotics *Bifidobacterium*, *Lactobacillus* and *Faecalibacterium*, and non-psychobiotics *Blautia*, *Roseburia* and *Akkermansia* genus (Hill-Burns et al., 2017). Another recent study found decreased *Blautia*, *Faecalibacterium* and *Ruminococcus*, and increased *Escherichia-Shigella*, *Streptococcus*, *Proteus*, and *Enterococcus* as in comparison with controls (Li et al., 2017).

In this context, by considering the most abundant GOs for each taxa, nine bacterial genera (*Lactobacillus*, *Bifidobacterium*, *Coprococcus*, *Prevotella*, *Ruminococcus*, *Escherichia*, *Streptococcus*, *Proteus*, and *Enterococcus*) are associated with potassium ion channels; three of them (*Faecalibacterium*, *Blautia*, *Roseburia*) are related to translational termination and RNA modification, and two (*Ruminococcus*, *Roseburia*) are also associated with axonogenesis. However, other functional associations could be found at the Table S4.

The *Methanobrevibacter* also have been found to influence the spliceosome at PD-associated brain substructures. We have not found any associations of this taxon with PD, however, most of the microbiota profiling projects are 16S-rRNA-based, and they missed archaea organisms.

Despite the extensive literature on PD and that we have found many coincidences for this disease, the results presented here could pave the way for novel hypotheses on PD pathophysiology.

4. CONCLUSIONS

In this work, we have presented an *in silico* framework to associate metaproteins with brain expression data through ontological labels. Also we have defined *a posteriori* GO slims based on semantic similarity clustering. This data-driven study suggests that microbiota could affect synapse and voltage-gated ion channels in brain structures, which have been related to movement disorders, like the basal ganglia. Beacuse of the GO associations, we can suggest that microbiota have an influence on DNA and RNA metabolism. Given the strong association of *Methanobrevibacter* with spliceosome GOs, we suggest that mechanisms involving miRNAs and mRNA catabolism may have a role in several brain structures. This last taxon along with *Dermabacter* were found associated with the MHC-I through the TAP pathway in the cerebellar cortex. We also found associations like *Paenisporosarcina* with histone modification, and with many other taxa, including known psychobiotics, as RNA modificators. Parkinson's disease was coincidently found associated to several taxa, brain structures, and functional slims related with neuronal communication, DNA/RNA metabolism and alterations in the MHC-I.

This work is a novel systems approach based on T2BS functional annotations, where we used large, specialized databases to discover possible mechanisms where the microbiota could influence specific brain regions. Our results could also inspire germ-manipulation studies to find therapeutic approaches on neurological movement disorders.

5. MATERIALS AND METHODS

5.1. Data Curation

Gastrointestinal tract microbiota proteome (metaproteome) of database (Reference Genome sequence data obtained from 300 subjects) was downloaded from the Human Microbiome Project website[1] as contigs (see **Figure 5**, database "HMPdb"). The human protein reference sequences (RefSeq-prot) database was downloaded from the NCBI ftp server[2] (see **Figure 5**, data "RefSeq-prot"). Also, post-mortem human brain RNA-sequencing dataset (donor H0351.2001) was downloaded from the Allen Brain Atlas web page[3] (see **Figure 5**, data "Allen exp."), which contains three or four replicates per brain substructure.

The metaproteome files were merged at the genus level to generate a single non-redundant file per taxon. These files were used as query for the Position Specific Iterative (PSI)-Blast local and the RefSeq-prot was used as database (see **Figure 5**, process "PSI-Blast"). PSI-Blast is an iterative version of protein blast to find highly conservative relationships between proteins. PSI-Blast parameters were set up to 10 iterations (maximum) and *e*-value threshold $\leq$ 0.05. The PSI-Blast results by taxa were obtained in one file each (see **Figure 5**, data "Human gene hits"). The human protein hits of the last iteration were extracted from the files and redundancies removed. Each list of non-redundant proteins was annotated with its geneID by using the GCRh38 database.

The human RNA-seq database at the Allen Brain Atlas contains normalized expression data on 22,318 genes. To see the normalization methods used go to documentation at brain-map.org. Genes not annotated in Entrez database or with zero counts in all samples were eliminated. Genes with CPM $\leq$ 0.5 in at least two replicates of the same brain sub-structure were also eliminated. We calculated the Euclidian distances between samples by using a multidimensional scaling with the function plotMDS of the edgeR library, scaling with the top 500 genes with larger log2-fold changes. Afterwards, we selected those genes within each substructure with differential expression compared to the mean across all samples by using the methods explained in Lun and Smyth (2015) using the edgeR library (McCarthy et al., 2012). For the latter step we first estimated the biological and technical variability of the reads by using

[1]https://www.hmpdacc.org/hmp/
[2]https://ftp.ncbi.nlm.nih.gov/refseq/H_sapiens/mRNA_Prot/
[3]http://human.brain-map.org/static/download

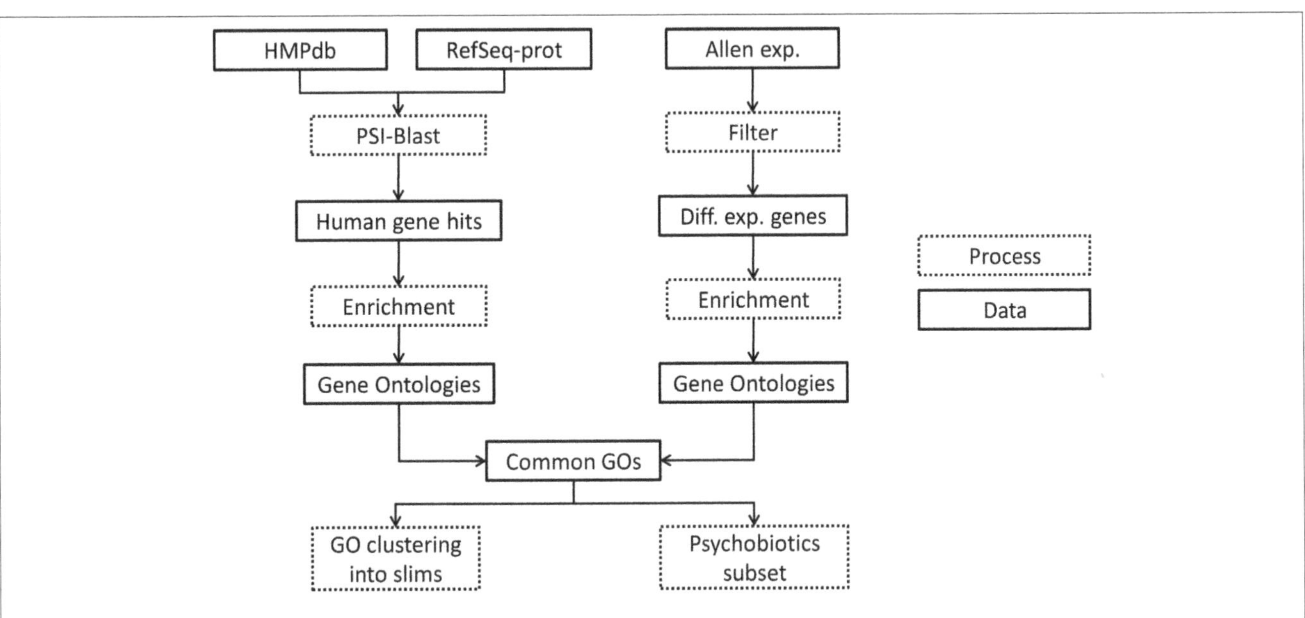

FIGURE 5 | Flowchart of the methodology used. Dotted boxes indicate processing steps and regular boxes are data downloaded or resulted from a process. HMPdb, Human Microbiome Project database; PSI, Position Specific Iterative; GO, Gene Ontology.

the glmQLFit function, which performs a gene-wise negative binomial generalized linear model with quasi-likelihood method (Lun and Smyth, 2015). Afterwards, we used a quasi-likelihood F-test (substructure CPMs vs. the mean CPMs) due to its rigid error rate control at including the uncertainty in the estimation of the dispersion. The multiple comparisons problem (which states that when many hypothesis are tested, the chance of erroneous conclusions increases) was corrected by Bonferroni method, and only the genes with $p \leq 0.05$ were preserved. Also, only genes with absolute log-fold change ≥ 1.5 were preserved (see **Figure 5**, process "Filter" and Data "Diff. exp. genes").

5.2. Gene Ontology Enrichment and Common Ontology

Each gene list associated to taxa or brain substructure was enriched using python's goatools[4] find_enrichment.py function to find the GOs statistically associated to the list of genes ($\alpha = 0.05$) (see **Figure 5**, process "Enrichment"). Ontologies with Bonferroni corrected $p \leq 0.05$ were selected. Statistically significant underrepresented GOs were discarded in the taxon associated gene lists. This resulted in a set of ontologies associated to each taxon and each brain sub-structure (see **Figure 5**, data "Gene Ontologies").

We annotated the T2BS common ontologies. This resulted in a T2BS association list of GOs with annotated genes (see **Figure 5**, data "Common GOs").

5.3. Analysis

For each pair of T2BS we calculated the Sorensen-Dice coefficient (similarity measure between two samples) and applied hierarchical clustering to observe the distribution of the common GOs. Also we applied Pearson's correlation (coefficient of linear correlation) to the number of genes found in each taxon to the number of common GO terms found in the same taxon.

From all of the GOs obtained, we calculated its semantic similarity by the goatools function semantic_similarity.py. This measure is defined as the reciprocal of the minimal number of branches (or edges) between two GO terms in the GO topology. It can also be defined as the reciprocal of the shortest path between two GO terms by using graph theory argot. We grouped GO terms with similar functions by manually curating clusters obtained by hierarchical clustering the semantic similarities between all GOs; to refer to these groups we use "slims" (see **Figure 5**, process "GO clustering into slims"). From the set of taxa we selected those known as psychobiotics according to literature to perform a deeper exploratory data analysis (see **Figure 5**, process "Psychobiotics subset").

[4]https://github.com/tanghaibao/goatools

AUTHOR CONTRIBUTIONS

AF and JM developed the main idea of the work, but the pipeline was finally designed by the three authors. The three authors participated in the figure design, discussion, and the final draft. AF performed the experiments, analyzed the results and wrote the initial draft of introduction, methods, and results. He also participated in the section 3 with an emphasis on the slims and Parkinson's disease. AM also participated in the discussion with an emphasis on the microbiota and psychobiotics. JM also participated in the discussion with a systems approach and edited the figures.

FUNDING

AF was supported through the doctorate scholarship to AF (award number 563065/301724) by the National Council of Science and Technology (CONACyT, Mexico).

ACKNOWLEDGMENTS

We acknowledge Rosana Farías for proofreading this work.

REFERENCES

Alam, R., Abdolmaleky, H. M., and Zhou, J.-R. (2017). Microbiome, inflammation, epigenetic alterations, and mental diseases. *Am. J. Med. Genet. B Neuropsychiat. Genet.* 174, 651–660. doi: 10.1002/ajmg.b.32567

Alural, B., Genc, S., and Haggarty, S. J. (2017). Diagnostic and therapeutic potential of microRNAs in neuropsychiatric disorders: past, present, and future. *Progr. Neuropsychopharmacol. Biol. Psychiatry* 73, 87–103. doi: 10.1016/j.pnpbp.2016.03.010

Baldessarini, R. (1996). *Goodman and Gilmans: The Pharmacological Basis of Therapeutics. 9th Edn.* New York, NY: McGraw-Hill Press, 399–430.

Barrett, E., Ross, R., O'Toole, P., Fitzgerald, G., and Stanton, C. (2012). γ-Aminobutyric acid production by culturable bacteria from the human intestine. *J. Appl. Microbiol.* 113, 411–417. doi: 10.1111/j.1365-2672.2012.05344.x

Bercik, P., Denou, E., Collins, J., Jackson, W., Lu, J., Jury, J., et al. (2011). The intestinal microbiota affect central levels of brain-derived neurotropic factor and behavior in mice. *Gastroenterology* 141, 599–609. doi: 10.1053/j.gastro.2011.04.052

Bierne, H. (2017). "Crsoss talk between bacteria and the host epigenetic machinery," in *Epigenetics of Infectious Diseases*, eds W. Doerfler and J. Casadesús (Cham: Springer), 113–158.

Borre, Y. E., O'Keeffe, G. W., Clarke, G., Stanton, C., Dinan, T. G., and Cryan, J. F. (2014). Microbiota and neurodevelopmental windows: implications for brain disorders. *Trends Mol. Med.* 20, 509–518. doi: 10.1016/j.molmed.2014.05.002

Bravo, J. A., Forsythe, P., Chew, M. V., Escaravage, E., Savignac, H. M., Dinan, T. G., et al. (2011). Ingestion of Lactobacillus strain regulates emotional behavior and central GABA receptor expression in a mouse via the vagus nerve. *Proc. Natl. Acad. Sci. U.S.A.* 108, 16050–16055. doi: 10.1073/pnas.1102999108

Carecchio, M., and Mencacci, N. E. (2017). Emerging monogenic complex hyperkinetic disorders. *Curr. Neurol. Neurosci. Rep.* 17:97. doi: 10.1007/s11910-017-0806-2

Cebrian, C., Loike, J. D., and Sulzer, D. (2014). Neuronal MHC-I expression and its implications in synaptic function, axonal regeneration and Parkinsons and other brain diseases. *Front. Neuroanat.* 8:114. doi: 10.3389/fnana.2014.00114

Chevalier, G., Suberbielle, E., Monnet, C., Duplan, V., Martin-Blondel, G., Farrugia, F., et al. (2011). Neurons are MHC class I-dependent targets for

CD8 T cells upon neurotropic viral infection. *PLoS Pathog.* 7:e1002393. doi: 10.1371/journal.ppat.1002393

Coppedè, F. (2012). Genetics and epigenetics of Parkinson's disease. *Sci. World J.* 2012:489830. doi: 10.1100/2012/489830

Desbonnet, L., Clarke, G., Traplin, A., OSullivan, O., Crispie, F., Moloney, R. D., et al. (2015). Gut microbiota depletion from early adolescence in mice: implications for brain and behaviour. *Brain Behav. Immun.* 48, 165–173. doi: 10.1016/j.bbi.2015.04.004

Devergnas, A., Piallat, B., Prabhu, S., Torres, N., Louis Benabid, A., David, O., et al. (2012). The subcortical hidden side of focal motor seizures: evidence from micro-recordings and local field potentials. *Brain* 135(Pt 7), 2263–2276. doi: 10.1093/brain/aws134

Diaz Heijtz, R., Wang, S., Anuar, F., Qian, Y., Björkholm, B., Samuelsson, A., et al. (2011). Normal gut microbiota modulates brain development and behavior. *Proc. Natl. Acad. Sci. U.S.A.* 108, 3047–3052. doi: 10.1073/pnas.1010529108

Dinan, T. G., and Cryan, J. F. (2016). Gut Instincts: microbiota as a key regulator of brain development, ageing and neurodegeneration. *J. Physiol.* 595, 489-503. doi: 10.1113/JP273106

Dinan, T. G., and Cryan, J. F. (2017). The microbiome-gut-brain axis in health and disease. *Gastroenterol. Clin. North Am.* 46, 77–89. doi: 10.1016/j.gtc.2016.09.007

Eskandarian, H. A., Impens, F., Nahori, M.-A., Soubigou, G., Coppee, J.-Y., Cossart, P., et al. (2013). A Role for SIRT2-dependent histone H3K18 deacetylation in bacterial infection. *Science* 341, 1238858–1238858. doi: 10.1126/science.1238858

Foster, J. A., Rinaman, L., and Cryan, J. F. (2017). Stress and the gut-brain axis: Regulation by the microbiome. *Neurobiol. Stress.* 7, 124-136. doi: 10.1016/j.ynstr.2017.03.001.

Friese, M. A., and Fugger, L. (2005). Autoreactive CD8+ T cells in multiple sclerosis: a new target for therapy? *Brain* 128(Pt 8), 1747–1763. doi: 10.1093/brain/awh578

Goddard, C. A., Butts, D. A., and Shatz, C. J. (2007). Regulation of CNS synapses by neuronal MHC class I. *Proc. Natl. Acad. Sci. U.S.A.* 104, 6828–6833. doi: 10.1073/pnas.0702023104

Hamon, M. A., and Cossart, P. (2008). Histone modifications and chromatin remodeling during bacterial infections. *Cell Host Microbe*, 4, 100–109. doi: 10.1016/j.chom.2008.07.009

Häsler, R., Sheibani-Tezerji, R., Sinha, A., Barann, M., Rehman, A., Esser, D., et al. (2016). Uncoupling of mucosal gene regulation, mRNA splicing and adherent microbiota signatures in inflammatory bowel disease. *Gut.* 66 2087–2097. doi: 10.1136/gutjnl-2016-311651

Hentze, M. W., and Kulozik, A. E. (1999). A perfect message: RNA surveillance and nonsense-mediated decay. *Cell* 96, 307–310. doi: 10.1016/S0092-8674(00)80542-5

Hill-Burns, E. M., Debelius, J. W., Morton, J. T., Wissemann, W. T., Lewis, M. R., Wallen, Z. D., et al (2017). Parkinson's disease and Parkinson's disease medications have distinct signatures of the gut microbiome. *Mov. Disord.* 32, 739–749. doi: 10.1002/mds.26942

Hoban, A. E., Stilling, R. M., M. Moloney, G., Moloney, R. D., Shanahan, F., Dinan, T. G., et al. (2017a). Microbial regulation of microRNA expression in the amygdala and prefrontal cortex. *Microbiome* 5:102. doi: 10.1186/s40168-017-0321-3

Hoban, A. E., Stilling, R. M., Moloney, G., Shanahan, F., Dinan, T. G., Clarke, G., et al. (2017b). The microbiome regulates amygdala-dependent fear recall. *Mol. Psychiatry.* doi: 10.1038/mp.2017.100. [Epub ahead of print].

Holzer, P., and Farzi, A. (2014). "Neuropeptides and the microbiota-gut-brain axis," in *Microbial Endocrinology: The Microbiota-Gut-Brain Axis in Health and Disease, Advances in Experimental Medicine and Biology*, eds M. Lyte and J. F. Cryan (New York, NY: Elsevier), chapter 9, 195–219.

Horiuchi, Y., Kimura, R., Kato, N., Fujii, T., Seki, M., Endo, T., et al. (2003). Evolutional study on acetylcholine expression. *Life Sci.* 72, 1745–1756. doi: 10.1016/S0024-3205(02)02478-5

Imbrici, P., Camerino, D. C., and Tricarico, D. (2013). Major channels involved in neuropsychiatric disorders and therapeutic perspectives. *Front. Genet.* 4:76. doi: 10.3389/fgene.2013.00076

Jiang, H., Ling, Z., Zhang, Y., Mao, H., Ma, Z., Yin, Y., et al. (2015). Altered fecal microbiota composition in patients with major depressive disorder. *Brain Behav. Immun.* 48, 186–194. doi: 10.1016/j.bbi.2015.03.016

Kelly, J. R., Borre, Y., O' Brien, C., Patterson, E., El Aidy, S., Deane, J., et al. (2016). Transferring the blues: depression-associated gut microbiota induces neurobehavioural changes in the rat. *J. Psychiatr. Res.* 82, 109–18. doi: 10.1016/j.jpsychires.2016.07.019

Keshavarzian, A., Green, S. J., Engen, P. A., Voigt, R. M., Naqib, A., Forsyth, C. B., et al. (2015). Colonic bacterial composition in Parkinson's disease. *Mov. Disord.* 30, 1351–1360. doi: 10.1002/mds.26307

Kim, T., Vidal, G. S., Djurisic, M., William, C. M., Birnbaum, M. E., Garcia, K. C., et al. (2013). Human LilrB2 is a β-amyloid receptor and its murine homolog PirB regulates synaptic plasticity in an Alzheimer's model. *Science* 341, 1399–1404. doi: 10.1126/science.1242077

Letellier, M., Willson, M. L., Gautheron, V., Mariani, J., and Lohof, A. M. (2008). Normal adult climbing fiber monoinnervation of cerebellar Purkinje cells in mice lacking MHC class I molecules. *Dev. Neurobiol.* 68, 997–1006. doi: 10.1002/dneu.20639

Li, W., Wu, X., Hu, X., Wang, T., Liang, S., Duan, Y., et al. (2017). Structural changes of gut microbiota in Parkinson's disease and its correlation with clinical features. *Sci. China. Life Sci.* 60, 1223–1233. doi: 10.1007/s11427-016-9001-4

Loke, Y. J., Hannan, A. J., and Craig, J. M. (2015). The role of epigenetic change in autism spectrum disorders. *Front. Neurol.* 6:107. doi: 10.3389/fneur.2015.00107

Lun, A. T., and Smyth, G. K. (2015). diffHic: a Bioconductor package to detect differential genomic interactions in Hi-C data. *BMC Bioinformatics* 16:258. doi: 10.1186/s12859-015-0683-0

Lyte, M. (2014). "Microbial endocrinology and the microbiota-gut-brain axis," in *Microbial Endocrinology: The Microbiota-Gut-Brain Axis in Health and Disease, 1st Edn*, eds M. Lyte and J. F. Cryan (New York, NY: Springer), chapter 1, 3–24.

MacFabe, D. F., Cain, N. E., Boon, F., Ossenkopp, K.-P., and Cain, D. P. (2011). Effects of the enteric bacterial metabolic product propionic acid on object-directed behavior, social behavior, cognition, and neuroinflammation in adolescent rats: relevance to autism spectrum disorder. *Behav. Brain Res.* 217, 47–54. doi: 10.1016/j.bbr.2010.10.005

Maqsood, R., and Stone, T. W. (2016). The gut-brain axis, BDNF, NMDA and CNS disorders. *Neurochem. Res.* 41, 2819–2835. doi: 10.1007/s11064-016-2039-1

McCarthy, D. J., Chen, Y., and Smyth, G. K. (2012). Differential expression analysis of multifactor RNA-Seq experiments with respect to biological variation. *Nucleic Acids Res.* 40, 4288–4297. doi: 10.1093/nar/gks042

McConnell, M. J., Huang, Y. H., Datwani, A., and Shatz, C. J. (2009). H2-Kb and H2-Db regulate cerebellar long-term depression and limit motor learning. *Proc. Natl. Acad. Sci. U.S.A.* 106, 6784–6789. doi: 10.1073/pnas.0902018106

Messaoudi, M., Lalonde, R., Violle, N., Javelot, H., Desor, D., Nejdi, A., et al. (2011). Assessment of psychotropic-like properties of a probiotic formulation (Lactobacillus helveticus R0052 and Bifidobacterium longum R0175) in rats and human subjects. *Br. J. Nutr.* 105, 755–764. doi: 10.1017/S0007114510004319

Meyer, K. D., Saletore, Y., Zumbo, P., Elemento, O., Mason, C. E., and Jaffrey, S. R. (2012). Comprehensive analysis of mRNA methylation reveals enrichment in 3' UTRs and near stop codons. *Cell* 149, 1635–1646. doi: 10.1016/j.cell.2012.05.003

Mourre, C., Manrique, C., Camon, J., Aidi-Knani, S., Deltheil, T., Turle-Lorenzo, N., et al. (2017). Changes in SK channel expression in the basal ganglia after partial nigrostriatal dopamine lesions in rats: functional consequences. *Neuropharmacology* 113(Pt A), 519–532. doi: 10.1016/j.neuropharm.2016.11.003

Mulder, I. E., Schmidt, B., Stokes, C. R., Lewis, M., Bailey, M., Aminov, R. I., et al. (2009). Environmentally-acquired bacteria influence microbial diversity and natural innate immune responses at gut surfaces. *BMC Biol.* 7:79. doi: 10.1186/1741-7007-7-79

Nair, V. D., and Ge, Y. (2016). Alterations of miRNAs reveal a dysregulated molecular regulatory network in Parkinson's disease striatum. *Neurosci. Lett.* 629, 99–104. doi: 10.1016/j.neulet.2016.06.061

Neufeld, K. M., Kang, N., Bienenstock, J., and Foster, J. A. (2011). Reduced anxiety-like behavior and central neurochemical change in germ-free mice. *Neurogastroenterol. Motil.* 23, 255–264. doi: 10.1111/j.1365-2982.2010.01620.x

Parashar, A., and Udayabanu, M. (2017). Gut microbiota: Implications in Parkinson's disease. *Parkinsonism Relat. Disord.* 38, 1–7. doi: 10.1016/j.parkreldis.2017.02.002

Parracho, H. M. R. T., Bingham, M. O., Gibson, G. R., and McCartney, A. L. (2005). Differences between the gut microflora of children with autistic spectrum disorders and that of healthy children. *J. Med. Microbiol.* 54(Pt 10), 987–991. doi: 10.1099/jmm.0.46101-0

Pereira, R. A., and Simmons, A. (1999). Cell surface expression of H2 antigens on primary sensory neurons in response to acute but not latent herpes simplex virus infection *in vivo*. *J. Virol.* 73, 6484–6489.

Prabowo, A. S., Iyer, A. M., Anink, J. J., Spliet, W. G. M., van Rijen, P. C., and Aronica, E. (2013). Differential expression of major histocompatibility complex class I in developmental glioneuronal lesions. *J. Neuroinflammation* 10:12. doi: 10.1186/1742-2094-10-12

Rea, K., Dinan, T. G., and Cryan, J. F. (2016). The microbiome: a key regulator of stress and neuroin flammation. *Neurobiol. Stress* 4, 23–33. doi: 10.1016/j.ynstr.2016.03.001

Rehfeld, J. F. (2014). Gastrointestinal hormones and their targets. *Adv Exp. Med. Biol.* 817, 157–175. doi: 10.1007/978-1-4939-0897-4_7

Reig-Viader, R., Sindreu, C., and Bayés, A. (2017). Synaptic proteomics as a means to identify the molecular basis of mental illness: are we getting there? *Prog. Neuropsychopharmacol. Biol. Psychiatry.* doi: 10.1016/j.pnpbp.2017.09.011. [Epub ahead of print].

Renthal, W., Maze, I., Krishnan, V., Covington, H. E., Xiao, G., Kumar, A., et al. (2007). Histone deacetylase 5 epigenetically controls behavioral adaptations to chronic emotional stimuli. *Neuron* 56, 517–529. doi: 10.1016/j.neuron.2007.09.032

Ribic, A., Flügge, G., Schlumbohm, C., Mätz-Rensing, K., Walter, L., and Fuchs, E. (2011). Activity-dependent regulation of MHC class I expression in the developing primary visual cortex of the common marmoset monkey. *Behav. Brain Funct.* 7:1. doi: 10.1186/1744-9081-7-1

Roeper, J. (2017). Closing gaps in brain disease-from overlapping genetic architecture to common motifs of synapse dysfunction. *Curr. Opin. Neurobiol.* 48, 45–51. doi: 10.1016/j.conb.2017.09.007

Rook, G. A. W., Raison, C. L., and Lowry, C. A. (2014). Microbiota, immunoregulatory old friends and psychiatric disorders. *Adv. Exp. Med. Biol.* 817, 319–356. doi: 10.1007/978-1-4939-0897-4_15

Sarkar, A., Lehto, S. M., Harty, S., Dinan, T. G., Cryan, J. F., and Burnet, P. W. (2016). Psychobiotics and the Manipulation of BacteriaGutBrain Signals. *Trends Neurosci.* 39, 763–781. doi: 10.1016/j.tins.2016.09.002

Scheperjans, F., Aho, V., Pereira, P. A. B., Koskinen, K., Paulin, L., Pekkonen, E., et al. (2015). Gut microbiota are related to Parkinson's disease and clinical phenotype. *Mov. Disord.* 30, 350–358. doi: 10.1002/mds. 26069

Seeburg, P. H., Single, F., Kuner, T., Higuchi, M., and Sprengel, R. (2001). Genetic manipulation of key determinants of ion flow in glutamate receptor channels in the mouse. *Brain Res.* 907, 233–243. doi: 10.1016/S0006-8993(01)02 445-3

Shatz, C. J. (2009). MHC Class I: an unexpected role in neuronal plasticity. *Neuron* 64, 40–45. doi: 10.1016/j.neuron.2009.09.044

Sudo, N., Chida, Y., Aiba, Y., Sonoda, J., Oyama, N., Yu, X.-N., et al. (2004). Postnatal microbial colonization programs the hypothalamic-pituitary-adrenal system for stress response in mice. *J. Physiol.* 558(Pt 1), 263–275. doi: 10.1113/jphysiol.2004.063388

Sullivan, P. F., Daly, M. J., and O'Donovan, M. (2012). Genetic architectures of psychiatric disorders: the emerging picture and its implications. *Nat. Rev. Genet.* 13, 537–551. doi: 10.1038/nrg3240

Tan, C. L., Plotkin, J. L., Veno, M. T., von Schimmelmann, M., Feinberg, P., Mann, S., et al. (2013). MicroRNA-128 governs neuronal excitability and motor behavior in mice. *Science* 342, 1254–1258. doi: 10.1126/science.1244193

Tillisch, K., Mayer, E., Gupta, A., Gill, Z., Brazeilles, R., Le Nevé, B., et al. (2017). Brain structure and response to emotional stimuli as related to gut microbial profiles in healthy women. *Psychos. Med.* 79, 905–913. doi: 10.1097/PSY.0000000000000493

Tsankova, N. M., Berton, O., Renthal, W., Kumar, A., Neve, R. L., and Nestler, E. J. (2006). Sustained hippocampal chromatin regulation in a mouse model of depression and antidepressant action. *Nat. Neurosci.* 9, 519–525. doi: 10.1038/nn1659

Vitaliti, G., Pavone, P., Mahmood, F., Nunnari, G., and Falsaperla, R. (2014). Targeting inflammation as a therapeutic strategy for drug-resistant epilepsies: an update of new immune-modulating approaches. *Hum. Vaccin. Immunother.* 10, 868–875. doi: 10.4161/hv.28400

Wahlstedt, H., Daniel, C., Enstero, M., and Ohman, M. (2009). Large-scale mRNA sequencing determines global regulation of RNA editing during brain development. *Genome Res.* 19, 978–986. doi: 10.1101/gr.089409.108

Wall, R., Cryan, J. F., Ross, R. P., Fitzgerald, G. F., Dinan, T. G., and Stanton, C. (2014). "Bacterial Neuroactive Compounds Produced by Psychobiotics," in *Microbial Endocrinology: The Microbiota-Gut-Brain Axis in Health and Disease. Advances in Experimental Medicine and Biology, 1st Edn*, eds M. Lyte and J. Cryan (New York, NY: Springer), chapter 10, 221–239.

Waszkielewicz, A. M., Gunia, A., Szkaradek, N., Sloczynska, K., Krupinska, S., and Marona, H. (2013). Ion channels as drug targets in central nervous system disorders. *Curr. Med. Chem.* 20, 1241–1285. doi: 10.2174/0929867311320100005

Wiley, N. C., Dinan, T. G., Ross, R. P., Stanton, C., Clarke, G., and Cryan, J. F. (2017). The microbiota-gut-brain axis as a key regulator of neural function and the stress response: implications for human and animal health. *J. Anim. Sci.* 95:3225. doi: 10.2527/jas.2016.1256

Wu, Z.-P., Bilousova, T., Escande-Beillard, N., Dang, H., Hsieh, T., Tian, J., et al. (2011). Major histocompatibility complex class I-mediated inhibition of neurite outgrowth from peripheral nerves. *Immunol. Lett.* 135, 118–123. doi: 10.1016/j.imlet.2010.10.011

Yogeeswari, P., Ragavendran, J. V., Thirumurugan, R., Saxena, A., and Sriram, D. (2004). Ion channels as important targets for antiepileptic drug design. *Curr. Drug Targets* 5, 589–602. doi: 10.2174/1389450043345227

Zheng, P., Zeng, B., Zhou, C., Liu, M., Fang, Z., Xu, X., et al. (2016). Gut microbiome remodeling induces depressive-like behaviors through a pathway mediated by the host's metabolism. *Mol. Psychiatry* 21, 786–96. doi: 10.1038/mp.2016.44

19

A New Age-Structured Multiscale Model of the Hepatitis C Virus Life-Cycle During Infection and Therapy with Direct-Acting Antiviral Agents

Barbara de M. Quintela[1], *Jessica M. Conway*[2], *James M. Hyman*[3], *Jeremie Guedj*[4], *Rodrigo W. dos Santos*[1], *Marcelo Lobosco*[1] *and Alan S. Perelson*[5*]

[1] FISIOCOMP Laboratory, PPGMC, Universidade Federal de Juiz de Fora, Juiz de Fora, Brazil, [2] Department of Mathematics and Center for Infectious Disease Dynamics, The Pennsylvania State University, State College, PA, United States, [3] Mathematics Department, Tulane University, New Orleans, LA, United States, [4] IAME, UMR 1137, Institut National de la Santé et de la Recherche Médicale, Université Paris Diderot, Sorbonne Paris Cité, Paris, France, [5] Theoretical Biology and Biophysics, Los Alamos National Laboratory, Los Alamos, NM, United States

***Correspondence:**
Alan S. Perelson
asp@lanl.gov

The dynamics of hepatitis C virus (HCV) RNA during translation and replication within infected cells were added to a previous age-structured multiscale mathematical model of HCV infection and treatment. The model allows the study of the dynamics of HCV RNA inside infected cells as well as the release of virus from infected cells and the dynamics of subsequent new cell infections. The model was used to fit *in vitro* data and estimate parameters characterizing HCV replication. This is the first model to our knowledge to consider both positive and negative strands of HCV RNA with an age-structured multiscale modeling approach. Using this model we also studied the effects of direct-acting antiviral agents (DAAs) in blocking HCV RNA intracellular replication and the release of new virions and fit the model to *in vivo* data obtained from HCV-infected subjects under therapy.

Keywords: computational biology, HCV, RNA, DAAs, differential equations

INTRODUCTION

Chronic hepatitis C virus (HCV) infection affects about 130–150 million people worldwide and is the primary cause of liver cirrhosis and liver cancer (WHO, 2016). HCV has a linear positive strand RNA molecule with ~9,600 nucleotides as its genome and has been classified as belonging to the genus *Hepacivirus* in the *Flaviridae* family (Appel et al., 2006; Gastaminza et al., 2008). For many years HCV replication was not completely understood due to the inability to culture virus *in vitro*. However, the development of an HCV cell culture (HCVcc) system has allowed investigation of the processes that govern HCV replication and other features of its life cycle (Appel et al., 2006; Elliot et al., 2009; Afzal et al., 2015). Moreover, new means of distinguishing and quantifying both positive and negative HCV RNA strands have been developed and improved (Bessaud et al., 2001; Craggs et al., 2001).

HCV primarily infects liver cells, called hepatocytes. After entry into a hepatocyte, the positive strand HCV RNA is uncoated and translated into a polyprotein from which all HCV proteins are produced. The HCV NS5B RNA-dependent RNA polymerase copies the positive HCV RNA into one or more HCV RNA negative strands. The nonstructural HCV proteins together with negative strand HCV RNA form replication complexes, the molecular machines responsible for producing more positive strands of HCV RNA (Quinkert et al., 2005). The newly produced positive strands can either be used for translation, replication or be assembled into virus particles and exported from the infected cell. How the decision among the options is made remains unclear (Appel et al., 2006; Elliot et al., 2009; Bisceglie, 2010). HCV RNA replication depends not only on HCV proteins but host factors also play an important role (Scheller et al., 2009; Jangra et al., 2010).

Guedj et al. (2013) developed an age-structured multiscale model of HCV infection and treatment including the dynamics of intracellular viral RNA (vRNA). The model has been analyzed mathematically and various approximate solutions derived (Rong et al., 2013; Rong and Perelson, 2013).

Age-structured models have been widely used to study the epidemiology of infectious diseases, such as HIV (Thieme and Castillo-Chavez, 1993), hepatitis C (Martcheva and Castillo-Chavez, 2003) and tuberculosis (Castillo-Chavez and Feng, 1997; Thieme and Castillo-Chavez, 2002). Nelson et al. (2004) presented an age-structured model of the dynamics of within host HIV. Gilchrist et al. (2004) used an age-structured model to explore how the intracellular HIV production rate influenced the virus' fitness. One advantage of using such an approach is the possibility of considering that individuals or cells with distinct ages could behave differently (Li and Brauer, 2008). Using that approach in modeling the dynamics of virus within a host allows a realistic representation of infection biology in which the rate of production and release of new virus is not constant but rather depends on the length of time a cell has been infected. Moreover, the model can also account for an infected cell death rate that depends on the time the cell has been infected.

The Guedj et al. (2013) age-structured multiscale model of HCV infection only considered the dynamics of positive strand HCV RNA. Guedj and Neumann (2010) studied the intracellular dynamics of both positive- and negative-strand viral RNA. They used ordinary differential equations to represent the number of positive-strands of viral RNA, available for transcription and translation, and the number of negative-strands of viral RNA or "replication units." Benzine et al. (2017) developed a more detailed ordinary differential equation model in which they distinguished positive strand HCV RNA used for translation, replication and viral assembly. However, both Guedj and Neumann (2010) and Benzine et al. (2017) did not consider that the number of positive and negative strands of viral RNA depend on how long a cell has been infected.

Here we used a three-equation age-structured model for intracellular HCV RNA dynamics, introduced by Quintela et al. (2017), which incorporated negative strand HCV RNA as well as the positive-strand HCV RNA available for translation and replication separately and validated the model by comparison to *in vitro* experiments. We then coupled this intracellular model to a well-established cell infection model and showed the model was able to fit *in vivo* viral load data obtained from patients treated with direct acting antiviral (DAA) therapy.

MATERIALS AND METHODS

Intracellular Model of HCV Replication

We developed a mathematical model to represent the intracellular replication of HCV shown schematically in **Figure 1**. The model allows the study of aspects such as translation of positive-strand HCV RNA after cell entry, transfer of the positive strand to the membranous web where it is used for replication, production of negative- and positive-strand HCV RNA within replication complexes and secretion of positive-strand RNA as virions. The replication of HCV RNA has been studied in detail c.f. (Chatel-Chaix and Bartenschlager, 2014; Li et al., 2015).

The system of ordinary differential equations used to represent the dynamics of intracellular infection over time is

$$\begin{cases} \frac{d}{da}R_t = \theta R_c - (\sigma + \rho(a) + \mu_t)R_t, \\ \frac{d}{da}R_c = \alpha R_m + \sigma R_t - (\theta + \rho(a) + \mu_c)R_c, \\ \frac{d}{da}R_m = r(1 - \frac{R_m}{R_{max}})R_c - \mu_c R_m, \end{cases} \tag{1}$$
$$R_t(0) = R_{t_0}, \quad R_c(0) = 0, \quad R_m(0) = 0,$$

where R_t represents positive strand HCV RNA used for translation, R_c represents positive strands within replication complexes used for replication, R_m represents minus (or negative) strand RNA and a represents the time a cell has been infected. Positive strand HCV RNA forms the viral genome. After cell entry, cellular machinery translates this positive strand RNA into a polyprotein in the cytoplasm (Shi and Lai, 2006). However,

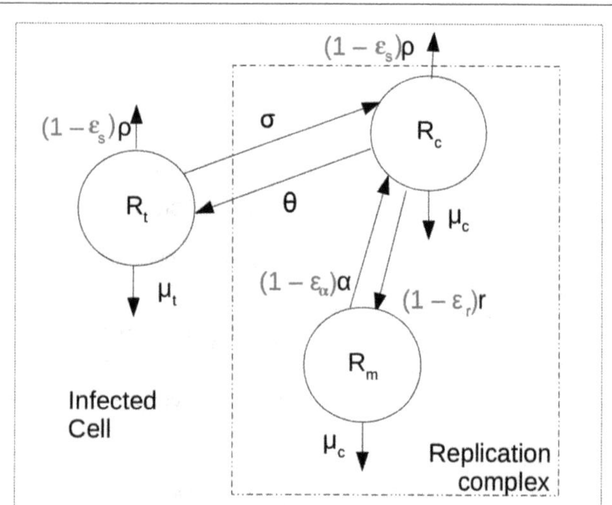

FIGURE 1 | Intracellular model scheme. After cell entry positive strand HCV RNA is available for translation, represented by R_t. It can be exported at rate ρ and decay at rate μ_t. Negative or minus strand HCV RNA (R_m) is produced at maximum rate r and forms the replication complexes that produce more positive strand RNA (R_c) at rate α. It is assumed that HCV RNA inside the replication complex in both orientations have the same decay rate μ_c. The positive strand HCV RNA available for translation is assumed to move into replication complexes at rate σ and from replication complexes at rate θ. The terms in red represent the action of therapy in blocking secretion and production of viral RNA.

after polyproteins are made the positive strand must also be used for replication and must be copied into minus stand RNA. We assume that the positive-strand HCV RNA used for translation (R_t in Equation 1) moves from the cytoplasm into what is called the membranous web and interacts with the proteins needed for replication to become a species we call R_c at rate σ per strand. We also assume the positive strand in the cytoplasm, R_t has a natural decay rate of μ_t per strand. Lastly, positive strands need to be assembled into virions which are then exported from the infected cell. Virion assembly occurs in association with cytosolic lipid droplets (Chatel-Chaix and Bartenschlager, 2014). As it is not clear whether the positive strand RNA in the membranous web needs first to be transported into the cytosol for viral assembly, we assume both R_t and R_c can be assembled into virions and exported at rate $\rho(a)$. The time-dependence of ρ will be discussed below. Further, we assume positive-strand HCV RNA in the replication complex (R_c) can move out of the replication complex and membranous web and back into the cytoplasm to become R_t at rate θ. More detailed models can be developed that separate virion assembly from secretion and that include a separate compartment of positive strand RNA used for virion assembly (cf. Benzine et al., 2017), but here for simplicity we have combined these steps.

Minus-strand HCV RNA (R_m) is formed in the replication complex by copying the positive strand R_c at maximum rate r. As in Guedj and Neumann (2010), it is assumed that host factors limit the replication of negative-strand RNAs, so that as the maximum number R_{max} is reached replication slows according to a logistic growth law. The positive strands in replication complexes, R_c, are copied from the negative strand template at rate α per template. We consider that both R_c and R_m are in the replication complex and decay at the same *per capita* rate μ_c.

In order to have a positive equilibrium when the model represents an established infection, the parameters need to satisfy the relations: $\phi_2 > \frac{\sigma\theta}{\phi_1}$ and $\alpha r > (\phi_2 - \frac{\sigma\theta}{\phi_1})\mu_c$ in which $\phi_1 = \theta + \rho + \mu_t$ and $\phi_2 = \sigma + \rho + \mu_c$.

Delay in Particle Assembly

Following translation and replication, positive-strand HCV RNA is assembled into a virus particle that can then be exported out of the cell (Lindenbach and Rice, 2013). Such assembly can not begin immediately after infection as viral proteins are needed as components of the virion and hence first need to be produced. The release of virus by an infected cell *in vitro* is observed approximately 12 h after infection (Keum et al., 2012).

To incorporate this biological delay, τ, we assume the viral secretion rate is a function of the length of time a cell has been infected, i.e., its age of infection. The function we use is

$$\rho(a) = \begin{cases} 0, & a < \tau \\ (1 - e^{-k(a-\tau)})\rho, & \text{otherwise,} \end{cases} \tag{2}$$

where $a = 0$ is the time of infection and the constant ρ is the maximum secretion rate. This functional form was chosen to avoid any discontinuities.

When we analyze *in vitro* experiments, the kinetics of secreted HCV RNA, R_s can be represented by the differential equation

$$\begin{cases} \frac{d}{da}R_s = \rho(a)(R_t + R_c) - c_s R_s \\ R_s(0) = 0, \end{cases} \tag{3}$$

where $\rho(a)$ is the secretion rate and c_s is the rate of clearance or degradation of secreted HCV RNA, which is estimated from the data.

Coupling of Multiple Scales

We also analyze *in vivo* data in which the effects of antiviral treatment on kinetics of HCV RNA levels in plasma are measured. To fit this data we introduced a new multiscale model depicted in **Figure 2**.

The intracellular portion of the multiscale model with treatment is represented by the following partial differential equations (PDEs) in which t represents clock time and a the age of an infected cell:

$$\begin{cases} \frac{\partial}{\partial t}R_t(a,t) + \frac{\partial}{\partial a}R_t(a,t) = \theta R_c - (\sigma + (1-\epsilon_s)\rho(a) + \kappa_t\mu_t)R_t, \\ \frac{\partial}{\partial t}R_c(a,t) + \frac{\partial}{\partial a}R_c(a,t) = (1-\epsilon_\alpha)\alpha R_m + \sigma R_t - \\ \qquad (\theta + (1-\epsilon_s)\rho(a) + \kappa_c\mu_c)R_c, \\ \frac{\partial}{\partial t}R_m(a,t) + \frac{\partial}{\partial a}R_m(a,t) = (1-\epsilon_r)r(1 - \frac{R_m}{R_{max}})R_c - \kappa_c\mu_c R_m, \end{cases}$$
$$R_t(0,t) = R_{t_0}, \quad R_t(a,0) = \overline{R}_t(a), \tag{4}$$
$$R_c(0,t) = 0, \quad R_c(a,0) = \overline{R}_c(a),$$
$$R_m(0,t) = 0, \quad R_m(a,0) = \overline{R}_m(a).$$

We have assumed that intracellular infection is initiated by the introduction of R_{t_0} positive HCV RNA strands into the cytoplasm of a cell. Typically, we shall assume that infection is the result of a single virion, carrying a single positive-strand HCV RNA, entering a cell, so that $R_{t_0} = 1$. Further, we shall assume that the individual's being treated with antivirals are chronically infected and have reached steady state in which $\overline{R}_t(a)$, $\overline{R}_c(a)$ and $\overline{R}_m(a)$ are the steady state distributions of positive-strand HCV RNA in translation and in replication complexes and negative-strand HCV RNA in replication complexes, respectively, in the absence of treatment and are given by the steady state solutions of the ODEs in Equation (1). Further, we let ϵ_α be the effectiveness of therapy in decreasing or blocking positive-strand RNA replication, ϵ_r the effectiveness of therapy in decreasing or blocking negative-strand RNA replication, and ϵ_s the effectiveness of therapy in decreasing or blocking secretion of positive-strand RNA, where for each of the ϵ's, $\epsilon = 1$ corresponds to a 100% effective drug and $\epsilon = 0$ corresponds to a completely ineffective or absent drug. Further κ_t is a factor by which therapy changes the degradation rate of positive-strand RNA used for translation and κ_c is the factor by which therapy changes the degradation rate of both positive and negative strand RNA in replication complexes.

To complete the multiscale model, we then coupled the intracellular model to an established HCV cellular infection

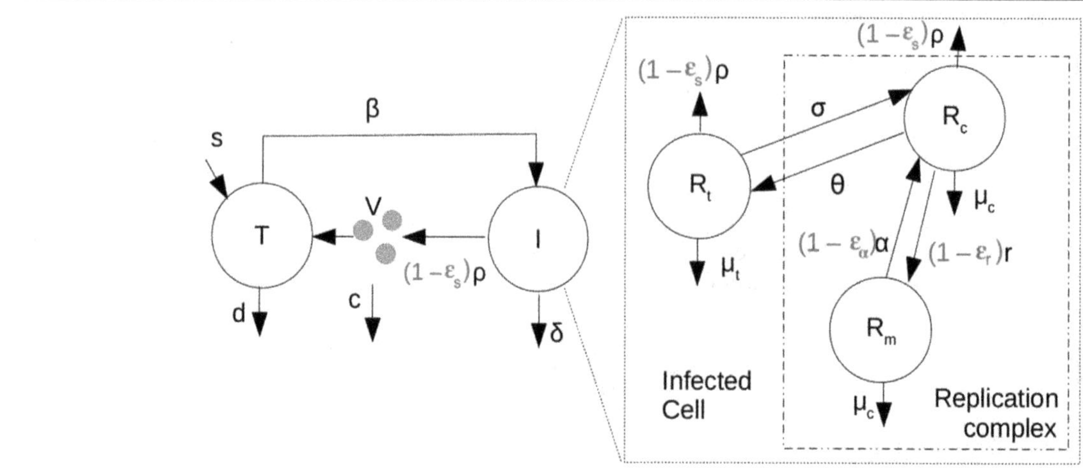

FIGURE 2 | Scheme representing the coupled multiscale model with therapy (parameters in red). T are target cells, I, infected cells and V, the HCV RNA concentration in plasma. Target cells become infected at rate β.

model (Equation 5) (Neumann et al., 1998; Canini and Perelson, 2014).

$$\begin{cases} \frac{d}{dt}T(t) = s - \beta V(t)T(t) - dT(t), \\ \frac{\partial}{\partial t}I(a,t) + \frac{\partial}{\partial a}I(a,t) = -\delta(a)I(a,t), \\ \frac{d}{dt}V(t) = (1-\epsilon_s)\int_0^\infty \rho(a)(R_t(a,t) + R_c(a,t))I(a,t)da - cV(t), \end{cases}$$
$$T(0) = T_0,$$
$$I(0,t) = \beta V(t)T(t), \qquad I(a,0) = \bar{I}(a),$$
$$V(0) = V_0, \tag{5}$$

in which, T are target cells, I, infected cells and V the HCV RNA concentration in plasma. Target cells become infected at rate β, have a constant source rate s and a natural per capita decay rate d. The parameter $\delta(a)$ represents the death rate of an infected cell of age "a" and the effects of therapy on the virus export are given by ϵ_s. Here for simplicity we shall only analyze the case in which $\delta(a)$ is a constant, δ. Virus in the plasma is cleared from the circulation at per capita rate c. Here we have assumed that at $t = 0$, the time therapy starts, the system is in steady state, where $\bar{I}(a)$ is the steady-state distribution of infected cells, which can be shown to be $\bar{I}(a) = \beta V_0 T_0 e^{-\delta a}$. $T_0 = \frac{c}{\beta N}$, where N is the steady state total amount of virus secreted by an infected cell over its lifetime, $N = \rho\int_0^\infty(\bar{R}_t(a) + \bar{R}_c(a)e^{-\delta a}da$, and $V_0 = \frac{s-dT_0}{\beta T_0}$. See Rong et al. (2013). The coupling between the intracellular and extracellular models occurs through the equation for V, the virus in the plasma. The amount of plasma virus depends on the number of infected cells and number of virions being packaged and exported per infected cell. This coupling has been used before (Guedj et al., 2013; Rong et al., 2013; Rong and Perelson, 2013).

Numerical Algorithms

The model equations were discretized in space, i.e., age, and integrated in time using the method of lines (MOL) approach (Sadiku and Obiozor, 2000; Shakeri and Dehghan, 2008) where the partial derivatives in age were approximated by finite-differences and the solution at the grid points was integrated along lines in time. We integrated the equations using the Matlab® ordinary differential equation Runge-Kutta solver *ode45*.

The domain was discretized on a uniform grid of 201 mesh points between ages 0 and 50 days, as it is unlikely for an infected cell to live longer than this. The boundary of domain at $a = 50$ was defined as a simple outflow boundary condition and was incorporated into the numerical solution by linearly extrapolating the solution to two buffer grid points outside the domain. The partial derivatives in age were approximated with fourth-order centered finite differences.

We verified the convergence of the numerical solution to an accuracy of 10^{-3} by varying the number of spatial grid points and the time integration error tolerance.

The simulation time was varied according to the length of time that virus was detected in plasma after therapy initiation in the data we analyzed. The computer run time were typically a few seconds for a single simulation using a laptop computer.

We used the Matlab® nonlinear optimization program *fmincon* to fit the solutions of the model to the experimental data by minimizing the L_2 norm of the residual difference between the model solution and the data. This routine was chosen due to the possibility of specifying lower and upper bounds for the parameters we wanted to estimate. The algorithm we used was *"interior-point"* as it satisfies the bounds at all iterations.

The data we fit to validate the model was obtained from different sources. We extracted *in vitro* data from Keum et al. (2012) and Binder et al. (2013) using the on-line tool WebPlotDigitizer (Rohatgi, 2016). We also fit clinical trial data from Guedj et al. (2013) that we had access to.

Because our models have a large number of parameters we numerically approximated the Hessian of the objective function at the optimal parameter values. At a minimum, the gradient of the objective function is zero. If an eigenvalue of the Hessian is zero at the minimum, then the gradient remains zero along the direction of the associated eigenvector. That is, the solution is not unique (identifiable) (Beck, 2014). Here, for each of the data sets we fit, at the optimum, all of the eigenvalues of the Hessian were positive, and the condition number was below 10^4, indicating that the parameters were locally identifiable.

RESULTS

Calibrating Intracellular Parameters in the Absence of Therapy

To validate the intracellular mathematical model, we first compared the results of Equation (1) to transfection experiments performed by Binder et al. (2013). In that paper the authors used two distinct cell lines to assess HCV RNA replication over 72 h: (a) Huh7-Lunet cells which are highly permissive to HCV RNA replication and (b) Huh7 cells (Huh7-lp) which presents lower levels of HCV RNA replication. They measured positive-strand and negative-strand RNA by strand specific quantitative Northern blotting. Binder et al. (2013) developed a complex mathematical model that included 13 molecular species with 16 parameters in two compartments: the cytoplasm and a replication compartment.

Using the three equation mathematical model, Equation (1), we were able to fit the dynamics of both positive and negative strand HCV RNA in both the high and low permissive cell lines (**Figure 3**). Our model was able to replicate the initial decay seen after transfection with both types of cells and the plateau during the 72 h measured (**Figures 3A,B**).

In fitting the data, the parameters used to describe the age-dependent virion export rate, $\rho(a)$, were fixed at $\rho = 0.1$ d^{-1}, $\tau = 0.5$ d^{-1} and $k = 0.8$ d^{-1}. We set τ at 0.5 d^{-1} based on the fact that Keum et al. (2012) could not detect any extracellular virus until 12 h post-infection. We further tested different values of τ and k and chose the values that gave the best fits to the data in both the Binder and Keum experiments. Choosing the export rate as a time-dependent function rather than a constant allowed us to have an initial delay followed by a smooth transition to the maximum export ρ. Regarding the maximum export rate, ρ, we at first chose the value estimated by Guedj et al. (2013) based on fitting *in vivo* data. However, using this value did not give good fits to the *in vitro* data. We then scanned through different values and chose the one giving the best fit. HCV uses the host cell export machinery and thus it is not surprising that these parameters differ between *in vitro* and *in vivo* systems.

The initial number of HCV positive strands introduced into these cells to initiate HCV replication in this *in vitro* system was $R_{t_0} = 4{,}000$ molecules cell^{-1}. Other parameters of the model were estimated using the *fmincon* routine in Matlab and are shown in **Table 1**.

Another form of validation we performed was testing the model predictions by comparing to positive-strand measurements using a replication deficient replicon (Binder et al., 2013). By setting the rate at which positive-strand RNA goes from use in translation to use in replication (σ) to zero we could compare the results obtained with the model to the measurements reported by Binder et al. (2013) Without replication, the initial amount of transfected HCV RNA decays exponentially and no negative-strand is formed. Further as Binder et al. show the decay of positive strand RNA is similar in both the high permissive and low permissive cell lines. We simulated the intracellular model with the parameters that were estimated for the highly-permissive cell line (**Table 1**) and the results are shown in **Figure 4**. The results using the parameters for the low permissive cell line are the same.

Sensitivity Analysis of the Intracellular Model

Forward sensitivity analysis was performed to estimate how the model solution is affected by small perturbations to each model parameter. The sensitivity index was defined as the ratio:

$$S_i = \frac{\delta J/J}{\delta p/p}, \qquad J, p \neq 0 \tag{6}$$

in which, J denotes a model output that depends on a parameter p, δ is some perturbation to the parameter p and δJ is the resulting perturbation to the output J.

The sensitivity index is a measure of the percentage of change in the output given a perturbation in each parameter. We varied by 10% the value of each parameter, while other parameters were kept the same, and calculated the sensitivity index of each parameter to the resulting value of R_t, R_c and R_m at 72 h (**Figure 5**). Positive values indicate an increase in the output given the increase in the parameter and negative values indicate that the output decreases as we increase the parameter.

The sensitivity index confirms that perturbing α, the positive-strand RNA replication rate, increases by more than 10% the amount of positive-strand RNA used for translation and in replication complexes. μ_t represents the natural decay rate of translated RNA and changes in that parameter decreases positive-strand RNA in translation and μ_c, the natural decay rate for both positive and negative strands in the replication complex, affects mainly the positive-strand RNA.

Calibrating the Intracellular Parameters for a Different *in Vitro* Experiment

We also compared the intracellular model to experiments *in vitro* performed by Keum et al. (2012) in which a high multiplicity of infection was used (MOI = 5 or 6) so that only one round of infection occurred. Theoretically, with an MOI of 5, 99.3% of cells should be infected with a least one infectious virion (Keum et al., 2012). A cell culture adapted HCV, JFH-m4, was incubated with Huh7.5.1 cells for 3 h to initiate infection. At subsequent times cells and supernatant were harvested to measure HCV RNA levels intra-cellularly and the amount secreted into the medium. Keum et al. quantified the number of positive and negative HCV RNA strands using real-time RT-PCR. As shown in **Figure 6** the number of cell-associated positive strands initially decreased reaching a minimum of about 1 positive strand per cell at 6 h post-infection (pi). Intracellular negative strand, which serves as a template for making new positive strands, was first detected at 6 h pi. Our model was able to reproduce the observed intracellular

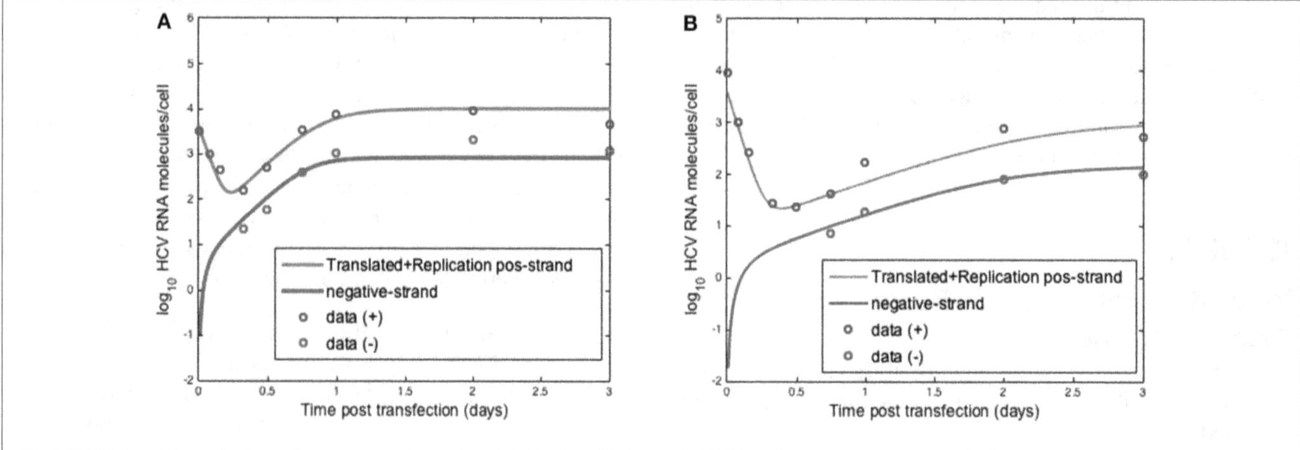

FIGURE 3 | HCV RNA replication. Circles represent experimental data from Binder et al. (2013) and lines show the results obtained with the model described herein with distinct sets of parameters for **(A)** high and **(B)** low permissive cells.

TABLE 1 | Model parameter values estimated for the *in vitro* transfection experiments in Binder et al. (2013).

Name	Huh7-Lunet	Huh7-lp	Unit	Biological meaning
α	60	20	Day^{-1}	R_c replication rate
μ_t	20	20	Day^{-1}	R_t natural decay rate
r	2.1	1	Day^{-1}	R_m replication rate
μ_c	3.4	1.7	Day^{-1}	Repl. complex decay rate
σ	0.3	0.1	Day^{-1}	Translation to repl. rate
θ	2.1	1.2	Day^{-1}	Repl. to translation rate
R_{max}	1000	200	Molecules cell^{-1}	Max. number of R_m

HCV RNA dynamics (**Figure 6**) as well as the dynamics of positive strand HCV RNA secreted into the media (**Figure 7**). As before we fixed the export rate with $\rho = 0.1$ d^{-1}, $\tau = 0.5$ d^{-1}, and $k = 0.8$ d^{-1}. The initial time $t_0 = 0$, $R_{t_0} = 12.8$ and no therapy was given (**Figure 7**). Other parameters were estimated and were found to be $\alpha = 30$ d^{-1}, $\mu_t = 24$ d^{-1}, $r = 3.18$ d^{-1}, $\mu_c = 1.05$ d^{-1}, $R_{max} = 100$ molecules, $\sigma = 0.1$ d^{-1} and $\theta = 1.2$ d^{-1}. As both the cell line and virus used in these experiments are different than the ones used by Binder et al. (2013), it is surprising that resulting parameters do not differ very much from those we estimated in the previous section for high and low-permissive cells.

In Vivo Effect of Therapy With an NS5A Inhibitor

We validated the coupled multiscale model by fitting Equations (4) and (5) to data obtained from patients treated with one dose of 10 or 100 mg of daclatasvir (DCV) (Guedj et al., 2013). DCV inhibits the action of the HCV NS5A protein, which has been shown to play an important role in HCV RNA replication and secretion (Lee, 2013; Scheel and Rice, 2013). This data was previously analyzed by Guedj et al. (2013) using a much simpler multiscale model that only considered HCV positive strand RNA dynamics.

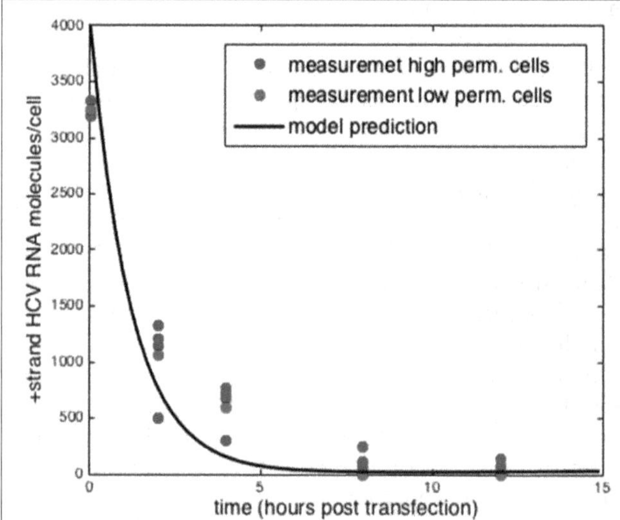

FIGURE 4 | Comparison to measurements of replication deficient HCV RNA in high and low permissive cells. Model prediction setting $\sigma = 0$ for both sets of parameters. Data taken from Binder et al. (2013).

We assumed that the parameters that represent *in vivo* infection dynamics are different from those we estimated for *in vitro* infection as both the virus and target cells are different. We also assumed that there was no superinfection, so that only one virus infects each cell. Using the same approach as for the intracellular model, we performed a sensitivity analysis of the coupled model parameters in order to determine how sensitive the predicted viral load is to each parameter. We chose to vary each parameter one at a time and compared how they affected the predicted viral load at day 2 on therapy.

The sensitivity index was calculated using Equation (6) and the results are shown in **Figure 8**. Intracellular parameters such as the replication and decay rates of HCV RNA, α, r, μ_c are the ones which the viral load is most sensitive to. The parameters that

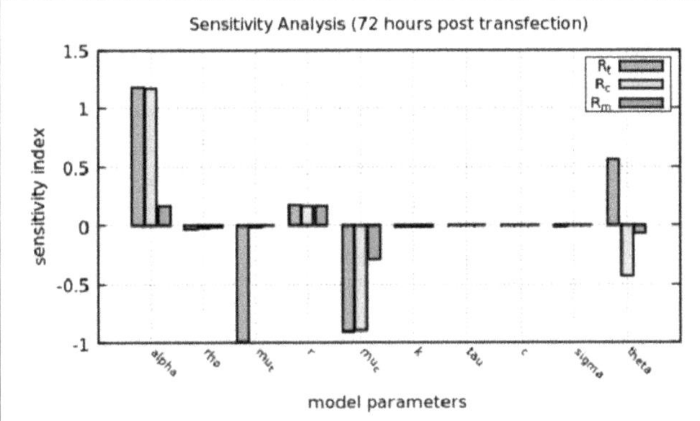

FIGURE 5 | Sensitivity analysis of the model at 72 h. The positive-strand RNA replication rate, α, the natural decay rates for positive-strand RNA used for translation and within replication complexes, μ_t and μ_c, respectively and the rate at which positive-strand RNA goes from replication complexes to the cytoplasm to be translated, θ, are the most sensitive parameters in the model.

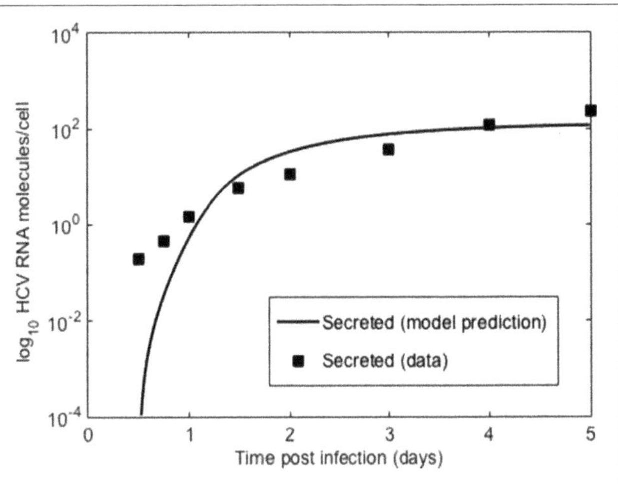

FIGURE 7 | Secreted HCV RNA. Data points from Keum et al. (2012) and lines are the model prediction based on Equation (1).

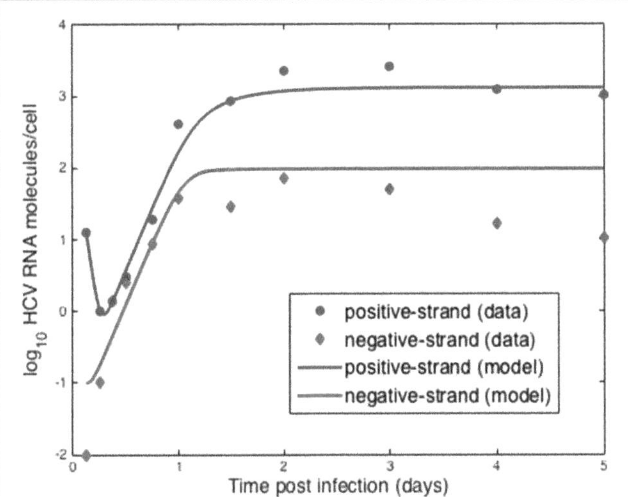

FIGURE 6 | Comparison of model results to *in vitro* infection data. Data points were extracted from Keum et al. (2012) and the lines were obtained by fitting the intracellular model to the data where we assumed the measured positive strands were the sum of the positive strands used for translation, R_t and in replication complexes, R_C. As before we fixed the export rate with $\rho = 0.1$ d^{-1}, $\tau = 0.5$ d^{-1}, and $k = 0.8$ d^{-1}. The initial time $t_0 = 0$. Based on the data we set $R_{t_0} = 12.8$. Other parameters were estimated and were found to be $\alpha = 30$ d^{-1}, $\mu_t = 24$ d^{-1}, $r = 3.18$ d^{-1}, $\mu_C = 1.05$ d^{-1}, $R_{max} = 100$ molecules, $\sigma = 0.1$ d^{-1} and $\theta = 1.2$ d^{-1}.

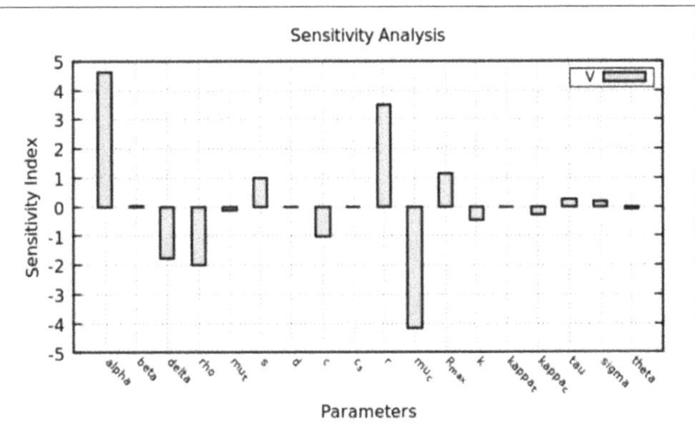

FIGURE 8 | Sensitivity analysis of the model at 2 days. The figure shows how much a perturbation of the parameters influence the viral load (V).

represents the export rate, ρ, and infected cell decay rate δ, are also important to define the viral load.

A baseline *in vivo* set of parameters was fixed based on the literature: $\alpha = 30$ d^{-1}, $\rho = 8.18$ d^{-1}, $\delta = 0.14$ d^{-1}, and c $= 22.3$ d^{-1} were taken from Rong et al. (2013) and $\epsilon_s = 0.998$ was taken from Guedj et al. (2013). The remaining parameters were estimated and their values are shown in **Table 2**.

Figures 9, 10 depict the results obtained with the multiscale model for each patient. We fixed the replication rate of positive strand HCV RNA $\alpha = 30$ d^{-1} and considered no enhancement in HCV RNA decay with therapy, $\kappa_t = \kappa_c = 1$. Our model predicted that initiation of therapy affects the replication of both positive and negative strands and that initially there is a slightly increase in the number of positive strand HCV RNAs used for translation (**Figure 10**). This increase is most likely due to the fact that DCV effectively blocks secretion of positive strands thus allowing them to accumulate in the cytoplasm. Therapy also blocks the appearance of new replication complexes, which only decrease in the presence of the drug (**Figure 10**).

DISCUSSION

HCV infection and treatment has been modeled using variants of the basic model of viral infection starting with the work of Neumann et al. (1998). This initial ordinary differential equation model was followed by others and various clinical applications were shown (Layden et al., 2003; Layden-Almer et al., 2003; Powers et al., 2003; Ribeiro et al., 2003; Dixit and Perelson, 2004; Dahari et al., 2005, 2006, 2007a,b; Shudo et al., 2008a,b; Dahari et al., 2009; Reluga et al., 2009). These models were all based on

TABLE 2 | Model parameters estimated from fitting *in vivo* patient data.

Param.	PAT 8	PAT 42	PAT 68	PAT 69	PAT 83	Mean	Range	Std	Conf.
δ	0.58	0.64	0.1	0.47	0.62	0.48	0.1–0.8	0.199	0.209
μ_t	0.89	0.89	0.88	0.89	0.89	0.89	0.8–1	0.004	0.004
r	1.49	1.1	5.08	2.24	1.61	2.3	1–6	1.435	1.506
μ_c	2.55	1.72	3.38	3.15	2.39	2.6	1–6	0.587	0.616
ϵ_α	0.928	0.909	0.992	0.936	0.924	0.937	0.9–0.99999	0.028	0.029
ϵ_r	0.47	0.12	0.61	0.36	0.29	0.37	0–0.99999	0.165	0.173

Mean values, range allowed for fitting, standard deviation and confidence interval (p = 0.05). We fixed $\alpha = 30\ d^{-1}$ and $\kappa_t = \kappa_c = 1$. The parameters ϵ_α and ϵ_r are unitless, other parameters units, per day.

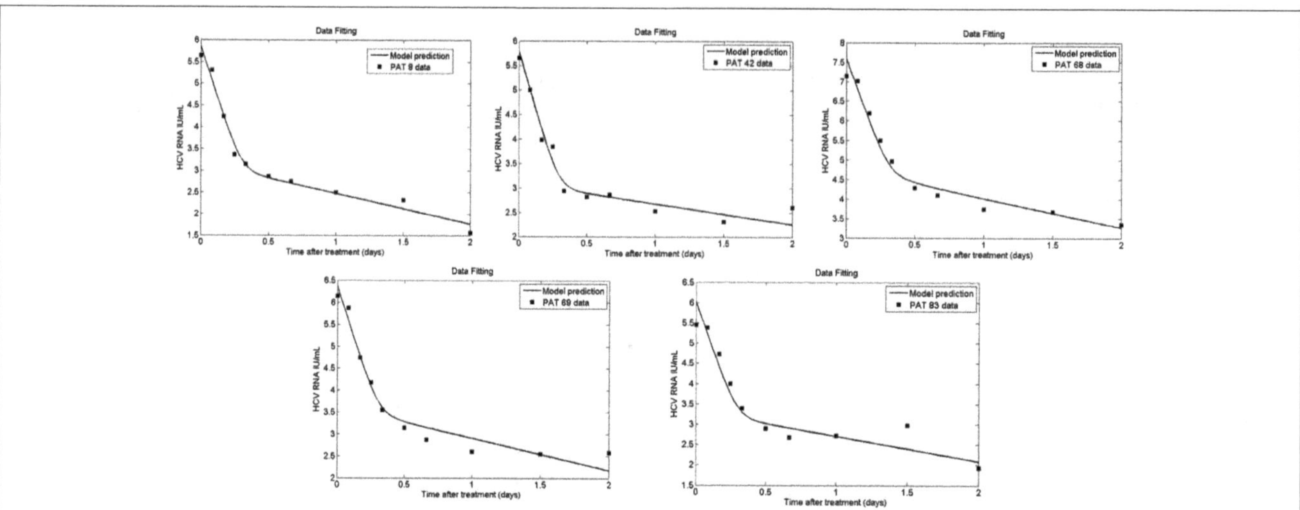

FIGURE 9 | Fit of coupled multiscale model (solid line) to patient viral load data (squares) from Guedj et al. (2013). All 5 patients were treated with one dose of 10 or 100 mg of daclatasvir. The best-fit parameters are shown in **Table 2**.

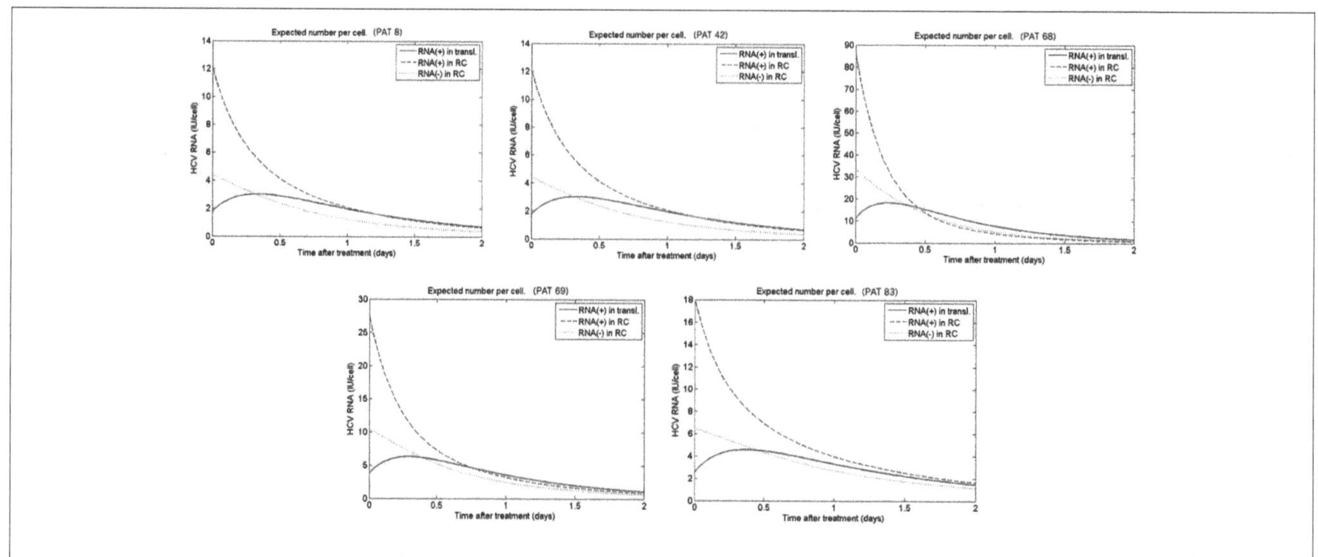

FIGURE 10 | Predicted intracellular HCV RNA obtained from fitting the patient data from Guedj et al. (2013). The best-fit parameters are shown in **Table 2**.

the standard treatment at the time using type I interferon alone or in combination with ribavirin. When new small molecule inhibitors of HCV replication, such as the protease inhibitor telaprevir, were introduced parameters that were thought to reflect the host response to infection, such as the loss rate of infected cells (Guedj and Perelson, 2011) and the clearance rate of free virus (Adiwijaya et al., 2009) were found to change with the drug being used. To make sense of these findings a multiscale model was introduced by Guedj et al. (2013) that showed that the protease inhibitor telaprevir and the HCV NS5A inhibitor daclatasvir affected both viral replication and viral production. The Guedj et al. model only included postive strand HCV RNA and did not distinguish between the various functions of this RNA. However, the model showed that to fully understand the modes of action of anti-HCV drugs one would need to develop more detailed models of the viral lifecycle and couple them to models of cellular infection. Here we have done just that.

As negative-strand HCV RNA is only synthesized during viral replication, it should be considered a more reliable marker of viral replication than positive-strand HCV RNA (Yuki et al., 2005). In this work, the dynamics of negative-strand HCV RNA during replication was added to a multiscale age-structured model of HCV infection to better represent the steps of HCV replication inside of infected cells. Moreover, the addition of positive-strand RNA used for translation to the model is a new feature that allowed us to understand the initial decay in positive strand HCV RNA observed in *in vitro* experiments (Keum et al., 2012; Binder et al., 2013) before viral replication expanded the population of positive strands. This pool of HCV RNA is also a possible target of therapy and hence it is valuable to represent it in models. Another novel feature of our model was that we modeled the rate of export of positive strand HCV RNA not as a constant but rather as an increasing function of the time a cell has been infected. In this way, the initial positive strand RNA used to infect a cell has time to replicate before it is assembled into virions. The intracellular model was fit to two different *in vitro* experiments and was able to account for the intracellular dynamics seen in both as well as for the amount of positive strand HCV RNA secreted as virions into the medium in the experiment by Keum et al. (2012).

A sensitivity analysis of both the intracellular model and the multiscale model was performed indicating that the results are more sensitive to some parameters than others. In particular, the viral load is sensitive to the choice of intracellular parameters. The choice of parameters to be estimated or fixed was based on the availability of their values in the literature and which were more influential in determining the viral load during the sensitivity analysis.

The multiscale model presented here was able to reproduce the viral load during therapy and also the intracellular concentrations of positive and negative strands of HCV RNA observed during *in vitro* transfection experiments. Interestingly, the estimates of some parameters made from *in vitro* experiments were similar to estimates made from patient data. For example, we estimated that the replication rate constant for negative strand HCV RNA in the highly permissive Huh7-Lunet cells was 2.1 d^{-1}, whereas our *in vivo* estimates varied between 1.1 d^{-1} and 5.1 d^{-1} with a mean of 2.3 d^{-1}. Similarly, we estimated that the rate of decay of replication complexes, μ_c in Huh7-Lunet cells was 3.4 d^{-1}, whereas our *in vivo* estimates ranged between 1.7 d^{-1} and 3.4 d^{-1}, with a mean of 2.6 d^{-1}. The estimate of the rate of decay of positive strands used for translation differed significantly between *in vivo* and *in vitro*, possibly due to more efficient depletion of positive strands *in vivo* by packaging into virions and secretion.

The model allows the effects of therapy to be estimated in terms of the targets: production of positive and negative stranded HCV RNA, secretion of new virions, and the enhancement in degradation of both strands of HCV RNA. Our estimate of the effectiveness of daclatasvir (DCV) treatment in blocking positive strand synthesis was between 0.91 and 0.99, whereas in Guedj et al. the mean was 0.99. More strikingly, we estimated that DCV was not nearly efficient in blocking negative strand synthesis, with estimates of ϵ_r ranging from 0.12 to 0.61 with a mean of 0.37. Thus, our model predicts that the NS5A inhibitor DCV is not very effective at blocking negative strand synthesis. This is consistent with the *in vitro* finding of McGivern et al. (2014) that NS5A inhibitors have no activity against preformed replication complexes and only inhibit the formation of new ones. If this is also true *in vivo*, then production of negative strand HCV RNA from existing replication complexes would continue in the presence of an NS5A inhibitor yielding a very low effectiveness of DCV in blocking this step of the HCV life cycle. However, preformed replication complexes also produce positive strands and why this production seems to be efficiently inhibited remains to be explained.

In summary, we have developed a new multiscale model of HCV replication and spread by cellular infection. The model is more realistic than the simple model developed by Guedj et al. (2013) that only contained positive strand RNA and more realistic than the prior model of Guedj and Neumann, which tracked positive strand RNA and replication complexes (Guedj and Neumann, 2010) but that was never fit to data. Here we showed that a model with positive strands used for translation separate from those used for replication as well as negative strands could fit both *in vitro* and *in vivo* data. More tests and refinement of the model may be needed, but it seems apparent that one does not need to introduce the complexity of the Binder model (Binder et al., 2013) or the earlier Dahari et al. model (Dahari et al., 2007c), both of which modeled HCV replication in enormous detail, in order to explain the *in vitro* and *on vivo* data analyzed here.

AUTHOR CONTRIBUTIONS

AP, JC, and JG contributed to conception and design of the study; BQ worked on the simulations, performed the statistical analysis and wrote the first draft of the manuscript; JH developed the MATLAB® solver and wrote sections of the manuscript. All authors contributed to manuscript revision, read and approved the submitted version.

FUNDING

Portions of this work were performed under the auspices of the U.S. Department of Energy under contract DE-AC52-06NA25396. This work was developed with the support of CAPES Proc. number 99999.002789/2014-00 and the Center for Nonlinear Studies, Los Alamos National Laboratory. AP acknowledges support from National Institutes Health grants R01-AI078881, R01-AI116868, R01-AI028433, and R01-OD011095. ML and RdS acknowledge support from UFJF, FAPEMIG, CNPq, and CAPES.

REFERENCES

Adiwijaya, B. S., Hare, B., Caron, P. R., Randle, J. C., Neumann, A. U., Reesink, H. W., et al. (2009). Rapid decrease of wild-type hepatitis C virus on telaprevir treatment. *Antivir. Ther.* 14, 591–595. Available online at: https://www.intmedpress.com/journals/avt/abstract.cfm?id=23&pid=88

Afzal, M. S., Alsaleh, K., Farhat, R., Belouzard, S., Danneels, A., Descamps, V., et al. (2015). Regulation of core expression during the hepatitis C virus life cycle. *J. Gen. Virol.* 96, 311–321. doi: 10.1099/vir.0.070433-0

Appel, N., Schaller, T., Penin, F., and Bartenschlager, R. (2006). From structure to function: new insights into hepatitis C virus RNA replication. *J. Biol. Chem.* 281, 9833–9836. doi: 10.1074/jbc.R500026200

Beck, A. (2014). *Introduction to Nonlinear Optimization: Theory, Algorithms, and Applications with MATLAB, Vol. 19 (Siam).* Natick, MA: The MathWorks, Inc..

Benzine, T., Brandt, R., Lovell, W. C., Yamane, D., Neddermann, P., de Francesco, R., et al. (2017). NS5A inhibitors unmask differences in functional replicase complex half-life between different hepatitis C virus strains. *PLoS Pathog.* 13:e1006343. doi: 10.1371/journal.ppat.1006343

Bessaud, M., Autret, A., Jegouic, S., Balanant, J., Joffret, M., and Delpeyroux, F. (2001). Development of a Taqman RT-PCR assay for the detection and quantification of negatively stranded RNA of human enteroviruses: evidence for false-priming and improvement by tagged RT-PCR. *J. Virol Methods* 153, 182–189. doi: 10.1016/j.jviromet.2008.07.010

Binder, M., Sulaimanov, N., Clausznitzer, D., Schulze, M., Huber, C. M., Lenz, S. M., et al. (2013). Replication vesicles are load- and choke-points in the hepatitis C virus lifecycle. *PLoS Pathog.* 9:e1003561. doi: 10.1371/journal.ppat.1003561

Bisceglie, A. M. D. (2010). *Essentials of Hepatitis C Infection*. London: Springer Healthcare.

Canini, L., and Perelson, A. S. (2014). Viral kinetic modeling: state of the art. *J. Pharmacokinet. Pharmacodyn.* 41, 431–443. doi: 10.1007/s10928-014-9363-3

Castillo-Chavez, C., and Feng, Z. (1997). To treat or not to treat: the case of tuberculosis. *JMB* 35, 629–656. doi: 10.1007/s002850050069

Chatel-Chaix, L., and Bartenschlager, R. (2014). Dengue virus- and hepatitis C virus-induced replication and assembly compartments: the enemy inside — caught in the web. *J. Virol.* 88, 5907–5911. doi: 10.1128/JVI.03404-13

Craggs, J. K., Ball, J. K., Thomson, B. J., Irving, W. L., and Grabowska, A. (2001). Development of a strand-specific RT-PCR based assay to detect the replicative form of hepatitis C virus RNA. *J. Virol Methods* 94, 111–120. doi: 10.1016/S0166-0934(01)00281-6

Dahari, H., Forns, X., Neumann, A. U., and Perelson, A. S. (2006). The extrahepatic contribution to HCV plasma viremia. *J. Hepatol.* 45, 459–464. doi: 10.1016/j.jhep.2006.07.004

Dahari, H., Lo, A., Ribeiro, R. M., and Perelson, A. S. (2007a). Modeling hepatitis C virus dynamics: liver regeneration and critical drug efficacy. *J. Theor. Biol.* 247, 371–381. doi: 10.1016/j.jtbi.2007.03.006

Dahari, H., Major, M., Zhang, X., Mihalik, K., Rice, C. M., Perelson, A. S., et al. (2005). Mathematical modeling of primary hepatitis C infection: non-cytolytic clearance and early blockage of virion production. *Gastroenterology* 128, 1056–1066. doi: 10.1053/j.gastro.2005.01.049

Dahari, H., Ribeiro, R. M., and Perelson, A. S. (2007b). Triphasic decline in HCV RNA during antiviral therapy. *Hepatology* 46, 16–21. doi: 10.1002/hep.21657

Dahari, H., Ribeiro, R. M., Rice, C. M., and Perelson, A. S. (2007c). Mathematical modeling of subgenomic hepatitis C viral replication in Huh-7 cells. *J. Virol.* 81, 750–760. doi: 10.1128/JVI.01304-06

Dahari, H., Shudo, E., Cotler, S. J., Layden, T. J., and Perelson, A. S. (2009). Modelling hepatitis C virus kinetics: the relationship between the infected cell loss rate and the final slope of viral decay. *Antiviral Ther.* 14, 459–464.

Dixit, N. M., Layden-Almer, J. E., Layden, T. J., and Perelson, A. S. (2004). Modelling how ribavirin improves interferon response rates in hepatitis C virus infection. *Nature* 432, 922–924. doi: 10.1038/nature03153

Elliot, R. M., Armstrong, V. J., and McLauchlan, J. (2009). "Structural molecular virology," in *Hepatitis C Virus*, eds P. Karaylannis, J. Main, and H. Thomas (International Medical Press).

Gastaminza, P., Cheng, G., Wieland, S., Zhong, J., Liao, W., and Chisari, F. V. (2008). Cellular determinants of hepatitis C virus assembly, maturation, degradation, and secretion. *J. Virol.* 82, 2120–2129. doi: 10.1128/JVI.02053-07

Gilchrist, M. A., Coombs, D., and Perelson, A. S. (2004). Optimizing within-host viral fitness: infected cell lifespan and virion production rate. *J. Theor. Biol.* 229, 281–288. doi: 10.1016/j.jtbi.2004.04.015

Guedj, J., Dahari, H., Rong, L., Sansone, N. D., Nettles, R. E., Cotler, S. J., et al. (2013). Modeling Shows that the NS5A inhibitor dacatasvir has two modes of action and yields a shorter estimate of the hepatitis C virus half-life. *Proc. Natl. Acad. Sci. U.S.A.* 110, 3991–3996. doi: 10.1073/pnas.1203110110

Guedj, J., and Neumann, A. (2010). Understanding hepatitis C viral dynamics with direct-acting antiviral agents due to the interplay between intracellular replication and cellular infection dynamics. *J. Theor. Biol.* 267, 330–340. doi: 10.1016/j.jtbi.2010.08.036

Guedj, J., and Perelson, A. S. (2011). Second-phase hepatitis C virus RNA decline during telaprevir-based therapy increases with drug effectiveness: implications for treatment duration. *Viral Hepatitis* 53, 1801–1808. doi: 10.1002/hep.24272

Jangra, R. K., Yi, M., and Lemon, S. M. (2010). Regulation of hepatitis C virus translation and infectious virus production by the MicroRNA miR-122. *J. Virol.* 84, 6615–6625. doi: 10.1128/JVI.00417-10

Keum, S., Park, S., Park, J., Jung, J., Shin, E., and Jang, S. (2012). The specific infectivity of hepatitis C virus changes through its life cycle. *Virol* 433, 462–470. doi: 10.1016/j.virol.2012.08.046

Layden, T. J., Layden, J. E., Ribeiro, R. M., and Perelson, A. S. (2003). Mathematical modeling of viral kinetics: a tool to understand and optimize therapy. *Clin. Liver Dis.* 7, 163–178. doi: 10.1016/S1089-3261(02)00063-6

Layden-Almer, J. E., Ribeiro, R. M., Wiley, T., Perelson, A. S., and Layden, T. J. (2003). Viral dynamics and response differences in HCV-infected African American and white patients treated with IFN and ribavirin. *Hepatology* 37, 1343–1350. doi: 10.1053/jhep.2003.50217

Lee, C. (2013). Daclatasvir: potential role in hepatitis C. *Drug Des. Dev. Ther.* 7, 1223–1233. doi: 10.2147/DDDT.S40310

Li, J., and Brauer, F. (2008). "Continuous-time age-structured models in population dynamics and epidemiology," in *Math Epidemiol, volume 1945 of Lecture Notes in Mathematics*, eds F. Brauer, P. van den Driessche, and J. Wu (Berlin; Heidelberg: Springer), 205–227.

Li, Y., Yamane, D., Masaki, T., and Lemon, S. M. (2015). The yin and yang of hepatitis C: synthesis and decay of hepatitis C virus RNA. *Nat. Rev. Microbiol.* 13, 554–558. doi: 10.1038/nrmicro3506

Lindenbach, B. D., and Rice, C. M. (2013). The ins and outs of hepatitis C virus entry and assembly. *Nat. Rev. Microbiol.* 11, 688–700. doi: 10.1038/nrmicro3098

Martcheva, M., and Castillo-Chavez, C. (2003). Diseases with chronic stage in population with varying size? *Math. Biosci.* 182, 1–25. doi: 10.1016/S0025-5564(02)00184-0

McGivern, D., Masaki, T., Williford, S., Ingravallo, P., Feng, Z., Lahser, F., et al. (2014). Kinetic analyses reveal potent and early blockade of hepatitis C virus assembly by NS5A inhibitors. *Gastroenterology* 147, 453–462. doi: 10.1053/j.gastro.2014.04.021

Nelson, P. W., Gilchrist, M. A., Coombs, D., Hyman, J. M., and Perelson, A. S. (2004). An age-structured model of HIV infection that allows for variations in the death rate of productively infected cells. *Math. Biosci.* 1, 267–288. doi: 10.3934/mbe.2004.1.267

Neumann, A. U., Lam, N., Dahari, H., Gretch, D., and Wiley, T. E. (1998). Hepatitis C viral dynamics *in vivo* and the antiviral efficacy of interferon-alpha therapy. *Science* 282, 103–107. doi: 10.1126/science.282.5386.103

Powers, K. A., Dixit, N. M., Ribeiro, R. M., Golia, P., Talal, A. H., and Perelson, A. S. (2003). Modeling viral and drug kinetics: hepatitis C virus treatment with pegylated interferon alpha-2b. *Semin. Liver Dis.* 23(Suppl. 1), 13–18. doi: 10.1055/s-2003-41630

Quinkert, D., Bartenschlager, R., and Lohmann, V. (2005). Quantitative analysis of the hepatitis C virus replication complex. *J. Virol.* 79, 13594–13605. doi: 10.1128/JVI.79.21.13594-13605.2005

Quintela, B. M., Conway, J. M., Hyman, J. M., Reis, R. F., dos Santos, R. W., Lobosco, M., et al. (2017). "An age-based multiscale mathematical model of the hepatitis C virus life-cycle during infection and therapy: including translation and replication," in *VII Latin American Congress on Biomedical Engineering CLAIB 2016, IFMBE Proceedings*, Vol. 60, eds I. Torres, J. Bustamante, and D. Sierra (Bucaramanga: Santander), 508–511.

Reluga, T., Dahari, H., and Perelson, A. S. (2009). Analysis of hepatitis C virus infection models with hepatocyte homeostasis. *SIAM J. Appl. Math* 69, 999–1023. doi: 10.1137/080714579

Ribeiro, R. M., Layden-Almer, J., Powers, K. A., Layden, T. J., and Perelson, A. S. (2003). Dynamics of alanine aminotransferase during hepatitis C virus treatment. *Hepatology* 38, 509–517. doi: 10.1053/jhep.2003.50344

Rohatgi, A. (2016). *WebPlotDigitizer: Web Based Tool to Extract Data from Plots, Images, and Maps*. Version 4.0. Available online at: https://automeris.io/WebPlotDigitizer

Rong, L., Guedj, J., Dahari, H., Coffield, D. J., Levi, M., Smith, P., et al. (2013). Analysis of hepatitis C virus decline during treatment with the protease inhibitor danoprevir using a multiscale model. *PLoS Comput. Biol.* 9:e1002959. doi: 10.1371/journal.pcbi.1002959

Rong, L., and Perelson, A. S. (2013). Mathematical analysis of multiscale models for hepatitis C virus dynamics under therapy with direct-acting antiviral agents. *Math. Biosci.* 245, 22–30. doi: 10.1016/j.mbs.2013.04.012

Sadiku, M. N. O., and Obiozor, C. N. (2000). A simple introduction to the method of lines. *Intl. J. Elect. Eng. Educ.* 37, 282–296. doi: 10.7227/IJEEE.37.3.8

Scheel, T. K. H., and Rice, C. M. (2013). Understanding the hepatitis C virus life cycle paves the way for highly effective therapies. *Nat. Med.* 19, 837–849. doi: 10.1038/nm.3248

Scheller, N., Mina, L., Galão, R., Chari, A., Giménez-Barcons, M., Noueiry, A., et al. (2009). Translation and replication of hepatitis C virus genomic RNA depends on ancient cellular proteins that control mRNA fates. *Proc. Natl. Acad. Sci. U.S.A.* 106, 13517–13522. doi: 10.1073/pnas.0906413106

Shakeri, F., and Dehghan, M. (2008). The method of lines for solution of the one-dimensional wave equation subject to an integral conservation condition. *Comput. Math. Appl.* 56, 2175–2188. doi: 10.1016/j.camwa.2008.03.055

Shi, S. T., and Lai, M. M. C. (2006). "HCV 5' and 3'UTR: when translation meets replication," in *Hepatitis C Viruses: Genomes and Molecular Biology*, ed S. L. Tan (Norfolk: Horizon Bioscience). Available online at: http://www.ncbi.nlm.nih.gov/books/NBK1624/

Shudo, E., Ribeiro, R. M., and Perelson, A. S. (2008a). Modeling the kinetics of hepatitis C RNA decline over four weeks of treatment with pegylated interferon alpha-2b. *J. Viral Hepat.* 15, 379–382. doi: 10.1111/j.1365-2893.2008.00977.x

Shudo, E., Ribeiro, R. M., Talal, A. H., and Perelson, A. S. (2008b). A hepatitis C viral kinetic model that allows for time-varying drug effectiveness. *Antiviral. Ther.* 13, 919–926. Available online at: https://www.intmedpress.com/journals/avt/abstract.cfm?id=107&pid=88

Thieme, H., and Castillo-Chavez, C. (1993). How may infection-age-dependent infectivity affect the dynamics of HIV/AIDS? *SIAM J. Appl. Math.* 53, 1337–1379. doi: 10.1137/0153068

Thieme, H., and Castillo-Chavez, C. (2002). A two-strain tuberculosis model with age infection. *SIAM J. Appl. Math.* 62, 1634–1656. doi: 10.1137/S003613990038205X

WHO (2016). *Guidelines for the Screening, Care and Treatment of Persons With Chronic Hepatitis C Infection*. Geneva: WHO. (Accessed July 8, 2016).

Yuki, N., Matsumoto, S., Tadokoro, K., Mochizuki, K., Kato, M., and Yamaguchi, T. (2005). Significance of liver negative-strand HCV RNA quantitation in chronic hepatitis C. *J. Hepatol.* 44, 302–309. doi: 10.1016/j.jhep.2005.10.014

Permissions

All chapters in this book were first published in ICSBAIM, by Frontiers; hereby published with permission under the Creative Commons Attribution License or equivalent. Every chapter published in this book has been scrutinized by our experts. Their significance has been extensively debated. The topics covered herein carry significant findings which will fuel the growth of the discipline. They may even be implemented as practical applications or may be referred to as a beginning point for another development.

The contributors of this book come from diverse backgrounds, making this book a truly international effort. This book will bring forth new frontiers with its revolutionizing research information and detailed analysis of the nascent developments around the world.

We would like to thank all the contributing authors for lending their expertise to make the book truly unique. They have played a crucial role in the development of this book. Without their invaluable contributions this book wouldn't have been possible. They have made vital efforts to compile up to date information on the varied aspects of this subject to make this book a valuable addition to the collection of many professionals and students.

This book was conceptualized with the vision of imparting up-to-date information and advanced data in this field. To ensure the same, a matchless editorial board was set up. Every individual on the board went through rigorous rounds of assessment to prove their worth. After which they invested a large part of their time researching and compiling the most relevant data for our readers.

The editorial board has been involved in producing this book since its inception. They have spent rigorous hours researching and exploring the diverse topics which have resulted in the successful publishing of this book. They have passed on their knowledge of decades through this book. To expedite this challenging task, the publisher supported the team at every step. A small team of assistant editors was also appointed to further simplify the editing procedure and attain best results for the readers.

Apart from the editorial board, the designing team has also invested a significant amount of their time in understanding the subject and creating the most relevant covers. They scrutinized every image to scout for the most suitable representation of the subject and create an appropriate cover for the book.

The publishing team has been an ardent support to the editorial, designing and production team. Their endless efforts to recruit the best for this project, has resulted in the accomplishment of this book. They are a veteran in the field of academics and their pool of knowledge is as vast as their experience in printing. Their expertise and guidance has proved useful at every step. Their uncompromising quality standards have made this book an exceptional effort. Their encouragement from time to time has been an inspiration for everyone.

The publisher and the editorial board hope that this book will prove to be a valuable piece of knowledge for researchers, students, practitioners and scholars across the globe.

List of Contributors

Humayra Tasnim and Justyna O. Sotiris
Moses Biological Computation Laboratory, Department of Computer Science, The University of New Mexico, Albuquerque, NM, United States

G. Matthew Fricke
Moses Biological Computation Laboratory, Department of Computer Science, The University of New Mexico, Albuquerque, NM, United States
UNM Center for Advanced Research Computing (CARC), The University of New Mexico, Albuquerque, NM, United States

Janie R. Byrum
The Cannon Laboratory, Molecular Genetics & Microbiology, The University of New Mexico, Albuquerque, NM, United States

Judy L. Cannon
The Cannon Laboratory, Molecular Genetics & Microbiology, The University of New Mexico, Albuquerque, NM, United States
Department of Pathology, The University of New Mexico, Albuquerque, NM, United States Autophagy, Inflammation, and Metabolism Center of Biomedical Research Excellence, The University of New Mexico, Albuquerque, NM, United States

Melanie E. Moses
Moses Biological Computation Laboratory, Department of Computer Science, The University of New Mexico, Albuquerque, NM, United States
Biology Department, The University of New Mexico, Albuquerque, NM, United States
Santa Fe Institute, Santa Fe, NM, United States

Ágnes Móréh
MTA Centre for Ecological Research, Danube Research Institute, Budapest, Hungary

András Szilágyi and István Scheuring
Evolutionary Systems Research Group, MTA Centre for Ecological Research, Tihany, Hungary
MTA-ELTE Theoretical Biology and Evolutionary Ecology Research Group, Institute of Biology, Eötvös Loránd University, Budapest, Hungary

Viktor Müller
Evolutionary Systems Research Group, MTA Centre for Ecological Research, Tihany, Hungary Department of Plant Systematics, Ecology and Theoretical Biology, Institute of Biology, Eötvös Loránd University, Budapest, Hungary

Ethan O. Romero-Severson
Theoretical Biology and Biophysics Group, Los Alamos National Laboratory, Los Alamos, NM, United States

Mario Castro
Grupo Interdisciplinar de Sistemas Complejos and DNL, Universidad Pontificia Comillas, Madrid, Spain Department of Applied Mathematics, School of Mathematics, University of Leeds, Leeds, United Kingdom

Naveen K. Vaidya
Department of Mathematics and Statistics, San Diego State University, San Diego, CA, United States

Ruy M. Ribeiro
Theoretical Biology and Biophysics Group, MS K710, Los Alamos National Laboratory, Los Alamos, NM, United States
Laboratório de Biomatemática, Faculdade de Medicina, Universidade de Lisboa, Lisboa, Portugal

Pinghuang Liu
Harbin Veterinary Research Institute, Chinese Academy of Agricultural Sciences, Harbin, China

Barton F. Haynes and Georgia D. Tomaras
Duke University School of Medicine, Durham, NC, United States

Alan S. Perelson
Theoretical Biology and Biophysics Group, MS K710, Los Alamos National Laboratory, Los Alamos, NM, United States

Stanca M. Ciupe
Department of Mathematics, Virginia Tech, Blacksburg, VA, United States

Christopher J. Miller
Department of Pathology, Microbiology, and Immunology, School of Veterinary Medicine, Center for Comparative Medicine and California National Primate Research Center, University of California, Davis, Davis, CA, United States

Neha Thakre and Frederik Graw
Centre for Modeling and Simulation in the Biosciences, BioQuant-Center, Heidelberg University, Heidelberg, Germany

Priyanka Fernandes
Parasitology Unit, Centre for Infectious Diseases, University Hospital, Heidelberg, Germany

Jonathan E. Forde
Department of Mathematics and Computer Science, Hobart and Williams Smith Colleges, Geneva, NY, United States

Ann-Kristin Mueller
Parasitology Unit, Centre for Infectious Diseases, University Hospital, Heidelberg, Germany
German Center for Infectious Diseases (DZIF), Heidelberg, Germany

Carolin Zitzmann and Lars Kaderali
Institute of Bioinformatics and Center for Functional Genomics of Microbes, University Medicine Greifswald, Greifswald, Germany

Marc Thilo Figge
Applied Systems Biology, Leibniz Institute for Natural Product Research and Infection Biology, Hans Knöll Institute (HKI), Jena, Germany
Faculty of Biological Sciences, Friedrich Schiller University Jena, Jena, Germany
Center for Sepsis Control and Care (CSCC), Jena University Hospital, Jena, Germany
Faculty of Biology and Pharmacy, Friedrich Schiller University Jena, Jena, Germany

Alexandre B. Pigozzo
Department of Computer Science, Federal University of São João Del-Rei, São João Del-Rei, Brazil

Dominique Missiakas
Department of Microbiology, University of Chicago, Chicago, IL, United States

Sergio Alonso
Department of Physics, Universitat Politècnica de Catalunya, Barcelona, Spain

Rodrigo W. dos Santos and Marcelo Lobosco
Graduate Program in Computational Modeling, Federal University of Juiz de Fora, Juiz de Fora, Brazil FISIOCOMP Laboratory, PPGMC, Universidade Federal de Juiz de Fora, Juiz de Fora, Brazil

Amanda P. Smith and Amber M. Smith
Department of Pediatrics, University of Tennessee Health Science Center, Memphis, TN, United States

David J. Moquin
Department of Internal Medicine, University of Tennessee Health Science Center, Memphis, TN, United States

Veronika Bernhauerova
Viral Populations and Pathogenesis Unit, Institut Pasteur, Paris, France

Richard A. Cangelosi
Department of Mathematics, Gonzaga University, Spokane, WA, United States

Elissa J. Schwartz
Department of Mathematics and Statistics, Washington State University, Pullman, WA, United States
School of Biological Sciences, Washington State University, Pullman, WA, United States

David J. Wollkind
Department of Mathematics and Statistics, Washington State University, Pullman, WA, United States

Anjali Garg, Bandana Kumari, Ravindra Kumar and Manish Kumar
Department of Biophysics, University of Delhi, New Delhi, India

Louis R. Joslyn and Elsje Pienaar
Department of Chemical Engineering, University of Michigan, Ann Arbor, MI, United States
Department of Microbiology and Immunology, University of Michigan Medical School, Ann Arbor, MI, United States

Robert M. DiFazio and JoAnne L. Flynn
Department of Microbiology and Molecular Genetics, University of Pittsburgh School of Medicine, Pittsburgh, PA, United States

Sara Suliman, Benjamin M. Kagina and Thomas J. Scriba
South African Tuberculosis Vaccine Initiative and Institute of Infectious Disease and Molecular Medicine, Division of Immunology, Department of Pathology, University of Cape Town, Cape Town, South Africa

Jennifer J. Linderman
Department of Chemical Engineering, University of Michigan, Ann Arbor, MI, United States

Denise E. Kirschner
Department of Microbiology and Immunology, University of Michigan Medical School, Ann Arbor, MI, United States

Yiding Yang
Department of Microbiology, University of Tennessee, Knoxville, TN, United States

Vitaly V. Ganusov
Department of Microbiology, University of Tennessee, Knoxville, TN, United States
National Institute for Mathematical and Biological Synthesis, University of Tennessee, Knoxville, TN, United States
Department of Mathematics, University of Tennessee, Knoxville, TN, United States

Assaf Amitai
Chemical Engineering, Massachusetts Institute of Technology, Cambridge, MA, United States
Institute for Medical Engineering and Science, Massachusetts Institute of Technology, Cambridge, MA, United States
Ragon Institute of MGH, MIT and Harvard, Cambridge, MA, United States

Luka Mesin and Gabriel D. Victora
Laboratory of Lymphocyte Dynamics, Rockefeller University, New York, NY, United States

Mehran Kardar
Physics, Massachusetts Institute of Technology, Cambridge, MA, United States

Arup K. Chakraborty
Chemical Engineering, Massachusetts Institute of Technology, Cambridge, MA, United States
Institute for Medical Engineering and Science, Massachusetts Institute of Technology, Cambridge, MA, United States
Ragon Institute of MGH, MIT and Harvard, Cambridge, MA, United States
Biological Engineering and Chemistry, Massachusetts Institute of Technology, Cambridge, MA, United States

Sandra Timme and Maria T. E. Prauße
Research Group Applied Systems Biology, Leibniz Institute for Natural Product Research and Infection Biology—Hans Knöll Institute, Jena, Germany Faculty of Biological Sciences, Friedrich Schiller University Jena, Jena, Germany

Kerstin Hünniger
Fungal Septomics, Septomics Research Center, Leibniz Institute for Natural Product Research and Infection Biology—Hans Knöll Institute, Friedrich Schiller University, Jena, Germany
Fungal Septomics, Leibniz Institute for Natural Product Research and Infection Biology, Hans Knöll Institute (HKI), Jena, Germany
Institute for Hygiene and Microbiology, University of Würzburg, Würzburg, Germany

Ines Leonhardt
Center for Sepsis Control and Care (CSCC), Jena University Hospital, Jena, Germany
Fungal Septomics, Septomics Research Center, Leibniz Institute for Natural Product Research and Infection Biology—Hans Knöll Institute, Friedrich Schiller University, Jena, Germany
Fungal Septomics, Leibniz Institute for Natural Product Research and Infection Biology, Hans Knöll Institute (HKI), Jena, Germany

Teresa Lehnert
Research Group Applied Systems Biology, Leibniz Institute for Natural Product Research and Infection Biology—Hans Knöll Institute, Jena, Germany
Center for Sepsis Control and Care (CSCC), Jena University Hospital, Jena, Germany

Oliver Kurzai
Center for Sepsis Control and Care (CSCC), Jena University Hospital, Jena, Germany
Fungal Septomics, Septomics Research Center, Leibniz Institute for Natural Product Research and Infection Biology—Hans Knöll Institute, Friedrich Schiller University, Jena, Germany
Institute for Hygiene and Microbiology, University of Würzburg, Würzburg, Germany
Fungal Septomics, Leibniz Institute for Natural Product Research and Infection Biology, Hans Knöll Institute (HKI), Jena, Germany

Adolfo Flores Saiffe Farías and J. Alejandro Morales
Computer Sciences Department, University of Guadalara, Guadalajara, Mexico

Adriana P. Mendizabal
Pharmacobiology Department, University of Guadalajara, Guadalajara, Mexico

Barbara de M. Quintela
FISIOCOMP Laboratory, PPGMC, Universidade Federal de Juiz de Fora, Juiz de Fora, Brazil

Jessica M. Conway
Department of Mathematics and Center for Infectious Disease Dynamics, The Pennsylvania State University, State College, PA, United States

James M. Hyman
Mathematics Department, Tulane University, New Orleans, LA, United States

Jeremie Guedj
IAME, UMR 1137, Institut National de la Santé et de la Recherche Médicale, Université Paris Diderot, Sorbonne Paris Cité, Paris, France

Index

Printed in the USA
CPSIA information can be obtained
at www.ICGtesting.com
JSHW051405091023
49903JS00006B/293